VASCULAR FACTORS IN ALZHEIMER'S DISEASE

ANNALS OF THE NEW YORK ACADEMY OF SCIENCES
Volume 903

VASCULAR FACTORS IN ALZHEIMER'S DISEASE

Edited by Raj N. Kalaria and Paul Ince

The New York Academy of Sciences
New York, New York
2000

Library of Congress Cataloging-in-Publication Data

Vascular factors in Alzheimer's disease / edited by Raj N. Kalaria and Paul Ince.
    p.; cm. — (Annals of the New York Academy of Sciences, ISSN 0077-8923; v. 903)
    Includes bibliographical references and index.
    ISBN 1-57331-251-7 (cloth : alk. paper) — ISBN 1-57331-252-5 (paper : alk. paper).
    1. Alzheimer's disease–Pathophysiology—Congresses. 2.
Brain—Blood-vessels—Congresses. 3. Cerebrovascular
disease—Pathophysiology—Congresses. I. Kalaria, Raj N. II. Ince, Paul. III. Series.
    [DNLM: 1. Alzheimer Disease—physiopathology—Congresses. 2. Alzheimer
Disease—etiology—Congresses. 3. Cerebral Amyloid Angiopathy—Congresses. 4.
Cerebrovascular Disorders—physiopathology—Congresses. 5.
Dementia—etiology—Congresses. 6. Dementia—physiopathology—Congresses. WT 155
V331 2000]
Q11 N5 vol. 903
[RC523]
500 s—dc21
[616.8'3107]   00-023955

GYAT / PCP
Printed in the United States of America
ISBN 1-57331-251-7 (cloth)
ISBN 1-57331-252-5 (paper)
ISSN 0077-8923

ANNALS OF THE NEW YORK ACADEMY OF SCIENCES
Volume 903
April 2000

VASCULAR FACTORS IN ALZHEIMER'S DISEASE[a]

Editors and Conference Chairs
RAJ N. KALARIA AND PAUL INCE

CONTENTS

Henryk Miroslaw Wisniewski, 1931–1999. *By* R.N. KALARIA AND A.E. OAKLEY xiii

Preface. *By* RAJ N. KALARIA xvii

Part I. Alzheimer's Disease: Vascular Concepts, Cellular Issues, and Genetics (Plenary Lectures)

Vascular Factors in Cognitive Impairment—Where Are We Now? *By* VLADIMIR HACHINSKI AND DAVID MUNOZ 1

Role of Perivascular Cells and Myocytes in Vascular Amyloidosis. *By* H.M. WISNIEWSKI, J. WEGIEL, A.W. VORBRODT, B. MAZUR-KOLECKA, AND J. FRACKOWIAK 6

Binswanger Disease: The History of a Silent Epidemic. *By* GUSTAVO C. ROMÁN 19

Cascading Glia Reactions: a Common Pathomechanism and Its Differentiated Control by Cyclic Nucleotide Signaling. *By* PETER SCHUBERT, TADAO MORINO, HIROFUMI MIYAZAKI, TADANORI OGATA, YOICHI NAKAMURA, CRISTINA MARCHINI, AND STEFANO FERRONI 24

Part II. Vascular Pathology in Alzheimer's Disease: Recent Developments

Linguistic Ability in Early Life and the Neuropathology of Alzheimer's Disease and Cerebrovascular Disease: Findings from the Nun Study. *By* D.A. SNOWDON, L.H. GREINER, AND W.R. MARKESBERY 34

Cerebrovascular Pathology in Alzheimer's Disease and Leukoaraiosis. *By* WILLIAM R. BROWN, DIXON M. MOODY, CLARA R. THORE, AND VENKATA R. CHALLA 39

[a]This volume contains the papers from a conference entitled *Vascular Factors in Alzheimer's Disease*, which was held in Slaley Hall, near Newcastle upon Tyne, UK on May 25–28, 1999.

Role of Blood Vessels in Producing Pathological Changes in the Brain with Alzheimer's Disease. *By* TAIHEI MIYAKAWA, TAKEMI KIMURA, SHINICHI HIRATA, NOBORU FUJISE, TSUNEHIKO ONO, KOKO ISHIZUKA, AND JUN NAKABAYASHI 46

Cerebrovasculature-mediated Neuronal Cell Death. *By* PAULA GRAMMAS, ULRICH REIMANN-PHILIPP, AND PAUL H. WEIGEL 55

Role of Aberrant Nitric Oxide Synthase-3 Expression in Cerebrovascular Degeneration and Vascular-mediated Injury in Alzheimer's Disease. *By* SUZANNE M. DE LA MONTE, YOON K. SOHN, DANNIE ETIENNE, JOANNY KRAFT, AND JACK R. WANDS 61

Similar Ultrastructural Breakdown of Cerebrocortical Capillaries in Alzheimer's Disease, Parkinson's Disease, and Experimental Hypertension: What is the Functional Link? *By* ESZTER FARKAS, GINEKE I. DE JONG, ETELKA APRÓ, ROB A.I. DE VOS, ERNST N.H. JANSEN STEUR, AND PAUL G.M. LUITEN 72

Distribution of Amyloid β_{42} in Relation to the Cerebral Microvasculature in an Elderly Cohort with Alzheimer's Disease. *By* A.J. THOMAS, C.M. MORRIS, I.N. FERRIER, AND R.N. KALARIA 83

Part III. Cerebral Amyloid Angiopathy and Factors Regulating Cerebral Amyloidosis

Cerebrovascular Smooth Muscle Cell Surface Fibrillar Aβ: Alteration of the Proteolytic Environment in the Cerebral Vessel Wall. *By* WILLIAM E. VAN NOSTRAND, JERRY MELCHOR, MATTHEW WAGNER, AND JUDIANNE DAVIS 89

Aβ Vasoactivity: An Inflammatory Reaction. *By* DANIEL PARIS, TERRENCE TOWN, TIMOTHY PARKER, JAMES HUMPHREY, AND MICHAEL MULLAN 97

Cerebral Amyloid Angiopathy: Accumulation of Aβ in Interstitial Fluid Drainage Pathways in Alzheimer's Disease. *By* ROY O. WELLER, ADRIAN MASSEY, YU-MIN KUO, AND ALEX E. ROHER 110

Traumatic Brain Injury Elevates the Alzheimer's Amyloid Peptide $A\beta_{42}$ in Human CSF: A Possible Role for Nerve Cell Injury. *By* M.R. EMMERLING, M.C. MORGANTI-KOSSMANN, T. KOSSMANN, P. F. STAHEL, M.D. WATSON, L.M. EVANS, P.D. MEHTA, K. SPIEGEL, Y.-M. KUO, A.E. ROHER, AND C.A. RABY 118

Prospects for Noninvasive Imaging of Brain Amyloid β in Alzheimer's Disease. *By* R.P. FRIEDLAND, J. SHI, J.C. LaMANNA, M.A. SMITH, AND G. PERRY 123

A Newly Formed Amyloidogenic Fragment due to a Stop Codon Mutation Causes Familial British Dementia. *By* J. GHISO, R. VIDAL, A. ROSTAGNO, S. MEAD, T. RÉVÉSZ, G. PLANT, AND B. FRANGIONE . . 129

Relationship between Severe Amyloid Angiopathy, Apolipoprotein E Genotype, and Vascular Lesions in Alzheimer's Disease. *By* J.M. OLICHNEY, L.A. HANSEN, J.H. LEE, C.R. HOFSTETTER, R. KATZMAN, AND L.J. THAL 138

Plasma β-Amyloid Peptide, Transforming Growth Factor-β1, and Risk for Cerebral Amyloid Angiopathy. *By* STEVEN M. GREENBERG, HYUN-SOON CHO, HEATHER C. O'DONNELL, JONATHAN ROSAND, ALAN Z. SEGAL, LINDA H. YOUNKIN, STEVEN G. YOUNKIN, AND G. WILLIAM REBECK 144

The Effect of Iron and Aluminum on Transferrin and Other Serum Proteins as Revealed by Isoelectric Focusing Gel Electrophoresis. *By* S.J. VAN RENSBURG, M.E. CARSTENS, F.C.V. POTOCNIK, AND J.J.F. TALJAARD 150

Aβ Vasoactivity *in Vivo*. *By* ZHIMING SUO, GEORGE SU, ANDON PLACZEK, AMY KUNDTZ, JAMES HUMPHREY, FIONA CRAWFORD, AND MIKE MULLAN 156

Cytochemistry of Intraplatelet Ca++ Spots as a Peripheral Marker of Age-related Brain Impairment. *By* CARLO BERTONI-FREDDARI, TIZIANA CASOLI, PATRIZIA FATTORETTI, LUCIANO GALEAZZI, GIUSEPPINA DI STEFANO, NATASCIA BELARDINELLI, EUGENIO PUCCI, AND MARIO SIGNORINO 164

Part IV. Apolipoprotein E and Genetics in Cerebral Amyloid Angiopathy and Alzheimer's Disease

Lipoproteins in the Central Nervous System. *By* MARY JO LaDU, CATHERINE REARDON, LINDA VAN ELDIK, ANNE M. FAGAN, GUOJUN BU, DAVID HOLTZMAN, AND GODFREY S. GETZ 167

Apolipoprotein E Genotype and Cerebral Amyloid Angiopathy-related Hemorrhage. *By* MARK O. MCCARRON AND JAMES A.R. NICOLL 176

Apolipoprotein E, Smooth Muscle Cells and the Pathogenesis of Cerebral Amyloid Angiopathy: the Potential Role of Impaired Cerebrovascular Aβ Clearance. *By* REINHARD PRIOR, GÜNTHER WIHL, AND BRITTA URMONEIT 180

Amyloid-β-induced Degeneration of Human Brain Pericytes Is Dependent on the Apolipoprotein E Genotype. *By* MARCEL M. VERBEEK, WILLIAM E. VAN NOSTRAND, IRENE OTTE-HÖLLER, PIETER WESSELING, AND ROBERT M.W. DE WAAL 187

Earlier Age of Onset of Alzheimer's Disease in Patients with Both the Transferrin C2 and Apolipoprotein E-ε4 Alleles. *By* S.J. VAN RENSBURG, F.C.V. POTOCNIK, J.N.P. DE VILLIERS, M.J. KOTZE, AND J.J.F. TALJAARD 200

Inherent Abnormalities in Energy Metabolism in Alzheimer Disease: Interaction with Cerebrovascular Compromise. *By* JOHN P. BLASS, REX KWAN-FU SHEU, AND GARY E. GIBSON 204

Insulin Effects on Glucose Metabolism, Memory, and Plasma Amyloid Precursor Protein in Alzheimer's Disease Differ According to Apolipoprotein-E Genotype. *By* SUZANNE CRAFT, SANJAY ASTHANA, GERARD SCHELLENBERG, LAURA BAKER, MONIQUE CHERRIER, ADAM A. BOYT, RALPH N. MARTINS, MURRAY RASKIND, ELAINE PESKIND, AND STEPHEN PLYMATE 222

Part V. VAD: Clinical Aspects, Vascular Lesions, and Imaging

Interface between Vascular Dementia and Alzheimer Syndrome: Nosologic Redefinition. *By* V. OLGA EMERY, EDWARD X. GILLIE, AND JOSEPH A. SMITH ... 229

Which Vascular Lesions Are of Importance in Vascular Dementia? *By* MARGARET M. ESIRI ... 239

Severity of Cardiovascular Disease, Apolipoprotein E Genotype, and Brain Pathology in Aging and Dementia. *By* IRINA ALAFUZOFF, SEPPO HELISALMI, ARTO MANNERMAA, AND HILKKA SOININEN ... 244

Can PET Data Differentiate Alzheimer's Disease from Vascular Dementia? *By* KEN NAGATA, HIROSHI MARUYA, HIROMICHI YUYA, HIROO TERASHI, YASUNORI MITO, HARUHISA KATO, MIKA SATO, YUICHI SATOH, YASUHITO WATAHIKI, YUTAKA HIRATA, ERIKO YOKOYAMA, AND JUN HATAZAWA ... 252

Limitations of Clincal Criteria for the Diagnosis of Vascular Dementia in Clinical Trials: Is a Focus on Subcortical Vascular Dementia a Solution? *By* TIMO ERKINJUNTTI, DOMENICO INZITARI, LEONARDO PANTONI, ANDERS WALLIN, PHILIP SCHELTENS, KENNETH ROCKWOOD, AND DAVID W. DESMOND ... 262

Part VI. Vasculopathies and CADASIL

CADASIL: Hereditary Arteriopathy Leading to Multiple Brain Infarcts and Dementia. *By* MATTI VIITANEN AND HANNU KALIMO ... 273

Skin Biopsy Value and Leukoaraiosis. *By* M.M. RUCHOUX, P. BRULIN, E. LETEURTRE, AND C.A. MAURAGE ... 285

Hereditary Vascular Dementia Linked to Notch 3 Mutations: CADASIL in British Families. *By* N.J. THOMAS, C.M. MORRIS, F. SCARAVILLI, J. JOHANSSON, M. ROSSOR, R. DE LANGE, D. ST CLAIR, J. NICOLL, C. BLANK, A. COULTHARD, K. BUSHBY, P.G. INCE, D. BURN, AND R.N. KALARIA ... 293

Linear Relation between Cerebral Phosphocreatine Concentration and Memory Capacities during Permanent Brain Vessel Occlusions in Rats. *By* KONSTANZE PLASCHKE, SEONG-WOOK YUN, EIKE MARTIN, SIEGFRIED HOYER, AND HUBERT J. BARDENHEUER ... 299

Part VII. Transgenic Animal and *In Vitro* Models: Vascular Effects

Mechanisms of Cerebrovascular Amyloid Deposition: Lessons from Mouse Models. *By* PATRICK BURGERMEISTER, MICHAEL E. CALHOUN, DAVID T. WINKLER, AND MATHIAS JUCKER ... 307

Alzheimer's Disease–like Cerebrovascular Pathology in Transforming Growth Factor-β1 Transgenic Mice and Functional Metabolic Correlates. *By* T. WYSS-CORAY, C. LIN, D. VON EUW, E. MASLIAH, L. MUCKE, AND P. LACOMBE ... 317

The Role of Apolipoprotein E in the Deposition of β-Amyloid Peptide during Ischemia-Reperfusion Brain Injury: A Model of Early Alzheimer's Disease. *By* Ryszard Pluta ... 324

Alterations of Alzheimer's Disease in the Cholesterol-fed Rabbit, Including
Vascular Inflammation: Preliminary Observations. *By* D. LARRY
SPARKS, YU-MIN KUO, ALEX ROHER, TIM MARTIN, AND
RONALD J. LUKAS 335

Animal Model of Alzheimer-like Vascular Pathology and Inflammatory
Reaction. *By* J. RHODIN, T. THOMAS, M. BRYANT, AND E.T. SUTTON . 345

Vascular Endothelium Is a Site of Free Radical Production and Inflammation
in Areas of Neuronal Loss in Thiamine-deficient Brain. *By* NOEL Y.
CALINGASAN AND GARY E. GIBSON 353

Marked Hippocampal Neuronal Damage without Motor Deficits after Mild
Concussive-like Brain Injury in Apolipoprotein E-deficient Mice. *By*
SEOL-HEUI HAN AND SEUNG-YUN CHUNG 357

Part VIII. Cholinergic Mechanisms and Vascular Pathology

Cortical Cholinergic Denervation Elicits Vascular Aβ Deposition. *By*
ALEX E. ROHER, YU-MIN KUO, PAMELA E. POTTER, MARK R.
EMMERLING, ROBERT A. DURHAM, DOUGLAS G. WALKER,
LUCIA I. SUE, WILLIAM G. HONER, AND THOMAS G. BEACH 366

β-Amyloid Excitotoxicity in Rat Magnocellular Nucleus Basalis: Effect of
Cortical Deafferentation on Cerebral Blood Flow Regulation and
Implications for Alzheimer's Disease. *By* TIBOR HARKANY,
BOTOND PENKE, AND PAUL G.M. LUITEN 374

Effect of a Memory-Enhancing Drug, AIT-082, on the Level of Synaptophysin. *By* D.K. LAHIRI, Y.-W. GE, AND M.R. FARLOW 387

Differentiated Cerebrovascular Effects of Physostigmine and Tacrine in
Cortical Areas Deafferented from the Nucleus Basalis Magnocellularis
Suggest Involvement of Basalocortical Projections to Microvessels. *By*
PHILIPPE PERUZZI, DOMINIQUE VON EUW, AND PIERRE LACOMBE . . . 394

**Part IX. Cardiovascular Risk Factors and Vascular
Pathophysiology in Dementia**

Plasma Total Homocysteine and Cognitive Performance in a Volunteer
Elderly Population. *By* M. BUDGE, C. JOHNSTON, E. HOGERVORST,
C. DE JAGER, E. MILWAIN, S.D. IVERSEN, L. BARNETSON, E. KING,
AND A.D. SMITH 407

Cardiovascular and Other Risk Factors for Alzheimer's Disease and
Vascular Dementia. *By* JOHN S. MEYER, GAIANE M. RAUCH, RONALD
A. RAUCH, ANWARUL HAQUE, AND KATE CRAWFORD 411

Critically Attained Threshold of Cerebral Hypoperfusion: Can It Cause
Alzheimer's Disease? *By* J.C. DE LA TORRE 424

The Renin Angiotensin System and Alzheimer's Disease. *By* PHILIPPE
AMOUYEL, FLORENCE RICHARD, CLAUDINE BERR, ISABELLE DAVID-
FROMENTIN, AND NICOLE HELBECQUE 437

Neurocardiovascular Instability, Hypotensive Episodes, and MRI Lesions in
Neurodegenerative Dementia. *By* CLIVE BALLARD, JOHN O'BRIEN,
BOB BARBER, PHILIP SCHELTENS, FIONA SHAW, IAN MCKEITH, AND
ROSE ANNE KENNY 442

β-Amyloid Vasoactivity and Proinflammation in Microglia Can Be Blocked by cGMP-Elevating Agents. *By* DANIEL PARIS, TERRENCE TOWN, TIMOTHY PARKER, JAMES HUMPHREY, AND MICHAEL MULLAN 446

β-Amyloid Fragment 25–35 Induces Changes in Cytosolic Free Calcium in Human Platelets. *By* LUCIANO GALEAZZI, TIZIANA CASOLI, SERGIO GIUNTA, PATRIZIA FATTORETTI, NATASCIA GRACCIOTTI, UGO CASELLI, AND CARLO BERTONI-FREDDARI 451

Part X. White Matter Lesions and Dementia

Vascular Involvement in Cognitive Decline and Dementia: Epidemiologic Evidence from the Rotterdam Study and the Rotterdam Scan Study. *By* MONIQUE M.B. BRETELER 457

Relevance of White Matter Changes to Pre- and Poststroke Dementia. *By* FLORENCE PASQUIER, HILDE HÉNON, AND DIDIER LEYS 466

Corpus Callosum Measurement as an *in Vivo* Indicator for Neocortical Neuronal Integrity, but not White Matter Pathology, in Alzheimer's Disease. *By* HARALD HAMPEL, STEFAN J. TEIPEL, GENE E. ALEXANDER, BARRY HORWITZ, PIETRO PIETRINI, HANNS HIPPIUS, HANS-JÜRGEN MÖLLER, MARK B. SCHAPIRO, AND STANLEY I. RAPOPORT 470

Contrast-enhanced MRI of White Matter Lesions in Patients with Blood-Brain Barrier Dysfunction. *By* LARS-OLOF WAHLUND AND LENA BRONGE 477

The Association between White Matter Lesions on Magnetic Resonance Imaging and Noncognitive Symptoms. *By* JOHN O'BRIEN, ROBERT PERRY, ROBERT BARBER, ANIL GHOLKAR, AND ALAN THOMAS 482

Neuropathological Findings in the Very Old: Results from the First 101 Brains of a Population-based Longitudinal Study of Dementing Disorders. *By* J.H. XUEREB, C. BRAYNE, C. DUFOUIL, H. GERTZ, C. WISCHIK, C. HARRINGTON, E. MUKAETOVA-LADINSKA, M.A. MCGEE, A. O'SULLIVAN, D. O'CONNOR, E.S. PAYKEL, AND F.A. HUPPERT 490

Leukoaraiosis at Presentation and Disease Progression during Follow-up in Histologically Confirmed Cases of Dementia. *By* R. CLARKE, C. JOACHIM, M. ESIRI, J. MORRIS, H. BUNGAY, A. MOLYNEUX, M. BUDGE, C. FROST, E. KING, L. BARNETSON, AND A.D. SMITH 497

Part XI. Diagnostic, Preventative, and Treatment Strategies in Alzheimer's Disease and Vascular Dementia

Vascular Actions of Estrogen and Alzheimer's Disease. *By* T. THOMAS AND J. RHODIN 501

Subcortical Vascular Dementia as a Specific Target for Clinical Trials. *By* DOMENICO INZITARI, TIMO ERKINJUNTTI, ANDERS WALLIN, TEODORO DEL SER, MARCO ROMANELLI, AND LEONARDO PANTONI .. 510

The Diagnosis of "Mixed" Dementia in the Consortium for the Investigation of Vascular Impairment of Cognition (CIVIC). *By* K. ROCKWOOD, C. MACKNIGHT, C. WENTZEL, S. BLACK, R. BOUCHARD, S. GAUTHIER, H. FELDMAN, D. HOGAN, A. KERTESZ, AND P. MONTGOMERY FOR THE CIVIC INVESTIGATORS 522

Glial Modulating and Neurotrophic Properties of Propentofylline and Its
Application to Alzheimer's Disease and Vascular Dementia. *By*
GARTH E. RINGHEIM 529

Investigating the Natural Course and Treatment of Vascular Dementia and
Alzheimer's Disease: Parallel Study Populations in Two Randomized,
Placebo-Controlled Trials. *By* BARBARA KITTNER, PETER PAUL
DE DEYN, AND TIMO ERKINJUNTTI 535

Preliminary Results from an MRI/CT-Based Database for Vascular
Dementia and Alzheimer's Disease. *By* PHILIP SCHELTENS AND
BARBARA KITTNER 542

Alzheimer's Disease and Vascular Dementia: Some Points of Confluence.
By HEDDA AGÜERO-TORRES AND BENGT WINBLAD 547

INDEX OF CONTRIBUTORS 553

Sponsorship was received from:

- BAYER AG
- EISAI LIMITED
- G.J. LIVANOS TRUST (ALZHEIMER'S REPORTS)
- HOECHST MARRION ROUSSEL
- JANSSEN PHARMACEUTICA
- NOVARTIS PHARMA AG
- PARKE-DAVIS
- PFIZER INC.
- SMITH KLINE BEECHAM PHARMACEUTICALS
- ZENECA
- MEDICAL RESEARCH COUNCIL
- INSTITUTE FOR BRAIN AND BLOOD VESSELS, AKITA JAPAN
- INSTITUTE FOR HEALTH OF THE ELDERLY
- UNIVERSITY OF NEWCASTLE UPON TYNE

Henryk Miroslaw Wisniewski, 1931–1999

Alzheimer's disease (AD) researchers and neuropathologists worldwide will appreciate the prolific scientific contributions of Dr. Henryk Wisniewski. Until his death on September 5, 1999, Henry had been a productive and creative researcher for almost 40 years having authored or coauthored some 650 papers. He made several seminal contributions not only to AD but to other degenerative conditions of the nervous system. In particular he carried out pioneering studies on the ultrastructure of neuritic plaques, tangles, and cerebral vessels affected by amyloid angiopathy. He also explored plaque pathogenesis and the role of microglia, perivascular cells, and myocytes in amyloid beta formation in man, monkey, and dog. Remarkably, other topics in his earlier contributions included the blood-brain barrier, scrapie mice, mechanisms of chronic relapsing demyelination, and experimental allergic encephalomyelitis, subacute sclerosing encephalitis, Landry-Guillain-Barre and Steele-Richardson-Olszewski syndromes, Pick disease, phenylketonuria, hydrocephalus and aluminium and spindle inhibitors induced encephalomyelopathy. These studies have withstood the test of time and set the stage for subsequent studies by many research groups. This characteristic multidisciplinary approach was developed from his early days in the 1960s at the Albert Einstein College of Medicine in Dr. Robert Terry's laboratory when he interacted with biochemists, molecular biologists, immunologists, neuroanatomists, brain imagers, and clinicians as well as psychologists and psychiatrists.

Up to his untimely departure, Henryk Wisniewski had been Director of the New York State Institute for Basic Research in Developmental Disabilities, generally known as the IBR. He assumed the IBR directorship in 1976 and assembled a multidisciplinary team of scientists most of whom are now internationally known and have their own successful research programs. Henry also attracted several international visiting scientists and neuropathologists to work for periods of time at the IBR. His enthusiasm and energy resulted in one of the largest integrated programs at the IBR focusing on age-associated changes and performance among adults with mental retardation. In 1995 together with Dr. M. Janicki he edited a book entitled *Aging and Developmental Disabilities: Issues and Approaches.* This book drew the general public's and health providers' attention to the fact that like the rest of the population individuals with mental retardation age and are affected by old age diseases including AD.

Dr. Wisniewski's entrepreneurial skills were also to be evident in his busy life. Recognizing the importance of monoclonal antibodies in research and diagnosis of AD, he encouraged the IBR scientists to initiate production of antibodies against the proteins involved in the pathogenesis of AD and prion dementias. Dr. K.S. Kim's research resulted in production of the most sensitive and specific antibodies for detecting human amyloid beta protein. Two of these antibodies 4G8 reactive to the 17–24 residue of amyloid beta, and 6E10, reactive to the 1–17 residue to human amyloid beta are used extensively by scientists throughout the world. IBR scientists have also produced antibodies that detect Alzheimer type of neurofibrillary tangles and prion proteins. These antibodies have enabled many scientists led by the IBR immunologist Dr. P.D. Mehta to assay body fluids and develop laboratory diagnostic tests for diseases of the nervous system.

Under Henry's direction, the IBR is also remembered as the base for a highly successful series of international conferences. It is now more than 12 years since Khalid Iqbal, Bengt Winblad, and Al Snider have convened biennial meetings on AD and related disorders that have now become so popular for clinicians and researchers alike. Indeed, Henry will be missed at these international jamborees.

Henry received many accolades and honorary degrees. He is listed in Marquis's *Who's Who in America?* and in *American Men and Women in Science*, but perhaps the best testimony of his contributions to our knowledge of degenerative diseases of the nervous system was evident when Henry was named among the neuropathologists of the 20th Century in 1990 at the XI International Congress of Neuropathology in Kyoto, Japan.

With respect to this volume, it is particularly gratifying that Henryk Wisniewski was able to contribute as a special lecturer. Dr Wisniewski had a particular interest in the identification of nonneuronal cells involved in beta-amyloidosis. In earlier work, Henry and his colleagues showed that cerebral vessels affected by amyloid and dyshoric angiopathy allowed the identification of smooth muscle cells in small and large vessels and perivascular cells and capillaries as a source of amyloid-beta. Most recently, Henry and his associates reported that smooth muscle cells in tissue culture produce both fibrillar and nonfibrillar amyloid deposits. The vascular cell system as Wisniewski and others (RNK and see this volume) have shown may represent a potential model in which therapeutic agents might be tested for the efficacy of preventing beta-amyloidosis in AD.

Perhaps outside USA and his home in Poland where he was born and studied at the Medical Schools in Gdansk and Warsaw, Henry will be particularly remembered by several individuals in Newcastle upon Tyne. Henry was director of the then Medical Research Council (MRC) Demyelinating Diseases Unit in Newcastle from 1974–1976 in between his posts at the Albert Einstein College of Medicine and the IBR. During his time in Newcastle he made many friends and came to know a number of dementia researchers who are still active today affiliated with the present MRC Neurochemical Pathology Unit. Despite his reduced activities curtailed by poor health, Henry traveled to what would be his last international meeting in May 1999 at Slaley Hall near Newcastle. Although Henry might have seemed softened at times, he was as engaging, controversial, and flamboyant as ever. A pleasure to have seen him once again in his old stomping grounds in the bright Northumberland Spring.

Those who are promoting the vascular field in AD research will particularly remember Henry. Perhaps memories of his long speeches and his strong views on certain aspects of AD pathogenesis that irritated many will be quickly forgotten when one recalls that Henry was indeed an inspiration and a testament to what hard work and devotion to science can bring. There is no doubt that Henry would have given many more interesting lectures, voiced controversial ideas, and written papers germane to the current research in AD had he lived into the new millennium.

R.N. Kalaria
A.E. Oakley

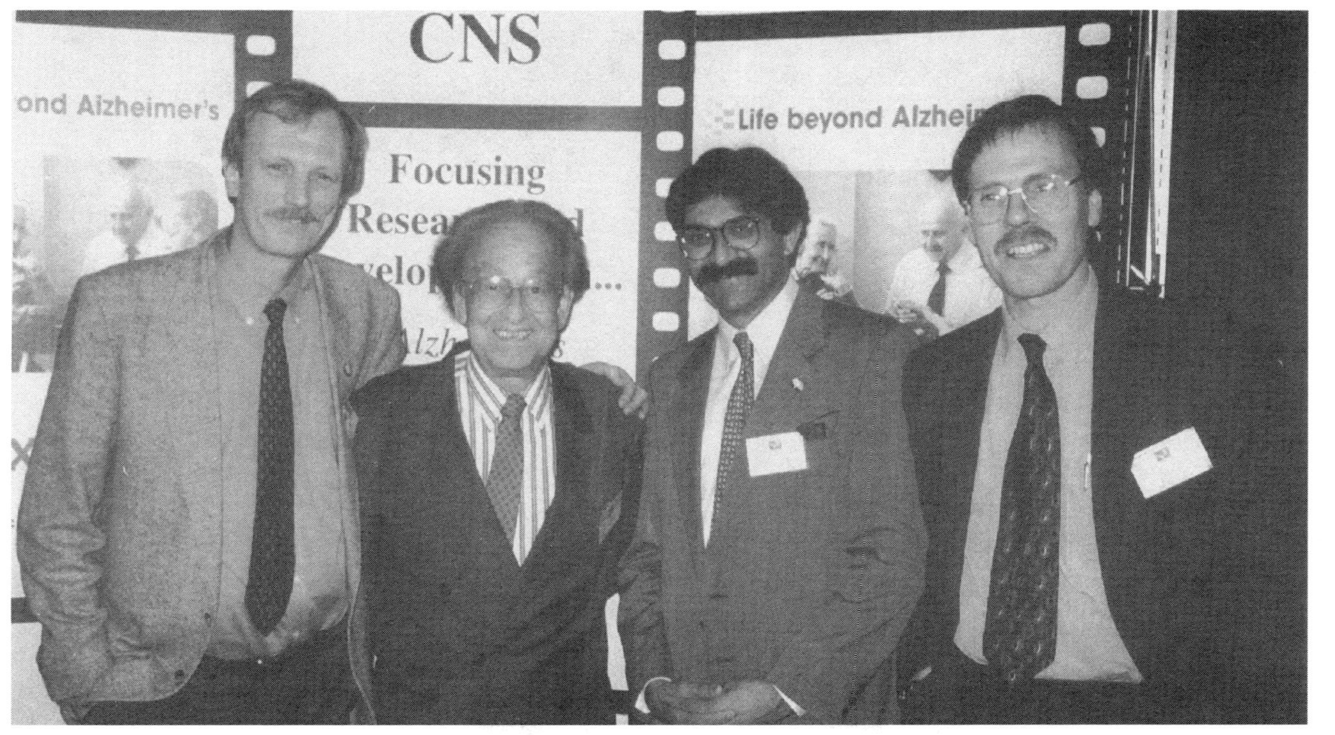

Conference organizers (left to right): Mr. Arthur Oakley (Conference Manager), Professor Henryk Wisniewski (1931–1999), Professor Raj Kalaria, and Dr. Paul Ince.

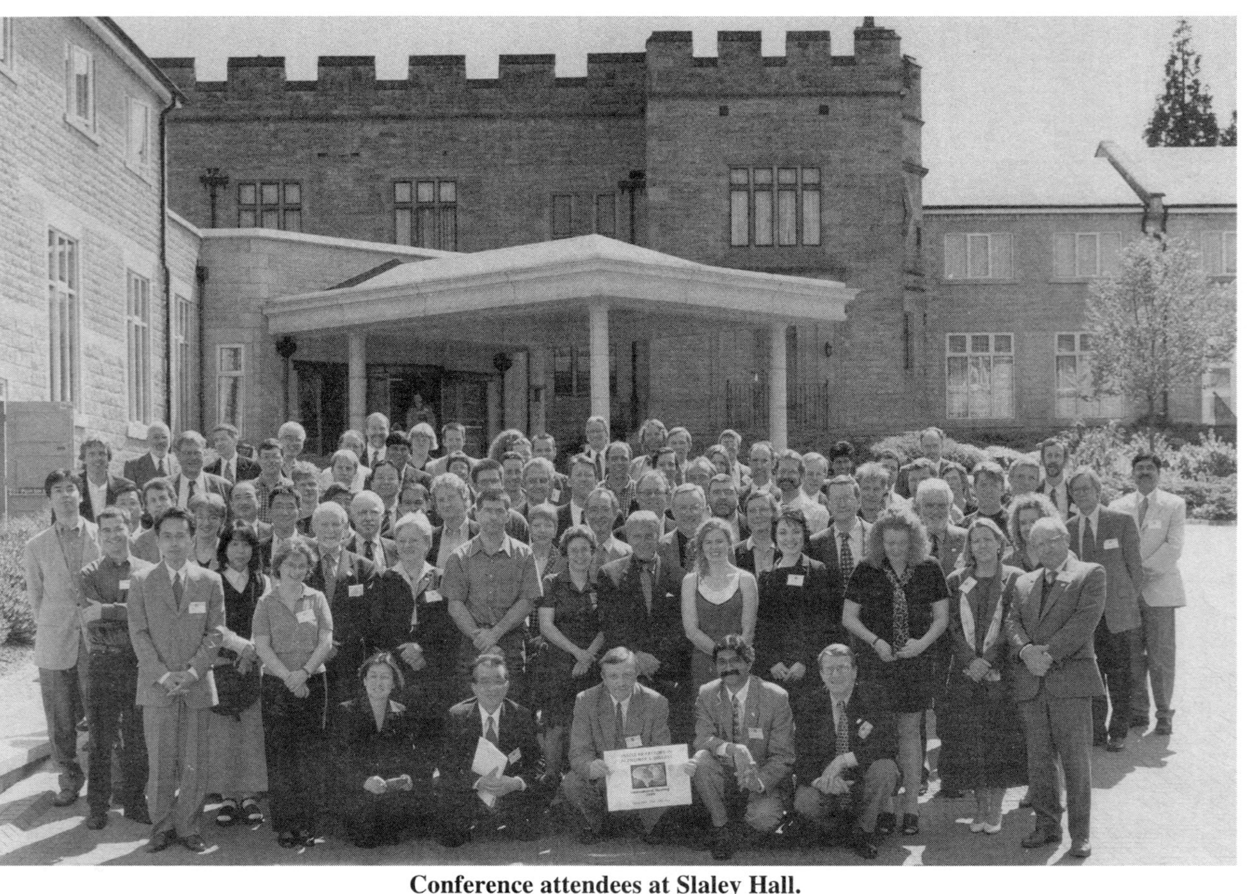

Conference attendees at Slaley Hall.

Preface

Acceptance of new vistas in science is almost always faced with difficulty invariably because they come ahead of their time. Neither the science nor the scientist prevails until the time is right. The search for the cause of Alzheimer's disease continues strongly despite 90 years plus since Alzheimer described the case of Auguste D. in 1907. This past "Decade of the Brain," has clearly witnessed significant advances in Alzheimer's disease, which have sprung from new ideas. Is failure in vascular integrity a causal factor in Alzheimer's disease? This volume testifies that many researchers believe so and have invested much time and effort to these ends. Indeed, vascular influences that relate to cerebrovascular abnormalities or vascular pathophysiology have rapidly gained importance in the cause and progression of Alzheimer's disease. Serious thinking on these issues is readily evident from the contents of this volume on the role of brain vascular pathology and cardiovascular factors in Alzheimer's disease. These monographs represent a considerable advancement since the last proceedings published by the Academy on this subject.[1] One can truly hope that research grant support for this important field of dementia will continue to increase in tandem with what now appears to be of phenomenal interest.

This volume will be of use and interest to many. It singly addresses several pertinent epidemiological, clinical, genetic, and pathological issues to establish the role of vascular factors in the etiopathogenesis of Alzheimer's disease. Indeed, the scope of the presentations extends beyond what the theme of the volume suggests and perhaps rightly so. Many cases of dementia lie in the "border zone" and present with pathologies associated with both Alzheimer's disease and vascular dementia. Therefore, the distinction between entities defined by the clinical criteria and pathological stance need to be resolved. Since we like to "box" items we do not know where to place cases with mixed or fuzzy pathologies or clearly understand common features like white matter lesions or microinfarcts in the etiology of dementia. We may accept that white matter lesions contribute to dementia occurring in stroke, but we are uncertain whether these matter or are predictive for Alzheimer's disease. Appropriately the suggested prospective studies involving assessments at multiple time points would be necessary to underpin this important pathological feature of the ageing brain.

In addition to novel and inspiring ideas with respect to cerebral pathology, animal models, risk factors for dementia, and diagnostic issues, several papers tackle questions related to the dynamics, origin and mobilization of amyloid-beta and its modulation by apolipoprotein E. Nonneuronal cells including myocytes associated with arterial vessels and perivascular cells are likely additional sources of fibrillar and nonfibrillar amyloid-beta, but it is intriguing that purely neuronal amyloid-beta may cause cerebral amyloid angiopathy, at least in one transgenic mouse with brain amyloidosis. On the other hand, the accumulation of cerebral amyloid and vascular deposition in Alzheimer patients may solely be due to clogging of the vascular routes leading to the brain's lymphatic drainage pathways. Interestingly, the cerebral microvasculature itself may be responsible for producing undesirables such as nitric oxide or proteinacious toxins that may cause injury to perivascular neurons.

The volume also presents several timely issues relating to the brain amyloid angiopathies, vasculopathies, and familial forms of vascular dementia including cerebral autosomal dominant arteriopathy with subcortical infarcts and leukoencephalopathy. The existence of a new missense mutation in the amyloid precursor protein associated with hereditary cerebral hemorrhage of the Italian type is of interest. However, it is exciting to fathom the familial disorder originally described by Worster-Drought *et al.*[2] as a British type of cerebral amyloid angiopathy with neurofibrillary changes. This type of dementia dubbed as familial British dementia (or FBD) is caused by a mutation in the stop codon of a novel gene (*BRI*) and, needless to say, the product of the gene forms characteristic amyloid fibrils associated with the cerebral vasculature.

As several papers show we have sufficient information to seriously consider the need for preventative measures to protect the vascular system such that we can counter senile dementia. The OPTIMA study suggests that plasma concentrations of total homocysteine are increased in Alzheimer patients and that homocysteine might be used as an independent predictor of cognitive decline in the elderly. While the cardiovascular anomalies may be corrected by supplementing with folate, these observations highlight the timely view that drug companies need to now seriously embark on trials to test whether existing lipid or cholesterol lowering drugs are efficacious to deter cognitive decline in the elderly. Intervention studies with β-hydroxy-β-methylglutaryl coenzyme A (HMG-CoA) reductase inhibitors (e.g., pravastatin) or low dose estrogen could be beneficial to preserve cognitive function. Meanwhile, treatment with anticholinesterases in both Alzheimer's disease and vascular dementia may continue to be explored. A few papers remind us why the cholinergic connection should still be pursued. Impairment in the cholinergic innervation associated with the cerebral vasculature might be important in the pathogenesis. Even though cholinergic deficits are apparent in the cholesterol fed rabbit, it is also a viable model to investigate vascular inflammatory mechanisms associated with cerebral amyloidosis.

Newcastle has had a strong tradition in dementia research, where Bernard Tomlinson, Gary Blessed, and Martin Roth "rediscovered" Alzheimer's disease and linked the critical volume of cerebral infarction to dementia in the elderly. With respect to the latter we are now enlightened that microinfarction rather than macroinfarction is critical to dementia, and the lesion likely also increases the burden of Alzheimer's disease. There is no doubt that this volume provides an impetus for such tradition to continue in Newcastle as it profoundly does to those who have contributed from other renowned institutions. We believe the recently established "Medical Research Council-University Centre Development for Clinical Brain Ageing" under the directorship of Professor James Edwardson should afford greater opportunities to pursue these new vistas. Although centuries prior to these developments, can we boast that "the cultural flowering focus of language had found its sharpest focus in the far northern kingdom of Northumbria?" Here on the outermost edge of the then civilized world sprang forth England's first great poet, the monastic Caedmon, first great historian, the Venerable Bede the monk from Jarrow famed by writing *The Ecclesiastical History of the English People*, and first great scholar Alcuin of York, keeper of Charlmagne's palace school and a progenitor of the Renaissance!

Finally, Paul Ince and I take this opportunity to offer our sincere appreciation for the scientific contributions and of course to our sponsors comprising several organizations without whose support this volume and indeed the conference would not have been possible. We are also indebted to several individuals at the Medical

Research Council Unit, the Institute for the Health of the Elderly, and the University of Newcastle upon Tyne. Of these we mention Arthur Oakley who has assisted us ever so willingly and tirelessly to achieve success in every task. Newcastle had the good fortune to be at the center of the focus perhaps compliant with Simeon Potter's notation in *Our Language*[3] that "The light of learning then shone more brightly in Northumbria than anywhere else in Europe."

We would also like to thank Barbara M. Goldman for taking on this book and all the staff at the office of the *Annals* of The New York Academy of Sciences. I particularly express gratitude to Justine Cullinan, Marion L. Garry, and Cook Kimball who were extremely accommodating and patiently worked with us through all the stages in the production of this volume.

Raj N. Kalaria

REFERENCES

1. DE LA TORRE, J.C. & V. HACHINSKI. 1997. Cerebrovascular pathology in Alzheimer's disease. Ann. N.Y. Acad. Sci. **826.**
2. WORSTER-DROUGHT, C. *et al.* 1940. A familial form of presenile dementia with spastic paralysis. Brain **63:** 237–254.
3. POTTER, S. 1976. Our Language. Penguin Books. London.

Vascular Factors in Cognitive Impairment— Where Are We Now?

VLADIMIR HACHINSKI[a,c] AND DAVID MUNOZ[a,b]

[a]*Department of Clinical Neurological Sciences and* [b]*Department of Pathology, University of Western Ontario, London, Ontario, Canada N6A 5A5*

INTRODUCTION

Medicine advances by swaying between extremes. Thirty years ago, "atherosclerosis" was almost synonymous with dementia, now "Alzheimer's disease" is. However, a minority of investigators have noted vascular components of Alzheimer's disease, and they got together at the first conference on the cerebrovascular pathology of Alzheimer's disease in 1996 to explore these systematically.[1] Since then, their efforts have had some resonance, but much remains to be sorted out before we can tackle the upcoming epidemic of cognitive impairment.

OBSOLESCENCE OF CURRENT CONCEPTS OF DEMENTIA

All commonly used criteria for dementia have been developed by consensus and opinion, and it shows. At one point, when there was no hope for treatment or prevention, the validity or otherwise of the definitions and criteria did not matter, because nothing could be done about cognitive impairment. That is beginning to change. Most definitions of dementia require that the patient be incapable of self sufficiency. By that time it is too late to do anything except provide symptomatic treatment regardless of the etiology of the dementia. Moreover, for each patient considered demented, there are two individuals with cognitive impairment short of dementia (CIND).[2] The cornerstone of all criteria of dementia is memory impairment. This criterion works very well for Alzheimer's disease, where memory is an early and constant feature, but it seldom helps in identifying individuals with cognitive impairment on a vascular bases. About 80% of all strokes occur in the carotid artery distribution, only 20% affecting the vertebrobasilar system, which supplies the hippocampi. While strokes in the medial temporal lobes cause memory impairment, it usually takes bilateral lesions for serious and permanent memory problems. Strokes affecting cognition occur most commonly in the frontobasal systems that subserve judgement, planning, and emotion, features seldom tested in cognitive screens.

The most fundamental problem with current criteria of dementia is that they do not work. In the Canadian study of Health and Aging, which is both a population-

[c]Address for correspondence: Dr. Vladimir Hachinski, Department of Clinical Neurological Sciences, University of Western Ontario, London, Ontario, Canada N6A 5A5. Tel.: (519) 663-3652; fax: (519) 663-3910.
e-mail: Rebecca.Nott@LHSC.ON.CA

and institution-based study, 1879 subjects were identified as demented by consensus. Then six commonly used criteria of dementia were applied to the same subjects. Little overlap emerged, and a surprising 10-fold difference separated the least and the most sensitive criteria. According to ICD-10 criteria, 3.1% of the population over the age of 65 years is demented, by DSM-III criteria 29.1% are![3] This makes a huge difference to the individual, health planners, and investigators. An individual labeled as demented cannot drive a car, make a will, or look after his or her affairs. A health planner will submit a vastly different budget if expecting 3.1% or 29.1% of the population over 65 years to be demented. Investigators trying to interpret the findings of the researchers using other criteria are open to gross misinterpretations, since the populations are likely to differ in very significant ways. Moreover, knowledge cannot be built upon common bases in the presence of discordances of this magnitude.

ASCERTAINMENT AND CLASSIFICATION BIASES

Dementia series tend to come from memory clinics, where patients with Alzheimer's disease prevail. Even in epidemiological studies the definitions require that the patient have memory impairment and hence even among cases labeled "vascular" cases with Alzheimer's disease plus vascular lesions will predominate. If patients have a stroke severe enough to cause physical impairment, this gets the most of the attention, cognition seldom being examined. Those having a stroke only affecting cognition but sparing memory may not come to medical attention at all.

Most clinicopathological series claim an accuracy of about 90%. However, only patients who die come to autopsy, typically 7–8 years after the diagnosis of Alzheimer's disease is made. If one includes the 23% of patients who initially are diagnosed as Alzheimer's disease who do not deteriorate cognitively and survive in the denominator, the accuracy drops considerably.[4] This has many implications. What do the patients who do not deteriorate have? Should one make an initial diagnosis of "cognitive syndrome" to permit the possibility that the diagnosis of Alzheimer's disease is wrong and to allow for the family to adapt if it is right? What are the implications for clinical trials of entering patients who could not respond to medication?

Beyond these considerations, the connection of vascular factors with Alzheimer's disease rests on three lines of evidence: epidemiological studies of association of vascular risk factors with dementia, high prevalence of progressive dementia poststroke, and modulation of the clinical manifestations of pathologically diagnosed Alzheimer's disease by cerebral infarcts.

VASCULAR RISK FACTORS IN DEMENTIA

Hypertension, diabetes, smoking, and atrial fibrillation are well recognized risk factors for stroke and multiinfarct dementia. As discussed elsewhere in this volume, now it appears that they may also be risk factors for dementia diagnosed clinically as Alzheimer's disease. Moreover, preliminary evidence suggests that treating hypertension may decrease or delay dementia. High cholesterol, high plasma homocysteine levels, and low folate levels are also associated with Alzheimer's disease, although it remains to be seen whether the mechanism of action of these putative risk factors involves blood vessels.

DEMENTIA POST-STROKE

About one quarter of patients suffering a stroke are found to be demented three months later. This represents a risk more than 9 times greater than in the general population, after adjusting for age, education, and race. If impairment in cognitive domains, rather than dementia, is considered, almost half of patients under 65 years of age, and three quarters of those over 75 are affected.[5] Interestingly only a minority seem to deteriorate from multiinfarct dementia. Some have had prior cognitive impairment, and a majority progress like Alzheimer's disease. In fact, among patients remaining cognitively intact a few months after stroke, the risk of developing delayed dementia rises over that of the general population 6 times in hospital-based studies,[6] and 9 times in population-based studies.[7] Strokes may well precipitate, aggravate, or accelerate a preexisting process or predisposition.

COEXISTENCE AND POSSIBLE INTERACTION
FOR STROKE AND ALZHEIMER'S DISEASE

For too long Alzheimer's disease and dementia on a vascular basis were considered as antonymous. Some classifications do not even allow for a "mixed" category. Snowden *et al.*[8] have shown that among elderly nuns having the pathological diagnosis of "Alzheimer's disease" only 57% were demented. Among those having the pathological diagnosis of Alzheimer's disease plus cortical infarcts 75% were demented, and among those having pathological Alzheimer's disease and small infarcts in the subcortical areas, 93% were demented. Clearly the effects of Alzheimer's disease are potentiated by strokes, since "lesions in the brain do not add up, they multiply."[9]

In a clinical pathological study addressing the question of education and dementia, no difference was found in the progression of dementia once diagnosed among individuals with a primary education, secondary education, and college or university education. Similarly, the degree of brain atrophy and the presence of senile plaques and neurofibrillary tangles was comparable among the educational groups. However, the least-educated patients had a significantly higher prevalence of lacunar infarcts, white matter lesions, macroscopic infarcts, and other vascular lesions than the other two groups with higher education.[10] Some of the reported higher prevalence of dementia among the poorly educated may be accounted for by the higher prevalence of vascular lesions. Moreover, the prevalence of infarcts in addition to Alzheimer's disease increases with age, and thus the interaction is most relevant in the group with the highest prevalence and incidence of dementia.

VASCULAR MECHANISMS IN ALZHEIMER'S DISEASE

How could vascular abnormalities short of extensive infarcts influence the course of Alzheimer's disease? We lack enlightening clues. Several mechanisms come to mind: ischemia, inflammation, and alterations of the blood-brain barrier, the gateway to the brain.

As discussed elsewhere in this volume, amyloid deposits in cortical and leptomeningeal arteries have long been recognized, but are relatively scarce in Alzheimer's disease, are often severe in cases of hemorrhagic congophilic angiopathy in the absence of dementia, and have not been shown to relate to the clinical expression of Alzheimer's disease. The demonstration of the vasoactive properties of amyloid suggest the possibility of a wider and more ubiquitous role. Reductions in cerebral blood flow and metabolism and increases in oxygen extraction have been reported in Alzheimer's disease. However, it is unclear whether these are causes or consequences of Alzheimer's disease. Moreover, none of the alterations in cerebral blood flow and metabolism have reached critical levels. The concept of chronic ischemia is often invoked, but proof has remained elusive. The actions of estrogen and statins on the endothelium may be relevant. Collagenosis of veins may play a role in leukoaraiosis and thus perhaps cognitive impairment.

THE NEED FOR A NEW APPROACH

We need to take a pragmatic conceptual retreat before we are ready to advance at an accelerated pace. We need to identify potential patients long before they are demented, including symptomless individuals at high risk of developing cognitive impairment. When subjects have cognitive impairment, this should be characterized clinically and by a commonly agreed minimum of standardized tests.[11] The assessment should also include a minimum set of demographic, medical, and neurological characteristics. Imaging of the brain and DNA banking should be carried out whenever feasible. Rather than seeking a clinical opinion about etiology, progression of clinical, neuropsychological, and imaging parameters should be recorded in a quantitative fashion.

If data are recorded in a modular form, they can be reformatted into working criteria, updated and reanalyzed. With standardized data and the ability to analyze for genetic factors as knowledge grows, we would continue to learn from the same set of patients. Updates and corrections should be regular features of longitudinal studies, and autopsies should be secured whenever possible. Clinical trials can already begin, focusing on mechanisms that may be common to a number of causes of cognitive impairment such as glutamate release, oxidative stress, apoptosis, and inflammation. Each trial will narrow the target and bring us closer to a treatment. Effective treatments are already available for vascular risk factors, some with potential for acting via more than one mechanism, such as the statins that lower cholesterol and probably also act on the vascular endothelium. We must learn by doing.

CONCLUSION

Historically and by definition vascular risk factors predisposed to stroke and vascular dementia. Their presence was often used as an exclusion criterion for diagnosing Alzheimer's disease, and hence no relationship was found, by definition. It took several longitudinal studies to establish that hypertension, diabetes, atrial fibrillation, and smoking are risk factors for dementia, including Alzheimer's disease. Preliminary data suggest that treating these risk factors may prevent or delay dementia.

It is also becoming evident that strokes and ischemic processes not only coexist with but may precipitate or potentiate Alzheimer's disease. We still do not know how these factors act nor how they may relate to the vascular components of Alzheimer's disease. The important point is that they do, and this provides new avenues for research and potential treatment. We are still at that bewildering stage that follows discovery but precedes true understanding.

REFERENCES

1. DE LA TORRE, J. & V. HACHINSKI, Eds. 1997. Cerebrovascular Pathology in Alzheimer's Disease. Annals of the New York Academy of Sciences. Vol. 826. The New York Academy of Sciences. New York.
2. EBLY, E.M., D.B. HOGAN & I.M. PARHAD. 1995. Cognitive impairment in the nondemented elder: results from the Canadian Study of Health and Aging. Arch. Neurol. **52:** 612–619.
3. ERKINJUNTTI, T., T. OSTBYE, R. STEENHUIS & V. HACHINSKI. 1997. The effect of different diagnostic criteria on the prevalence of dementia. N. Engl. J. Med. **337:** 1667–1674.
4. BOWLER, J.V., D.G. MUNOZ, H. MERSKEY & V. HACHINSKI. 1998. Fallacies in the pathological confirmation of the diagnosis of Alzheimer's disease. J. Neurol. Neurosurg. Psychiatry **64:** 18–24.
5. TATEMICHI, T.K., D.W. DESMOND, Y. STERN, M. PAIK, M. SANO & E. BAGIELLA. 1994. Cognitive impairment after stroke: frequency, patterns and relationship to functional abilities. JNNP **57:** 202–207.
6. TATEMICHI, T.K., M. PAIK, E. BEGIELLA, D.W. DESMOND, Y. STERN, M. SANO, W.A. HAUSER & R. MAYEUX. 1994. Risk of dementia after stroke in a hospitalized cohort: results of a longitudinal study. Neurology **44:** 1885–1896.
7. KOKMEN, E., J.P. WHISNANT, W.M. O'FALLON, C.-P. CHU & C.M. BEARD. 1996. Dementia after ishemic stroke: a population-based study in Rochester, Minnesota. Neurology **46:** 154–159.
8. SNOWDEN, D.A., L.H. GRENER, J.A. MORTIMER, K.P. RILEY, P.A. GREINER & W.R. MARKESBERY. 1997. Brain infarction and the clinical expression of Alzheimer's disease: the nun study. JAMA **277:** 813–817.
9. HACHINSKI, V. 1983. Multi-infarct dementia (Symposium on Cerebrovascular Disease) *In* Neurology Clinicals. Vol. 1, No. 1, 27–36.
10. DEL SER, T., V. HACHINSKI, H. MERSKEY & D.G. MUNOZ. 1999. An autopsy-verified study of the effect of education on degenerative dementia. Brain **122:** 2309–2319.
11. HACHINSKI, V.C. 1992. Preventable senility: a call for action against the vascular dementias. Lancet **340:** 645–648.

Role of Perivascular Cells and Myocytes in Vascular Amyloidosis

H.M. WISNIEWSKI, J. WEGIEL, A.W. VORBRODT, B. MAZUR-KOLECKA, AND J. FRACKOWIAK

New York State Institute for Basic Research in Developmental Disabilities, Staten Island, New York 10314, USA

ABSTRACT: Amyloidogenic processing of amyloid-β precursor protein (APP) by cells of the brain is the major pathologic component of Alzheimer's disease. Amyloid-β (Aβ) is of heterogenous origin. Perivascular cells of monocyte-macrophage-microglial cell lineage produce fibrillar Aβ in the wall of capillaries, whereas parenchymal microglial cells produce fibrillar Aβ in the parenchyma of gray matter. Fibrillar Aβ deposition by perivascular cells leads to endothelial cell degeneration and death, obliteration of affected capillaries, and reduction of the length of the vascular network. These changes cause local ischemia with neuronal degeneration and death. Smooth muscle cells are the source of Aβ in the tunica media of parenchymal and leptomeningeal arteries and veins. Fibrillar Aβ in the tunica media of leptomeningeal and parenchymal vessels causes degeneration and necrosis of smooth muscle cells and leads to multiple cortical hemorrhages. Smooth muscle cells isolated from blood vessels with amyloid deposits secrete Aβ and accumulate nonfibrillar Aβ intracellularly. The amyloidogenic processing of APP can be enhanced by apolipoprotein E, reduced by transthyretin, and modulated by several cytokines.

In elderly individuals and some species of animals, as well as victims of Alzheimer disease (AD), there are two types of vascular amyloidosis: one affecting larger meningeal and parenchymal vessels; the other, capillaries and precapillaries. The latter condition is also called dyshoric angiopathy. In dyshoric angiopathy, the perivascular cells appear to be the source and cause of amyloid-β (Aβ) fibrillization. As in microglia,[1] the process of fibrillization appears to be a cell membrane-associated phenomenon.[2] In electron microscopy pictures at higher magnification, one can see amyloid fibrils streaming out of the deep infoldings of the cytoplasmic membranes of perivascular cells (FIG. 1). Depending on the distribution of the perivascular cells along the vessel wall and the amount of amyloid fibril deposits, a broad spectrum of morphological forms of fibril arrangement is possible ranging from focal, semicircular deposits to circular, tuberous deposits and fully developed single or confluent amyloid stars (FIG. 2).

In areas where the amyloid fibers break through the glia-limiting membrane, some dystrophic response from the neuropil is visible. In our experience, the amyloid stars that are formed within the wall of the vessel and afterward "grow" into the neuropil are always surrounded by a narrow rim of astrocytic processes. This configuration is in contrast to the stars of the classical plaques of the neuropil, whose surface is covered only partially by astrocytes and which show many wisps of amy-

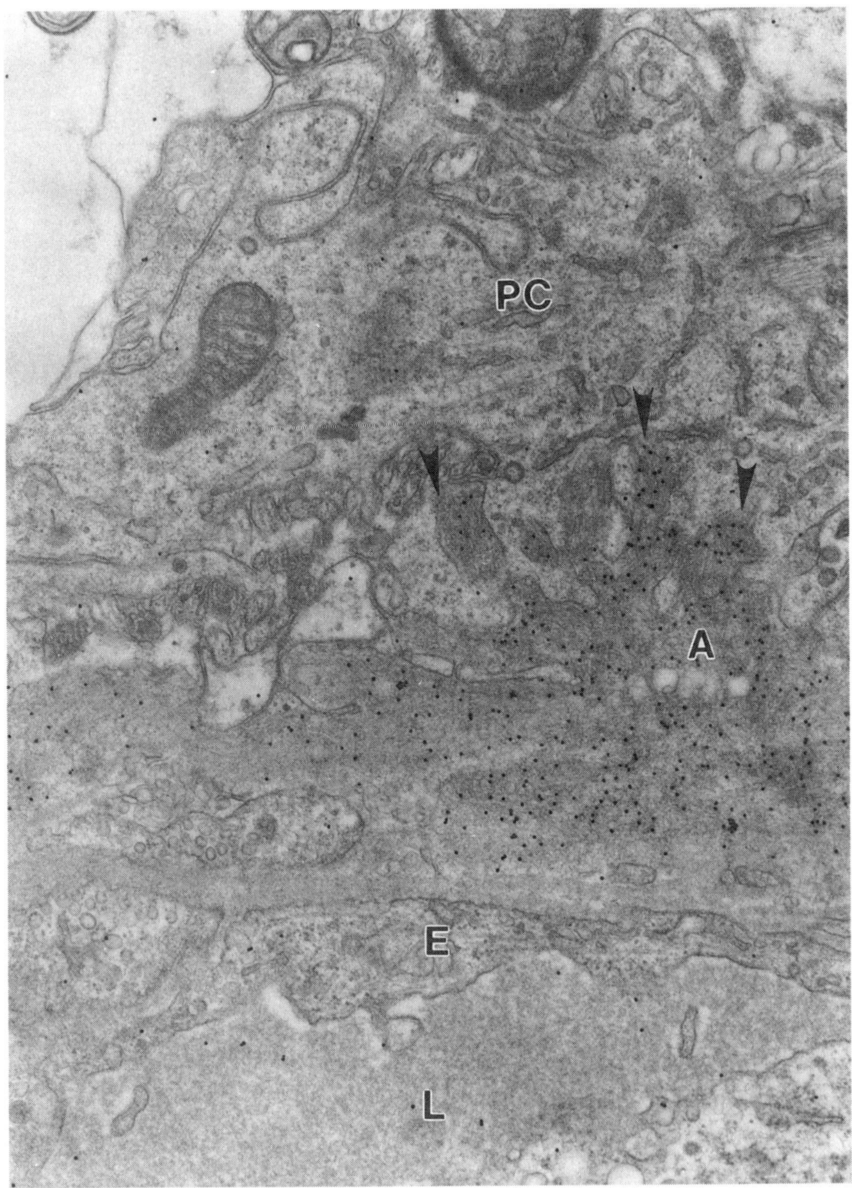

FIGURE 1. Perivascular cell (PC) with fibrillar amyloid streaming from deep cytoplasmic channels (*arrows*). A, amyloid deposit in the basal lamina; L, lumen of the capillary vessel; E, endothelial cell. Amyloid immunolabeled with mAb 4G8 (17–24 aa).

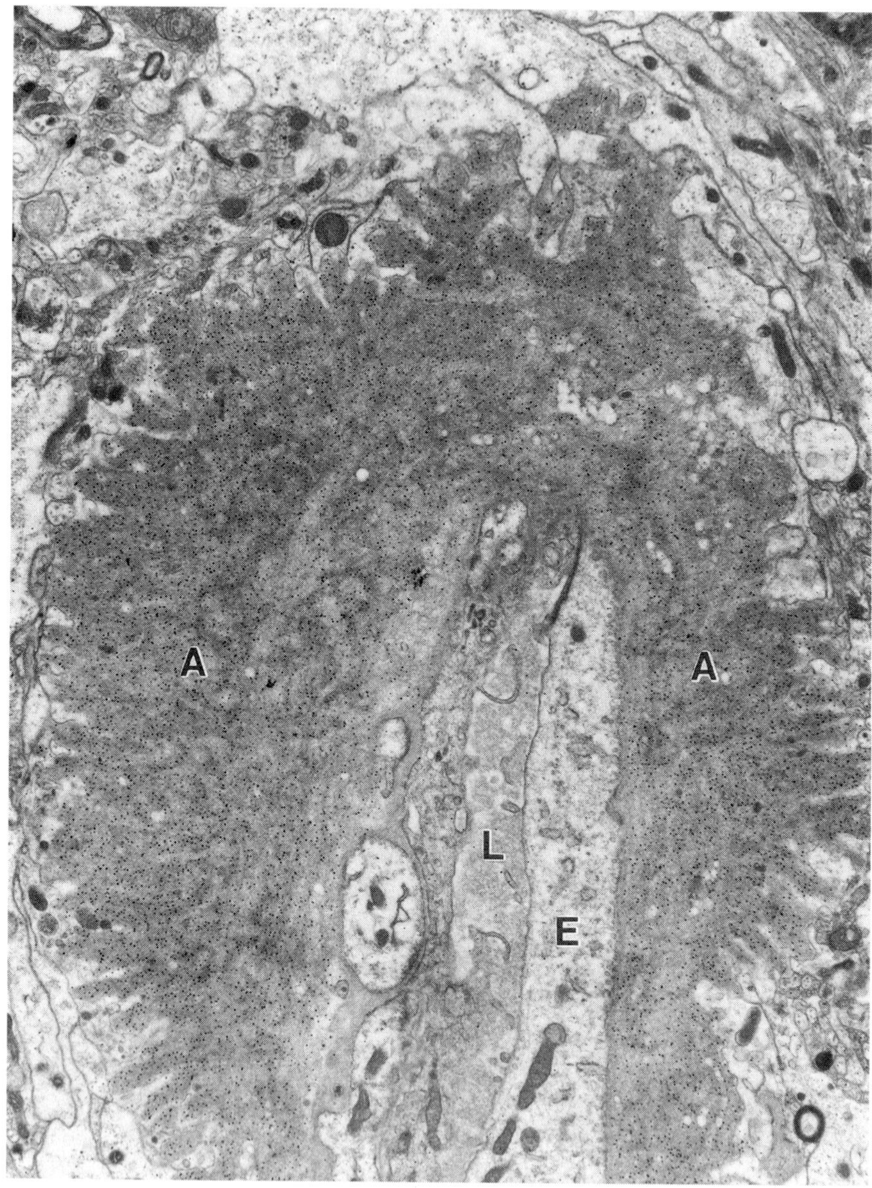

FIGURE 2. Confluent amyloid (A) deposit in the wall of the capillary vessel. E, endothelial cell; L, lumen of the capillary.

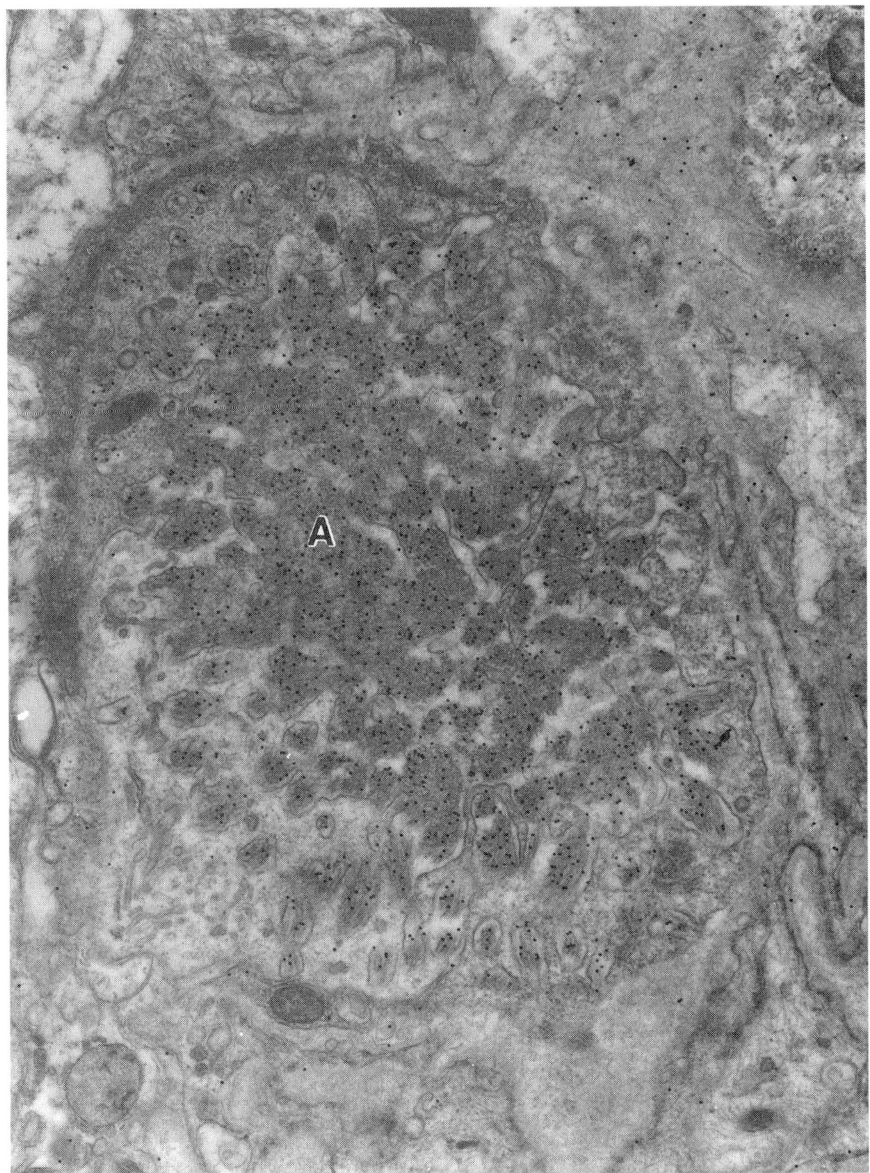

FIGURE 3. Tangential cut of the perivascular amyloid star (A) recalls burned-out plaque.

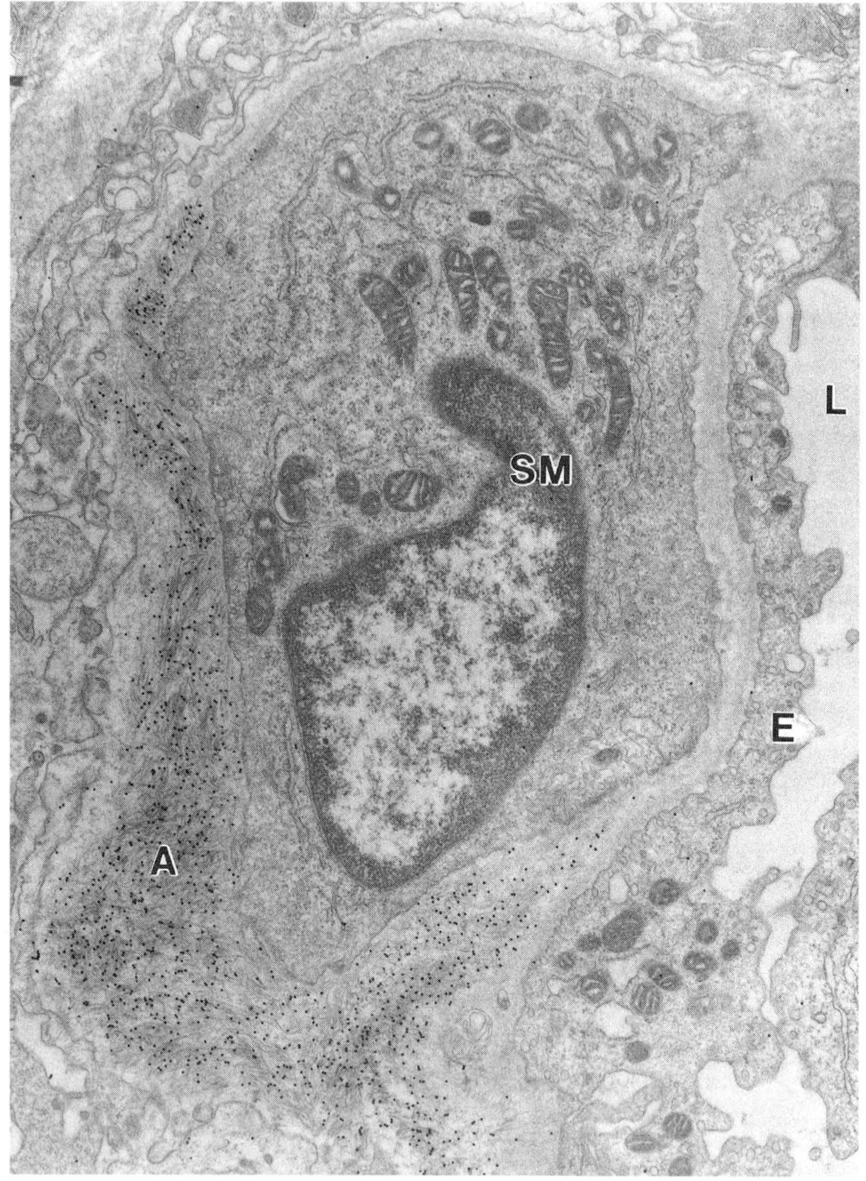

FIGURE 4. Fibrillar amyloid (A) in the tunica media of arteriole is the product of smooth muscle cell (SM). L, lumen of the artery; E, endothelial cell.

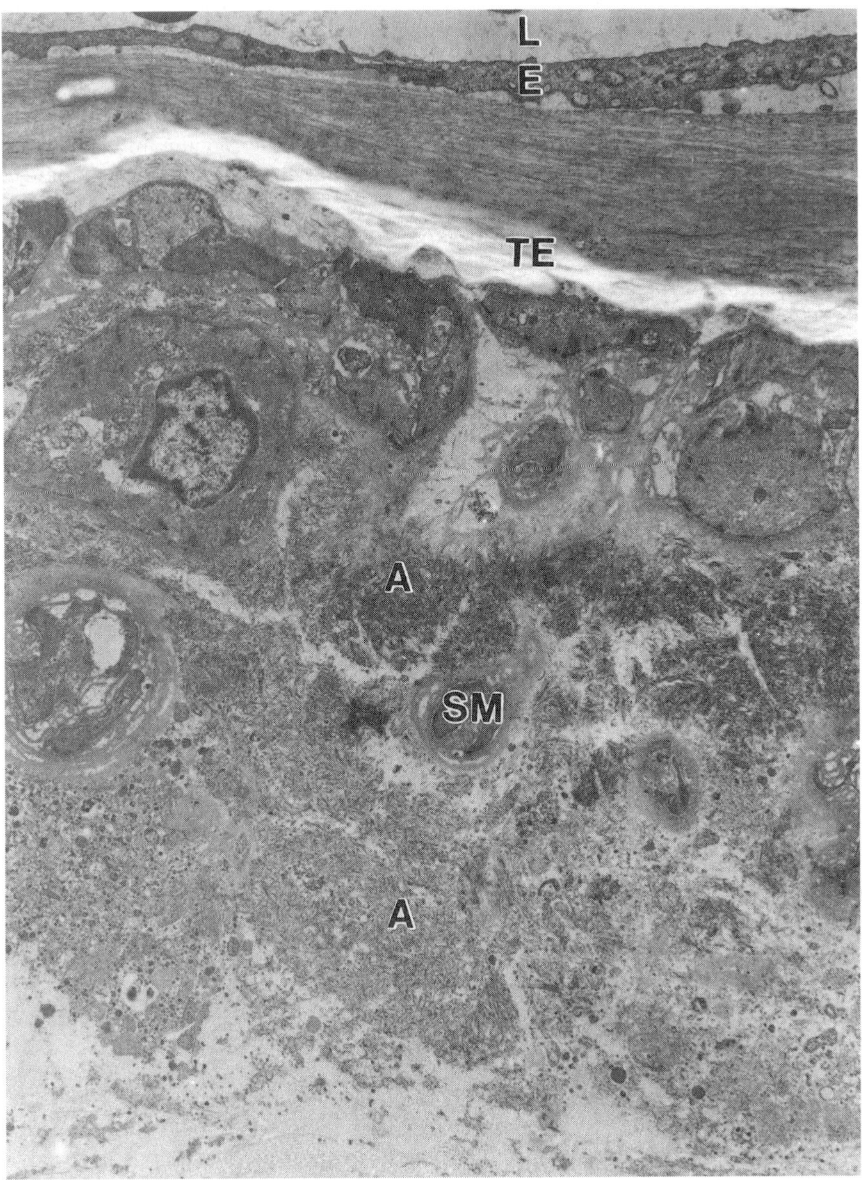

FIGURE 5. External zone of the tunica media of artery with degenerated smooth muscle cells (SM) and cell debris surrounded by fibrillar and partially degraded amyloid (A). Better preservation of smooth muscle cells in internal zone of the tunica media, which is later affected by amyloidosis. L, lumen of the artery; E, endothelial cell; TE, tunica elastica; A, adventitia.

loid fibrils infiltrating the neuropil.[1] Tangential cuts of the perivascular amyloid stars (FIG. 3), accompanied by minimal or no neuritic response, have a similar appearance to that of burned-out or amyloid plaques that have a small number of degenerating and dystrophic neurites. Only reconstruction using serial sections allows classification of the type of lesion.[3]

The amount of amyloid deposited had an impact on the endothelium and the lumen of the affected vessels. Many of the vessels with multiple amyloid stars were obliterated. Vessels with amyloid stars and tuberous amyloid deposits contained both degenerating endothelia and completely destroyed basal lamina. The extensive astrogliosis and the many neurons in various stages of degeneration seen in these areas therefore appear to be the result of ischemic changes.

On the basis of changes somewhat similar to those described in this paper, Ishii[4,5] and Miyakawa and co-workers[6,7] concluded that all plaques arise from the vessel wall. In our experience, as well as that of other investigators studying human and monkey brains,[8,9] only a part of the plaques comes from the vessel wall.

However, the morphology of cells that are engaged in the formation of amyloid fibrils, as well as the fact that their bodies lie in part under an external layer of vascular basal lamina and in part in the neuropil, suggests that the microglia that make amyloid fibrils in the neuropil are derived from the vessel wall.

In large vessels at early stages of amyloidogenesis, β-protein immunoreactive material is present at the light microscopic level in the vascular tunica media in the cytoplasm of myocytes or extracellularly between smooth muscle cells. The sites of β-protein deposition exhibit increased immunoreactivity for C-terminal fragments of Aβ-precursor protein. The cells around small β-protein deposits express actin, myosin, and vimentin, but most lack another smooth muscle-specific protein— desmin. These muscle cells often have swollen nuclei and express the proliferating cell nuclear antigen.[10] At more advanced stages of amyloidosis, the tunica media is replaced by amyloid deposits with only scanty smooth muscle cells. Macrophages and leukocytes are not present at the sites of amyloid formation. The results indicate that the cells engaged in the formation of vascular amyloid are proliferate and degenerate.

Ultrastructural study of the leptomeningeal vessels affected by amyloid angiopathy shows that Aβ deposits in the media of arteries and arterioles are produced by smooth muscle cells. It appears that the soluble β-protein secreted by sarcolemmal vesicles of the muscle cells polymerizes into amyloid fibrils in the basal lamina (FIG. 4). Myocytes trapped in amyloid deposits degenerate and die. The most common and severe degeneration of smooth muscle cells is seen in the external and medial zone of the vascular media. In more advanced stages of amyloidotic changes, the internal zone of the media also is involved. The media of vessels with severe changes consists of amyloid deposits and cell debris. Amyloid fibrils around the dead myocytes also undergo degradation (FIG. 5). Amyloid masses lose their fibrillar appearance and become floccular, granular, amorphous, proteinous material; however, this material is continually positive in immunostaining for Aβ. This study suggests that amyloid formation by smooth muscle cells involves a secretory pathway of Aβ. Our data indicate that the smooth muscle cell secretes nonfibrillar β-protein and that conversion of non-fibrillar into fibrillar Aβ takes place in the environment of the basement membrane.

In our material, aged dogs very rarely show perivascular cells producing dyshoric angiopathy. However, large amyloidogenic vessels, the product of myocytes, is a

TABLE 1. Numerical density of amyloid-positive vessels in neocortex of nondemented elderly individuals and of individuals with sporadic AD

Region	Numerical Density (n/mm^2)	
	Nondemented Elderly (mean age: 75 years) ($n = 5$)	Alzheimer Disease (mean age: 79 years) ($n = 20$)
Frontal	0.18 (0.34)	0.59 (2.15)
Temporal	0.18 (0.34)	0.34 (0.96)
Parietal	0.18 (0.27)	0.45 (1.41)
Occipital	0.44 (0.60)	1.07 (2.90)
Limbic	0.12 (0.23)	0.50 (1.81)
Insular	0.08 (0.15)	0.31 (0.87)

Values in parentheses indicate standard deviation.

common old-age–associated pathology. It appears that the same is true in transgenic Karen Hsiao and Karen Duff mice.

TOPOGRAPHY OF AMYLOID-POSITIVE VESSELS

Amyloid-positive vessels are common findings in nondemented elderly individuals. The numerical density of amyloid-positive vessels, immunostained with antibody (mAb) 4G8 (17–24 aa; number of amyloid-positive vascular profiles per square millimeter), is almost identical in frontal, temporal, and parietal cortices (0.18/mm^2) and is insignificantly lower in the limbic (0.12/mm^2) and insular (0.08/mm^2) cortices. Higher numerical density of amyloid-positive vessels was found in the occipital cortex (0.44/mm^2) of nondemented elderly persons.

The numerical density of amyloid-positive vessels in AD is from two to three times more than in the control group; however, no correlation exists between the numerical density of amyloid-positive cortical vessels and the age of AD subjects or the stage (GDS FAST) of AD. This lack of correlation and the lack of correlation between the amount of parenchymal plaques and amyloid-positive vessels suggest that vascular amyloidosis develops separately from parenchymal amyloidosis. Insignificant differences in the numerical density of amyloid-positive vessels in neocortical regions with a different blood supply suggest that the onset and progression of amyloidosis is not attributed to a specific brain artery.

The amount of amyloid-positive vessels is associated with genetic factors. Amyloid angiopathy is about two times more severe in the brains of individuals with Down syndrome (DS) than in sporadic AD, which indicates that the trisomy increases amyloidogenic amyloid-β precursor protein (APP) processing by smooth muscle cells. However, the pattern of distribution of amyloid-positive vessels is similar in both sporadic AD and in DS. Striking differences in the onset, progression, and topographic pattern of amyloid angiopathy are seen in the brains of individuals with the Polish P117L presenilin-1 (PS1) mutation. The presence of severe amyloid an-

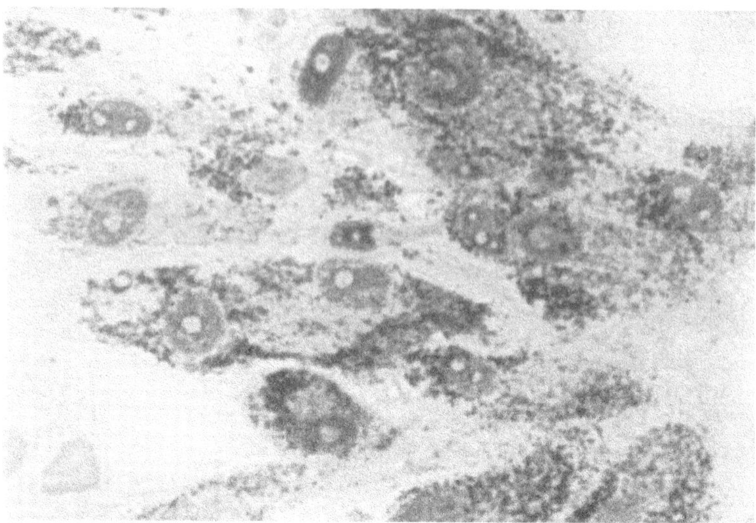

FIGURE 6. Vascular smooth muscle cells isolated from amyloid-affected blood vessels from a 17-year-old dog in the fourth passage. Cells contain cytoplasmic deposits immunoreactive for Ab with mAb 4G8. Magnification: 620×.

giopathy in the brains of people who die in the fourth decade of life after six to seven years of the clinical course of AD suggests that the PS1 mutation accelerates the onset and progression of amyloid angiopathy. The numerical density of amyloid-positive vessels is ten times greater in the brains of people with the PS1 mutation than in those of people with sporadic AD. Remarkable topographic differences in the numerical density of amyloid-positive vessels, with almost 91% of amyloid load in the cerebellar leptomeningeal vessels, indicate that the topography of amyloid deposition is genetically controlled.[11]

CELL CULTURE MODEL OF β-AMYLOIDOSIS

The amyloidogenic pathology of vascular smooth muscle cells can be transferred into cell culture. Myocytes, cultured from amyloidosis-affected brain-blood vessels, reveal certain features of amyloidogenic pathology:

(1) Accumulation of intracellular Aβ deposits, typically nonfibrillar and occasionally fibrillar deposits, demonstrated by immunocytochemical staining at the light microscopy (FIG. 6) and electron microscopy levels.[12–15] The increased cellular levels of Aβ also were confirmed by ELISA and immunoblotting[14,16,17] (FIG. 7A,B).

(2) Increased secretion of Aβ, shown by ELISA,[14,16,17] immunoblotting, and immunoprecipitation[13] (FIG. 7C).

(3) Altered processing of APP: increased intracellular retention of mature amyloid precursor protein 770, as demonstrated by metabolic labeling.[17]

A. Intracellular accumulation of Aβ (immunocytochemical staining)

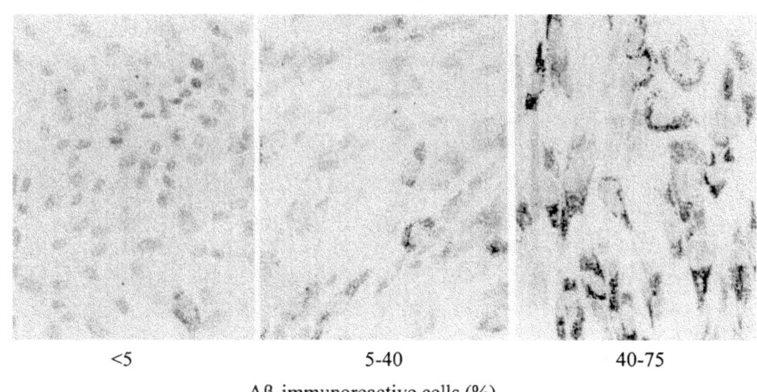

B. Intracellular accumulation of Aβ (ELISA)

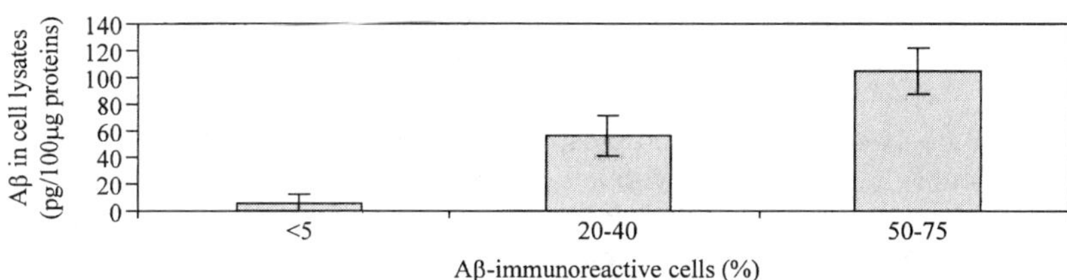

C. Secretion of Aβ (ELISA)

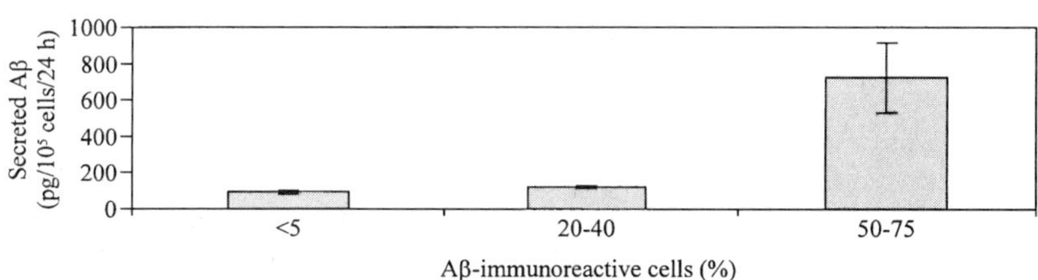

FIGURE 7. Stages of amyloidogenic pathology in cultures of vascular smooth muscle cells—initial, intermediate, and advanced—as detected by immunocytochemistry and ELISA.

Characterization of the above parameters allows us to estimate the level of cell involvement in β-amyloidogenic pathology.

Characterization of numerous cell strains isolated from brain-blood vessels affected by amyloid angiopathy of each individual human and canine case revealed prominent differences regarding their involvement in amyloidogenic processes. These results reflect a variability in the involvement of myocytes in amyloid formation *in vivo*. It is well known that amyloid formation is a focal process; thus, the blood vessels contain altered myocytes and apparently normal cells. By culturing cells from small fragments of vessels, we were able to obtain populations that were enriched in cells with certain levels of pathological changes.

Myocytes in which extensive Aβ accumulation takes place reveal several features of cell senescence: lowered mitochondrial activity, low proliferation rate, and tendency to detach from the culture surface.[15] Some cells with abundant Aβ deposits were shown to undergo apoptosis (unpublished data). Cell senescence induced by the prolonged culture of cells derived from a young individual also leads to intracellular accumulation of Aβ.[13] These data confirm the link between the processes of aging and β-amyloidogenesis.

Using cultured myocytes from blood vessels with amyloid angiopathy from dog brains, we created the first cell culture model to study β-amyloidosis.[12,13,15] This model appears useful for studying the mechanisms of amyloidogenic pathology, as well as for quick and easily reproducible screening studies of potential drugs that may interfere with the secretion, accumulation, and fibrillization of Aβ, and may reduce the cytotoxic effects of Aβ.

In the smooth muscle culture model, we found that deposition of Aβ can be enhanced by Alzheimer disease risk factors[14,17,18] and modulated by Aβ carriers—enhanced or stimulated by apolipoprotein E[14,17,18] and reduced by transthyretin.[14,18] The amyloidogenic process is modulated also by monokines secreted by activated microglia.[16] Cytokines such as interleukin-1, interleukin-6, tumor necrosis factor-α, transforming growth factor-β, and prostaglandin E1,[19] were shown to reduce the accumulation of Aβ in myocytes with amyloidogenic pathology. In contrast, cytokines (particularly, transforming growth factor-β) may also increase the sensitivity of myocytes to some amyloidogenic factors, for example, to apolipoprotein E (unpublished data). Further studies will provide more insight into the complex interactions of various cytokines and other factors in the development of amyloidogenic pathology.

AMYLOID ANGIOPATHY AND BLOOD-BRAIN BARRIER CHANGES

Our studies[20] showed that vessels affected by cerebral amyloid angiopathy (dyshoric and myocyte-type vessels) showed increased blood-brain barrier (BBB) permeability to endogenous albumin. Regardless of the nature of the protein forming amyloid deposits, Aβ or prion protein, the segments of blood vessels affected by amyloid deposits showed increased BBB permeability. This increased permeability appears to be the result of the disturbance of the structural integrity of the vascular wall by the fibrillized amyloid deposits (degenerative changes in the endothelium, myocytes, and the basement membrane). Increased BBB permeability may have both negative and positive effects on the course and treatment of AD; the negative is allowing all nondesirable compounds (e.g., excitatory amino acids) into the brain; the positive is that drugs used to affect polymerization and defibrillization of the amyloid deposits can more readily enter the brain and affect the rate of deposition of Aβ protein.

ACKNOWLEDGMENT

This research was supported by Grant No. PO1 AG04220 from the National Institute on Aging, National Institutes of Health.

REFERENCES

1. WISNIEWSKI, H.M., J. WEGIEL, K.C. WANG, M. KUJAWA & B. LACH. 1989. Ultrastructural studies of the cells forming amyloid fibers in classical plaques. Can. J. Neurol. Sci. **16:** 535–542.
2. WISNIEWSKI, H.M., J. WEGIEL, K.C. WANG & B. LACH. 1992. Ultrastructural studies of the cells forming amyloid in the cortical vessel wall in Alzheimer's disease. Acta Neuropathol. **84:** 117–127.
3. WISNIEWSKI, H.M., A.B. JOHNSON, C.S. RAINE, W.J. KAY & R.D. TERRY. 1970. Senile plaques and cerebral amyloidosis in aged dogs. A histochemical and ultrastructural study. Lab. Invest. **23:** 287–296.
4. ISHII, T. 1958. Histochemistry of the senile changes of the brain of the senile dementia. Psychiatr. Neurol. Jpn. **60:** 768–781.
5. ISHII, T. 1969. Enzyme histochemical studies of senile plaques and the plaque-like degeneration of arteries and capillaries (Scholz). Acta Neuropathol. (Berl.) **14:** 250–260.
6. MIYAKAWA, T. 1986. The relationship between amyloid fibrils around cerebral blood vessels and senile plaques, and ultrastructure of amyloid fibrils. International Symposium on Dementia and Amyloid. Neuropathology (Suppl.) **3:** 37–48.
7. MIYAKAWA, T., A. SHIMOJI, R. KUMAMOTO & Y. HIGUCHI. 1982. The relationship between senile plaques and cerebral blood vessels in Alzheimer's disease and senile dementia. Morphological mechanism of senile plaque production. Virchows Arch. B **40:** 121–129.
8. KAWAI, M., R.N. KALARIA, S.I. HARIK & G. PERRY. 1990. The relationship of amyloid plaques to cerebral capillaries in Alzheimer's disease. Am. J. Pathol. **137:** 1435–1446.
9. MANDYBUR, T.I. 1986. Cerebral amyloid angiopathy: the vascular pathology and complications. J. Neuropathol. Exp. Neurol. **45:** 79–90.
10. WISNIEWSKI, H.M., J. FRACKOWIAK, A. ZOLTOWSKA & K.S. KIM. 1994. Vascular β-amyloid in Alzheimer's disease angiopathy is produced by proliferating and degenerating smooth muscle cells. Amyloid: Int. J. Exp. Clin. Invest. **1:** 8–16.
11. WEGIEL, J., H.M. WISNIEWSKI, I. KUCHNA, M. TARNAWSKI, E. POPOVITCH, J. KULCZYCKI, W.K. DOWJAT & T. WISNIEWSKI. 1998. Cell-type specific enhancement of amyloid-β deposition in a novel presenilin-1 mutation (P117L). J. Neuropathol. Exp. Neurol. **57:** 831–838.
12. FRACKOWIAK, J., B. MAZUR-KOLECKA, J. WEGIEL, K.S. KIM & H.M. WISNIEWSKI. 1995. Culture of canine vascular myocytes as a model to study production and accumulation of β-protein by cells involved in amyloidogenesis. *In* Research Advances in Alzheimer's Disease and Related Disorders. K. Iqbal, J.A. Mortimer, B. Winblad & H.M. Wisniewski, Eds.: 747–754. J. Wiley & Sons. Chichester, England.
13. FRACKOWIAK, J., B. MAZUR-KOLECKA, H.M. WISNIEWSKI, A. POTEMPSKA, R.T. CARROLL, M.R. EMMERLING & K.S. KIM. 1995. Secretion and accumulation of Alzheimer β-protein by cultured vascular smooth muscle cells from old and young dogs. Brain Res. **676:** 225–230.
14. MAZUR-KOLECKA, B., J. FRACKOWIAK, R.T. CARROLL & H.M. WISNIEWSKI. 1997. Accumulation of Alzheimer amyloid-β peptide in cultured myocytes is enhanced by serum and reduced by cerebrospinal fluid. J. Neuropathol. Exp. Neurol. **56:** 263–272.
15. WISNIEWSKI, H.M., J. FRACKOWIAK & B. MAZUR-KOLECKA. 1995. In vitro production of β-amyloid in smooth muscle cells isolated from amyloid angiopathy-affected vessels. Neurosci. Lett. **183:** 120–123.
16. FRACKOWIAK, J., B. MAZUR-KOLECKA, R.T. CARROLL, A. CHAUHAN & H.M. WISNIEWSKI. 1997. Factors secreted by activated microglia and monocytes reduce amyloidogenesis in vascular smooth muscle cells. NeuroReport **8:** 2259–2263.
17. MAZUR-KOLECKA, J. FRACKOWIAK, J. KRZESLOWSKA, N. RAMAKRISHNA, T. HASKE, M. EMMERLING, W. ZHANG, K.S. KIM & H.M. WISNIEWSKI. 1999. Apolipoprotein E alters metabolism of AβPP in cells engaged in β-amyloidosis. J. Neuropathol. Exp. Neurol. **58:** 288–295.

18. MAZUR-KOLECKA, B., J. FRACKOWIAK & H.M. WISNIEWSKI. 1995. Apolipoproteins E3
    and E4 induce, and transthyretin prevents accumulation of the Alzheimer's β-amy-
    loid peptide in cultured vascular smooth muscle cells. Brain Res. **698:** 217–222.
19. MAZUR-KOLECKA, B., J. FRACKOWIAK, H. LE VINE III, T. HASKE & H.M. WISNIEWSKI.
    1997. Factors produced by activated macrophages reduce accumulation of Alzheimer's
    β-amyloid protein in vascular smooth muscle cells. Brain Res. **760:** 255–260.
20. WISNIEWSKI, H.M., A.W. VORBRODT & J. WEGIEL. 1997. Amyloid angiopathy and
    blood-brain barrier changes in Alzheimer's disease. Ann. N.Y. Acad. Sci. **826:**
    161–172.

Binswanger Disease: The History of a Silent Epidemic

GUSTAVO C. ROMÁN[a]

Department of Medicine/Neurology, University of Texas School of Medicine at San Antonio, San Antonio, Texas 78284-7883, USA

INTRODUCTION

The question, "Binswanger's disease: Does it exist?"[1] has been answered affirmatively. This senile brain disease of vascular origin is characterized by the presence of ischemic periventricular leukoencephalopathy that typically spares the arcuate subcortical U-fibers.[2] However, intense controversy still surrounds its clinical manifestations, pathophysiology, and prevalence. The descriptive but cumbersome "periventricular leukoencephalopathy," and a dozen other synonyms,[3] have been replaced by the concise term leukoaraiosis (Greek for "white rarefaction"), proposed as a radiological expression—a purely descriptive and noncommittal name in terms of pathogenesis—applied to white matter hypodensities on brain CT scans,[4] changes usually visualized as hyperintensities on MRI scans.[5] Unfortunately, leukoaraiosis is often used interchangeably with Binswanger disease. In this sense the use of this term should be discouraged since "leukoaraiosis is neither a disease nor even a specific indicator of white matter ischemia,"[1] and one can hardly study the pathophysiology, symptomatology, and natural history of a radiologic image.[6,7]

OTTO BINSWANGER

The biography of Otto Binswanger has been reviewed by Schneider & Wieczorek[8] and Román.[9] He was born in 1852 in Münsterlingen (Switzerland), studied in Heidelberg and Zürich, and graduated in medicine from Göttingen. His earliest interests were in pathology, and he was a disciple of von Recklinhausen in Strassburg, and of Theodor Meynert at the Neurological Institute in Vienna. After graduation he combined pathology and psychiatry, first under Ludwig Meyer in Göttingen, and then he succeeded C. Weigert at the Pathology Institute in Breslau. In 1880. he was appointed chief physician of the Psychiatry and Neurology clinic at the famous Charité Hospital in Berlin, where he worked with Wernicke and Pick. In 1882, Binswanger went to University of Jena (Germany), where he would spend the rest of his career. He became Professor of Psychiatry in 1891 and twice served as Rector of the University of Jena. In 1893, he published a book on the histopathology of syphilitic general paralysis,[10] and a year later described the subcortical leukoen-

[a]Address for correspondence: Gustavo C. Román, MD, FACP, FRSM (Lond.), Professor of Medicine/Neurology, The University of Texas Health Sciences Center at San Antonio, 7703 Floyd Curl Drive, San Antonio, Texas 78284-7883. Tel.: (210) 617-5161; fax: (210) 567-4659.
e-mail: romang@uthscsa.edu

cephalopathy that bears his name.[11] His students included Oskar Vogt, K. Brodmann, and Hans Berger, the discoverer of electroencephalography. Binswanger died on July 15, 1929.

ARTERIOSCLEROTIC DEMENTIA

The initial concept of vascular dementia was formulated by Emil Kraepelin in the 1910 edition of his famous Lehrbuch der Psychiatrie,[12] under the name Das arteriosklerotische Irresein [arteriosclerotic insanity/psychosis]. This concept was based on the clinicopathological correlations undertaken by Binswanger[10,11] and Alois Alzheimer[13-17] with the main purpose of separating from syphilitic dementia paralytica—then, a leading cause of dementia—other forms of senile and presenile dementia.[18] In a review of "mental disorders of arteriosclerotic origin" Alzheimer[17] mentioned: "In 1894, Binswanger and this reviewer [Alzheimer] first described arteriosclerotic brain atrophy [degeneration] and emphasized the need to differentiate it from [syphilitic] paralysis." Alzheimer also coined the name "Binswanger's disease" for the "subcortical arteriosclerotic encephalopathy" described in 1894 by his colleague.[19] Alzheimer and Binswanger had correctly concluded that "arteriosclerotic dementia" represented a large clinicopathological spectrum. The lesions illustrated in Kraepelin's chapter on Das arteriosklerotische Irresein[12] included: arteriosclerotic brain degeneration, characterized by multiple lacunar strokes and état criblé associated with severe arteriosclerosis of small and large blood vessels; senile cortical atrophy, probably granular atrophy and laminar necrosis; periventricular white matter atrophy or Binswanger disease; perivascular gliosis or wedge-shaped lesions resulting from large vessel ischemia; and, combinations of lesions. Alzheimer[17] considered dementia post-apoplexiam as the result of "preexisting arteriosclerotic hemispheric foci"—probably lacunes—rather than due to large strokes.

EARLY HISTORY

According to J.-J. Hauw,[20,21] prior to Binswanger's description of "subcortical arteriosclerotic encephalopathy," Maxime Durand-Fardel [1816–1899]—the father of gerontology—in his Traité Clinique et Pratique des Maladies des Vieillards,[22] described a condition he named atrophie interstitielle du cerveau (interstitial atrophy of the brain) consisting of: "an alteration of the cerebral pulp...[that] seems quite different from the infarct proper. ... It does not seem to be due to a change in the consistency of the brain but to a rarefaction of the pulp ... a mere interstitial atrophy. ... If a section is performed at the center of the changes, it can be seen that the white matter is rarefied. ... We do not know any symptom characteristic of this change." Durand-Fardel[23] was also the first to describe in 1842 a condition frequently seen in MRI in the elderly, état criblé, the dilatation of perivascular spaces around cerebral arterioles; he suggested that this "sieve-like state" was due to vascular congestion, i.e., an effect of arterial hypertension.[24] He was among the first to write a modern book on ischemic stroke[25] and to use the term lacune—coined by Dechambre[26] in

1838[27,28]—in its modern sense of a small, healed ischemic infarct. After Binswanger's report,[11] Pierre Marie[29] described a remarkably similar clinical condition, état lacunaire, emphasizing the presence of multiple lacunes. The syndrome included mild residual hemiparesis—lacunes were considered the most common cause of hemiparesis in the elderly[30]—, a peculiar gait (marche à petits pas), dysarthria, pseudobulbar palsy, and in some cases, astasia-abasia. Extrapyramidal features, such as inexpressive facies, slowness of movement, axial rigidity, loss of postural reflexes, and frequent falls were also commonly observed. Dementia was not a salient feature, but some intellectual deficit was considered to be constant in état lacunaire.[28,29] In addition to lacunes, ventricular dilatation and lesions of the white matter were observed and Thurel[31] described these lesions as having the appearance of a moth-eaten rag (aspect d'étoffe mitée). In 1926, Foix and Chavany[32] described the histological appearance of these "ilots de sclerose disséminés" in the white matter as follows: "The stains for fibrillary neuroglia show that in these islands of sclerosis the glial proliferation forms a dense network with perivascular preponderance. Axonal lesions are very important in these islands of neuroglia. There is substitution of the noble neurological elements destroyed, by a richly cellular neuroglial tissue."

CONTEMPORARY HISTORY

The arrival of modern brain imaging rediscovered these long-forgotten lesions of the periventricular white matter in the elderly and stirred much controversy regarding their nature.[33] Most studies now agree that these periventricular, distal-territory, white matter lesions in the elderly brain are of ischemic-hypoxic cause. The existence of a genetic form of this disease, familial Binswanger[34,35] or CADASIL,[36] offers a natural model for the sporadic Binswanger-type form of vascular dementia. CADASIL is a systemic autosomal dominant microarteriopathy mapped to chromosome 19q12 as a mutation of the Notch 3 gene[37–39] whose clinical expression is limited to the central nervous system. CADASIL not only confirmed the existence of nonfamilial sporadic cases of Binswanger disease, but provided support to the concept of a continuum of lesions ranging from mild, asymptomatic white-matter lesions (WMLs) to full-blown ischemic leukoencephalopathy with lacunes and dementia. This concept is important, since the presence of pausi- or asymptomatic WMLs and lacunes in the elderly may be a formal indication to identify and treat risk factors (i.e., hypertension, orthostatic hypotension, cardiac disease, diabetes mellitus, hyperfibrinogenemia), in order to prevent the development of senile vascular dementia of the Binswanger type.

CONCLUSION

White-matter lesions (leukoaraiosis) and lacunar strokes—the key components of Binswanger disease—are a common problem in the elderly population, affecting perhaps one third of normal subjects age 65 and older, and about 50% of those with Alzheimer's disease. Therefore, I wholeheartedly agree with Jan van Gijn's[40] statement that we are in the midst of "a silent epidemic" of Binswanger disease.

REFERENCES

1. BOGOUSSLAVSKY, J., Ed. 1996. Binswanger's disease: Does it exist? Cerebrovasc. Dis. **6:** 255–263.
2. ROMÁN, G.C. 1987. Senile dementia of the Binswanger type: a vascular form of dementia in the elderly. JAMA **258:** 1782–1788.
3. BROWN, M.M. 1995. Leukoaraiosis. *In* Lacunar and Other Subcortical Infarctions. G. Donnan, B. Norrving, J. Bamfortd & J. Bogousslavsky, Eds.: 181–198. Oxford University Press. Oxford.
4. HACHINSKI, V.C., P. POTTER & H. MERSKEY. 1986. Leuko-araiosis: an ancient term for a new problem. Can. J. Neurol. Sci. **13:** 533–534.
5. FAZEKAS, F., R. SCHMIDT, G. FAZEKAS & P. KAPELLER. 1994. The relevance of white matter changes to vascular dementia. *In* Vascular Dementia. D. Leys & P. Scheltens, Eds.: 133–154. ICG Publications. Dordrecht, the Netherlands.
6. PANTONI, L. & J.H. GARCÍA. 1995. The significance of cerebral white matter abnormalities 100 years after Binswanger's report: a review. Stroke **26:** 1293–1301.
7. PANTONI, L. & J.H. GARCÍA. 1997. Cognitive impairment and cellular/vascular changes in the cerebral white matter. Ann. N.Y. Acad. Sci. **826:** 92–102.
8. SCHNEIDER, R. & V. WIECZOREK. 1991. Otto Binswanger. J. Neurol. Sci. **103:** 61–63.
9. ROMÁN, G.C. 1992. Historical aspects: from Alzheimer to Binswanger. *In* Vascular Dementia. G.C. Román, Ed. New Issues in Neurosciences **4:** 83–85.
10. BINSWANGER, O. 1893. Die pathologische Histologie der Grosshirnrindenerkrankung bei der Allgemeinen Progressiven Paralyse. Gustav Fischer. Jena.
11. BINSWANGER, O. 1894. Die Abgrenzung der allgemeinen progressiven Paralyse (Referat, erstattet auf der Jahres versammlung des Vereins Deutscher Irrenärtzte zu Dresden am 20 Sept. 1894). Berl. Klin. Wochenschr. **31:** 1103–1105, 1137–1139, 1180–1186.
12. KRAEPELIN, E. 1910. Das arteriosklerotische Irresein. *In* Psychiatrie. Ein Lehrbuch für Studierende und Ärzte. Vol. II, Chapter VII. Das senile und präsenile Irresein.: 554–593. Verlag von Johann Ambrosius Barth. Leipzig.
13. ALZHEIMER, A . 1894. Die arteriosklerotische Atrophie des Gehirns. Neurologisches Zentralblatt **13:** 765–768.
14. ALZHEIMER, A. 1895. Die arteriosklerotische Atrophie des Gehirns. Allgemeine Zeitschrift für Psychiatrie und psychisch-gerichtliche Medicin **52:** 809–812.
15. ALZHEIMER, A. 1898. Neuere Arbeiten über die Dementia senilis und die auf atheromatöser Gefässerkrankung basierendenn Gehirnkrankheiten. Monatsschrift für Psychiatrie und Neurologie **3:** 101–115.
16. ALZHEIMER, A. 1899. Beitrag zur pathologischen Anatomie der Seelenstörungen des Greisenalters. Neurol. Zentralblatt **18:** 95–96.
17. ALZHEIMER, A. 1902. Die Seelenstörungen auf arteriosklerotischer Grundlage. Allgemeine Zeitschrift für Psychiatrie und psychisch-gerichtliche Medicin **59:** 695–711.
18. MAST, H., T.K. TATEMICHI & J.P. MOHR. 1995. Chronic brain ischemia: the contributions of Otto Binswanger and Alois Alzheimer to the mechanisms of vascular dementia. J. Neurol. Sci. **132:** 4–10.
19. BLASS, J.P., S. HOYER & R. NITSCH. 1991. A translation of Otto Binswanger's article: "The delineation of the generalized progressive paralyses." Arch. Neurol. **48:** 961–972.
20. HAUW, J-J. 1988. Leuko-araiosis: the brain interstitial atrophy (atrophie interstitielle du cerveau) of Durand-Fardel. Arch. Neurol. **45:** 140.
21. HAUW, J-J. 1995. The history of lacunes. *In* Lacunar and Other Subcortical Infarctions. G. Donnan, B. Norrving, J. Bamfortd & J. Bogousslavsky, Eds.: 3–15. Oxford University Press. Oxford.
22. DURAND-FARDEL, M. 1854. Traité Clinique et Pratique des Maladies des Vieillards.: 25. Baillière. Paris.
23. DECHAMBRE, A. 1838. Mémoire sur la curabilité du ramollissement cérébral. Gazette Médicale (Paris) **6:** 305–314.
24. DURAND-FARDEL, M. 1842. Mémoire sur une altération particulière de la substance blanche. Gazette Médicale (Paris) **10:** 23–26, 33–38.
25. ROMÁN, G.C. 1987. Cerebral congestion: a vanished disease. Arch. Neurol. **44:** 444–448.

26. DURAND-FARDEL, M. 1843. Traité du Ramollissement du Cerveau. Baillière. Paris.
27. ROMÁN, G.C. 1986. The original description of lacunes. Neurology **36**: 85.
28. ROMÁN, G.C. 1986. Lacunae cerebri: the early history of a peculiar form of cavitation of the brain. Neurology **36**(Suppl.1): 213.
29. MARIE, P. 1901. Des foyers lacunaires de désintégration et de différents autres états cavitaires du cerveau. Revue de Médecine (Paris) **21**: 281–298.
30. FERRAND, J. 1902. Essay sur l'hémiplégie des Vieillards. Les lacunes de Désintégration Cerebrale. Rousset. Paris.
31. THUREL, R. 1929. Les Pseudobulbaires. Étude Clinique et Anatomopathologique. Paris: Thesis Medicine No. 55.
32. FOIX, C.H. & M. CHAVANY. 1926. Palilalia syllabique: sclerose intracérébrale en foyers disseminés. Rev. Neurol. (Paris) **1**: 61–72.
33. ROMÁN, G.C. 1996. From UBOs to Binswanger's disease. Impact of MRI on VaD research. Stroke **27**: 1269–1273.
34. VAN BOGAERT, L. 1955. Encéphalopathie sous-corticale progressive (Binswanger) à évolution rapide chez deux soeurs. Med. Hellen. **24**: 961–972.
35. GUTIÉRREZ-MOLINA, M., A. CAMINER RODRÍGUEZ, C. MARTÍNEZ GARCÍA *et al*. 1994. Small arterial granular degeneration in familial Binswanger's syndrome. Acta Neuropathol. (Berlin) **87**: 8–105.
36. BOUSSER, M.-G. & E. TOURNIER-LASSERVE. 1994. Summary of the Proceedings of the First International Workshop on CADASIL. Paris, May 19–21, 1993. Stroke **25**: 704–707.
37. TOURNIER-LASSERVE, E., A. JOUTEL, J. MELKI *et al*. 1993. Cerebral autosomal dominant arteriopathy with subcortical infarcts and leukoencephalopathy maps to chromosome 19q12. Nat. Genet. **3**: 256–259.
38. JOUTEL, A., C. CORPECHOT, A. DUCROS *et al*. 1996. Notch3 mutations in CADASIL, a hereditary adult-onset condition causing stroke and dementia. Nature **383**: 707–710.
39. JOUTEL, A., K. VAHEDI, C. CORPECHOT *et al*. 1997. Strong clustering and stereotyped nature of Notch3 mutations in CADASIL patients. Lancet **350**: 1511–1515.
40. VAN GIJN, J. 1998. Leukoaraiosis and vascular dementia. Neurology **51**(Suppl. 3): S3–S8.

Cascading Glia Reactions: a Common Pathomechanism and Its Differentiated Control by Cyclic Nucleotide Signaling

PETER SCHUBERT,[a,e] TADAO MORINO,[a] HIROFUMI MIYAZAKI,[b] TADANORI OGATA,[b] YOICHI NAKAMURA,[b] CRISTINA MARCHINI,[c] AND STEFANO FERRONI[d]

[a]*Department of Neuromorphology, Max Planck Institute of Neurobiology, Martinsried, Germany*

[b]*Departments of Physiology and Orthopaedic Surgery, Ehime University, Japan*

[c]*Department of Pharmacology, University of Camerino, Italy*

[d]*Department of Physiology, University of Bologna, Italy*

ABSTRACT: A pathological glia activation, stimulated by inflammatory proteins, β-amyloid, or brain ischemia, is discussed as a common pathogenic factor for progressive nerve cell damage in vascular and Alzheimer dementia. A critical point seems to be reached, if the cytokine-controlled microglial upregulation causes a secondary activation of astrocytes which loose the negative feedback control, are forced to give up their physiological buffering function, and may add to neuronal damage by the release of nitric oxide (NO) and by promoting toxic β-amyloid formation. A strengthening of the cyclic adenosine-5′,3′-monophosphate (cAMP) signaling exerted a differential inhibition of the stimulatory cytokines tumor necrosis factor-α (TNF-α) and interleukin-1β (IL-1β) released from cultured rat microglia, but maintained the negative feedback signal IL-6; cAMP inhibited also the release of free oxygen radicals (OR) but not of NO. Reinforcement of the NO-induced cyclic guanosine monophosphate (cGMP) increase by blockade of the phosphodiesterase (PDE) subtype-5 with propentofylline counterbalanced the toxic NO action that causes with OR neuronal damage by peroxynitrate formation. In rat cultured astrocytes, a prolonged cAMP elevation favored cell differentiation, the expression of a mature ion channel patter, and an improvement of the extracellular glutamate uptake. Cyclic AMP signaling could be strengthened by PDE blockade and by raising extracellular adenosine, which stimulates A_2 receptor-mediated cAMP synthesis. Via an A_1 receptor-mediated effect, elevated adenosine was found to overcome a deficient intracellular calcium mobilization resulting from an impaired muscarinic signaling at pathologically decreased acetylcholine concentrations. We suggest that pharmaca, which elevate extracellular adenosine and/or block the degradation of cyclic nucleotides, may be used to counteract glia-related neuronal damage in dementing processes.

[e]Address for correspondence: Peter Schubert, MD., Head of the Electrophysiological Laboratory in the Department of Neuromorphology, Max Planck Institute of Neurobiology, am Klopferspitz 18a, 82152 Martinsried, Germany. Tel.: +49-89-8578-3689; fax: +49-89-8995-0088.

e-mail: schubert@neuro.mpg.de

INTRODUCTION

Glial cells are cells with a Janus face: supportive and potentially destructive. In particular, the astrocytes fulfill a number of physiological tasks prerequisite for the regular function of neurons. But in conjunction with a pathological microglial activation, they may add to nerve cell damage. Thus, astrocytes are an essential element of the blood-brain barrier providing a protective shield, and they significantly add to the maintenance of the extracellular ion homeostasis by buffering neuronally released excitotoxic transmitters and potassium ions. They are able to produce trophic factors, which support neuronal growth and survival. Activated microglia seem to play a role in determining the architecture of the central nervous system during development as well. But it is unclear whether microglia cells in the adult brain exert a physiological function if they are in a resting state. They represent, however, highly sensitive immunocompetent cells, which are in standby position and may adopt powerful weapons upon pathological activation.[1] This, again, reflects a Janus-faced event, which may be part of a meaningful response of the brain-intrinsic immune system that defends against foreign aggressors or helps to clear up cellular debris by the phagocytotic action of microglia-derived macrophages. But if the pathological glia activation escapes its vigorous endogenous control, it may turn into an auto-aggressive pathomechanism that contributes to secondary neuronal damage occurring, e.g., after brain trauma, ischemia or during the course of neurodegenerative diseases.

PATHOGENIC MECHANISMS OF A CASCADING GLIAL CELL ACTIVATION

Reactive microglia are able to release glutamate.[2] This increases the risk of excitotoxic neuronal damage, which will further be aggravated if elevated extracellular glutamate leads to an excessive membrane depolarization of astrocytes and to an impairment of their physiological buffer function. The most powerful microglial weapon is presumably the oxidative burst causing the release of extraordinary high amounts of free oxygen radicals.[3] They form, in conjunction with nitric oxide (NO), the highly aggressive peroxynitrites. The probability of glia-related oxidative damage is further increased by the release of tumor necrosis factor-α (TNF-α), a microglial cytokine that has been reported to cause NO-induced nerve cell death *in vitro*.[4] A critical point seems to be reached if the pathological conditions allow a cascading glial cell activation that is not restricted to microglia but also involves the astrocytes. When astrocytes are forced by the microglial cytokine interleukin-1β (IL-1β) to undergo secondary activation, they not only have to give up physiological functions coupled to their mature differentiated state, but may even cooperate with microglia in enhancing oxidative stress. Choi's group has shown that stimulation of astrocytes with the microglial cytokine IL-1β and interferon-γ potentiated neuronal injury by activation of the inducible NO synthase.[5] The damage produced by the pathologically increased NO production of astrocytes resulted from an increased peroxynitrite formation in the presence of oxygen radicals, as can be provided by activated microglia and microglia-derived macrophages. Thus, the neurotoxic potential of a pathological glia activation seems to be determined by functional interactions between microglia and astrocytes.

A pathogenic role of a cascading microglia/astrocyte activation in neurodegenerative diseases is supported by their almost obligatory presence in the periphery of β-amyloid plaques in the brains of Alzheimer disease patients.[6] Only the dense core plaques, associated with dying neurons, but not the diffuse amyloid deposits were apolipoprotein E (ApoE)-positive.[7,8] Reactive astrocytes have been identified to be the brain endogenous producers of those inflammatory chaperones, like ApoE, which promote the formation of toxic β-amyloid.[9,10] An upregulated expression of the amyloid precursor protein (APP) in activated glial cells can be expected to potentiate the pathologically β-amyloid load,[11] particularly since free oxygen radicals, released at large amounts from reactive microglial cells, are known to aggravate the pathological APP processing by C-terminal oxidation.[12] It follows that a cascading glial cell activation, involving microglia and astrocytes, may largely contribute to the formation of toxic β-amyloid, which can be regarded as common pathogenic factor for the deleterious plaque formation in Alzheimer disease as well as for the amyloid angiopathy contributing to vascular dementia.

TRIGGERS OF GLIAL CELL REACTIONS

Besides of the direct cytotoxicity exerted by β-amyloid,[13] its genetically favored generation may be one of the triggers that initiates pathological glia activation. There is evidence that plaque-derived β-amyloid provides a docking site for microglia, which then are stimulated to transform from quiescent to neurotoxic cells. As a consequence, they secrete a lipophilic amine (Ntox), which was found to aggravate glutamate-induced excitotoxic damage of neurons, presumably by modifying the N-methyl-D-aspartate (NMDA) receptor function.[14]

Another trigger, which effectively activates microglia, is brain ischemia—the primary pathogenic factor of vascular dementia and also known to intensify the dementing process in Alzheimer disease. An ischemia-induced energy breakdown leads to adenosine triphosphate (ATP) degradation and disturbance of the ion homeostasis. The resulting extracellular potassium rises can be expected to elicit a strong depolarizing inward current through microglia-specific potassium channels,[15] followed by a massive calcium influx that may serve as a trigger for consecutive cell activation.[16] There is evidence that the ATP breakdown product, adenosine, participates in activating resting microglia by stimulating the arachidonic acid pathway via Gs protein-coupled A_2 receptors.[17] Since microglia have complement receptors as well, activation of the classical complement cascade by initial cell damage and reactive brain inflammation could be another possible trigger.[18]

Following experimental brain ischemia, an obvious microglial activation is already seen within the first hours, reflected by the initiation of cell proliferation and by the expression of specific surface antigens.[19] Among those, the expression of the major histocompatibility (MHC)-complexes enables these brain intrinsic glial cells to communicate with the general blood cell-linked immune system. Reactive changes of astrocytes—characterized by a marked cell hypertrophy, increased glial fibrillary acidic protein (GFAP) content, and retraction of processes—were not seen before the second day after transient brain ischemia.[20] This underlines that the pathogenetically significant activation of astrocytes is a secondary event in a cascade that starts with the activation of microglia.

ENDOGENOUS CONTROL OF GLIAL REACTIONS

There is evidence that astrocytes—via the cytokine transforming growth factor-β (TGF-β)—exert a negative feedback regulation of activated microglial cell functions.[21] This serves presumably as an important endogenous mechanism by which the dangerous peroxynitrite production can be controlled and restricted to the microglia. In order to specify the working parameters of this astrocyte-related control system, we recently studied the NO generation in cultured rat glial cells using lipopolysaccharide (LPS) and interferon-γ as pathological stimulators. The observed powerful inhibitory effect of astrocytes on the massive microglial NO release turned out to be dependent on the astrocytic differentiation state. Conditioned medium, which had been harvested from confluent and low proliferative rat astrocyte cultures, effectively inhibited microglial NO release. But if we used astrocyte-conditioned medium from nondifferentiated and highly proliferative cultures, which resembled pathologically activated astrocytes, the inhibitory effect was largely reduced or missing (unpublished data).

This suggests that a powerful endogenous control of the potentially neurotoxic NO release from activated microglia can be overrun, if the astrocytes are forced to

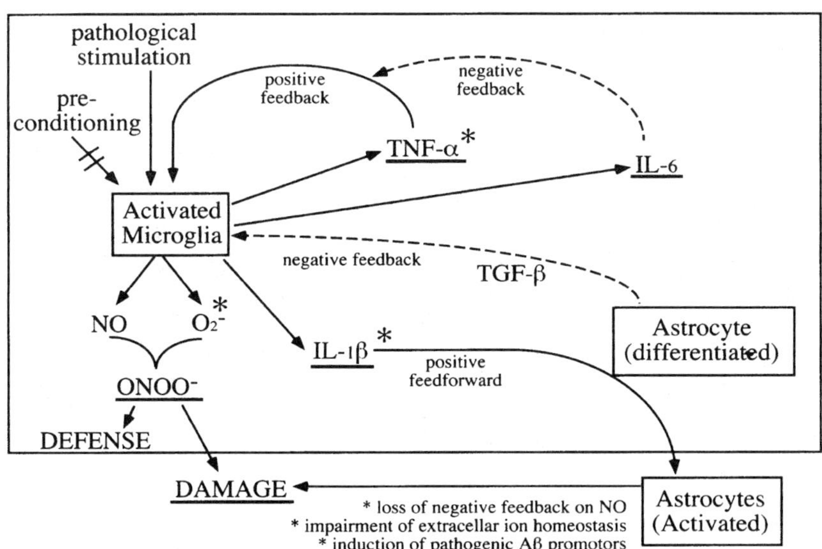

FIGURE 1. Endogenous control of a cascading activation of microglial cells and astrocytes.

undergo dedifferentiation upon pathological activation. Whether or not such a cascading glial activation occurs depends on the level of microglial activation. This is a graded response controlled by the interplay of cytokines that are released from microglia and astrocytes (FIG. 1). Among those, TNF-α acts as a positive feedback signal, which helps to reinforce glial cell activation (see also Ref. 22). As a consequence, the reactive microglia may reach an upgraded level of activation, which enables them to produce IL-1β, the cytokine promoting the feed-forward activation of astrocytes (see FIG. 1). This escalating cascade, however, is also under inhibitory control, e.g., by the cytokine IL-6, which has been shown to exert a negative feed back on TNF-α signaling.[23]

It follows that an inhibition of the stimulatory signals and the maintenance or reinforcement of the inhibitory signal loops may be a possible strategy to prevent an escalating microglial activation that leads to the critical secondary activation of astrocytes. Another chance of interference would be a conditioning of reactive microglial cells that brings them back into a less activated state or the induction of cellular apoptosis. The latter represents a commonly used emergency control by which non-adequately activated and dangerous immune-effective cells can be eliminated.

INDUCTION OF MICROGLIAL APOPTOSIS BY ADENOSINE AND PRECONDITIONING BY REINFORCED cAMP SIGNALING

Immature microglial cells, obtained from the brains of newly born rats, maintain in culture their activated state, which allows them to proliferate and to transform *in vitro* spontaneously into free radical-generating macrophages. They may therefore provide a reliable model to investigate the pathological properties of microglial cells in relation to their activation state and to test possible modes of interference. Similar to immune-activated cells of the general defense system, cultured microglia were sensitive to apoptosis, and adenosine was found to be an effective trigger.[24] The induction of apoptosis, verified by terminal deoxynucleotidyl transferase-mediated deoxyuridine triphosphate-biotin nick end labeling (TUNEL) staining, DNA ladder formation, and quantitative measurements of intracellular DNA fragmentation, required elevated concentrations of adenosine up to 10 micromolar. This raises the possibility to eliminate potentially neurotoxic microglia by pharmaca, which increase extracellular adenosine by blocking its cellular reuptake.

The sensitivity of microglial cells to adenosine-induced apoptosis is apparently related to the degree of activation and was lost when the microglial cells had been brought into a less proliferative state. This could be achieved by several days' pretreatment with the membrane-permeable dibutyryl-cAMP or with propentofylline (Aventis), a selective phosphodiesterase (PDE) inhibitor. The findings suggest that conditioning of microglial cells by prolonged strengthening of the cAMP-dependent signaling brings them into a less activated and probably less dangerous state, which no longer requires the emergency control by inducible apoptosis. Such a preconditioning also reduced the capacity of cultured microglia to generate NO in response to pathological stimulation (unpublished).

DIFFERENTIAL CONTROL OF CYTOKINE AND OXYGEN RADICAL RELEASE FROM MICROGLIA BY cAMP

Acute strengthening of the cAMP signaling was found to alter the pattern of microglia-released cytokines in a way that can be expected to reduce the neurotoxic power and to add to neuroprotection. Specifically, the LPS-induced release of TNF-α and IL-1β from cultivated rat microglia was markedly inhibited by treatment with dibutyryl-cAMP or propentofylline, whereas the IL-6 release was unaffected or even increased.[25] This means that those cytokines, which tend to stimulate a cascading glial reaction, are suppressed, whereas the negative feedback control remains functioning (see FIG. 1).

Interestingly, such a differential modulation by cAMP was also observed for the stimulated release of NO and oxygen radicals. The latter were significantly depressed, but not the NO release. This should protect against oxidative neuronal damage by preventing the NO-stimulated formation of toxic peroxynitrates, which depends on the availability of oxygen radicals.

GUIDING THE AMBIGUOUS ACTION OF NITRIC OXIDE INTO A cGMP-LINKED PROTECTION

Nitric oxide is an ambivalent molecular signal. It serves as substrate for the formation of toxic peroxynitrate, and it stimulates the cyclic guanosine monophosphate (cGMP) synthesis by guanylcyclase. Mimicking a pathologically increaeased NO load by treatment with nitroprusside caused nerve cell death in microglia-containing

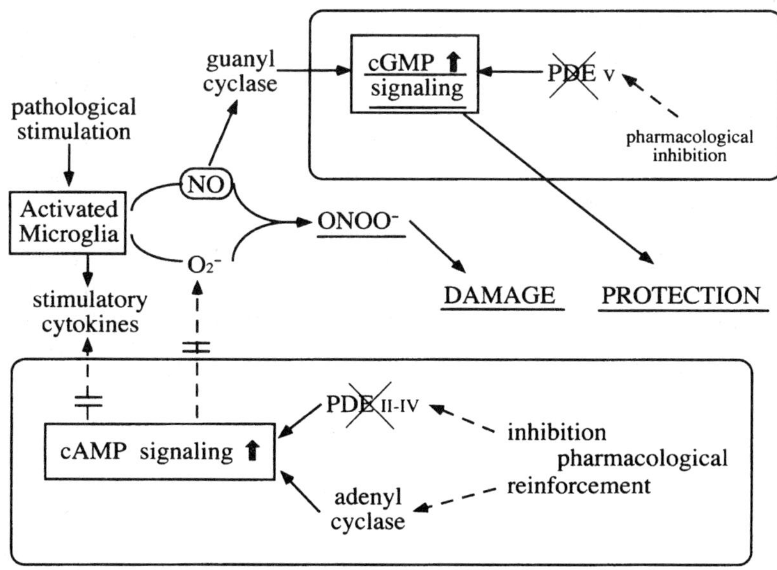

FIGURE 2. Modes of pharmacological interference.

cultures of spinal cord neurons. The damage was prevented in the presence of oxygen radical scavengers indicating that peroxynitrate formation is the NO-induced pathomechanism that can be inhibited by depressing concomitant oxygen radical generation. Protection could further be achieved by strengthening the cGMP-enhancing NO path, i.e., by treatment with the PDE inhibitor propentofylline, which blocks the cGMP degrading subtype-5.[26] Accordingly, protection was seen in the presence of membrane-permeable cGMP analogues.

Taken together, these findings suggest that oxidative neuronal damage resulting from the release of NO and oxygen radicals from pathologically activated glial cells can be counteracted in two ways: the one is to strengthen cAMP signaling, which can be expected to depress microglial activation, their transformation into macrophages, and the related free radical generation; the other is a pharmacologically supported shift of the ambivalent NO action from the peroxynitrate-generating path to a preferential formation of cGMP, which can further be increased by pharmacological blockade of cGMP degradation (see FIG. 2).

MAINTENANCE OF PHYSIOLOGICAL ASTROCYTE FUNCTIONS

A strengthening of cAMP signaling not only reduces the risk of secondary astrocyte activation by microglial IL-1β release, but also seems to influence the astrocytic activation state directly. Cultured astrocytes from the embryonic rat brain resemble pathologically activated astrocytes. This is indicated by a high proliferation rate, a nondifferentiated phenotype lacking cell processes, and an immature ion channel pattern. A prolonged treatment with dibutyryl-cAMP for several days favored the formation of process-rich stellate cells and also induced the new expression of specific potassium and chloride ion channels.[27] These channels belong to the repertoire of mature astrocytes and are required to stabilize the membrane potential and the physiological buffering function of astrocytes. Accordingly, the capacity for the uptake of extracellular glutamate could be improved in astrocyte cultures by a prolonged rise of intracellular cAMP. This was achieved by treatment with an adenosine analogue in conjunction with the PDE-blocker propentofylline (Ogata *et al.*, manuscript in preparation). Treatment with propentofylline has further been reported to increase the release of nerve growth factor from astrocytes.[28]

We conclude from such observations that a prolonged pharmacological strengthening of the cAMP-dependent signaling may help to bring back pathologically activated astrocytes into a more differentiated state. This is supposed to recover physiological astrocyte functions, i.e., the maintenance of the extracellular ion homeostasis, the feedback control of activated microglial functions, and the release of trophic factors, but to reduce the contribution of reactive astrocytes to oxidative damage or to β-amyloid related toxicity.

CONCLUDING REMARKS

Evidence is increasing that the concomitant pathological activation of glial cells plays a pathogenic role for the generation of progressive nerve cell damage in Alzheimer and vascular dementia. Therefore, an interference with the escalating activation of microglial cells and with the deleterious secondary involvement of astrocytes could provide a target for the pharmacological treatment. The complex pathomechanism implicating several interwoven vicious circles, which overrun the endogenous control of the glia-related immune system, is not completely clarified. We therefore think, it is a good strategy to focus on a central point of the molecular signaling chains that mediate the alterations of glial cell properties upon pathological stimulation. Such a bottleneck, where the receptor-mediated input from different agonists merges before being transduced to the diverse cellular effectors, is the sophisticated information processing at the second messenger level. There is evidence that the interplay of the second messengers calcium and cAMP is altered in dementing processes. Thus, the Gs-protein coupled synthesis of cyclic nucleotides has been reported to be impaired in Alzheimer disease,[29] and brain ischemia has been found to upregulate those metabotropic glutamate receptors that favor an intracllular calcium mobilization and an inhibition of the cAMP synthesis.

One may speculate that such an imbalance of the second messengers and a reduced cAMP signaling plays a role in executing pathological glial cell functions. This could explain the observed inhibitory effect of a pharmacologically strengthened cAMP signaling on the cytokine-controlled microglial upregulation, on secondary astrocyte reactions, and on related potentially neurotoxic functions. An effcctive and prolonged intracellular increase of cAMP and cGMP may be achieved by treatment with the respective PDE inhibitors. In addition, an elevation of the extracellular adenosine concentration up to a level that stimulates the A_2 receptor-mediated cAMP synthesis in glial cells can be obtained by pharmaca blocking the uptake of adenosine from the extracellular space. In recent experiments on cultured rat cortical astrocytes, elevated adenosine was also found to overcome a deficient intracellular calcium mobilization that resulted from pathologically reduced acetylcholine concentrations (manuscript in preparation). Since the latter represents a key symptom of Alzheimer disease, the restoration of a deficient muscarinergic signaling by adenosine raising pharmaca may provide a complimentary treatment, in addition to the conventional use of acetylcholinesterase inhibitors (for details, see reviews in Refs. 30 and 31).

REFERENCES

1. BANATI, R.B., J. GEHRMANN, P. SCHUBERT & G.W. KREUTZBERG. 1993. Cytotoxicity of microglia. Glia **7:** 111–118.
2. KLEGERIS, A. & P.L. McGEER. 1994. Inhibition of respiratory burst in macrophages by complement receptor blockade. J. Neuroimmunol. **260:** 273–277.
3. BANATI, R., P. SCHUBERT, G. ROTHE, J. GEHRMANN, K.A. RUDOLPHI, G. VALET & G.W. KREUTZBERG. 1994. Modulation of intracellular formation of reactive oxygen intermediates in peritoneal macrophages and microglia/brain macrophages by propentofylline. J. Cereb. Blood Flow Metab. **14:** 145–149.
4. MEDA, L., M.A. CASSATELLA & I. SZENDREI. 1995. Activation of microglial cells by β-amyloid protein and interferon-γ. Nature **374:** 647–650.
5. HEWETT, S.J., C.A. CSERNANSKY & D.W. CHOI. 1994. Selective potentiation of NMDA induced neuronal injury following induction of astrocytic iNOS. Neuron **13:** 487–494.
6. McGEER, P.L., T. KAWAMATA, D. WALKER, H. ABYAMA, I. TOYAMA & E.G. McGEER. 1993. Microglia in degenerative neurological disease. Glia **7:** 84–92.
7. WISNIEWSKY, T. & B. FRANGIONE.1992. Apolipoprotein E: a pathological chaperone in patients with cerebral amd systemic amyloid. Neurosci. Lett. **135:** 235–238.

8. SHENG, J.G., R.E. MRAK & W.S. GRIFFIN. 1996. Apolipoprotein E distribution among different plaque types in Alzheimer disease: implications for its role in plaque progression. Neuropathol. Appl. Neurobiol. **22:** 334–341.

9. MA, J., A. YEE, H.B. BREWER, S. DAS & H. POTTER. 1994. Amyloid-associated proteins alpha 1-antichymotrypsin and apolipoprotein E promote assembly of beta-protein into filaments. Nature **372:** 92–94.

10. BOWMAN, B.H., F. YANG, J.M. BUCHANAN, G.S. ADRIAN & A.O. MARTINEZ. 1996. Human APOE protein localized in brains of transgenic mice. Neurosci. Lett. **219:** 57–59.

11. FORLONI, G., F. DEMICHELI, S. GIORGI, C. BENDOTTI & N. ANGERETTI. 1992. Expression of amyloid precursor protein mRNAs in endothelial, neuronal and glial cells: modulation by interleukin-1. Mol. Brain Res. **16:** 128–134.

12. DYRCKS, T., E. DYRCKS, C.L. MASTERS & K. BEYREUTHER. 1993. Amyloidogenicity of rodent and human β A_4 sequences. FEBS Lett. **324:** 231–236.

13. BEHL, C., J.B. DAVIS, R. LESLEY & D. SCHUBERT. 1994. Hydrogen peroxide mediates amyloid β protein toxicity. Cell **77:** 817–827.

14. GIULLIAN, D. 1998. A strategy for identifying immunosuppressive therapies for Alzheimer disease. Alzheimer Dis. Assoc. Disord. **12**(Suppl. 2): 7–14.

15. KETTENMANN, H., D. HOPPE, K. GOTTMANN, R. BANATI & G.W. KREUTZBERG. 1990. Cultured microglia have a distinct pattern of membrane channels different from peritoneal macrophages. J. Neurosci. Res. **26:** 278–287.

16. ILLES, P., W. NÖRENBERG & P.J. GEBICKE-HAERTER. 1996. Molecular mechanisms of microglial activation. Neurochem. Int. **1:** 13–26.

17. FIEBICH, B.L., K. BIBER, K. LIEB, D. VAN CALKER, M. BERGER, J. BAUER & P.J. GEBICKE-HAERTER. 1996. Cyclooxygenase-2 expression in rat microglia is induced by adenosine A_{2a}-receptors. Glia **18:** 152–160.

18. AKIYAMA, H. & P.L. MCGEER. 1990. Brain microglia constitutively express β-2 integrins. J. Neuroimmunol. **30:** 81–93.

19. MORIOKA, T., A.N. KALEHUA & W.J. STREIT. 1991. The microglial reaction in the rat dorsal hippocampus following transient forebrain ischemia. J. Cereb. Blood Flow Metab. **10:** 850–859.

20. DELEO, J., L. TÓTH, P. SCHUBERT, K. RUDOLPHI & G.W. KREUTZBERG. 1987. Ischemia-induced neuronal cell death, calcium accumulation and glial response in the hippocampus of the gerbil and protection by the xanthine derivative HWA 285. J. Cereb. Blood Flow Metab. **7:** 745–752.

21. VINCENT, V.A.M., F.J.H. TILDERS & A.M. VAN DAM. 1997. Inhibition of endotoxin-induced oxide synthase production in microglial cells by the presence of astroglial cells: a role for transforming growth factor β. Glia **19:** 190–198.

22. WEKERLE, H., C. LININGTON, H. LASSMANN & R. MEYERMANN. 1986. Cellular immune reactivity within the CNS. TINS **9:** 271–277.

23. ADERKA, D., J.M. LE & J. VILEK. 1989. IL-6 inhibits LPS-induced tumor necrosis factor production in cultured human monocytes. J. Immunol. **143:** 3517–3523.

24. OGATA, T. & P. SCHUBERT. 1996. Programmed cell death in microglia is controlled by extracellular adenosine. Neurosci. Lett. **218:** 91–94.

25. SI, Q., Y. NAKAMURA, T. OGATA, K. KATAOKA & P. SCHUBERT. 1998. Differential regulation of microglial activation by propentofylline via cAMP signaling. Brain Res. **812:** 97–104.

26. OGATA, T., S. KOHGAMI, H. OKUMURA, T. SHIBATA, Y. NAKAMURA, K. KATAOKA & P. SCHUBERT. 1998. Nitric oxide-induced neurotoxicity is inhibited by propentofylline via cyclic GMP elevation [Abstract]. Neurobiol. Aging **19:** S255.

27. FERRONI, S., C. MARCHINI, P. SCHUBERT & C. RAPISARDA. 1995. Two distinct inward rectifying conductances are expressed in cultured rat cortical astrocytes after long term dibutyryl-cyclic-AMP treatment. FEBS Lett. **267:** 319–325.

28. SHINODA, J., Y. FURUKAWA & S. FURUKAWA. 1990. Stimulation of nerve growth factor synthesis/secretion by propentofylline in cultured mouse astroglial cells. Biochem. Pharmacol. **39:** 1813–1816.

29. O'NEILL, C., C.J. FOWLER, B. WINBLAD & R.F. COWBURN. 1994. G-protein coupled signal transduction systems in the Alzheimer's disease brain. Biochem. Soc. Trans. **22:** 167–171.

30. SCHUBERT, P., K. RUDOLPHI, F. FREDHOLM & Y. NAKAMURA. 1994. Modulation of nerve and glial cell function by adenosine—role in the development of ischemic brain damage. Int. J. Biochem. **26:** 1227–1236.
31. SCHUBERT, P., T. OGATA, H. MIYAZAKI, C. MARCHINI, S. FERRONI & K. RUDOLPHI. 1998. Immuno-reactions of glial cells in Alzheimer's disease and possible sites of interference. J. Neural Transm. Suppl. **54:** 167–174.

Linguistic Ability in Early Life and the Neuropathology of Alzheimer's Disease and Cerebrovascular Disease

Findings from the Nun Study

D.A. SNOWDON,[a,b] L.H. GREINER,[a] AND W.R. MARKESBERY[a,c]

[a]*Sanders-Brown Center on Aging, and* [b]*Department of Preventive Medicine,*
College of Medicine, University of Kentucky, Lexington, Kentucky 40536-0230, USA

[c]*Departments of Pathology and Neurology, University of Kentucky,*
Lexington, Kentucky 40536-0230, USA

ABSTRACT: Findings from the Nun Study indicate that low linguistic ability in early life has a strong association with dementia and premature death in late life. In the present study, we investigated the relationship of linguistic ability in early life to the neuropathology of Alzheimer's disease and cerebrovascular disease. The analyses were done on a subset of 74 participants in the Nun Study for whom we had handwritten autobiographies completed some time between the ages of 19 and 37 (mean = 23 years). An average of 62 years after writing the autobiographies, when the participants were 78 to 97 years old, they died and their brains were removed for our neuropathologic studies. Linguistic ability in early life was measured by the idea (proposition) density of the autobiographies, i.e., a standard measure of the content of ideas in text samples. Idea density scores from early life had strong inverse correlations with the severity of Alzheimer's disease pathology in the neocortex: Correlations between idea density scores and neurofibrillary tangle counts were –0.59 for the frontal lobe, –0.48 for the temporal lobe, and –0.49 for the parietal lobe (all p values < 0.0001). Idea density scores were unrelated to the severity of atherosclerosis of the major arteries at the base of the brain and to the presence of lacunar and large brain infarcts. Low linguistic ability in early life may reflect suboptimal neurological and cognitive development, which might increase susceptibility to the development of Alzheimer's disease pathology in late life.

BACKGROUND

We have proposed that linguistic ability in early life reflects important aspects of cognitive ability, neurocognitive development, and brain reserve.[1] Our findings from the Nun Study indicate that low linguistic ability in early life has a strong relationship to poor cognitive function and the risk of dementia,[1] as well as to a reduced life expectancy.[2] It is not known why low linguistic ability in early life is associated with the risk of dementia and premature death in late life, although preliminary evidence suggests that Alzheimer's disease may play a role.[1]

In the present study, we investigated the relationship of low linguistic ability in early life to the neuropathology of Alzheimer's disease and cerebrovascular disease. Women included in this analysis were participants in the Nun Study, a longitudinal study of aging and Alzheimer's disease.[1,3,4] Cognitive and physical function were assessed annually, and all participants agreed to brain donation at death. At the first exam given between 1991 and 1993, the 678 participants were 75 to 102 years old. The present analysis was conducted on a subset of 74 participants for whom we had handwritten autobiographies from early life, and all of whom had died.

LINGUISTIC MEASURES

In September 1930, the leader of the School Sisters of Notre Dame religious congregation in North America requested that each sister write a short sketch of her life and include parentage, interesting and edifying childhood events, schools attended, and influences that led her to the convent. Handwritten autobiographies were found in the archives of two convents participating in the Nun Study, that is, one in Baltimore, Maryland, and the other in Milwaukee, Wisconsin.

Two indicators of linguistic ability were derived from each autobiography: idea density[5,6] and grammatical complexity.[7] Our prior studies indicated that only low idea density had strong and consistent associations with the risk of dementia and premature death.[1,2] Thus, only findings on idea density are presented in this report.

Idea density was defined as the average number of ideas expressed per ten words for the last ten sentences of each autobiography. Ideas corresponded to elementary propositions, typically a verb, adjective, adverb, or prepositional phrase. Complex propositions that stated or inferred causal, temporal, or other relationships between ideas also were counted. Without the linguistic coder's knowledge of the age or cognitive function of each sister during late life, each autobiography was scored for idea density. The following sentence from an autobiography illustrates the method used to compute idea density: "I was born in Eau Claire, Wis., on May 24, 1913 and was baptized in St. James Church." The ideas (propositions) expressed in this sentence were (1) I was born, (2) born in Eau Claire, Wis., (3) born on May 24, 1913, (4) I was baptized, (5) was baptized in church, (6) was baptized in St. James Church, and (7) I was born...and was baptized. There were 18 words or utterances in that sentence. The idea density for that sentence was 3.9 (i.e., 7 ideas divided by 18 words and multiplied by 10, resulting in 3.9 ideas per 10 words).

NEUROPATHOLOGIC MEASURES

Gross and microscopic examination of the participants' brains was performed by a neuropathologist who was blinded to the participants' cognitive test scores. Brain infarcts were identified by examining the intact brain and 1.5 cm thick coronal sections of the cerebral hemispheres, brain stem, and cerebellum. Infarcts visible to the naked eye were classified as either lacunar infarcts (<1.5 cm) or large infarcts (≥1.5 cm). The neuropathologist also classified the degree of atherosclerosis of the major arteries at the base of the brain (circle of Willis), with moderate defined as atherosclerotic plaques present in 25 to 50% of the vessel wall and severe defined as greater than 50%.

Senile plaques and neurofibrillary tangles were counted in the five most severely involved microscopic fields of the middle frontal gyrus (Brodmann area 9), inferior parietal lobule (areas 39/40), and middle temporal gyrus (area 21). The number of senile plaques (both diffuse and neuritic types) per 10× microscopic field and the number of neurofibrillary tangles per 20× microscopic field were determined using Bielschowsky stained sections. As described in detail elsewhere,[3] those who met our neuropathologic criteria for Alzheimer's disease had abundant senile plaques in at least one of three lobes of the neocortex (i.e., frontal, temporal, or parietal); some neuritic plaques in the neocortex; and some neurofibrillary tangles in the neocortex.

TABLE 1. Mean idea density of early life autobiographies by presence of neuropathologic conditions at autopsy for 74 participants in the Nun Study

Neuropathologic condition	Condition present at death	Unadjusted mean idea density of early life autobiographies within each convent		Adjusted mean idea density of early life autobiographies for both convents combined (95% CL)[a]	Number of participants in combined analyses
		Baltimore	Milwaukee		
Met neuropathologic criteria for Alzheimer's disease	Yes	4.3**	5.5**	4.9 (4.6–5.3)***	47
	No	5.2	7.1	6.1 (5.6–6.6)	27
Neurofibrillary tangles in frontal lobe of neocortex	Yes	4.1***	5.2***	4.7 (4.3–5.1)***	40
	No	5.2	7.0	6.1 (5.7–6.5)	34
Neurofibrillary tangles in temporal lobe of neocortex	Yes	4.3**	5.4**	4.9 (4.5–5.3)***	43
	No	5.2	6.8	6.0 (5.5–6.5)	31
Neurofibrillary tangles in parietal lobe of neocortex	Yes	4.3*	5.3**	4.8 (4.4–5.3)***	37
	No	5.0	6.8	5.9 (5.4–6.3)	37
Lacunar or large brain infarct	Yes	4.6	5.8	5.2 (4.7–5.8)	28
	No	4.7	6.1	5.4 (5.0–5.8)	46
Large brain infarct	Yes	3.9*	6.0	4.9 (4.1-5.6)	14
	No	4.8	6.0	5.5 (5.1-5.8)	60
Lacunar brain infarct	Yes	4.9	5.7	5.4 (4.8–6.0)	23
	No	4.5	6.1	5.3 (5.0–5.7)	51
Moderate to severe atherosclerosis of the circle of Willis	Yes	4.5	5.7	5.2 (4.7–5.7)	36
	No	4.7	6.4	5.5 (5.1–6.0)	38

[a]Variables adjusted in the analyses were age at death and location of convent (i.e., either Baltimore, Maryland or Milwaukee, Wisconsin). CL refers to confidence limits.

***$p \leq 0.001$ for difference in mean idea density between those with and those without neuropathologic condition.

**$p \leq 0.01$ value for difference in mean idea density between those with and those without neuropathologic condition.

*$p \leq 0.05$ for difference in mean idea density between those with and those without neuropathologic condition.

RESULTS

Each of the 74 participants wrote an autobiography some time between the ages of 19 and 37 (mean = 23 years). An average of 62 years after writing the autobiographies, when the participants were 78 to 97 years old, they died and their brains were removed for our neuropathologic studies.

Findings in TABLE 1 indicate that those who met our neuropathologic criteria for Alzheimer's disease had lower idea density scores for their autobiographies from early life than those who did not meet the criteria. The presence of neurofibrillary tangles in the frontal, temporal, or parietal lobe also was strongly associated with lower idea density scores from early life (TABLE 1). Correlations between idea density scores from early life and the mean neurofibrillary tangle counts were −0.59 for the frontal lobe, −0.48 for the temporal lobe, and −0.49 for the parietal lobe. p Values for each of these Spearman rank correlations were less than 0.0001, and each correlation was adjusted for age at death and the location of the convent (i.e., either Baltimore, Maryland or Milwaukee, Wisconsin). When the same correlation analyses were done using mean senile plaque counts as the outcome, the correlations with idea density scores from early life were −0.34 for the frontal lobe, −0.34 for the temporal lobe, and −0.31 for the parietal lobe (all three p values < 0.01).

Other findings suggest that there were no consistent associations between idea density scores and lacunar brain infarcts, large brain infarcts, or moderate to severe atherosclerosis of the major arteries at the base of the brain (TABLE 1).

COMMENT

Linguistic ability, measured an average of 62 years before death, appeared to be unrelated to cerebrovascular disease pathology present at autopsy. However, a strong inverse association was found between linguistic ability and Alzheimer's disease lesions in the neocortex of the brain. Low linguistic ability in early life may reflect suboptimal neurological and cognitive development which might increase susceptibility to the development of Alzheimer's disease pathology in late life.

ACKNOWLEDGMENTS

This study was funded by grants R01AG09862 (D.A.S.), K04AG00553 (D.A.S.), and 5P50AG05144 (W.R.M.) from the National Institute on Aging, and grants from the Abercrombie Foundation and the Kleberg Foundation. More information about the Nun Study may be obtained by visiting our web page: http://www.coa.uky.edu/nunnet

REFERENCES

1. SNOWDON, D.A., S.J. KEMPER, J.A. MORTIMER, L.H. GREINER, D.R. WEKSTEIN & W.R. MARKESBERY. 1996. Linguistic ability in early life and cognitive function and Alzheimer's disease in late life: findings from the Nun Study. JAMA **275:** 528–532.
2. SNOWDON, D.A., L.H. GREINER, S.J. KEMPER, N. NANAYAKKARA & J.A. MORTIMER. 1999. Linguistic ability in early life and longevity: findings from the Nun Study. *In*

The Paradoxes of Longevity. J.-M. Robine, B. Forette, C. Franchesci & M. Allard, Eds.: 103–113. Springer-Verlag. Berlin.
3. SNOWDON, D.A., L.H. GREINER, J.A. MORTIMER, K.P. RILEY, P.A. GREINER & W.R. MARKESBERY. 1997. Brain infarction and the clinical expression of Alzheimer disease: the Nun Study. JAMA **277:** 813–817.
4. SNOWDON, D.A. 1997. Aging and Alzheimer's disease: lessons from the Nun Study. Gerontologist **37:** 150–156.
5. KINTSCH, W. & J. KEENAN. 1973. Reading rate and retention as a function of the number of propositions in the base structure of sentences. Cognit. Psychol. **5:** 257–274.
6. TURNER, A. & E. GREENE. 1977. The construction and use of a propositional text base. University of Colorado Psychology Department. Boulder, CO.
7. CHEUNG, H. & S. KEMPER. 1992. Competing complexity metrics and adults' production of complex sentences. Appl. Psycholinguistics **13:** 53–76.

Cerebrovascular Pathology in Alzheimer's Disease and Leukoaraiosis

WILLIAM R. BROWN,[a,b,c,d] DIXON M. MOODY,[b,d] CLARA R. THORE,[b] AND VENKATA R. CHALLA[c,b]

Departments of [b]Radiology and [c]Pathology, and [d]Program in Neuroscience, Wake Forest University School of Medicine, Winston-Salem, North Carolina 27157, USA

ABSTRACT: A high percentage of patients with Alzheimer's disease (AD) show evidence of white matter degeneration known as leukoaraiosis (LA), which is due to chronic ischemia. We found that the periventricular veins tend to become occluded by multiple layers of collagen in the vessel walls in the elderly. This collagen deposition is particularly excessive in LA lesions. Therefore, it is present in the brains of many AD patients, along with other ischemia-causing cerebrovascular pathology. We found evidence that there is severe loss of oligodendrocytes in LA, due to extensive apoptosis. No evidence of inflammation was found in the LA lesions. In thick celloidin sections of AD brain, we have obtained detailed 3D views of small (early) deposits of amyloid (stained with β-amyloid antibody) around capillaries (stained with collagen IV antibody).

LEUKOARAIOSIS

LA is an age-related neurodegenerative condition that appears as an area of hyperintense signal in the white matter on magnetic resonance (MR) images. When severe, it can cause dementia.[1] It is characterized histologically by demyelination, loss of glial cells, and vacuolization (spongiosis) (FIG. 1).[2] Although the pathogenesis of LA is not yet fully established, it appears to be a multifactorial disease with several potentially overlapping pathogenic mechanisms, including cerebrovascular pathology, which contribute to white matter ischemia. The deep white matter, the area where LA is found, receives its blood supply from arteries or arterioles originating from the pial border zone, a region with an already perilous blood supply.[3] We believe that the more severe grades of LA, those in which the white patches are large and becoming confluent, represent chronic ischemia, albeit in an area of the brain that is more resistant to ischemia than the cortex. This is why the putative ischemic process is slow and clinically silent until the patient ultimately develops dementia. If ischemia is the cause of LA, this raises concern regarding possible overaggressive antihypertensive therapy. Furthermore, carotid stenosis of a severity currently considered not to be hemodynamically significant might result in poor irrigation of the deep white matter due to damping of the pulse pressure.

[a]Address for correspondence: Dr. William R. Brown, Department of Radiology, Wake Forest University School of Medicine, Winston-Salem, NC 27157. Tel.: (336) 716-2225; fax (336) 716-2029.

e-mail: brownb@rad.wfubmc.edu

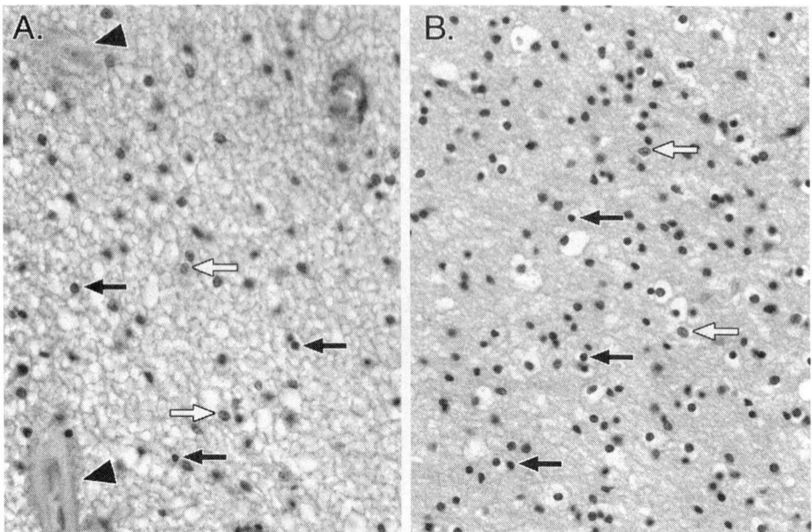

FIGURE 1. Comparison of the leukoaraiosis lesion (**A**) and an unaffected area in nearby white matter (**B**). Note that in the leukoaraiosis lesion oligodendrocytes (*solid arrows*) appear to be preferentially reduced in number compared to astrocytes which have slightly larger and less densely stained nuclei (*hollow arrows*). Also, note the veins with walls thickened by multiple layers of collagen (*arrowheads*). Hematoxylin and eosin staining.

Cerebral Vascular Pathology in Leukoaraiosis

Some pathological alterations of the brain arterial/arteriolar wall that might contribute to LA include *intimal* hyperplasia and atherosclerosis; *medial* fibrinoid necrosis, hyaline degeneration, arteriolosclerosis, lipohyalinosis, amyloidosis, and dissection; *adventitial* calcifications, siderosis, and Charcôt-Bouchard microaneurysms. Restriction of blood flow or impairment of autoregulation are features of most of these lesions. Less widely recognized is vascular tortuosity in the white matter. Our studies suggest that it would take hypertensive levels of pulsatile blood pressure to maintain flow in these vessels.[4] Some of these tortuous arterioles arise from the leptomeningeal arterial border zone which already has a precarious blood supply.

Periventricular Venous Collagenosis

In some cases with confluent LA, we found a striking degree of collagenous thickening in the walls of periventricular veins, resulting in narrowed lumina and even occlusion (FIG. 1).[5] Increased venous resistance could induce chronic edema in the deep white matter, perhaps leading to LA. With ordinary hematoxylin and eosin sections these vessels could be mistaken for hyalinized arterioles, but we have established that this material is collagen. These vessels have an apparently normal basement membrane as revealed by immunostaining for collagen IV, a thick layer of collagens I and III, and an outer membrane of collagen IV at the interface with the brain parenchyma.

ALZHEIMER'S DISEASE

Connection between Leukoaraiosis and Alzheimer's Disease

AD patients with LA have been reported to perform significantly worse on neuropsychological testing than those without LA. It has been estimated that one-third of all patients with the clinical diagnosis of AD could be suffering from a mixture of primary neurodegenerative disease and vascular dementia. It has been shown that LA is common in AD, and MRI studies have shown that LA is more prevalent in AD than in controls. Ultrastructural studies have shown collagen deposition in vessel walls in AD, as we have shown in LA. Our working hypothesis is that ischemia is fundamental to LA and contributory to AD. The very high prevalence of LA in AD could be coincidental, or it may suggest that many people are genetically susceptible to having cerebral ischemia, which may lead not only to LA, but also to AD.

Cerebral Vascular Pathology in Alzheimer's Disease

Before amyloid was found in AD, senility was thought to result from cerebrovascular pathology, i.e., "hardening of the arteries." In addition to amyloid angiopathy, there are other types of microvascular pathology, such as decreased microvascular density, string vessels, loss of endothelium, loss of the fine perivascular neural plexus, lumpy vessels, and tortuous arterioles. Some of these microvascular alterations have been found in regional and laminar patterns which parallel patterns of neuronal loss. The basal lamina constituents—laminin, collagen IV (FIG. 2), and heparan sul-

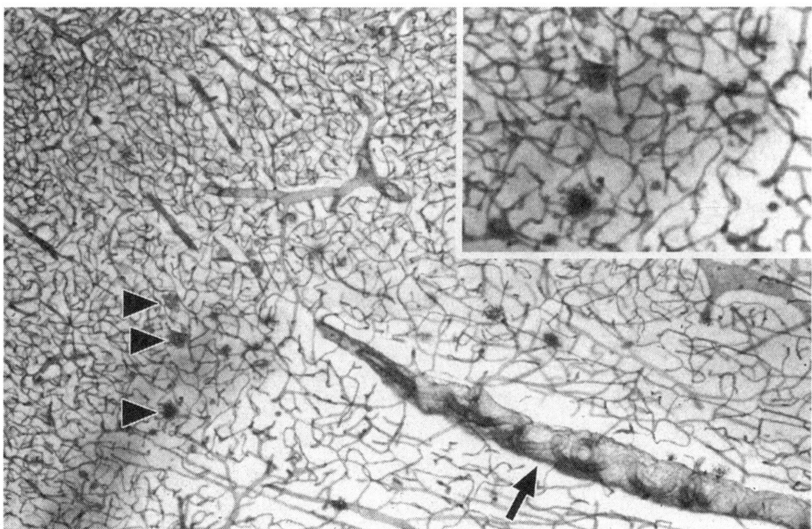

FIGURE 2. Staining with antibody to collagen IV, a basement membrane component, shows a tortuous arteriole (*arrow*) that appears to be in a "bag" within the white matter. Several Alzheimer's plaques (*arrowheads*), containing collagen IV can be seen in the cortex near the border with the white matter. **Inset:** Higher magnification of the plaques.

fate proteoglycan—have all been found in amyloid plaques, and it has been proposed that they may form a nidus for amyloidogenesis. It is unknown whether these basal lamina constituents represent remnants of vessels or become associated with amyloid without having been incorporated into a basal lamina. Apolipoprotein E has been found to play a significant role in AD and, like β-amyloid, it is a blood-borne molecule. A chronic leaky blood-brain barrier is a potential gateway for blood-borne molecules that might be capable of initiating or accelerating plaque formation, or causing other non-plaque-related cerebral injury. The investigation of vascular factors is important because there are new therapeutic approaches that could improve cerebral perfusion in AD.

Microvascular-associated Amyloid Plaque

Amyloid angiopathy has been reported to affect even the microvasculature, and some studies have suggested that amyloid plaques often form around vessels, but the degree to which this happens is not yet clear. To approach this question, we have developed a method that provides an excellent 3D view of the vessels and amyloid. We use 100-μm-thick celloidin sections with immunohistochemical staining for β-amyloid and the basement membrane constituent collagen IV. Very small (early) deposits of amyloid can be seen surrounding capillaries (FIG. 3). Studies to quantitatively determine the relation between vessels and plaque are under way.

Chronic Obstructive Pulmonary Disease and Amyloid Plaque

In studies of several cases of chronic obstructive pulmonary disease (COPD), we found a specific pattern of β-amyloid plaque formation. These plaques, which are of

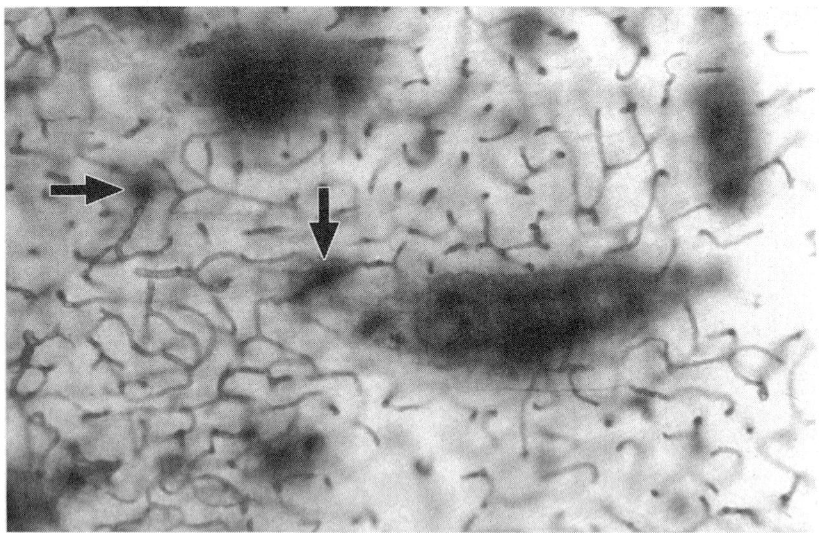

FIGURE 3. Staining with antibodies to collagen IV and β-amyloid shows amyloid deposition not only around larger vessels, but even down to the capillary level (*arrows*).

the diffuse rather than neuritic type, first appear deep in the sulcus and spread upward. We speculate that this pattern of amyloid deposition is related to the compression of veins leading out of the parenchyma and up the sulcus to the brain surface. In COPD, there is brain swelling that can cause the sulcus to swell closed and perhaps compress the enclosed veins. If this finding is confirmed, it would suggest that chronically impaired perfusion may somehow cause amyloid deposition.

APOPTOSIS IN LEUKOARAIOSIS AND BLOOD VESSEL WALLS

Because no obvious necrosis has been observed in LA lesions, we looked for apoptosis, which is a programmed cell death that occurs in a biochemical cascade, sometimes delayed for weeks.[6] It occurs in ischemia and plays an important role in neuronal cell death in stroke and neurodegeneration. Various triggering mechanisms converge on a final common pathway that results in DNA cleavage and protein destruction, but the cell remnants remain membrane enclosed. No inflammatory mediators are released, and the apoptotic bodies are phagocytosed with minimal toxicity to neighboring cells. Unlike necrosis, apoptosis can be halted.

Case Report

We investigated an LA lesion in a 70-year-old man who died of cardiac arrest.[7] His history included myocardial ischemia, atherosclerosis, hypercholesterolemia, hypertension, gout, insulin-dependent diabetes mellitus, 60 pack-years of smoking, pulmonary emphysema, and coronary artery bypass graft surgery. The autopsy report noted mild cerebral atrophy with multiple mildly stenotic atherosclerotic lesions in cerebral arteries. He was not reported to have dementia.

Results

MRI showed an LA lesion in a brain slice. Sections from this area, stained for Luxol Fast Blue, exhibited a pattern of demyelination corresponding to the lesion seen on MRI. Trichrome-stained sections revealed severe venous collagenosis in the lesion. TUNEL staining showed scattered, labeled brain parenchymal cells, as well as many labeled cells in vessel walls. Vessels of all sizes had labeled cells; those with excessive collagen did not have more of them. A moderate number of amyloid plaques was found in the overlying cortex, but there were very few in the hippocampus. TUNEL-positive parenchymal cells were counted in areas of the lesion, nearby white matter, and adjacent cortex. Apoptosis counts were 97.1 cells/cm^2 in the lesion, 38.0 cells/cm^2 in adjacent white matter, and 3.8 cells/cm^2 in the nearby cortex. Counts were greater in the lesion than the white matter ($p = .004$) or the cortex ($p < .001$). Double staining for TUNEL and the astrocyte marker GFAP showed a few double-stained cells in the cortex, but none in the white matter. Staining for interleukin-1α, a marker for activated microglia and macrophages, showed few positive cells in the white matter or cortex.

Discussion

Apoptosis appears to account for at least some of the cell loss seen in this LA lesion. Because no TUNEL-positive cells in the white matter stained with GFAP, the apoptotic cells were likely oligodendrocytes. This fits with the histological finding that LA lesions show demyelination with a profound loss of oligdendrocytes (FIG. 1). The paucity of activated microglia or macrophages in the LA lesion indicates that little or no inflammation was present. TUNEL-positive cells in the walls of blood vessels in human brains have been previously reported,[8–10] but their significance is unknown. They provide a convenient positive internal control for apoptosis, but they make the counting of labeled parenchymal cells more difficult. Because this LA lesion was distant from the lateral ventricle, and the most severe collagenosis "followed" the lesion away from the ventricle, we conclude that there is a mechanistic link between LA and venous collagenosis, rather than an incidental association.

SUMMARY AND CONCLUSIONS

Cerebral vascular pathology develops with aging, and certain aspects are pronounced in LA and perhaps in AD as well. LA results from chronic ischemia and involves loss of oligodendrocytes by apoptosis. AD is often associated with LA and cerebral vascular pathology that could cause chronic ischemia. Other factors that point to a potential vascular contribution to the development of AD include the finding of small (early) deposits of amyloid around capillaries, and vascular basement membrane components in amyloid plaques.

ACKNOWLEDGMENTS

This work was supported by NIH grant NS-20618 (D.M.M.).

REFERENCES

1. KOBARI, M., J.S. MEYER, M. ICHIJO & W.T. ORAVEZ. 1990. Leukoaraiosis: correlation of MR and CT findings with blood flow, atrophy, and cognition. Am. J. Neuroradiol. **11:** 273–281.
2. MUNOZ, D.G., S.M. HASTAK, B. HARPER, D. LEE & V.C. HACHINSKI. 1993. Pathologic correlates of increased signals of the centrum ovale on magnetic resonance imaging. Arch. Neurol. **50:** 492–497.
3. MOODY, D.M., M.A. BELL & V.R. CHALLA. 1990. Features of the cerebral vascular pattern that predict vulnerability to perfusion or oxygenation deficiency: an anatomic study. Am. J. Neuroradiol. **11:** 431–439.
4. MOODY, D.M., W.P. SANTAMORE & M.A. BELL. 1991. Does tortuosity in cerebral arterioles impair down-autoregulation in hypertensives and elderly normotensives? A hypothesis and computer model. Clin. Neurosurg. **37:** 372–387.
5. MOODY, D.M., W.R. BROWN, V.R. CHALLA & R.L. ANDERSON. 1995. Periventricular venous collagenosis: association with leukoaraiosis. Radiology **194:** 469–476.
6. CUMMINGS, M.C., C.M. WINTERFORD & N.I. WALKER. 1997. Apoptosis. Am. J. Surg. Pathol. **21:** 88–101.
7. BROWN, W.R., D.M. MOODY, C.R. THORE & V.R. CHALLA. 2000. Apoptosis in leukoaraiosis. Am. J. Neuroradiol. **21.** In press.

8. ADLE-BIASSETTE, H., Y. LEVY, M. COLOMBEL, *et al.* 1995. Neuronal apoptosis in HIV infection in adults. Neuropathol. Appl. Neurobiol. **21:** 218–227.
9. GRAY, F., F. CHRETIEN, H. ADLE-BISSETTE, *et al.* 1999. Neuronal apoptosis in Creutzfeld-Jacob disease. J. Neuropathol. Exp. Neurol. **58:** 321–328.
10. LUCASSEN, P.J., W.C.J. CHUNG, W. KAMPHORST & D.F. SWAAB. 1997. DNA damage distribution in the human brain as shown by in situ end labeling; area-specific differences in aging and Alzheimer's disease in the absence of apoptotic morphology. J. Neuropathol. Exp. Neurol. **56:** 887–900.

Role of Blood Vessels in Producing Pathological Changes in the Brain with Alzheimer's Disease

TAIHEI MIYAKAWA,[a] TAKEMI KIMURA, SHINICHI HIRATA, NOBORU FUJISE, TSUNEHIKO ONO, KOKO ISHIZUKA, AND JUN NAKABAYASHI

Department of Neuropsychiatry, Kumamoto University School of Medicine, 1-1-1 Honjo, Kumamoto 860-8556, Japan

ABSTRACT: Vascular factors have been shown to be highly involved in the deposition of the amyloid β-protein (Aβ) in the brain of Alzheimer's disease (AD). However, the detailed mechanism remains unknown. Here, we showed that more numerous deposits of Aβ_{40} and Aβ_{42} in the brain were found in AD patients than in controls. Together with evidence of no difference in the level of Aβ_{40} and Aβ_{42} in sera between sporadic AD and conrols, a certain dysfunction of the blood-brain barrier could induce an abnormal transport of Aβ from sera to the parenchyma in AD. In addition, vascular Aβ deposits and mature Aβ plaques stained by Congo red in AD brains contained more Aβ_{40} than Aβ_{42}, whereas Congo red-negative immature plaques mainly consisted of Aβ42. Our confocal laser scanning microscopy demonstrated an intimate relationship between Aβ_{40} and the vascular network. The amount of mature plaques but not that of immature plaques was reportedly correlated with the severity of dementia in AD patients. These results suggest that serum-derived Aβ_{40} and/or Aβ_{42} cause Aβ_{40} deposition in and around blood vessels through unknown but possible mechanisms such as (1) endocytosis of Aβ_{40}, (2) selective transport Aβ_{40} and Aβ_{42} into blood vessels and the parenchyma, respectively, and (3) proteolysis of Aβ_{42} into Aβ_{40} induced by a putative carboxyl dipeptidase in blood vessels including vascular feet, which is involved in Aβ fibrillation and cognitive deterioration in the patients. Therefore, the accumulation of Aβ_{40} associated with blood vessels may play a critical role in the development of AD.

INTRODUCTION

The deposition of the amyloid β-protein (Aβ) in the brain is a cardinal feature of Alzheimer's disease (AD). Aβ is a 4-kDa peptide consisting of 40–42 residues derived from a large protein, designated as the amyloid precursor protein (APP).[1] According to the difference of the carboxyl terminus of Aβ, it is classified into Aβ_{40} and Aβ_{42}. Until now, the mechanism of Aβ production inducing senile plaques has not yet been clearly determined. We have speculated that microvessels in the brain with AD play an important role in producing the morphological changes in the AD brain. In the present study, we examined the brain using Aβ-immunostaining and Congo-red staining. In addition, tissues of the brain were examined under confocal laser scanning microscopy and electron microscopy.

[a]Corresponding author. Tel.: +81 (96) 373-5183; fax: +81 (96) 362-8741.
e-mail: psychiat@kaiju.medic.kumamoto-u.ac.jp

MATERIALS AND METHODS

Materials

Tissues of cerebral temporal cortex were obtained at autopsy from 10 AD patients aged 70 to 100 years (mean $\pm$ SD, 81.9 $\pm$ 9.6) and 10 aged-matched nondemented individuals aged 60 to 85 years (80.1 $\pm$ 7.7). Patients with AD were diagnosed according to DSM-III-R[2] and the neuropathological criterion of AD.[3] None of these nondemented subjects had suffered from neurological disorders or systemic diseases affecting the central nervous system.

Antibodies

We used carboxyl-terminal end-specific monoclonal anti-Aβ such as MBC40 (raised against 32–40 amino acids) (1:20) and MBC42 (37–42) (1:100) and the polyclonal anti-Aβ including BC40 (33-40) (1:500) and BC42 (37-42) (1:500)[4] and a polyclonal anti-human collagen type IV (ICN Pharmaceuticals, 1:100).

Histochemical and Immunohistochemical Procedures

Five-micrometer-thick paraffin-embedded sections prepared from each formalin-fixed sample were immunostained and subjected to Congo red staining. For immunostaining, the sections were deparaffinized, immersed in 0.3% H_2O_2 in methanol, pretreated with formic acid for 1–3 min, incubated with 1% bovine serum albumin for 20 min, and then with each antibody at 4°C overnight. Sections were incubated with biotinylated goat anti-rabbit IgG (Vector, 1:500) for 30 min, followed by incubation with avidin-biotin-peroxidase complex (Vector). Visualization was achieved using diaminobenzidine. For the absorption experiment, the section was treated with those Aβ antisera in an excess of synthesized Aβ_{1-42} or Aβ_{1-40}.

Double Fluorescent Immunohistochemistry and Confocal Laser Scanning Microscopy

Formalin-fixed parahippocampal tissues of AD brains were cut into 50 μm-thick sections on a Vibratome (Technical Products International), immersed in 0.3% H_2O_2 in 80% methanol for 3 h, incubated in 1% bovine serum albumin for 3 h, and then in a mixture of two primary antibodies raised in different species: mouse monoclonal anti-Aβ antibody such as MBC40 or MBC42 and rabbit polyclonal anti-collagen type IV, at 4°C for 5 days. They were incubated in a mixture of Fluorescein Isothiocyanate-conjugated goat anti-rabbit IgG (Jackson Lab, 1:200) and Cy 5-conjugated donkey anti-mouse IgG (Jackson Lab, 1:200) overnight, and mounted in Vectashield (Vector) after rinsing. Sections were examined with a confocal laser scanning microscope (FLUOVIEW, Olympus) equipped with an argon-krypton laser using laser beams of 488 and 568 nm for excitation with appropriated filter sets.

Electron Microscopic Procedures

Parts of the cerebral cortex were removed from AD brains immediately after death, cut into small pieces, and immersed in 3% glutaraldehyde in phosphate buffer (pH 7.4) for 2 h. They were washed in phosphate buffer (pH 7.4) for 10 min, and then

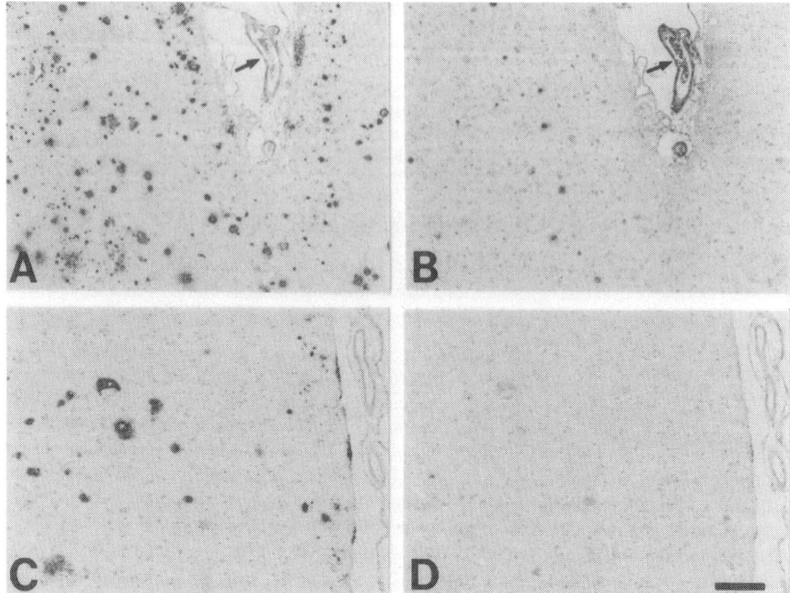

FIGURE 1. Immunostaining of serial sections reveals that deposits immunoreactive to BC42 (**A, C**) and BC40 (**B, D**) are found more in the cerebral cortex of a patient with Alzheimer's disease (AD) (**A, B**) than in that of a control (**C, D**), with BC42-immunoreactions being more prevalent. On the other hand, immunoreaction with BC40 in vascular Aβ deposits is more intensive than that with BC42 (*arrows* in **A** and **B**). Magnification ×130.

immersed for 2 h in 2.5% osmium tetroxide in phosphate buffer (pH 7.4). The tissues were dehydrated and embedded in epon. From the blocks, serial sections were stained with toluidine blue for light microscopy. Then 200-sheet meshes of serial thin sections (30–50 nm) were taken from each block and stained with uranyl acetate and lead acetate or with an alkaline bismuth solution. The sections were examined at 200 kV accelerated voltage in the electron microscope (2000EX, JEOL).

RESULTS

Histochemical and Immunohistochemical Findings

Extracellular deposition of Aβ was found in the parahippocampal cortex of all AD patients and 5 out of the 10 aged-matched nondemented subjects. Highly numerous deposits positive with BC42 and/or with BC40 in the brain were found, especially in AD brains, although the amount of deposits that reacted with BC42 was relatively more than that with BC40 (FIG. 1). Blood vessels that suffered from amyloid angiopathy more intensely reacted with BC40 than with BC42 (FIG. 1A, B). The Congo red-stained Aβ deposits and microvessels in the brain were shown to be positive with both of BC40 and BC42; however, the former immunoreaction was more prevalent than the latter (FIG. 2). Under confocal laser scanning microscopy, all

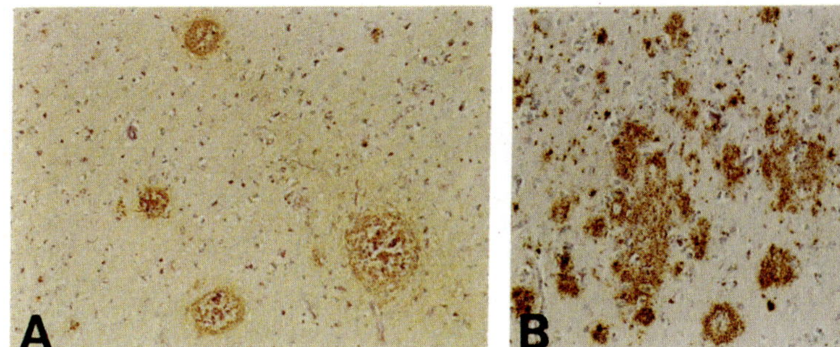

FIGURE 2. Double staining by Congo red and immunohistochemistry displays that most of BC40-reactive deposits (**A**) and little BC42-positive deposits (**B**) are accompanied with Congo red staining. Magnification ×100.

plaques and deposits stained with BC40 were found in and around microvessels positive for collagen type IV (Fig. 3A), whereas BC42-positive materials were almost always present in and around such microvessels, but some of them lacked any relationship to the blood vessels (Fig. 3B).

Electron Microscopic Findings

Examination of the epon-embedded serial sections stained with toluidine blue under light microscopy showed that almost all amyloid masses forming the cores of typical senile plaques seem to be deposited around microvessels (data not shown). However, some senile plaques lacked any relationship to the microvessels. Electron microscopy of typical senile plaques in close relation to microvessels showed that amyloid masses consisting of amyloid fibrils always existed around capillaries, with numerous amyloid fibrils projecting directly from the microvessels with amyloid angiopathy into the surrounding parenchyma (Fig. 4). Even when senile plaques seemed to have no relationship with the microvessels under light microscopy, electron microscopy almost always demonstrated degenerated or destroyed microvessels with amyloid angiopathy (Fig. 5).

DISCUSSION

Extracellular deposition of Aβ in the brain is an invariant characteristic of AD. It has been established that the cerebral Aβ deposition is closely involved in the development of AD. Many morphological studies on the mechanism of senile plaque production have been reported to date; however, the detailed mechanisms by which they are formed have not yet been clearly identified.

In 1938, Scholz[5] described plaque-like degeneration of arteries and capillaries (*drusige Entartung der Hirnarterien*) and considered that the core of senile plaques may consist of material that permeated from the blood vessels. In this context, Selkoe's laboratory demonstrated that Aβ was continuously produced in soluble form by a variety of cultured human cells under normal metabolic conditions,[6,7] sug-

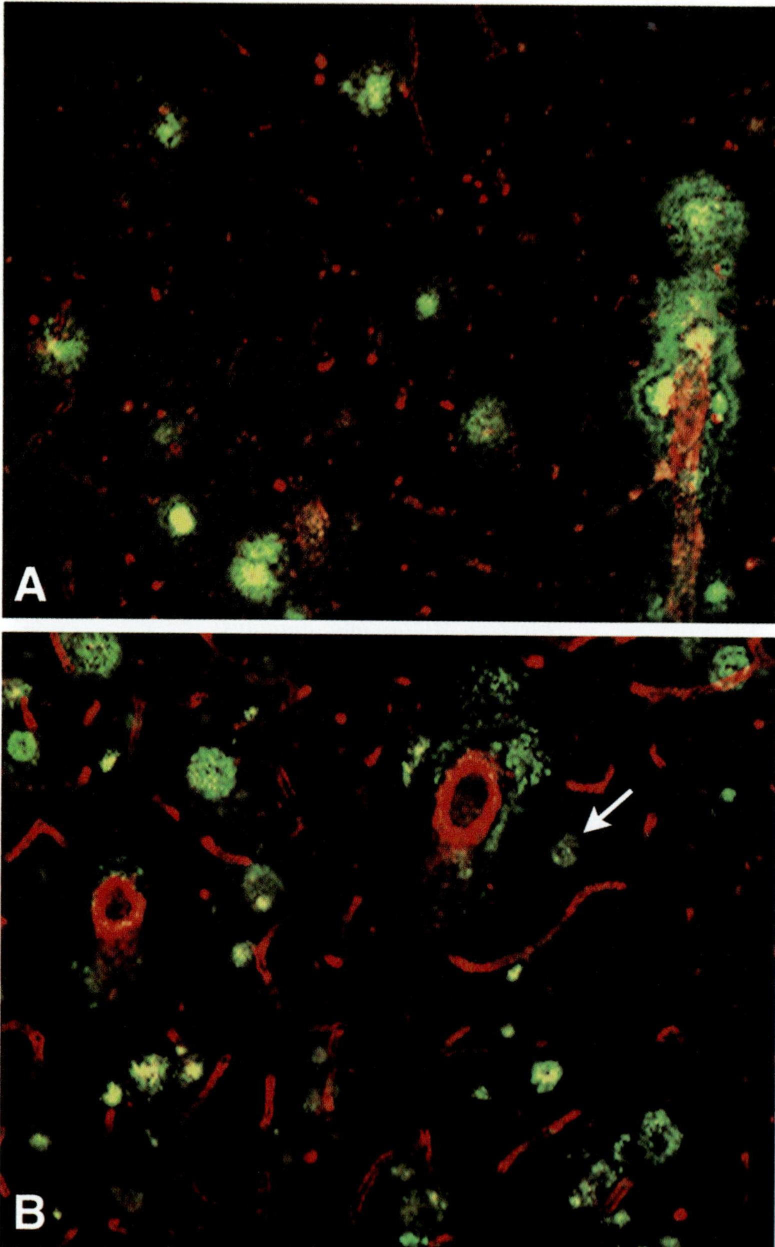

FIGURE 3. Confocal laser scanning microscopy shows that MBC40-positive (green) deposits are almost all associated with capillaries and blood vessels stained with anti-collagen type IV (red) (**A**), whereas a portion of MBC42-positive (green, *arrow in **B***) deposits have a lack of relationship to the vascular network. Magnification ×150.

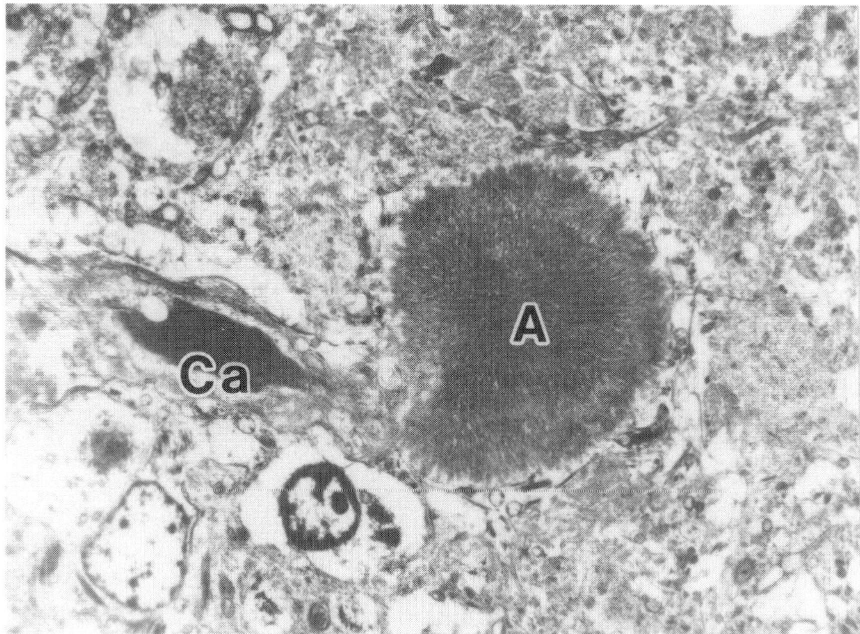

FIGURE 4. Amyloid mass (A) consisting of amyloid fibrils directly attaches to a degenerated capillary (Ca) with amyloid angiopathy. Numerous amyloid fibrils project into the surrounding parenchyma from the capillary. Magnification ×3,250.

gesting that several cellular sources may well contribute to the formation of senile plaques and vascular Aβ deposits through blood circulation. Together with evidence of no difference in the level of $A\beta_{40}$ and $A\beta_{42}$ in sera between sporadic AD and conrols,[8] our finding that more numerous deposits of $A\beta_{40}$ and $A\beta_{42}$ in the brain were found in AD patients than in controls has us to speculate that a certain dysfunction of the blood-brain barrier could induce an abnormal transport of Aβ from sera to the parenchyma in AD.

Our previous studies[9–13] and the current result obtained by electron microscopy showed that amyloid fibrils were present around the blood vessels with amyloid angiopathy in senile plaques and that all of the senile plaques contained at least some amyloid fibrils, which seemed to be produced at the basement membranes of capillary endothelial cells and spread into the surrounding parenchyma. These findings strongly suggest that amyloid fibrils forming senile plaques have a close relationship to microvessels.

This histochemical and immunohistochemical experiments revealed that vascular and perivascular Aβ deposits mainly composed of $A\beta_{40}$, but not diffuse $A\beta_{42}$-positive plaques, were stained with Congo red. In addition, using confocal laser scanning microscopy which enables us to clearly detect microvessels (FIG. 3) and precisely perform three-dimensional analysis between Aβ deposits and vascular network, we showed that all of the $A\beta_{40}$ deposits, but not all of the $A\beta_{42}$, occurred in and around the blood vessels. These findings suggest that $A\beta_{40}$ is significantly asso-

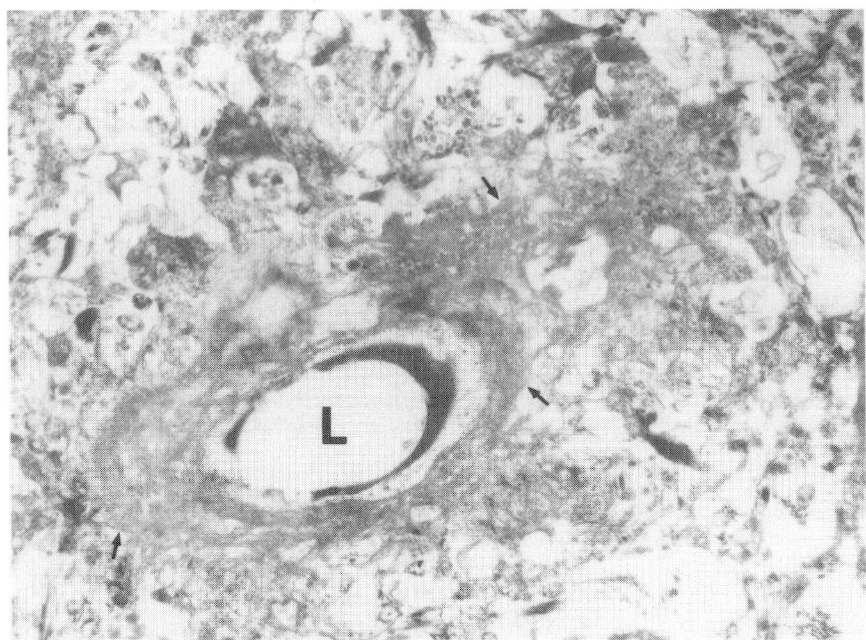

FIGURE 5. Many amyloid fibrils (*arrows*) originated from a degenerated capillary extended into the parenchyma. Note numerous degenerated neurites around the fibrils. L, lumen of capillary. Magnification ×4,100.

ciated with blood vessel-related $A\beta$ deposition, and its amyloid is likely to be a fibrillar structure, whereas a proportion of $A\beta_{42}$ deposits is neither aggregated nor has a relationship with blood vessels. Because both $A\beta_{40}$ and $A\beta_{42}$ were detected in sera, with $A\beta_{40}$ being highly prevalent,[14] serum-derived $A\beta_{40}$ and/or $A\beta_{42}$ cause $A\beta_{40}$ deposition in and around blood vessels through unknown but possible mechanisms (FIG. 6) such as (1) endocytosis of $A\beta_{40}$, (2) selective transport $A\beta_{40}$ and $A\beta_{42}$ into blood vessels and the parenchyma, respectively,[15] and (3) proteolysis of $A\beta_{42}$ into $A\beta_{40}$ induced by a putative carboxyl dipeptidase in blood vessels including vascular feet, which is involved in $A\beta$ fibrillation.

It has been established that diffuse plaques positive for $A\beta_{42}$ are an earlier immature form of senile plaques, whereas primitive and classic plaques are the mature form and mainly consist of $A\beta_{40}$. A part of long-lasting parenchymal $A\beta_{42}$ may be also metabolized into $A\beta_{40}$, which contributes to the maturation of senile plaques. In this connection, the amount of primitive and classic plaques, but not that of diffuse plaques, were reportedly correlated with the severity of dementia in AD patients.[16] Therefore, $A\beta_{40}$ accumulation certainly associated with blood vessels may play a critical role in the development into AD, which is supported by the evidence of a positive correlation between the amount of $A\beta_{40}$ in brain tissues from AD patients and the frequency of apolipoprotein E ϵ4 allele that accelerates the onset of AD.[17] In addition, a study by two-site enzyme immunoassay clearly showed that high lev-

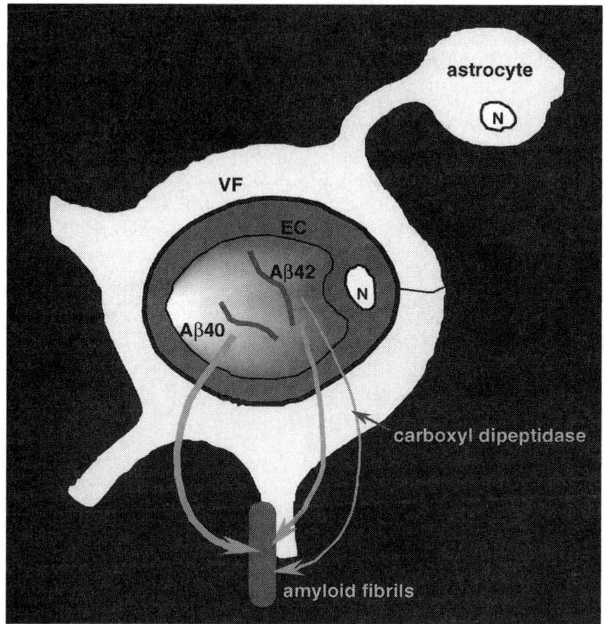

FIGURE 6. Putative mechanism of amyloid fibril production derived from serum Aβ. N, nucleus; VF, vascular feet; EC, endothelial cell.

els of $A\beta_{40}$ in the cerebral cortex were found to be associated with AD.[18] Elucidation of a detailed mechanism of $A\beta_{40}$ deposition in blood vessels and the parenchyma (e.g., the role of apolipoprotein E), using blood-brain barrier endothelial cell cultures and animals, could provide an insight into the development of useful treatment strategies against cognitive deterioration in AD.

ACKNOWLEDGMENT

We thank Dr. Haruyasu Yamaguchi (Gumma University) for giving us the antibodies used in this study.

REFERENCES

1. KANG, J. *et al.* 1987. The precursor of Alzheimer's disease amyloid A4 protein resembles a cell-surface receptor. Nature **325:** 733–736.
2. AMERICAN PSYCHIATRIC ASSOCIATION. 1987. DSM-III-R: Diagnostic and statistical manual of mental disorders, 3rd edit. revised. American Psychiatric Association, Washington, DC.
3. KHACHATURIAN, Z.S. 1985. Diagnosis of Alzheimer's disease. Arch. Neurol. **42:** 1097–1105.
4. YAMAGUCHI, H. *et al.* 1998. Immunohistochemical analysis of COOH-termini of amyloid beta protein (Aβ) using end-specific antisera for Aβ40 and Aβ42 in Alzheimer's disease and normal aging. Amyloid: Int. J. Exp. Clin. Invest. **2:** 7–16.

5. SCHOLZ, W. 1938. Studien zur Pathologie der Hirngefasse in Senium. *In* Proceedings of the Fifth International Congress of Neuropathology, Zurich.: 490–494.
6. KOSAKA, T. 1997. The βAPP717 Alzheimer mutation increases the percentage of plasma amyloid-β protein ending at Aβ42(43). Neurology **48:** 741–745.
7. HAASS, C. *et al.* 1992. Amyloid β-peptide is produced by cultured cells during normal metabolism. Nature **359:** 322–325.
8. SEUBERT, P. *et al.* 1992. Isolation and quantification of soluble Alzheimer's β-peptide from biological fluids. Nature **359:** 325–327.
9. MIYAKAWA, T. *et al.* 1974. Ultrastructure of capillary plaque-like degeneration in senile dementia: Mechanism of amyloid production. Acta Neuropathol. (Berl.) **29:** 229–236.
10. MIYAKAWA, T. & Y. UEHARA. 1979. Observations of amyloid angiopathy and senile plaques by the scanning electron microscope. Acta Neuropathol. (Berl.) **48:** 153–156.
11. MIYAKAWA, T. *et al.* 1982. The relationship between senile plaques and cerebral blood vessels in Alzheimer's disease and senile dementia. Morphological mechanism of senile plaque production. Virchows Arch. B Pathol. **40:** 121–129.
12. MIYAKAWA, T. *et al.* 1986. The relationship between amyloid fibrils around cerebral blood vessels and senile plaques, and ultrastructure of amyloid fibrils. *In* International Symposium on Dementia and Amyloid (Tokyo, Japan). Neuropathology **(Suppl. 3):** 37–48.
13. MIYAKAWA, T. 1997. Electron microscopy of amyloid fibrils and microvessels. Ann. N.Y. Acad. Sci. **826:** 25–34.
14. SUZUKI, N. *et al.* 1994. An increased percentage of long amyloid β-protein is secreted by familial amyloid β-protein precursor (βAPP717) mutants. Science **264:** 1336–1340.
15. MARTEL, C.L. *et al.* 1996. Blood-brain barrier uptake of the 40 and 42 amino acid sequences of circulating Alzheimer's amyloid β in guinea pigs. Neurosci. Lett. **206:** 157–160.
16. DELAÈRE, P. *et al.* 1991. Subtypes and differential laminar distributions of βA4 deposits in Alzheimer's disease: relationship with the intellectual status of 26 cases. Acta Neuropathol. (Berl.) **81:** 328–335.
17. ISHII, K. *et al.* 1997. Abeta$_{1-40}$ but not Abeta$_{1-42}$ levels in cortex correlate with apolipoprotein E epsilon4 allele dosage in sporadic Alzheimer's disease. Brain Res. **748:** 250–252.
18. FUNATO, H. *et al.* 1998. Quantitation of amyloid β-protein in the cortex during aging and in Alzheimer's disease. Am. J. Pathol. **152:** 1633–1640.

Cerebrovasculature-mediated Neuronal Cell Death

PAULA GRAMMAS,[a,c] ULRICH REIMANN-PHILIPP,[a,c] AND PAUL H. WEIGEL[b,c]

[a]*Departments of Pathology and* [b]*Biochemistry and Molecular Biology, and* [c]*Oklahoma Center for Neuroscience, University of Oklahoma Health Sciences Center, 975 N.E. 10th Street, Oklahoma City, Oklahoma 73104, USA*

ABSTRACT: The presence of significant vascular disease in patients with Alzheimer's disease (AD) and the recognition of the ApoE genotype as a risk factor for both coronary disease and AD support an association between AD and vascular disease. It is our hypothesis that brain microvessels contribute to the pathogenesis of AD by producing soluble factors that injure or kill neurons. In this study we report that AD microvessels produce factors that are noxious to neurons and that these vessels can evoke neuronal cell death *in vitro*. In these experiments, microvessels are isolated from the cerebral cortices of AD patients and non-demented elderly and young controls. Microvessels isolated from AD brains produce high levels of a known neurotoxin nitric oxide, compared to vessels from aged-matched controls. In addition, we demonstrate a direct neurotoxic effect of AD microvessels when co-cultured with primary rat cerebral cortical neurons. In contrast, vessels from elderly non-demented donors are less lethal, and brain vessels from younger donors are not neurotoxic. Similarly, AD vessels exhibit a dose-dependent toxicity in co-culture with the human neurons. Finally, treatment of AD microvessels with the protein synthesis inhibitor cycloheximide reduces AD vessel neurotoxicity, suggesting that the neurotoxic factor is a protein. These findings suggest that the cerebral microvasculature is a source of factors that can injure neurons and implicate a novel mechanism of vascular-mediated neuronal cell death in AD.

INTRODUCTION

Most patients with neuropathologically confirmed AD exhibit significant vascular disease.[1] Inheritance of the ApoE allele ε4 increases the risk of developing both atherosclerosis and late-onset AD.[2] This finding suggests a vascular component to the pathogenesis of neuronal degeneration in AD.[3] Several studies have shown a high correlation between hypertension and dementia.[4,5] There is growing evidence that in AD structural deformities of cerebral capillaries may lead to impaired cerebral perfusion and ultimately to neuronal dysfunction and death.[6] These data support the notion that vascular factors, traditionally thought to be important for the development of stroke and vascular dementia, also play a role in the pathogenesis of AD.

We have previously demonstrated a spectrum of biochemical defects in receptors and signaling pathways in cerebral microvessels in AD brains.[7–10] Our laboratory and others have documented that brain endothelial cells express an "activated phenotype" demonstrating characteristics of endothelium in inflammation, including expression of leukocyte adhesion molecules[11] and the monocyte chemoattractant protein CAP37.[12] It is our hypothesis that in AD an abnormal, pathologically altered brain endothelium produces factors that are toxic to neurons.

In this study, we report that microvessels isolated from AD brains produce large amounts of nitric oxide, a known neurotoxin, and that AD vessels, through secretion of as-yet-unidentified proteins, cause neuronal cell death *in vitro*.

METHODS

Human Microvessel Isolation

Human autopsy brain specimens were obtained ~6–11 h postmortem and frozen at −70°C until dissection. Microvessels were isolated from pooled temporal, parietal, and frontal cortices, filtered through a 210 µm sieve, and collected on a 53 µm sieve, as previously described.[7] Microvessels were then resuspended in Dulbecco's modified Eagle's medium (DMEM), containing 10% fetal calf serum (FCS) and 10% dimethylsulfoxide, and stored in liquid nitrogen until used.

NOS Activity

NOS activity was assayed by measuring the conversion of [^{3}H]arginine to [^{3}H]citrulline, as previously described.[13] Confirmation that the production of citrulline was mediated specifically by NOS was demonstrated using the NOS inhibitor, N^{G}Nitro-L-arginine methyl ester (10 µM), which markedly decreased the production of [^{3}H]citrulline.

Neuronal Cell Cultures

Cerebral cortices were isolated from 17-day fetal rats, dissociated, and seeded in polylysine-coated plates containing DMEM with 5% horse serum, as previously described.[14] The human neuronal cell line HCN-1A was obtained from ATCC and maintained in DMEM with 5% horse serum.

Determination of Neuronal Cell Death

Cell death was determined by release of cytoplasmic lactate dehydrogenase (LDH), as previously described.[14] Data were expressed as a percent of total LDH released by treatment with 1% Triton X-100 added to the same well. Vascular LDH release, determined for microvessel-containing inserts placed in wells without neuronal cells, was subtracted from each co-culture point. Each point was performed in duplicate. Data presented are means ± standard error of the mean. Statistical analysis between two groups was performed using the Student's *t* test.

RESULTS

The ability of control and AD brain microvessels to produce nitric oxide was determined by measuring NOS activity. Production of citrulline, the stable co-product produced by the conversion of arginine to nitric oxide, was significantly ($p < 0.001$) higher in AD microvessels compared to controls (FIG. 1).

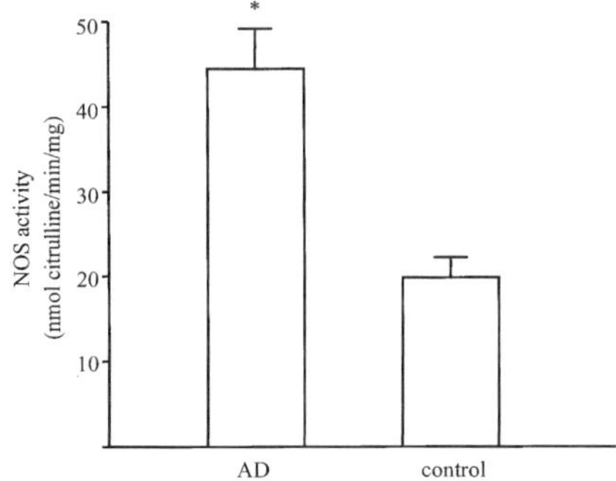

FIGURE 1. AD microvessels over-produce nitric oxide. AD and control microvessel (n = 6) supernatants (150 µg) were incubated with [^{3}H]arginine for 30 min at 37°C. [^{3}H]citrulline measured (∗) significantly different than control.

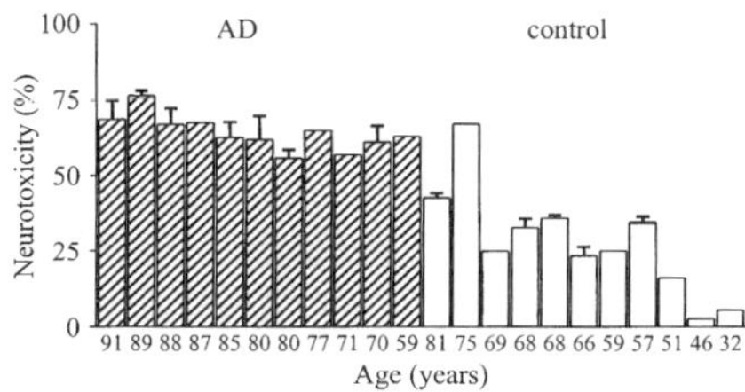

FIGURE 2. AD microvessels cause lethal injury to rat neurons in culture. Microvessels (200 µg) were washed and resuspended in media, added to Millipore filter inserts and co-cultured in 24-well plates with primary rat neuronal cultures at 37°C. After 4 h, 100 µl aliquots were assayed for LDH. Each bar represents a separate case (at least the average of duplicates). Cases shown with error bars are representative of four separate co-culture assays.

Results of experiments where microvessels from AD brains were co-cultured with primary rat neuronal cultures showed that AD-derived microvessels caused neuronal cell death (FIG. 2). Eleven separate AD cases were examined and although the amount of cytotoxicity varied, all were significantly ($p < 0.01$) above assay background (10–20%). The effect on non-AD vessels on neurons was variable and age-dependent. Microvessels from younger patients (<60 years) produced little cytotoxicity, whereas those from older patients caused some injury. A comparison between two individuals, an AD patient (70 years) and an age-matched control (68 years) showed significantly ($p < 0.02$) higher cytotoxicity with the AD-derived vessels. Increasing concentrations of AD microvessels (25–200 µg) co-cultured with the human neuronal cell line HCN-1A evoked a dose-dependent increase in neuronal cell death measured at 24 h (FIG. 3).

Incubation of AD microvessels with the protein synthesis inhibitor cycloheximide partially inhibited the appearance of the neurotoxin in vessel-conditioned media. Ten micromolar cycloheximide decreased the appearance of the toxic factor by 60% (FIG. 4).

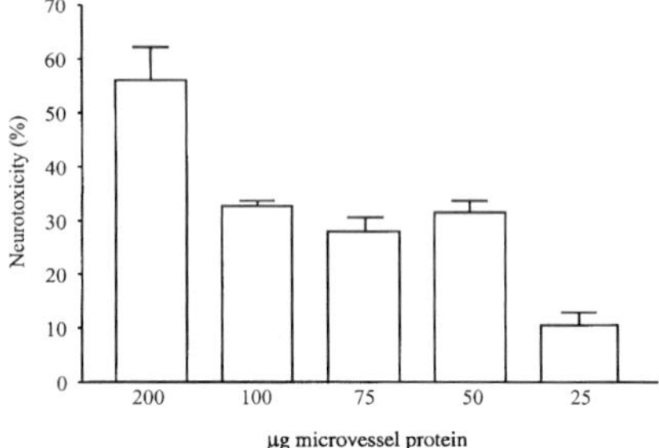

FIGURE 3. AD microvessels evoke human neuronal cell death in a dose-dependent manner. Microvessels (25–200 µg) were washed and resuspended in media, added to Millipore filter inserts and co-cultured in 24-well plates with HCN-1A cells at 37°C. After 24 h, 100 µl aliquots were assayed for LDH (n = 4).

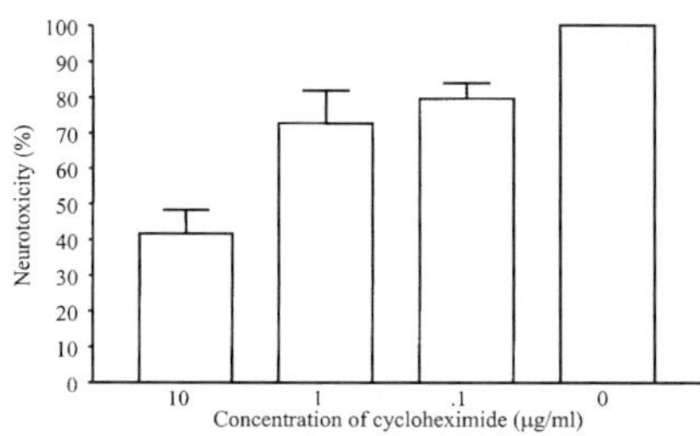

FIGURE 4. AD microvessel neurotoxicity is partially inhibited by cycloheximide. AD microvessels were treated with cycloheximide (0.1–10 µg/ml) for 24 h and microvessel-conditioned media (conditioned media toxicity similar to that evoked by co-culture[14]) added to primary rat cultures and LDH assayed after 24 h. Note that in the absence of cycloheximide, toxicity is defined as 100%, and data are expressed as neurotoxicity as a percent of 100 (n = 2).

DISCUSSION

Perturbations of brain microvascular endothelium are closely linked to the pathophysiology of several neuroinflammatory, neuroinfectious, and neurodegenerative disease states.[15] Indeed, biochemical defects in receptors and signaling pathways,[7–10] as well as active functions of the blood-brain barrier, such as glucose transport and metabolism, have been shown to be abnormal in AD.[16,17] In this study and in previous work,[13] we demonstrated that AD microvessels overproduce nitric oxide. Elevated vascular production of nitric oxide, a potentially neurotoxic mediator in the brain, may contribute to neuronal injury and death in AD. In our recent paper[14] and in this current study, which demonstrates that AD microvessels evoke neuronal cell death *in vitro*, the vasculature is implicated as an important mediator of neurodegeneration in this disease.

Considerable evidence exists that inflammatory molecules and mechanisms are involved in the pathogenesis of neurodegeneration in AD.[18,19] Endothelial cells are important regulators of the inflammatory process, secreting numerous and diverse molecules.[20] The notion that damaged or abnormal endothelial cells contribute inflammatory mediators to the AD disease process is supported by our data showing that "injury" of cultured endothelial cells by amyloid-β evokes expression of the multifunctional inflammatory protein CAP37 in these cells.[12] AD microvessels appear to be functionally abnormal, producing factors that cause neuronal (both rat and human) cell death in a dose-dependent manner.

Neurodegenerative diseases, such as AD, are characterized by damage to selective neuronal populations. The mechanisms triggering neuronal cell death could be related to the appearance of a neurotoxin and/or loss of neuroprotective proteins.[21] Our data demonstrating that AD microvessel neurotoxicity is partially inhibited by cycloheximide suggest that the vasculature may be a source of neurotoxic proteins in AD. Whether the neurotoxic factor is known or unique, the demonstration that AD brain microvessels produce soluble factors that injure or kill neurons shows that the cerebral microcirculation is a novel, unexplored source of neurotoxic factors in AD, and a heretofore unrecognized target for therapeutic intervention in this disorder.

ACKNOWLEDGMENTS

This work was supported in part by an Alzheimer's Association Zenith Award and the Presbyterian Health Foundation. Dr. P. Grammas is the recipient of the Alfred M. Shideler Professorship in Experimental Pathology.

REFERENCES

1. SPARKS, D.L. 1997. Coronary artery disease, hypertension, ApoE, and cholesterol: a link to Alzheimer's disease? Ann. N.Y. Acad. Sci. **826:** 128–146.
2. STRITTMATTER, W.J., A.M. SAUNDERS, D. SCHMECHEL, M. PERICAK-VANCE, J. ENGHILD, G.S. SALVESEN & A.D. ROSES. 1993. Apolipoprotein E: high-activity binding to β-amyloid and increased frequency of type 4 allele in late-onset familial Alzheimer's disease. Proc. Natl. Acad. Sci. USA **90:** 1977–1981.
3. MATTSON, M.P. 1997. Advances fuel Alzheimer's conundrum. Nature Gen. **17:** 254–256.
4. SKOOG, I. 1997. The relationship between blood pressure and dementia: a review. Biomed. Biopharmacother. **51:** 367–375.
5. TARISKA, P., V. KLEIN, G. PANCZEL, J. VITRAI, J. KNOLMAYER, A. MESAROS, K. URBANICS & E. KISS. 1997. Vascular disease risk factors and findings in patients with Alzheimer's disease. Arch. Gerontol. Geriatr. **25:** 237–243.
6. DE LA TORRE, J.C. 1997. Hemodynamic consequences of deformed microvessels in the brain in Alzheimer's disease. Ann. N.Y. Acad. Sci. **826:** 75–91.
7. GRAMMAS, P., A.E. ROHER & M.J. BALL. 1991. Decreased α-adrenergic receptors at the blood-brain barrier in Alzheimer's disease. *In* Alzheimer's Disease: Basic Mechanisms, Diagnosis and Therapeutic Strategies. K. Iqbal, D.R.C. McLachlan, B. Winblad & H.M. Wisniewski, Eds.: 129–136. John Wiley & Sons, Ltd. Chichester, England.
8. GRAMMAS, P., A. ROHER & M.J. BALL. 1994. Increased accumulation of cAMP in cerebral microvessels in Alzheimer's disease. Neurobiol. Aging **15:** 113–116.
9. GRAMMAS, P., P. MOORE, T. BOTCHLET, O. HANSON-PAINTON, D.E. COOPER, M.J. BALL & A. ROHER. 1995. Cerebral microvessels in Alzheimer's have reduced protein kinase C activity. Neurobiol. Aging **16:** 563–569.
10. CASHMAN, R.E. & P. GRAMMAS. 1995. cAMP-dependent protein kinase in cerebral microvessels in aging and Alzheimer's disease. Mol. Chem. Neuropathol. **26:** 247–258.
11. FROHMAN, E.M., T.C. FROHMAN, S. GUPTA, A. DE FOURGEROLLES & S. VAN DEN NOORT. 1991. Expression of intercellular adhesion molecule I (ICAM-1) in Alzheimer's disease. J. Neurol. Sci. **106:** 105–111.

12. PEREIRA, H.A., P. KUMAR & P. GRAMMAS. 1996. Expression of CAP37, a novel inflammatory mediator in Alzheimer's disease. Neurobiol. Aging **17:** 753–759.
13. DORHEIM, M.A., W.R. TRACEY, J.S. POLLOCK & P. GRAMMAS. 1994. Nitric oxide is elevated in Alzheimer's brain microvessels. Biochem. Biophys. Res. Commun. **205:** 659–665.
14. GRAMMAS, P., P. MOORE & P.H. WEIGEL. 1999. Alzheimer's disease brain microvessels kill neurons in vitro. Am. J. Pathol. **154:** 337–342.
15. ANDJELKOVIC, A.V. & J.S. PACHTER. 1998. Central nervous system endothelium in neuroinflammatory, neuroinfectious, and neurodegenerative disease. J. Neurosci. Res. **51:** 423–430.
16. KALARIA, R.N. & S.I. HARIK. 1989. Reduced glucose transporter at the blood-brain barrier in cerebral cortex in Alzheimer's disease. J. Neurochem. **53:** 1083–1088.
17. MARCUS, D.L. & M.L. FREEDMAN. 1997. Decreased brain glucose metabolism in microvessels from patients with Alzheimer's disease. Ann. N.Y. Acad. Sci. **826:** 248–253.
18. ROGERS, J., S. WEBSTER, L.F. LUE, L. BRACHOVA, W.H. CIVIN, M. EMMERLING, B. SHIVERS, D. WALKER & P. MCGEER. 1996. Inflammation and Alzheimer's disease pathogenesis. Neurobiol. Aging **17:** 681–686.
19. FIALA, M., L. ZHANG, X. GAN, B. SHERRY, D. TAUB, M.C. GRAVES, S. HAMA, D. WAY, M. WEINLAND, M. WITTE, D. LORTON, Y.M. KUO & A.E. ROHER. 1998. Amyloid-beta induces chemokine secretion and monocyte migration across a human blood-brain barrier model. Mol. Med. **7:** 480–489.
20. POBER, J.S. 1998. Activation and injury of endothelial cells by cytokines. Pathol. Biol. **46:** 159–163.
21. TAKEDA, A., M. MALLORY, M. SUNDSMO, W. HONER, L. HANSEN & E. MASLIAH. 1998. Abnormal accumulation of NACP/α-synuclein in neurodegenerative disorders. Am. J. Pathol. **152:** 367–372.

Role of Aberrant Nitric Oxide Synthase-3 Expression in Cerebrovascular Degeneration and Vascular-mediated Injury in Alzheimer's Disease

SUZANNE M. DE LA MONTE,[a] YOON K. SOHN, DANNIE ETIENNE, JOANNY KRAFT, AND JACK R. WANDS

MGH East Cancer and Cardiovascular Research Centers, Departments of Pathology and Medicine, Massachusetts General Hospital, Harvard Medical School, Boston, Massachusetts 02129, USA

ABSTRACT: Nitric oxide (NO) is an important signaling molecule that is generated through the catalytic activity of nitric oxide synthase (NOS). In the brain, NO mediates neuronal survival, synaptic plasticity, vascular smooth muscle relaxation, and endothelial cell permeability. Previous studies demonstrated aberrant expression of the NOS-III gene in neurons and glial cells in brains with Alzheimer's disease (AD). Since NOS-III is also expressed in vascular cells, and cerebrovascular disease (CVD) frequently complicates the pathology of AD, we investigated the role of NOS-III in relation to CVD in AD. Vasculopathy in AD+CVD was characterized by thickening and hyalinization of the media of small and medium-size vessels, variable degrees of β-amyloid (Aβ) deposition, and increased apoptosis of vascular smooth muscle and endothelial cells, particularly involving white matter vessels. These abnormalities were correlated with reduced levels of NOS-III expression in cerebral vessels. Double-labeling studies demonstrated that the low levels of cerebrovascular NOS-III were associated with increased levels of the pro-apoptosis gene product, p53 in smooth muscle and endothelial cells, suggesting a role for altered NOS-III expression in AD-associated vascular degeneration. Constitutively reduced cerebrovascular NOS-III expression and NO production could also lead to cerebral hypoperfusion due to impaired vasodilation responses, and diminished capacity to remove respiratory waste products and toxins from the extracellular space due to reduced capillary permeability. The role for phosphodiesterases as modulators of NOS activity is discussed, as these molecules represent potential therapeutic targets given their cell type and cyclic nucleotide specificities of action.

CEREBROVASCULAR PATHOLOGY AS A CONTRIBUTING FACTOR IN ALZHEIMER'S-TYPE DEMENTIA

Studies published within the last 3 to 4 years demonstrated that cerebrovascular disease (CVD) substantially contributes to the clinical manifestations and progres-

[a]Address for correspondence: Dr. S. M. de la Monte, Departments of Medicine and Pathology, Rhode Island Hospital, Brown University School of Medicine, 55 Claverick Street, Providence, RI 02903. Tel.: (401) 444-7364; fax: (401) 444-2939.
e-mail: delamonte@hotmail.com

sion of Alzheimer's disease (AD) such that AD+CVD may account for 20 to 40 percent of clinical AD.[1–3] CVD in AD includes hemispheric and microscopic infarcts, lacunes, hippocampal sclerosis, leukoaraiosis, microvasculopathy with cribriform change, and incomplete infarction of subcortical white matter.[1–11] Analysis of cases from the MGH-ADRC brain bank archives revealed that AD+CVD cases were not distinguished clinically from AD, but their brains had significantly lower densities of neurofibrillary tangles compared with uncomplicated AD.[12] Since neurofibrillary tangles are a major correlate of dementia in AD, it is unlikely that dementia in the AD+CVD group was caused by the AD lesions alone. On the other hand, in a study published by Snowdon *et al.*,[9] cerebral infarction in the absence of sufficient neuropathological criteria for AD was only weakly correlated with cognitive impairment. In AD+CVD, vascular lesions were distributed in structures that are typically damaged by AD neurodegeneration, in addition to the basal ganglia, thalamus, and cerebral white matter. However, we observed no examples in which CVD alone was associated with AD-type dementia. Most likely, dementia in AD+CVD is due to the combined effects of AD plus vascular lesions with prominent involvement of corticolimbic structures and pathways by both disease processes. In addition to structural lesions, CVD may contribute to cognitive deterioration by causing disruption of the blood-brain barrier,[13,14] facilitating inadvertent development of autoantibodies to central nervous system (CNS) cells,[15] or impairing cerebral blood flow, metabolic rate of oxygen consumption, and oxygen extraction.[16,17]

INCREASED APOPTOSIS OF CEREBROVASCULAR ENDOTHELIAL AND SMOOTH MUSCLE CELLS IN ALZHEIMER'S DISEASE

Apoptosis was assessed by the terminal deoxynucleotidyl transferase-mediated deoxyuridine triphosphate-biotin nick end labeling (TUNEL) assay and by immunostaining to detect the p53 pro-apoptosis gene product. Both methods revealed increased labeling of vascular endothelial cells and smooth muscle cells of medium and small size cortical, white matter, and leptomeningeal vessels in AD ($n = 20$) relative to control ($n = 9$) brains. In the white matter, thin-walled venules and capillaries also exhibited increased apoptosis in AD. White matter vascular apoptosis was associated with perivascular hemosiderin deposits, attrition of perivascular tissue, and pallor of myelin staining. Vascular endothelial cell degeneration and apoptosis could lead to impaired integrity of the blood-brain barrier with attendant exposure of axons to serum proteins and toxins. Vascular smooth muscle cell apoptosis could impair vascular responsiveness to changes in hemodynamics and chemotaxic stimuli, leading to hypoperfusion injury.

POTENTIAL ROLE FOR β-AMYLOID ANGIOPATHY IN APOPTOSIS OF CEREBROVASCULAR CELLS IN AD

Histological sections of frontal and temporal lobe were double-labeled to colocalize p53 with β-amyloid (Aβ) in vascular smooth muscle and endothelial cells. Control brains had little or no p53 or Aβ immunoreactivity. In AD, three patterns of labeling were observed in leptomeningeal and cortical vessels: 1) Aβ immunoreactivity only; Aβ plus p53; or p53 only. The Aβ immunoreactivity was localized in vascular smooth muscle cells and in the peri-adventitia, whereas p53 immunoreactivity was detected in endothelial and/or smooth muscle cells with or without associated Aβ immunoreactivity. In cerebral white matter, thin-walled venules and capillaries manifested reduced or absent immunoreactivity for p53 and no detectable Aβ. Brains with AD+CVD had nearly twofold higher densities of leptomeningeal and cortical vessels with Aβ plus p53 or p53-only immunoreactivity relative to AD, suggesting that vascular cell apoptosis was more relevant to the neuropathology of AD+CVD than AD.

With cerebral amyloid angiopathy, the frequencies of intracerebral hemorrhage as well as ischemic infarction are increased.[18] *In vitro* treatment of cerebrovascular smooth muscle cells with Aβ$_{1-42}$ peptide results in cellular degeneration with intracellular accumulations of amyloid precursor protein.[19] Experimental exposure to Aβ results in vascular disruption with damage to endothelial and smooth muscle cells, and transvascular migration of leukocytes.[20,21] Since experimental Aβ-induced vascular degeneration is preventable by treatment with free radical scavenger agents,[20] CVD and perhaps dementia associated with AD+CVD could be reduced with antioxidants. Importantly, the results of recent clinical trials suggest that cognitive function in patients with early AD may be preserved or improved following treatment with EGb 761,[22-25] the essential antioxidant compound present in *Gingko biloba*. On the other hand, the finding of p53-positive Aβ-negative vessels suggests yet another abnormality may be responsible for some aspects of CVD in AD.

POSITIVE AND NEGATIVE EFFECTS OF NITRIC OXIDE AND NITRIC OXIDE SYNTHASE EXPRESSION IN THE CENTRAL NERVOUS SYSTEM

Nitric oxide (NO) or nitrogen monoxide is a diffusable inter- and intracellular signaling molecule[26] that has diverse effects on the physiological function of smooth muscle cells, platelets, neurons, inflammatory and immune cells, and hepatocytes. NO is generated from NO synthases (NOSs) through the oxidation of a guanidino nitrogen of L-arginine. Three NOS isoforms have been identified and divided into two functional classes, constitutive and inducible. The two constitutive isoforms, initially identified in neurons (nNOS; NOS-I) and endothelial cells (NOS-III, NOS-III), are stimulated to synthesize NO by calcium/calmodulin signaling.[27,28] NOS-I and NOS-III are expressed in central nervous system (CNS) neurons.[27-29] The inducible NOS isoform (iNOS, NOS-II) has been detected in many cell types, typically after stimulation with lipopolysaccharide or cytokines. In the nervous system, NOS-II expression has been localized mainly in cytokine-activated astrocytes, inflammatory cells, and microglia.[30-33]

In the nervous system, high levels of NO can be either detrimental or beneficial to cell viability and function. NO is a free radical and its cytotoxic effects are due to peroxynitrite ($OONO^-$) formation and nitration of tyrosine residues in proteins,[34-37] or the generation of superoxides.[35,36,38] Calcium activation of NOS and NO production also mediate CNS glutamate excitotoxic metabolic injury,[39,40] ischemia,[41] and some forms of neurodegeneration.[42] NO-mediated cytotoxicity also occurs in vasogenic edema,[43] infection,[31,44] inflammatory demyelination,[45] and trauma.[46] In addition, NO can cause growth cone collapse[47] and inhibit neuronal regeneration following injury.[48]

The adverse effects of NO can be blocked by inhibiting NOS,[28,48,49] enhancing the expression of superoxide dismutase,[50] treating cells with free radical scavengers,[51] repletion of growth factors required for posttraumatic neuronal regeneration,[52,53] or impairing NOS gene expression.[54,55] However, abolishment of NOS activity and NO production is probably not a viable therapeutic approach, as there is ample evidence that NO has important normal physiological functions in some neurons. For example, NO plays a key role in synaptic plasticity and long-term potentiation,[29,56] an index of increased synaptic strength associated with learning and memory. In some neurons, neurite outgrowth is promoted by exposure to NO donor compounds or increased NOS activity.[57] In the mature CNS and differentiated neurons, basal NOS activity can be important for maintaining the structural integrity of synapses.[58–60] Therefore, in some circumstances or in specific subtypes of neurons, high levels of NO can be cytotoxic, whereas in others, NO may be required to maintain synaptic integrity or facilitate the structural modification of synapses required for learning and memory.

ABERRANT NITRIC OXIDE SYNTHASE-III (NOS-III) GENE EXPRESSION IN ALZHEIMER'S DISEASE

Impaired synaptic plasticity and cell death probably represent the underlying basis of dementia in AD. Apoptosis associated with increased levels of pro-apoptosis gene products such as p53 and Bax is an important mechanism of cell loss in AD.[61–63] In previous studies, we demonstrated aberrantly increased neuronal and glial expression of NOS-III in AD, with high levels of gene expression distributed in structural targets of neurodegeneration.[64,65] In AD, glial cells with increased NOS-III gene expression and immunoreactivity were prominently distributed in cortical Layers V and VI, the subcortical U-fibers, and central white matter, and characterized as $A_2B_5^+$ with double-labeling studies. $A_2B_5^+$ glial cells correspond to Type 2 protoplasmic astrocytes or oligodendrocytes,[66,67] cells responsible for maintaining the functional integrity of axons and dendrites in the CNS. Therefore, abnormal gene expression in glial cells may be linked to white mater fiber loss and synaptic disconnection in AD. Recently, we demonstrated altered NOS-III expression in vascular smooth muscle and endothelial cells of small and medium size cerebral vessels in AD. In AD and AD+CVD, the leptomeningeal, cortical, and white matter vessels exhibited reduced NOS-III mRNA and protein expression. In contrast, control brains had readily detected NOS-III expression in vascular smooth muscle and endothelial cells throughout the tissue sections. Together, these studies indicate that aberrant NOS-III expression is a feature of several different cell types and therefore could impair a number of distinct CNS functions in AD. Constitutively low levels of NOS-III expression and NO production could result in cerebral hypoperfusion due to reduced vascular smooth muscle relaxation and attendant impairment of vasodilation responses, and diminished capacity to remove extracellular toxins and waste products of respiration due to reduced vascular permeability. Both processes could lead to ischemic injury, leukoaraiosis, and rarefaction of white matter secondary to incomplete infarction in AD+CVD.

ABERRANT NOS-III EXPRESSION AND p53-ASSOCIATED NEURONAL AND GLIAL CELL APOPTOSIS IN AD

Double-labeling studies were used to colocalize NOS-III and p53 (nuclear) to assess the role of NOS-III expression in p53-mediated apoptosis in AD. In control brains, NOS-III was seldom colocalized with p53 due to the infrequent cellular labeling with the p53 antibody. In AD, increased nuclear p53 immunoreactivity was observed in neurons that either had strikingly increased or else, no detectable NOS-III immunoreactivity. In contrast, high levels of NOS-III in glial cells were frequently colocalized with p53, whereas glial cells with no detectable NOS-III expression (similar to control) were also p53-negative. The p53-immunoreactive glial cells were abundantly distributed in the cerebral cortex and deep cerebral white matter. With respect to the vasculature, reduced NOS-III expression in cerebrovascular cells was frequently associated with increased nuclear p53 expression. In the leptomeninges, cerebral cortex, and deep white matter, NOS-III-negative/p53-positive vascular smooth muscle and endothelial cells were detected frequently. Therefore, high levels of NOS-III expression were associated with p53-mediated apoptosis proneness in some neurons and most glial cells, whereas low levels of NOS-III expression in cerebral vessels were correlated p53-mediated apoptosis in AD+CVD. These results are consistent with the known diametrically opposing actions of NO since in some cell populations, high levels of NO mediate cell survival and optimum function, whereas in others, NO can be cytotoxic and cause apoptosis. Since NO is an important mediator of vascular smooth muscle responsiveness and vascular permeability, the strikingly reduced levels of cerebrovascular NOS-III expression could represent an important mechanism of cerebral hypoperfusion and impaired homeostasis of the extracellular fluid environment in AD. Accumulation of toxin could lead to degeneration of axons and dendrites, and impaired function of both neurons and glial cells.

MECHANISMS OF NITRIC OXIDE-INDUCED FUNCTIONAL MODULATION OF VASCULAR SMOOTH MUSCLE AND ENDOTHELIAL CELLS

Nitric oxide causes relaxation of vascular smooth muscle cells and vasodilation leading to increased blood flow. Transgenic mice depleted of the NOS-III gene, although relatively spared of the excitotoxic effects of high levels of NO in the perifocal zone,[41] exhibit increased intracerebral hemorrhage, suggesting that global inhibition of NOS-III would not be an acceptable therapeutic strategy. However, some of the downstream signaling pathways may be cell type specific and therefore provide more realistic and safer targets for intervention. The vascular smooth muscle responses to NO are mediated through activation of soluble guanylate cyclase and attendant increased levels of cyclic guanosine monophosphate (cGMP). Downstream signaling involves activation of cGMP-dependent protein kinases,[68] and probably phospholipase C and nuclear factor-κB (NFκB).[69–71] A number of vasoactive molecules such as Relaxin peptide hormone cause vasodilation by activating NOS catalytic activity and increasing local levels of NO and cGMP. Vasodilatation is associated with a change in smooth muscle cell shape due to reorganization of the actin cytoskeleton.

NOS-induced vasodilatation and neurotransmission are regulated in part by phosphodiesterases (PDEs). PDEs catalyze the hydrolysis of 3'-5'-cyclic nucleotides to nucleoside 5'-monophosphates. There are at least 10 different isoforms of PDE, each with different specificities with regard to cell type, substrate, kinetics, regulatory properties, immunologic properties, and response to antagonists. For example, PDE2 and PDE4 regulate degradation of cyclic adenosine-5',3'-monophosphate (cAMP) such that increased expression results in inhibition of NOS catalytic activity, and specific inhibitors of these PDE isoforms lead to increased levels of cAMP, NOS phosphorylation via cAMP-dependent protein kinase, inhibition of NOS catalytic activity, and reduced levels of NO production. In contrast, PDE3 and PDE5 inhibit cGMP and thereby reduce the effects of NO-activated guanylate cyclase and lower the levels of cGMP-dependent protein kinase activity. Inhibitors of PDE3 and PDE5 enhance the actions of NO and NOS. Within this loop there is considerable cross talk in that cGMP can both inhibit PDE3 and stimulate PDE2 to potentiate the actions of NO.

Another important action of NO is to regulate permeability of endothelial cells. Endothelial cells express PDE2, -3, and -4 and cGMP. Activation of adenylate cyclase or inhibition of PDE blocks hyperpermeability of vessels exposed to H_2O_2. The mechanism involves NO activation of cGMP in endothelial cells.[72] Similarly, treatment with inhibitors of NOS exacerbate H_2O_2-induced vascular hyperpermeability. Vascular endothelial growth factor (VEGF)-induced hyperpermeability of coronary venules is inhibited by inhibitors of NOS, and antagonists of phospholipase C (PLC) or protein kinase C.[71] Phospholipase C activates NOS and guanylate cyclase, leading to increased levels of cGMP and cGMP-dependent protein kinase. Histamine-induced venular hyperpermeability to macromolecules such as albumin is also mediated through the PLC-NOS-guanylate cyclase cascade,[73] and correspondingly, inhibition of NOS or guanylate cyclase blocks histamine-induced hyperpermeability.

In the rat brain, the cGMP generating enzyme, guanylate cyclase is expressed in glial cells and pericytes surrounding cerebral vessels, and NOS-III enzyme is localized in endothelium and neurites innervating larger brain vessels.[74] Therefore, NO-induced cGMP and cGMP-dependent protein kinase signaling may help regulate cerebral perfusion, maintenance of blood-brain barrier integrity, and vascular permeability. However, the same signaling pathways may mediate neuronal and glial cell apoptosis and cerebrovascular degeneration in the context of constitutively increased expression of NOS-III or high levels of NO production. Therefore, expression and activity of specific PDEs may have a critical role in modulating NO-induced apoptosis in a number of cell types within the CNS.

Previous studies demonstrated PDE modulation of pulmonary vascular responses to NO,[75] indicating that the adverse effects of aberrantly increased NOS-III expression may be abrogated by increasing PDE activity. Correspondingly, reduced PDE expression and enzyme activity could lead to increased apoptosis in cells that have normal levels of NOS-III enzyme activity, since some of the actions of NO are mediated through cGMP and cGMP-dependent protein kinase. Inhibition of PDE increases cGMP levels, and cGMP can directly signal downstream pathways involved in NO-induced apoptosis through activation of cGMP-dependent protein kinase.[76] Current efforts are focused on analyzing the expression of guanylate cyclase, cGMP-dependent protein kinase, and various isoforms of PDE in relation to AD, AD+CVD, and normal aging. The expectation is that apoptosis and degeneration of cells will be dictated by both the intactness of endogenous regulatory responses to NO and capacity of cells to divert excess NO production away from pathways that lead to formation of potent free-radical oxidants such as peroxynitrite.

REFERENCES

1. CRYSTAL, H.A., D.W. DICKSON, M.J. SLIWINSKI, R.B. LIPTON, E. GROBER, N.H. MARKS & P. ANTIS. 1993. Pathological markers associated with normal aging and dementia in the elderly. Ann. Neurol. **34:** 566–573.
2. DICKSON, D.W., P. DAVIES, C. BEVONA, H.K. VAN, S.M. FACTOR, E. GROBER, M.K. ARONSON & H.A. CRYSTAL. 1994. Hippocampal sclerosis: a common pathological feature of dementia in very old (> or = 80 years of age) humans. Acta Neuropathol. (Berl.) **88:** 212–221.
3. FRISONI, G.B., A. BELTRAMELLO, G. BINETTI, A. BIANCHETTI, C. WEISS, A. SCURATTI & M. TRABUCCHI. 1995. Computed tomography in the detection of the vascular component in dementia. Gerontology **41:** 121–128.
4. DE LA TORRE, J. 1994. Impaired brain microcirculation may trigger Alzheimer's disease. Neurosci. Biobehav. Rev. **18:** 397–401.
5. INCE, P.G., F.K. MCARTHUR, E. BJERTNESS, A. TORVIK, J.M. CANDY & J.A. EDWARDSON. 1995. Neuropathological diagnoses in elderly patients in Oslo: Alzheimer's disease, Lewy body disease, vascular lesions. Dementia **6:** 162–168.
6. KAWAMURA, J., J.S. MEYER, Y. TERAYAMA & S. WEATHERS. 1992. Leuko-araiosis and cerebral hypoperfusion compared in elderly normals and Alzheimer's dementia. J. Am. Geriatr. Soc. **40:** 375–380.
7. NAGY, Z., M.M. ESIRI, K.A. JOBST, J.H. MORRIS, E.M. KING, B. MCDONALD, C. JOACHIM, S. LITCHFIELD, L. BARNETSON & A.D. SMITH. 1997. The effects of additional pathology on the cognitive deficit in Alzheimer disease. J. Neuropathol. Exp. Neurol. **56:** 165–170.
8. PASQUIER, F. & D. LEYS. 1997. Why are stroke patients prone to develop dementia? J. Neurol. **244:** 135–142.
9. SNOWDON, D.A., L.H. GREINER, J.A. MORTIMER, K.P. RILEY, P.A. GREINER & W.R. MARKESBERY. 1997. Brain infarction and the clinical expression of Alzheimer disease. The Nun Study [see comments]. JAMA **277:** 813–817.
10. VICTOROFF, J., W.J. MACK, S.A. LYNESS & H.C. CHUI. 1995. Multicenter clinicopathological correlation in dementia. Am. J. Psychiatry **152:** 1476–1484.
11. ZAHNER, B., C.J. LANG, A. ENGELHARDT, P. THIERAUF & B. NEUNDORFER. 1995. A case of Alzheimer's disease with extensive focal white matter changes. Dementia **6:** 294–300.
12. ETIENE, D., J. KRAFT, N. GANJU, T. GOMEZ-ISLA, B. GEMELLI, B.T. HYMAN, E.T. HEDLEY-WHYTE, J.R. WANDS & S.M. DE LA MONTE. 1998. Cerebrovascular pathology contributes to the heterogeneity of Alzheimer's disease. J. Alzheimer Dis. **1:** 48–56.
13. TOMIMOTO, H., I. AKIGUCHI, T. SUENAGA, M. NISHIMURA, H. WAKITA, S. NAKAMURA & J. KIMURA. 1996. Alterations of the blood-brain barrier and glial cells in white-matter lesions in cerebrovascular and Alzheimer's disease patients [see comments]. Stroke **27:** 2069–2074.
14. TOMIMOTO, H., I. AKIGUCHI, H. WAKITA, T. SUENAGA, S. NAKAMURA & J. KIMURA. 1997. Regressive changes of astroglia in white matter lesions in cerebrovascular disease and Alzheimer's disease patients. Acta Neuropathol. (Berl.). **94:** 146–152.

15. LOPEZ, O.L., B.S. RABIN, F.J. HUFF, D. REZEK & O.M. REINMUTH. 1992. Serum autoantibodies in patients with Alzheimer's disease and vascular dementia and in nondemented control subjects. Stroke **23:** 1078–1083.

16. NAGATA, K., R.J. BUCHAN, E. YOKOYAMA, Y. KONDOH, M. SATO, H. TERASHI, Y. SATOH, Y. WATAHIKI, M. SENOVA, Y. HIRATA & J. HATAZAWA. 1997. Misery perfusion with preserved vascular reactivity in Alzheimer's disease. Ann. N.Y. Acad. Sci. **826:** 272–281.

17. TOHGI, H., H. YONEZAWA, S. TAKAHASHI, N. SATO, E. KATO, M. KUDO, K. HATANO & T. SASAKI. 1998. Cerebral blood flow and oxygen metabolism in senile dementia of Alzheimer's type and vascular dementia with deep white matter changes. Neuroradiology **40:** 131–137.

18. OLICHNEY, J.M., L.A. HANSEN, C.R. HOFSTETTER, M. GRUNDMAN, R. KATZMAN & L.J. THAL. 1995. Cerebral infarction in Alzheimer's disease is associated with severe amyloid angiopathy and hypertension. Arch. Neurol. **52:** 702–708.

19. VAN NOSTRAND, W.E., S.J. DAVIS & I.S. SAPORITO. 1996. Amyloid beta-protein induces the cerebrovascular cellular pathology of Alzheimer's disease and related disorders. Ann. N.Y. Acad. Sci. **777:** 297–302.

20. THOMAS, T., G. THOMAS, C. MCLENDON, T. SUTTON & M. MULLAN. 1996. beta-Amyloid-mediated vasoactivity and vascular endothelial damage [see comments]. Nature **380:** 168–171.

21. THOMAS, T., E.T. SUTTON, M.W. BRYANT & J.A. RHODIN. 1997. *In vivo* vascular damage, leukocyte activation and inflammatory response induced by beta-amyloid. J. Submicrosc. Cytol. Pathol. **29:** 293–304.

22. HAASE, J., P. HALAMA & R. HORR. 1996. [Effectiveness of brief infusions with *Ginkgo biloba* special extract EGb 761 in dementia of the vascular and Alzheimer type]. Z. Gerontol. Geriatr. **29:** 302–309.

23. HORR, R. & M. KIESER. 1998. [*Ginkgo biloba* special extract EGb 761—an anti-dementia drug]. Fortschr. Med. **116:** 39–40.

24. KANOWSKI, S., W.M. HERRMANN, K. STEPHAN, W. WIERICH & R. HORR. 1996. Proof of efficacy of the *Ginkgo biloba* special extract EGb 761 in outpatients suffering from mild to moderate primary degenerative dementia of the Alzheimer type or multi-infarct dementia. Pharmacopsychiatry **29:** 47–56.

25. LE BARS, P.L., M.M. KATZ, N. BERMAN, T.M. ITIL, A.M. FREEDMAN & A.F. SCHATZBERG. 1997. A placebo-controlled, double-blind, randomized trial of an extract of *Ginkgo biloba* for dementia. North American EGb Study Group [see comments]. JAMA **278:** 1327–1332.

26. SCHMIDT, H. & U. WALTER. 1994. NO at work. Cell **78:** 919–925.

27. BREDT, D. & S. SNYDER. 1994. Transient nitric oxide synthase neurons in embryonic cerebral cortical plate, sensory ganglia, and olfactory epithelium. Neuron **13:** 301–313.

28. KLATT, P., K. SCHMIDT, G. URAY & B. MAYER. 1993. Multiple catalytic functions of brain nitric oxide synthase. Biochemical characterization, cofactor requirement, and the role of Nw-hydroxy-L-arginine as an intermediate. J. Biol. Chem. **268:** 14781–14787.

29. DINERMAN, J., T. DAWSON, M. SCHELL, A. SNOWMAN & S. SNYDER. 1994. Endothelial nitric oxide synthase localized to hippocampal pyramidal cells: implications for synaptic plasticity. Proc. Natl. Acad. Sci. USA **91:** 4214–4218.

30. BOJE, K. & P. ARORA. 1992. Microglial-produced nitric oxide and reactive nitrogen oxides mediate neuronal cell death. Brain Res. **587:** 250–256.

31. KOPROWSKI, H., Y. ZHENG, E. HEBER-KATZ, N. FRASER, L. RORKE, A. FU, C. HANLON & B. DIETZXCHOLD. 1993. *In vivo* expression of inducible nitric oxide synthase in experimentally induced neurologic diseases. Proc. Natl. Acad. Sci. USA **90:** 3024–3027.

32. MERRILL, J., L. IGNARRO, M. SHERMAN, J. MELINEK & T. LANE. 1993. Microglial cell cytotoxicity of oligodendrocytes is mediated through nitric oxide. J. Immunol. **151:** 2132–2141.

33. VODOVOTZ, Y., M. LUCIA, K. FLANDERS, L. CHESTER, Q. XIE, T. SMITH, J. WEIDNER, R. MUMFORD, R. WEBBER, C. NATHAN, A. ROBERTS, C. LIPPA & M. SPORN. 1996. Inducible nitric oxide synthase in tangle-bearing neurons of patients with Alzheimer's disease. J. Exp. Med. **184:** 1425–1433.

34. XIA, Y., V. DAWSON, T. DAWSON, S. SNYDER & J. ZWEIER. 1996. Nitric oxide synthase generates superoxide and nitric oxide in arginine-depleted cells leading to peroxynitrite-mediated cellular injury. Proc. Natl. Acad. Sci. USA **93:** 6770–6774.

35. LIPTON, S., Y. CHOI, Z. PAN, S. LEIN, H. CHEN, N. SUCHER, J. LOSCALZO, D. SINGLE & J. STAMLER. 1993. A redox-based mechanism for the neuroprotective and neurodestructive effects of nitric oxide and related nitroso-compounds. Nature **364:** 626–632.

36. LEIST, M., E. FAVA, C. MONTECUCCO & P. NICOTERA. 1997. Peroxynitrite and nitric oxide donors induce neuronal apoptosis by eliciting autocrine excitotoxicity. Eur. J. Neurosci. **9:** 1488–1498.

37. STAMLER, J. 1994. Nitration and related target interactions of nitric oxide [review]. Cell **78:** 931–936.

38. POU, S., W. POU, D. BREDT, S. SNYDER & G. ROSEN. 1992. Generation of superoxide by purified brain nitric oxide synthase. J. Biol. Chem. **267:** 24173–24176.

39. CULCASI, M., M. LAFON-CAZAL, S. PIETRI & J. BOCKAERT. 1994. Glutamate receptors induce a burst of superoxide via activation of nitric oxide synthase in arginine-depleted neurons. J. Biol. Chem. **269:** 12589–12593.

40. WOLF, G., G. HENSCHKE & S. WURDIG. 1993. Glutamate agonist-induced hippocampal lesion and nitric oxide synthase/NADPH-diaphorase: a light and electron microscopical study in the rat. Neurosci. Lett. **161:** 49–52.

41. HUANG, A., P. HUANG, N. PANAHIAN, T. DALKARA, M. FISHMAN & M. MOSKOWITZ. 1994. Effects of cerebral ischemia in mice deficient in neuronal nitric oxide synthase. Science **265:** 1883–1885.

42. NORRIS, P., H. WALDVOGEL, R. FAULL, D. LOVE & P. EMSON. 1996. Decreased neuronal nitric oxide synthase messenger RNA and somatostatin messenger RNA in the striatum of Huntington's disease. Neuroscience **72:** 1037–1047.

43. OURY, T., C. PIANTADOSI & J. CRAPO. 1993. Cold-induced brain edema in mice: involvement of extracellular superoxide dismutase and nitric oxide. J. Biol. Chem. **268:** 15394–15398.

44. ZHENG, Y., M.-H. SCHAFER, E. WEIHE, H. SHENG, S. CORISEDO, Z. FU, H. KOPROWSKI & B. DIETZSCHOLD. 1993. Severity of neurological signs and degree of inflammatory lesions in the brains of rats with Borna disease correlated with induction of nitric oxide synthase. J. Virol. **67:** 5786–5791.

45. HOOPER, D., O. BAGASRA, J. MARINI, A. ZBOREK, S. OHNISHI, R. KEAN, J. CHAMPION, A. SARKER, L. BOBROSKI, J. FARBERT, T. AKAIKE, H. MAEDA & H. KOPROWSKI. 1997. Prevention of experimental allergic encephalomyelitis by targeting nitric oxide and peroxynitrite: implications for the treatment of multiple sclerosis. Proc. Natl. Acad. Sci. USA **94:** 2528–2533.

46. WU, W., F. LIUZZI, F. SCHINCO, A. DEPTO, Y. LI, J. MONG, T. DAWSON & S. SNYDER. 1994. Neuronal nitric oxide synthase is induced in spinal neurons by traumatic injury. Neuroscience **61:** 719–726.

47. HESS, D., S. PATTERSON, D. SMITH & J. SKENE. 1994. Neuronal growth cone collapse and inhibition of protein fatty acylation by nitric oxide. Nature **366:** 562–565.

48. MESENGE, C., C. VERRECCHIA, M. ALLIX, R. BOULU & M. PLOTKINE. 1996. Reduction of the neurological deficit in mice with traumatic brain injury by nitric oxide synthase inhibitors. J. Neurotrauma **13:** 11–16.

49. NISHIKAWA, T., J. KIRSCH, R. KOEHLER, D. BREDT, S. SNYDER & R. TRAYSTMANN. 1993. Effect of nitric oxide synthase inhibition on cerebral blood flow and injury volume during focal ischemia in cats. Stroke **24:** 1717–1724.

50. GRISCAVAGE, J., J. FUKUTO, Y. KOMORI & L. IGNARRO. 1994. Nitric oxide inhibits neuronal nitric oxide synthase by interacting with the heme prosthetic group. Role of tetrahydrobiopterin in modulating the inhibitory action of nitric oxide. J. Biol. Chem. **269:** 21644–21649.

51. OSGAWA, N. 1994. Free radicals and neural cell damage. Rinsho Shinkeigaku **34:** 1266–1268.

52. NOVIKOV, L., L. NOVIKOVA & J. KELLERTH. 1995. Brain-derived neurotrophic factor promotes survival and blocks nitric oxide synthase experession in adult rat spinal motoneurons after ventral root avulsion. Neurosci. Lett. **200:** 45–48.

53. LI, L., W. WU, L. LIN, M. LEI, R. OPPENHEIM & L. HOUENOU. 1995. Rescue of adult mouse motoneurons from injury-induced cell death by glial cell line-derived neurotrophic factor. Proc. Natl. Acad. Sci. USA **92:** 9771–9775.

54. DAWSON, V., V. KIZUSHI, P. HUANG, S. SNYDER & T. DAWSON. 1996. Resistance to neurotoxicity in cortical cultures from neuronal nitric oxide synthase-deficient mice. J. Neurosci. **16:** 2479–2487.

55. FERRIERO, D., D. HOLTZMAN, S. BLACK & R. SHELDON. 1996. Neonatal mice lacking neuronal nitric oxide synthase are less vulnerable to hypoxic-ischemic injury. Neurobiol. Dis. **3:** 64–71.

56. NOWICKY, A. & L. BINDMAN. 1993. The nitric oxide synthase inhibitor, N-monomethyl-L-arginine blocks induction of a long-term potentiation-like phenomenon in rat medial frontal cortical neurons *in vitro*. J. Neurophysiol. **70:** 1255–1259.

57. PEUNOVA, N. & G. ENIKOLOPOV. 1995. Nitric oxide triggers a switch to growth arrest during differentiation of neuronal cells. Nature **375:** 68–73.

58. FARINELLI, S., D. PARK & L. GREENE. 1996. Nitric oxide delays the death of trophic factor-deprived PC12 cells and sympathetic neurons by a cGMP-mediated mechanism. J. Neurosci. **16:** 2325–2334.

59. WARD, S., C. SHUTTLEWORTH & J. KENYON. 1994. Dorsal root ganglion neurons of embryonic chicks contain nitric oxide synthase and respond to nitric oxide. Brain Res. **648:** 249–258.

60. YEZIERSKI, R., S. LIU, G. RUENES, R. BUSTO & W. DIETRICH. 1996. Neuronal damage following intraspinal injection of a nitric oxide synthase inhibitor in the rat. J. Cereb. Blood Flow Metab. **16:** 996–1004.

61. DE LA MONTE, S.M., Y.K. SOHN, N. GANJU & J.R. WANDS. 1998. p53- and CD95-associated apoptosis in neurodegenerative diseases. Lab. Invest. **158:** 1001–1009.

62. DE LA MONTE, S.M., Y.K. SOHN & J.R. WANDS. 1997. Correlates of p53- and Fas (CD95)-mediated apoptosis in Alzheimer's disease. J. Neurol. Sci. **152:** 73–83.

63. SU, J.H., G. DENG & C.W. COTMAN. 1997. Bax protein expression is increased in Alzheimer's brain: correlations with DNA damage, Bcl-2 expression, and brain pathology. J. Neuropathol. Exp. Neurol. **56:** 86–93.

64. SOHN, Y.K., N. GANJU, K.D. BLOCH, J.R. WANDS & S.M. DE LA MONTE. 1999. Neuritic sprouting with aberrant expression of the nitric oxide synthase III gene in neurodegenerative diseases. J. Neurol. Sci. **162:** 133–151.

65. DE LA MONTE, S. & K. BLOCH. 1997. Aberrant expression of the constitutive endothelial nitric oxide synthase gene in Alzheimer's disease. Mol. Chem. Neuropathol. **30:** 139–159.

66. NOBLE, M. 1994. The O-2A lineage: from rats to humans. Recent Res. Cancer Res. **145:** 67–75.

67. RAFF, M., E. ABNEY, J. COHEN, R. LINDSAY & M. NOBLE. 1983. Two types of astrocytes in cultures of developing rat white matter: differences in morphology, surface gangliosides, and growth characteristics. J. Neurosci. **3:** 1289–1300.

68. KOCH, K., H. LAMBRECHT, M. HABERECHT, D. REDBURN & H. SCHMIDT. 1994. Functional coupling of a Ca^{2+}/calmodulin dependent nitric oxide synthase and a soluble guanylyl cyclase in vertebrate photoreceptor cells. EMBO J. **13:** 3312–3320.

69. BANI, D., P. FAILLI, M.G. BELLO, C. THIEMERMANN, T. BANI SACCHI, M. BIGAZZI & E. MASINI. 1998. Relaxin activates the L-arginine-nitric oxide pathway in vascular smooth muscle cells in culture. Hypertension **31:** 1240–1247.

70. BERK, B.C., M.A. CORSON, T.E. PETERSON & H. TSENG. 1995. Protein kinases as mediators of fluid shear stress stimulated signal transduction in endothelial cells: a hypothesis for calcium-dependent and calcium-independent events activated by flow. J. Biomech. **28:** 1439–1450.

71. WU, H.M., Y. YUAN, D.C. ZAWIEJA, J. TINSLEY & H.J. GRANGER. 1999. Role of phospholipase C, protein kinase C, and calcium in VEGF-induced venular hyperpermeability. Am. J. Physiol. **276:** H535–H542.

72. SUTTORP, N., S. HIPPENSTIEL, M. FUHRMANN, M. KRULL & T. PODZUWEIT. 1996. Role of nitric oxide and phosphodiesterase isoenzyme II for reduction of endothelial hyperpermeability. Am. J. Physiol. **270:** C778–785.

73. YUAN, Y., H.J. GRANGER, D.C. ZAWIEJA, D.V. DEFILY & W.M. CHILIAN. 1993. Histamine increases venular permeability via a phospholipase C-NO synthase-guanylate cyclase cascade. Am. J. Physiol. **264:** H1734–H1739.
74. POEGGEL, G., M. MULLER, I. SEIDEL, L. RECHARDT & H.G. BERNSTEIN. 1992. Histochemistry of guanylate cyclase, phosphodiesterase, and NADPH- diaphorase (nitric oxide synthase) in rat brain vasculature. J. Cardiovasc. Pharmacol. **20:** S76–S79.
75. SANCHEZ, L.S., S.M. DE LA MONTE, G. FILIPPOV, R.C. JONES, W.M. ZAPOL & K.D. BLOCH. 1998. Cyclic-GMP-binding, cyclic-GMP-specific phosphodiesterase (PDE5) gene expression is regulated during rat pulmonary development. Pediatr. Res. **43:** 163–168.
76. CHICHE, J.D., S.M. SCHLUTSMEYER, D.B. BLOCH, S.M. DE LA MONTE, J.D. ROBERTS, JR., G. FILIPPOV, S.P. JANSSENS, A. ROSENZWEIG & K.D. BLOCH. 1998. Adenovirus-mediated gene transfer of cGMP-dependent protein kinase increases the sensitivity of cultured vascular smooth muscle cells to the antiproliferative and pro-apoptotic effects of nitric oxide/cGMP. J. Biol. Chem. **273:** 34263–34271.

Similar Ultrastructural Breakdown of Cerebrocortical Capillaries in Alzheimer's Disease, Parkinson's Disease, and Experimental Hypertension

What is the Functional Link?

ESZTER FARKAS,[a,d] GINEKE I. DE JONG,[a] ETELKA APRÓ,[a] ROB A.I. DE VOS,[b] ERNST N.H. JANSEN STEUR,[c] AND PAUL G.M. LUITEN[a]

[a]Department of Animal Physiology, Graduate School of Behavioral and Cognitive Neurosciences, University of Groningen, Groningen, the Netherlands

Departments of [b]Pathology and [c]Neurology, Medisch Spectrum Twente, Enschede, the Netherlands

ABSTRACT: The brain, as an intensely active organ, is highly dependent on a sufficient nutrient and oxygen availability in order to reach its optimal working capacity. It is well known that the vital supply of energy substrates is provided by the circulatory system, which splits up into a fine, terminal capillary network in target tissues. These capillaries are considered as important sites, since the actual nutrient trafficking takes place through their walls. That is why an intact, preserved structure of the microvessels is crucial to fulfill their function. Since the brain is known to be particularly vulnerable to suboptimal oxygen and glucose delivery, the intact morphology of capillaries is of paramount importance.

Several observations have indicated that the cerebral capillary ultrastructure is damaged in Alzheimer's disease (AD). Curiously, the regional cerebral blood flow of AD patients is also significantly lower than in age-matched control individuals. Based on these data, it has been suggested that the decreased blood supply and the cerebrovascular alterations contribute to the development of dementia. However, we have observed similar capillary damage in Parkinson's disease patients and chronically hypertensive rats in addition to AD cases, as presented here. These findings indicate that cerebral capillary damage is not exclusive for AD but occurs under other neurodegenerative disorders and hypertension, as well. We hypothesize that ultrastructural abnormalities of cerebral capillaries are causally related to decreased cerebral blood flow and create a condition that favors neurodegenerative mechanisms including the development of dementia.

[d]Address for correspondence: Eszter Farkas, Department of Animal Physiology, University of Groningen, P.O.B. 14, 9750 AA Haren, the Netherlands. Tel.: +31-50-363-2363; fax: +31-50-363-5202.
e-mail: E.FARKAS@biol.rug.nl

INTRODUCTION

Cerebrovascular structural abnormalities have frequently been reported in demented patients diagnosed to have Alzheimer's disease (AD).[1–4] Capillary damage in AD brains consistently occurs in the form of capillary basement membrane thickening and collagen type IV accumulation, also known as fibrosis. These pathological alterations implicate several functional consequences: the thickening of the basement membrane can physically hinder nutrient transport to the neural tissue or the clearance of potentially toxic waste products from the brain, and may structurally affect the efficacy of important carrier systems of the blood-brain barrier. For example, a decreased density of glucose transporter sites supports the last assumption and suggests reduced glucose availability in the affected brain regions.[5–7] Hence, the imposed metabolic crisis may be reflected by data indicating decreased cerebral glucose uptake and oxygen utilization in Alzheimer brains.[8–10]

However, the observed cerebral capillary damage is not exclusive for AD. Similar ultrastructural alterations of the cerebral microvessel walls were described in aging and experimental cerebral hypoperfusion in rats.[11,12] Cerebral hypoperfusion has drawn major attention in AD research, too. Regional cerebral blood flow measured by single photon emission computed tomography (SPECT) in AD patients demonstrated significant decrease in the hippocampal formation and temporal cortex, regions first and most severely affected in the disease.[13–16] Interestingly, cerebral hypoperfusion was also found to coincide with hypertension due to possible high blood pressure-related lack of autoregulation of cerebral blood flow or atherosclerosis.[17,18] Supportive experimental evidence was obtained in spontaneously hypertensive rats where the observed reduced cerebral blood flow was reported to coincide with an additional tendency for poor learning skills.[19,20]

In the present study, we give an overview of the structural alterations of brain capillaries in neurodegenerative diseases and hypertensive rats and attempt to establish a comparison in the light of cerebral hypoperfusion.

CEREBROVASCULAR PATHOLOGY
IN NEURODEGENERATIVE DISEASES

The condition of cerebrocortical capillaries of AD and Parkinson's disease (PD) patients was investigated in postmortem samples from the cingulate cortex. The patients were selected based on neurological diagnosis and subsequent standard neuropathological characterization (Braak staging, Consortium to Establish a Registry for Alzheimer's Disease (CERAD) scale, Lewy body score, and substantia nigra pathology).[21–24] The PD cases were further differentiated based on the presence of neuropathological alterations characteristic of AD. Thus, four separate groups were established: an AD group ($n = 5$), a PD group without AD-like neuropathology ($n = 6$), a PD group with AD-like neuropathology (PDd, $n = 4$), and controls ($n = 5$).

The samples were processed for electron microscopic analysis: the tissue was imbedded in glycid ether and cut to ultrathin sections. The sections were mounted on copper grids and contrasted with 5% aqueous uranyl acetate and Reynolds lead solution. The analysis was performed with a Philips 200 electron microscope (EM).

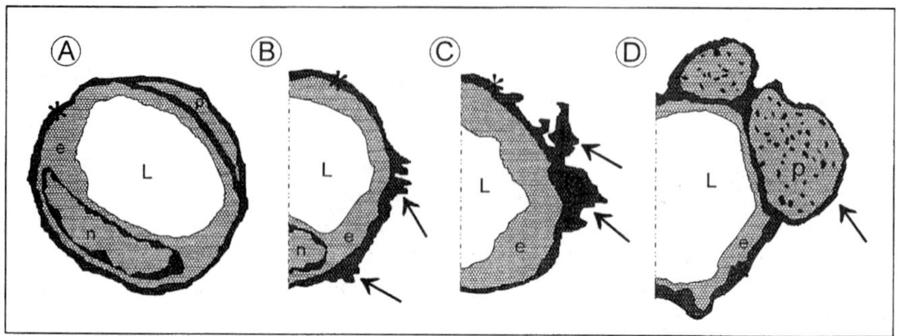

FIGURE 1. Schematic drawings demonstrating the ultrastructural abnormalities of cerebral capillaries. (**A**) An intact vessel; (**B**) basement membrane thickening (BMT); (**C**) collagen accumulation in the basement membrane (fibrosis); (**D**) degenerative pericyte. *, basement membrane; e, endothelial cell; L, capillary lumen; n, endothelial nucleus; p, pericyte.

We focused on deviations of the capillary walls and defined the following criteria. (1) When the basement membrane (BM) demonstrated local thickening exceeding double width compared to an intact BM segment of the same capillary, or showed duplications or branching, we considered the abnormality as basement membrane thickening (BMT) (FIG. 1B). (2) The appearance and accumulation of collagen fibers in the BM, occasionally invading the cytoplasm of an embraced pericyte, were taken to be fibrosis (FIG. 1C). (3) Membranous inclusion bodies and swollen pericytic profiles indicated pericytic degeneration (FIG. 1D). One hundred capillaries per case were screened, and the percentage of capillaries with any of the above-described abnormalities was calculated.

The data show that the percentage of microvessels with BMT and fibrosis has considerably increased in AD as well as in PD and PDd (FIG. 2). The occurrence of BMT was almost three times higher in the neurological diseases than in controls pointing to an obvious and remarkable increase of BMT (FIG. 2A). Similar tendency was observed in fibrosis, but the individual variance prevented statistical significance (FIG. 2B). In contrast, the percentage of capillaries with degenerating pericytes was found comparable in all groups (FIG. 2C) suggesting no specific involvement of pericytic degeneration in the pathology of AD or PD. Thus, the capillary wall, specifically the basement membrane, appears to be the major site of cerebrovascular damage in the investigated neurodegenerative disorders.

CEREBROVASCULAR PATHOLOGY IN HYPERTENSION

The effects of hypertension were investigated on the cerebral capillaries of the frontoparietal cortex of Wistar-Kyoto (WKY, $n = 6$) and spontaneously hypertensive stroke-prone rats (SHR-SP, $n = 6$). Blood pressure measurements were taken on the tail on every fourth week for a period of 20 weeks, starting when the animals were 40 weeks old. On the 60th week, the rats were perfused with 2% paraformaldehyde,

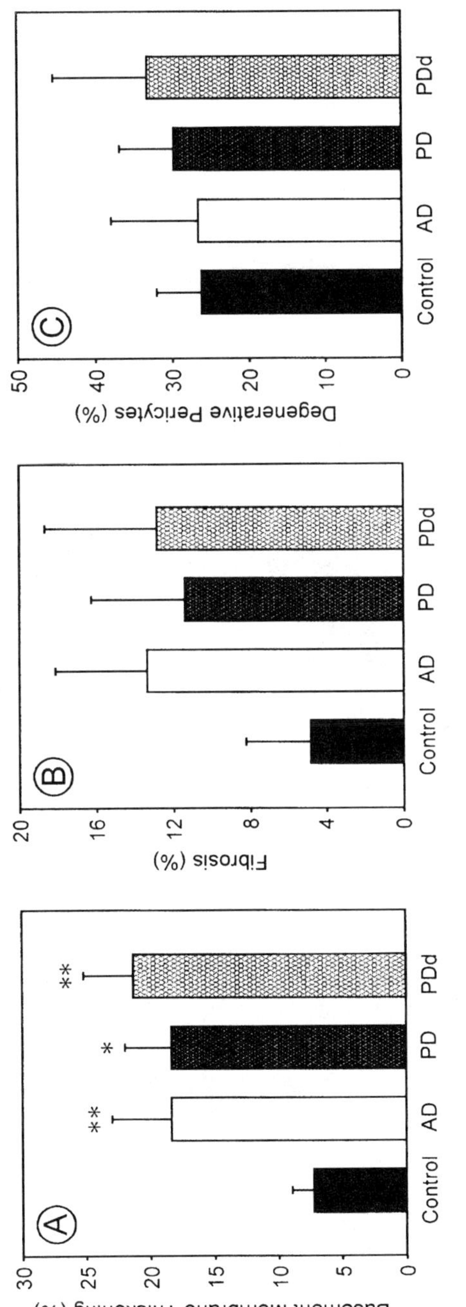

FIGURE 2. Cerebral capillary damage in Alzheimer's disease (AD) and Parkinson's disease with or without Alzheimer-like neuropathology (PDd and PD, respectively). (**A**) Percentage of capillaries with basement membrane thickening (BMT); (**B**) percentage of capillaries with fibrosis; (**C**) percentage of capillaries with degenerative pericytes. $*p < 0.05$, $**p < 0.02$.

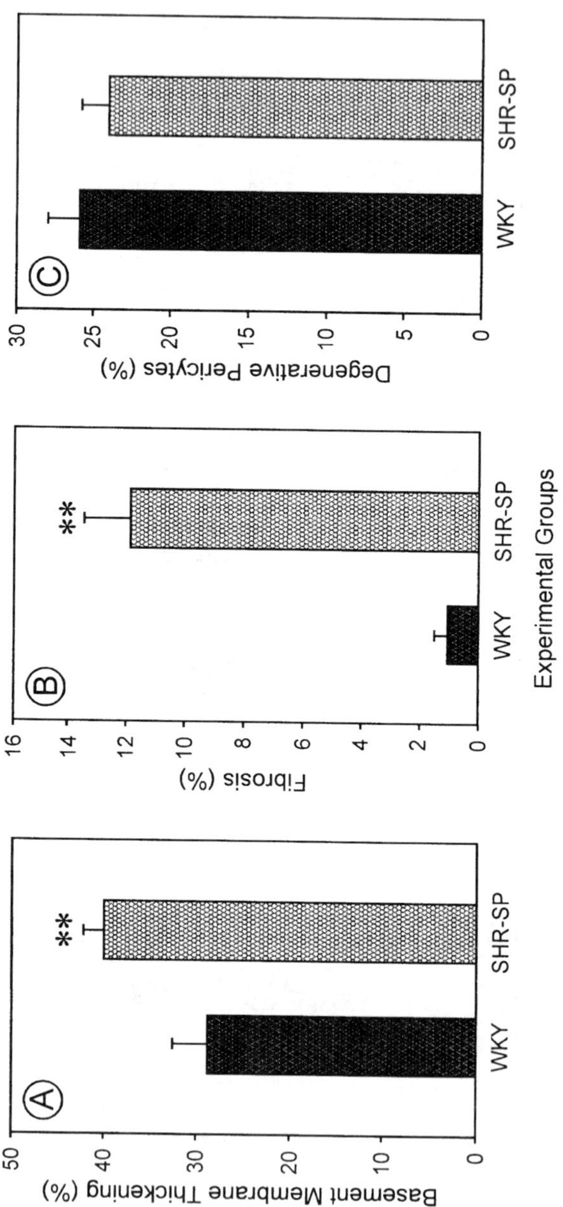

FIGURE 3. Cerebral capillary breakdown in spontaneously hypertensive rats at 60 weeks of age. (**A**) Percentage of capillaries with basement membrane thickening (BMT); (**B**) percentage of capillaries with fibrosis; (**C**) percentage of capillaries with degenerative pericytes. WKY, Wistar-Kyoto rats (control); SHR-SP, spontaneously hypertensive stroke-prone rats. *$p < 0.05$, **$p < 0.01$.

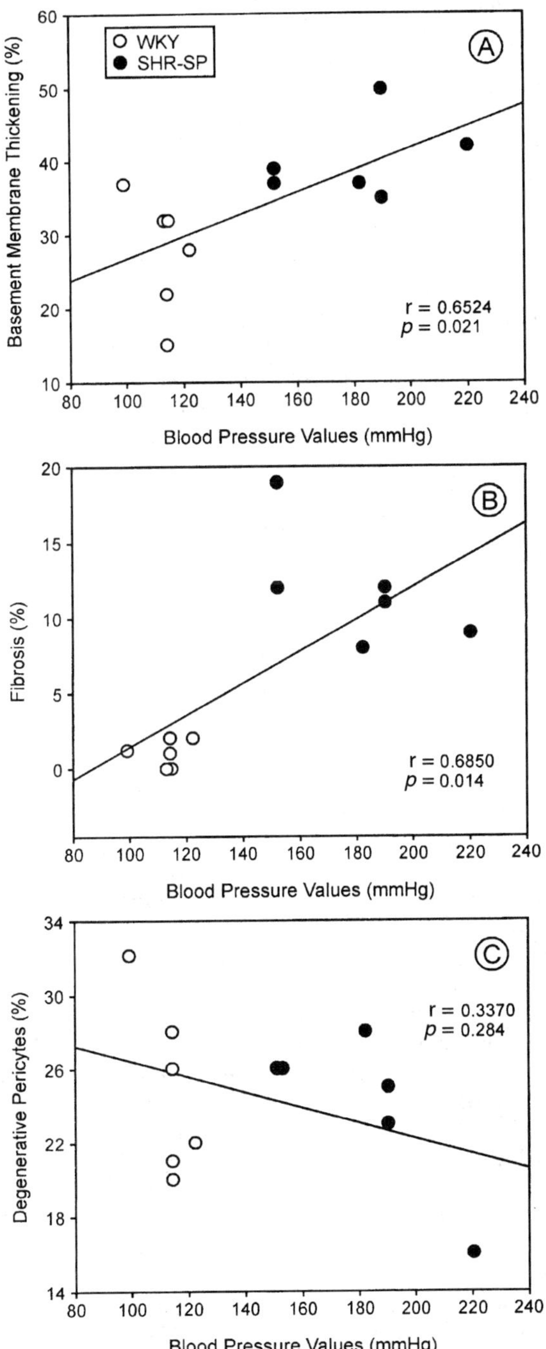

FIGURE 4. *Caption on following page.*

0.05% glutaraldehyde, and 0.2% picric acid in 0.1 M phosphate buffer. The brains were cut on a vibratome at 50 μm, and the slices were routinely embedded in glycid ether. Ultrathin sections were prepared of the frontoparietal cortex, mounted on 200 mesh copper grids, and contrasted for EM analysis.

For the examination of microvessels, we followed the guidelines described above for the human samples, thus, the same three categories of capillary abnormalities were established: basement membrane thickening (BMT), fibrosis, and degenerative pericytes. The percentage of capillaries with abnormal features was expressed as percentages of the total number of capillaries encountered.

The cortical capillaries of hypertensive animals suffered considerable damage. The frequency of BMT increased with 25% in the SHR-SP group (FIG. 3A), while the individual capillaries were endowed with more advanced forms of BMT compared to the alterations observed in the WKY group. Usually, larger segments of a particular capillary demonstrated clearly more pronounced alterations in the SHR-SP animals. Fibrosis, which was nearly absent in normotensive controls, increased remarkably in the hypertensive cases (FIG. 3B). At the same time, the condition of pericytes proved to be unaffected by high blood pressure (FIG. 3C). The occurrence of capillaries with BMT or fibrosis correlated with the blood pressure values taken before perfusion (FIG. 4A and 4B), whereas, pericytic degeneration showed no such relationship (FIG. 4C).

DISCUSSION

Here we have shown that neurological conditions such as AD and PD are accompanied by a progressive degeneration of cerebrocortical capillary wall ultrastructure in a similar manner. Furthermore, comparable microvessel damage was observed in the frontoparietal cortex of chronically hypertensive rats. FIGURE 5 demonstrates typical examples of these degenerative features.

The microanatomical capillary damage observed here and previously by others[1–4] coincides with alteration of additional, functional vascular factors in AD and possibly in PD. For example, clinical measurements of regional cerebral blood flow by the noninvasive SPECT method have indicated that AD is accompanied by a decreased regional cerebral blood flow in the hippocampal formation and temporal cortex.[13–16] This phenomenon was also described in the temporal cortex of PD patients,[25,26] but the data coming from different research groups is not uniform on this issue.[27] The theory that the vascular ultrastructural changes, like those described in the present study, and reduced cerebral blood flow are functionally related was tested in an animal model. Experimental cerebral hypoperfusion was created by a bilateral carotid artery occlusion (2VO),[12,28,29] which yields to 25–30% reduction of regional cerebral blood flow,[29] corresponding well with the values recorded in AD. Subsequently, the condition of hippocampal capillaries was examined, and a significant increase of BMT and fibrosis was found.[12] Therefore, we propose that hypo-

---

FIGURE 4. Correlation between blood pressure values and the different types of capillary damage. WKY, Wistar-Kyoto rats (control); SHR-SP, spontaneously hypertensive stroke-prone rats.

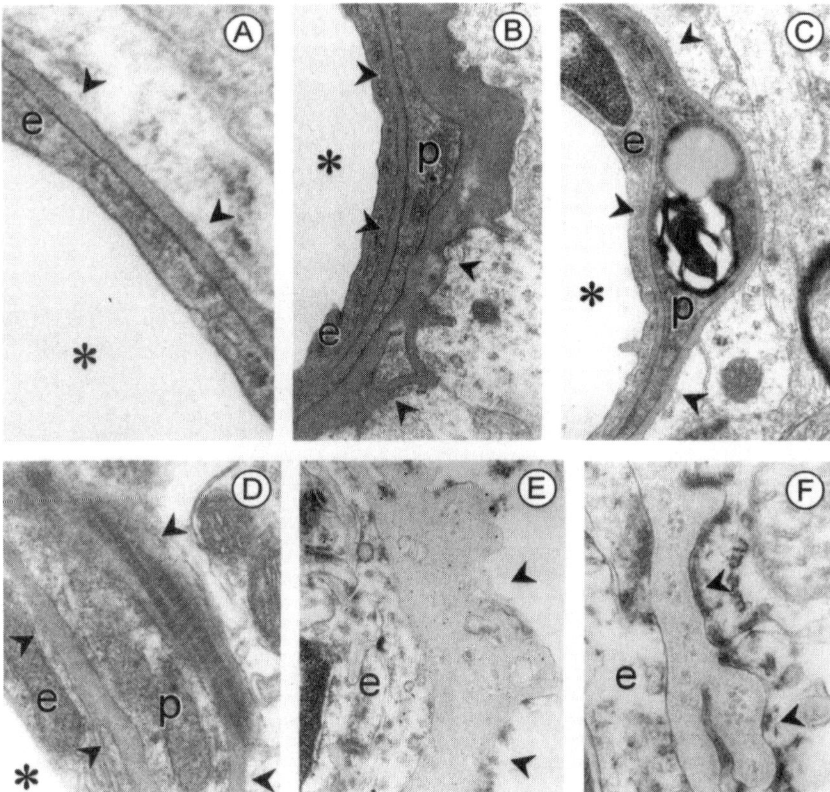

FIGURE 5. Computer images of electron microscopic photographs taken of cerebral capillaries in rat and human samples. **(A)** An intact capillary wall of a WKY rat; **(B)** basement membrane thickening (BMT) of an SHR-SP rat; **(C)** an early stage of pericytic degeneration of an SHR-SP rat; **(D)** longitudinal view of collagen bundles in the basement membrane of an SHR-SP rat; **(E)** BMT in an AD sample; **(F)** collagen fibers in cross section in the basement membrane of an AD patient. *, capillary lumen; e, endothelial cell; p, pericytic profile; *arrowheads*, basement membrane.

perfusion is a causal factor in the development of capillary alterations observed in the 2VO model, and possibly in AD and PD.

Reduced cerebral blood flow was also recorded in hypertensive patients by positron emission tomography (PET) and the ^{133}Xe-inhalation method.[17,18] In addition, parallel experiments revealed a comparable hypertension-induced cerebral hypoperfusion in spontaneously hypertensive rats.[19,20] Our own findings in the hypertensive animals show that the cerebral capillary wall is damaged in a similar fashion to hypoperfused rats, as well as to AD/PD patients: the basement membrane is thickened and contains collagen deposits. Fibrosis gives a considerable contribution to aberrations in the hypertensive animals, which is, nonetheless, more pronounced and uniform among cases than either in experimental hypoperfusion or the

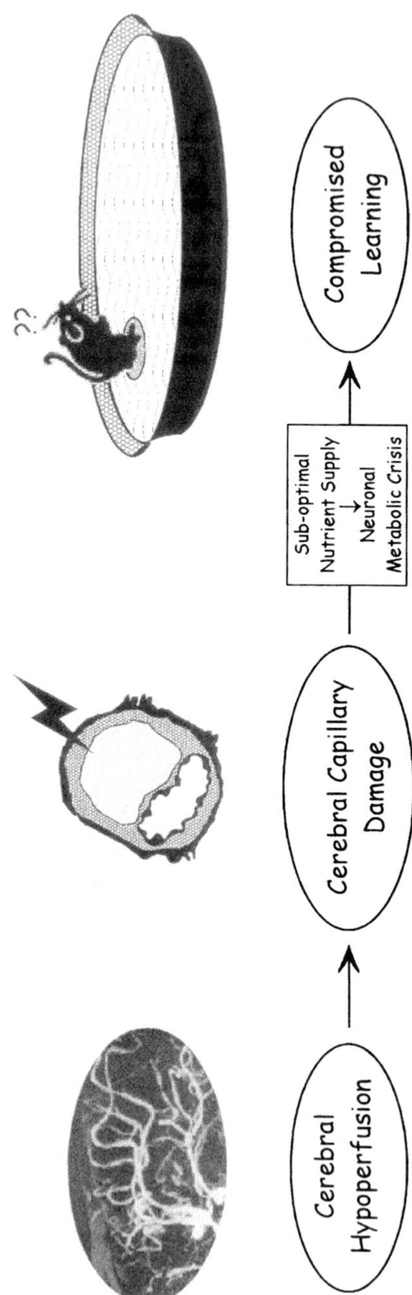

FIGURE 6. Causal events of cerebrovascular parameters leading to mild cognitive disorders.

here presented neurological diseases (AD or PD). At the same time, the increase in BMT appears higher in 2VO rats and AD/PD than in a hypertensive condition. We suggest that these differences emerge due to different stages and degree of cerebral hypoperfusion. BMT and fibrosis are thought to be in a functional relationship, and their relative ratio can change in the course of time as pointed out by De Jong *et al.* in aging rats.[11]

Our hypothesis that the same mechanisms are involved in the generation of capillary damage in the 2VO model of cerebral hypoperfusion, spontaneous hypertension in SHR-SP rats, and AD/PD finds support in the following behavioral data. Both 2VO rats and SHR-SP animals were independently tested in the Morris water maze and radial arm maze for their learning skills.[12,28–32] The experiments provided corresponding results in the sense that both the 2VO animals and the SHR-SP rats performed worse than their controls in the learning paradigms. By putting the findings into a sequential order, we may speculate that cerebral hypoperfusion gives rise to cerebrocapillary damage, which, in turn, is responsible for a mild decay of learning skills probably by preventing the optimal transport of sufficient nutrients to the neural tissue and subsequent neuronal dysfunction.

In conclusion, we propose that cerebral hypoperfusion is a mild but persistently prevailing condition shared by neurological disorders—AD or PD—and chronic hypertension, and that the constantly low flow rate triggers pathologic malformations of the cerebral capillary walls. This chain of degenerative events may be an underlying mechanism of mild memory deficits in chronic hypertension and PD, and probably contributes to a largely enhanced cognitive failure preestablished by numerous additional neuropathological factors in AD (FIG. 6).

REFERENCES

1. PERLMUTTER, L.S. & H.C. CHUI. 1990. Microangiopathy, the vascular basement membrane and Alzheimer's disease. Brain Res. Bull. **24:** 677–686.
2. CLAUDIO, L. 1996. Ultrastructural features of the blood-brain barrier in biopsy tissue from Alzheimer's disease patients. Acta Neuropathol. **91:** 6–14.
3. KALARIA, R.N. 1996. Cerebral vessels in aging and Alzheimer's disease. Pharmacol. Ther. **72**(3): 193–214.
4. BUÉE, L., P.R. HOF & A. DELACOURTE. 1997. Brain microvascular changes in Alzheimer's disease and other dementias. Ann. N.Y. Acad. Sci. **826:** 7–24.
5. HARIK, S.I. 1992. Changes in the glucose transporter of brain capillaries. Can. J. Physiol. Pharmacol. **70**(Suppl.): S113–S117.
6. HORWOOD, N. & D.C. DAVIES. 1994. Immunolabelling of hippocampal microvessel glucose transporter protein is reduced in Alzheimer's disease. Virchows Arch. **425**(1): 69–72.
7. MOORADIAN, A.D., H.C. CHUNG & G.N. SHAH. 1997. GLUT-1 expression in the cerebra of patients with Alzheimer's disease. Neurobiol. Aging **18**(5): 469–474.
8. RAPOPORT, S.I., B. HORWITZ, C.L. GRADY *et al.* 1991. Abnormal brain glucose metabolism in Alzheimer's disease, as measured by position emission tomography. Adv. Exp. Med. Biol. **291:** 231–248.
9. FUKUYAMA, H., M. OGAWA, H. YAMAUCHI *et al.* 1994. Altered cerebral energy metabolism in Alzheimer's disease: a PET study. J. Nucl. Med. **35**(1): 1–6.
10. BLESA, R., E. MOHR, R.S. MILETICH *et al.* 1996. Cerebral metabolic changes in Alzheimer's disease: neurobehavioral patterns. Dementia **7**(5): 239–245.
11. DE JONG, G.I., H. DE WEERD, T. SCHUURMAN *et al.* 1990. Microvascular changes in aged rat forebrain. Effects of chronic nimodipine treatment. Neurobiol. Aging **11**(4): 381–389.

12. DE JONG, G.I., E. FARKAS, C.M. STIENSTRA *et al.* 1999. Cerebral hypoperfusion yields capillary damage in hippocampus CA1 that correlated to spatial memory impairment. Neuroscience **91**(1): 203–210.
13. DEKOSKY, S.T., W.J. SHIH, F.A. SCHMITT *et al.* 1990. Assessing utility of single photon emission computed tomography (SPECT) scan in Alzheimer disease: correlation with cognitive severity. Alzheimer Dis. Assoc. Disord. **4**(1): 14–23.
14. EBERLING, J.L., W.J. JAGUST, B.R. REED & M.G. BAKER. 1992. Reduced temporal lobe blood flow in Alzheimer's disease. Neurobiol. Aging **13**: 483–491.
15. O'BRIEN, J.T., S. EAGGER, G.M. SYED *et al.* 1992. A study of regional cerebral blood flow and cognitive performance in Alzheimer's disease. J. Neurol. Neurosurg. Psychiatry **55**: 1182–1187.
16. OHNISHI, T., H. HOSHI, S. NAGAMACHI *et al.* 1995. High-resolution SPECT to assess hippocampal perfusion in neuropsychiatric diseases. J. Nucl. Med. **36**: 1163–1169.
17. NOBILI, F., G. RODRIGUEZ, S. MARENCO *et al.* 1993. Regional cerebral blood flow in chronic hypertension. A correlative study. Stroke **24**(8): 1148–1153.
18. NAKANE, H., S. IBAYASHI, K. FUJII *et al.* 1995. Cerebral blood flow and metabolism in hypertensive patients with cerebral infarction. Angiology **46**(9): 801–810.
19. FUJISHIMA, M., S. IBAYASHI, K. FUJII & S. MORI. 1995. Cerebral blood flow and brain function in hypertension. Hypertens. Res. **18**(2): 111–117.
20. KATSUTA, T. 1997. Decreased local cerebral blood flow in young and aged spontaneously hypertensive rats. Fukuoka Igaku Zasshi **88**(3): 65–74.
21. BRAAK, H. & E. BRAAK. 1991. Neuropathological stageing of Alzheimer-related changes. Acta Neuropathol. **82**: 239–259.
22. MIRRA, S.S., A. HEYMAN, D. MCKEEL *et al.* 1991. The consortium to establish a registry for Alzheimer's disease (CERAD). Part II. Standardization of the neuropathologic assessment of Alzheimer's disease. Neurology **41**: 479–486.
23. DE VOS, R.A.I., E.N. JANSEN, F.C. STAM *et al.* 1995. 'Lewy body disease': clinicopathological correlations in 18 consecutive cases of Parkinson's disease with and without dementia. Clin. Neurol. Neurosurg. **97**: 13–22.
24. MCKEITH, I.G., D. GALASKO, K. KOSAKA *et al.* 1996. Consensus guidelines for the clinical and pathologic diagnosis of dementia with Lewy bodies (DLB): Report of the consortium on DLB international workshop. Neurology **47**: 1113–1124.
25. KAWABATA, K., H. TACHIBANA & M. SUGITA. 1991. Cerebral blood flow and dementia in Parkinson's disease. J. Geriatr. Psychiatry Neurol. **4**(4): 194–203.
26. VARMA, A.R., P.R. TALBOT, J.S. SNOWDEN *et al.* 1997. A 99mTc-HMPAO single-photon emission computed tomography study of Lewy body disease. J. Neurol. **244**(6): 349–359.
27. BISSESSUR, S., G. TISSINGH, E.C. WOLTERS & P. SCHELTENS. 1997. rCBF SPECT in Parkinson's disease with mental dysfunction. J. Neural Transm. Suppl. **50**: 25–30.
28. DE LA TORRE, J.C., T. FORTIN, G.A. PARK *et al.* 1992. Chronic cerebrovascular insufficiency induces dementia-like deficits in aged rats. Brain Res. **582**: 186–195.
29. NI, J., H. OHTA, K. MATSUMOTO & H. WATANABE. 1994. Progressive cognitive impairment following chronic cerebral hypoperfusion induced by permanent occlusion of bilateral carotid arteries in rats. Brain Res. **653**: 231–236.
30. PAPPAS, B.A., J.C. DE LA TORRE, C.M. DAVIDSON *et al.* 1996. Chronic reduction of cerebral blood flow in the adult rat: late-emerging CA1 cell loss and memory dysfunction. Brain Res. **708**: 50–58.
31. WYSS, J.M., G. FISK & T. VAN GROEN. 1992. Impaired learning and memory in mature spontaneously hypertensive rats. Brain Res. **592**: 135–140.
32. OHTA, H., H. NISHIKAWA, H. KIMURA *et al.* 1997. Chronic cerebral hypoperfusion by permanent internal carotid ligation produces learning impairment without brain damage in rats. Neuroscience **79**(4): 1039–1050.

Distribution of Amyloid β_{42} in Relation to the Cerebral Microvasculature in an Elderly Cohort with Alzheimer's Disease

A.J. THOMAS,[a] C.M. MORRIS, I.N. FERRIER, AND R.N. KALARIA

Wolfson Research Centre, Institute for Health of the Elderly, Newcastle General Hospital, Newcastle upon Tyne NE4 6BE, United Kingdom

Department of Psychiatry, University of Newcastle, Newcastle upon Tyne NE4 6BE, United Kingdom

ABSTRACT: Amyloid β (Aβ) deposits and neurofibrillary pathology are characteristic features of Alzheimer's disease (AD). The association of Aβ with cerebral vessels is an intriguing feature of AD. While some degree of cerebral Aβ angiopathy involving the leptomeninges and intraparenchymal vessels occurs in almost all cases of AD, the proportion of microvessels within a neocortical region containing deposits of Aβ peptide is not known. In this study, we examined a cohort of clinically and pathologically evaluated AD cases to assess the percentage of cerebral microvessels in the temporal cortex and parahippocampal gyrus associated with the predominant, Aβ_{42} form of the peptide. We also assessed whether the distribution and burden of amyloid was related to apolipoprotein E (*APOE*) genotype. Using double immunostaining methods, we surprisingly found that at least 40% of the microvessels in the two brain regions contained Aβ_{42} deposits. There was no correlation of such localization with *APOE* genotype, however, $\varepsilon 4$ homozygotes revealed a greater burden of Aβ_{40}. These observations suggest that high proportions of cortical microvessels are associated with Aβ_{42}, which may affect microvascular function.

INTRODUCTION

The questions of origin and pattern of deposition of brain amyloid β (Aβ) have intrigued Alzheimer's disease (AD) researchers for a decade. Recent advances[1,2] have demonstrated the predominance of Aβ_{42}, the longer more pathogenic form of Aβ compared to the more soluble Aβ_{40}. Few previous studies have examined the exact relationship between Aβ deposition and the cerebral microvasculature. We have suggested that cerebral microvessels are closely associated with Aβ deposits in AD.[3,4] However, microvessels were most abundantly localized in and within a 10-μm circumference of the deposit, although the contact with the vessels could not be discounted to be by chance alone.[4] Aβ deposits rather than neurofibrillary tangles or remaining neurons were also associated with degenerated cerebral microvessels.[5,6] Miyakawa and colleagues[7,8] have emphasized and elegantly demonstrated by elec-

[a]Address for correspondence: Dr. Alan J. Thomas, Wolfson Research Centre, Institute for Health of Elderly, Newcastle General Hospital, Westgate Road, Newcastle upon Tyne NE4 6BE, UK. Tel.: (0191) 273 8811; fax: (0191) 272-5291.
e-mail: a.j.thomas@ncl.ac.uk

tron microscopy that both intact and degenerated microvessels are associated with Aβ deposits. Contact of aggregated Aβ with vascular elements or cerebral Aβ angiopathy may also be detrimental to cerebrovascular function.[9–12]

In this study, we examined the distribution of $A\beta_{42}$ containing cerebral microvessels in the temporal cortex and parahippocampal gyrus of AD patients from a cohort of elderly Norwegians. This cohort has been prospectively assessed and diagnosed for AD using the CERAD criteria.[13] In a previous study on this cohort, Morris *et al.*[14] had demonstrated significant densities of senile plaques and abundant neurofibrillary pathology, though up to 20% of the cases also showed Lewy bodies and cerebral infarctions.[13] We selected all individuals in this cohort who met the CERAD criteria for probable or definite AD and from whom tissue was available in the relevant areas. We also determined whether there were regional differences between forms of Aβ deposited in cerebral vessels and whether this was correlated apolipoprotein E (*APOE*) genotype.

MATERIALS AND METHODS

Brain tissue was obtained from elderly Norwegian patients who met CERAD diagnostic criteria for probable or definite AD.[13] We selected to study the temporal cortex and the parahippocampal gyrus from 50 individuals. The mean age of the patients was 85.74 (± 0.87). There were 14 men and 36 women. The *APOE* genotype of each individual in this cohort was also determined.[14]

Immunocytochemical localization of selected antigens in paraffin embedded tissue sections was carried out essentially as described previously.[2,15] We used specific antibodies (kind gift from Prof. H. Mori, Osaka, Japan) to detect $A\beta_{40}$ fragments (terminating at the residue valine-40) and $A\beta_{42}$ fragments (terminating at residues alanine-42/threonine-43) which have been well characterized previously.[2] Double immunolabeling was carried out to study the relationship between $A\beta_{42}$ deposits and the cerebral microvasculature localized with antibodies to collagen IV (1:100 dilution; Sigma).

For morphometric analysis five images were captured from each area of the grey matter using a Zeiss Axioplan 2 light microscope and a JVC CCD camera. The images were captured in a pseudorandom manner.[6] This simply involved moving the section to focus on an adjacent field of the grey matter and then focusing the image on the computer monitor. Each image was analyzed using ImagePro Plus software to determine the Aβ burden or load by measuring the area of Aβ stained with one color (diaminobezidine) against the total area of each image. In double immunolabeled sections the microvessels were stained blue-grey, Aβ plaques were brown, and the Aβ within or bound to vessels was revealed separately as a purplish color. We particularly concentrated on $A\beta_{42}$ and determined the proportion of vessels containing deposits of this peptide for each image and calculated an average for each section. The mean score of five images from each grey matter area per section was then used for statistical comparisons. Statistical analysis was carried out using SPSS (version 7.5) to look for Pearson correlations, and differences between the *APOE* genotype groups were tested for using the Mann-Whitney U test.

TABLE 1. Forms of Aβ load in the temporal cortex and parahippocampal gyrus of AD subjects

Brain Region	Aβ(40)	Aβ(42)
Temporal Cortex	1.38 ($\pm$ 0.19)	5.28 ($\pm$ 0.41)
Parahippocampal Gyrus	0.93 ($\pm$ 0.10)	5.97 ($\pm$ 0.31)

NOTE: Numbers show mean ($\pm$SEM) Aβ burden (arbitary units) in 50 individuals. There were no statistical differences between regions, but there was significantly greater amount of Aβ_{42} in both brain regions (p <0.001).

RESULTS AND DISCUSSION

The mean Aβ_{40} burden was much lower than Aβ_{42} burden in both the temporal and parahippocampal areas (TABLE 1). There were no apparent regional differences in burden.[14] Consistent with previous studies,[1,2] Aβ_{42} deposition was 4–5-fold greater than the more soluble Aβ_{40}. Although a large proportion of the Aβ_{42} deposits was either in close proximity to or contained cerebral microvessels,[4,5] upon double immunolabeling we found that a high percentage of the cerebral vessels also contained the Aβ_{42} (FIG. 1). In the temporal neocortex this was determined to be 39.62% ($\pm$ 1.19), whereas in the parahippocampal gyrus it was 43.34% ($\pm$ 1.02). There were no differences between the Aβ_{42} deposition in the vessels in these two areas. The association of Aβ_{40} was not specifically determined, although there were many microvessels containing this peptide.

In further analysis, we examined the relationship between Aβ burden and *APOE* genotype. In accord with our previous study[15] we found that the frequency of the

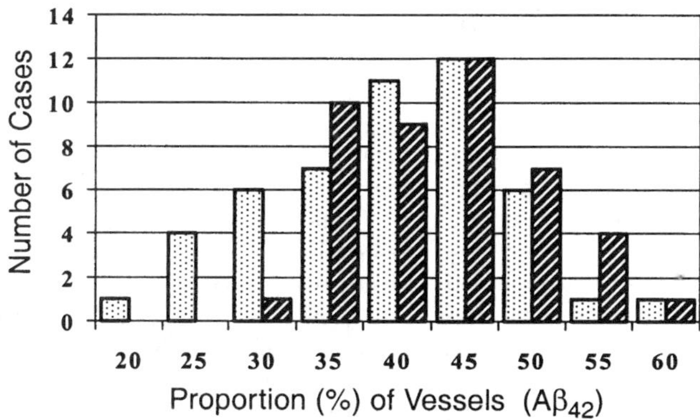

FIGURE 1. Proportion of microvessels with Aβ_{42} in temporal cortex from 50 AD cases and in parahippocampal gyrus from 44 cases. The histograms represent the number of cases with percentage of total vessels with Aβ_{42} in temporal cortex (*stippled columns*) and parahippocampal gyrus (*striated*). The mean ($\pm$ SEM) percentage of vessels containing Aβ_{42} was 39.6 ($\pm$ 1.2) and 43.3 ($\pm$ 0.96), respectively. The proportions represent the number of vessels containing or associated with Aβ_{42} over the total number of vessels in each case determined by taking the average number of vascular profiles immunostained by collagen IV in five different fields.

TABLE 2. The distribution of Aβ burden in two brain regions in relation to the presence of single or double copies of the APOE e4 allele

APOE ε4	$A\beta_{40}$	$A\beta_{42}$
2 alleles		
Temporal cortex	2.92 (± 0.89)	7.03 (± 1.13)
Parahippocampal gyrus	1.68 (± 0.31)*	5.86 (± 1.32)
1 allele		
Temporal cortex	1.16 (± 0.26)	5.11 (± 0.56)
Parahippocampal gyrus	0.83 (± 0.13)	6.11 (± 0.53)
No allele		
Temporal cortex	1.17 (± 0.15)	4.95 (± 0.69)
Parahippocampal gyrus	0.87 (± 0.16)	5.84 (± 0.32)

NOTE: Numbers show mean Aβ burden (± SEM) in 50 individuals.

*There was significantly increased $A\beta_{40}$ load in ε4 homozygotes compared to ε4 heterozygotes and cases without ε4 allele ($p < 0.05$).

APOE ε4 allele frequency in this sample of the cohort was 36%, whereas that of ε2 was 7%. There were no ε2/ε2 genotypes, and the numbers of cases of the five other genotypes (%) were determined to be as follows: 4 were ε2/ε3 (8%), 3 were ε2/ε4 (6%), 16 as ε3/ε3 (32%), 21 as ε3/ε4 (42%) and 6 as ε4/ε4 (12%). Interestingly, 20 (40%) of the 50 cases had no APOE ε4 allele. In this study, we did not detect any clear correlation between $A\beta_{42}$ load in either temporal cortex or parahippocampal gyrus and APOE genotype (TABLE 2). This was independent of whether Aβ was within or not associated with the microvessels. However, there was a significant excess of $A\beta_{40}$ in APOE ε4 homozygotes compared with heterozygotes ($p = 0.003$; Mann Whitney U Test) and those with no ε4 ($p = 0.03$; Mann Whitney U Test) in the parahippocampal gyrus but not apparent in the temporal neocortex. This is somewhat at variance with our previous observations,[15] although in this study we examined a much smaller sample.

We found greater deposition of $A\beta_{42}$ than $A\beta_{40}$ in both parenchyma and cerebral microvessels in the temporal and parahippocampal gyrus in a cohort of elderly Norwegians with AD. A *post hoc* examination of the amyloid loads by APOE group consisting of ε4 heterozygotes, ε4 homozygotes, and those not possessing an ε4 allele revealed that ε4 homozygotes had significantly more $A\beta_{40}$ than the other two groups. We also observed that $A\beta_{42}$ was heavily deposited in the cerebral microvessels in both areas of the brain and that surprisingly 40% of the microvessels contained this longer more pathogenic form of the peptide. Such distribution of Aβ peptide was not significantly related to APOE genotype. Thus possession of an ε4 allele was not associated with an increased amount of Aβ in the vessels in either the parahippocampal gyrus or the temporal neocortex. The localization of $A\beta_{42}$ peptide or deposits in cerebral vessels may occur by several mechanisms.[16–20] Aβ could be synthesized by vascular cells and deposited *in situ*,[16–18] or it could be derived from the brain parenchyma en route to being eliminated[21] in the lumen rather than extracted from the circulation. Nevertheless, our observations suggest that surprisingly high proportions of cortical microvessels contain or are associated with $A\beta_{42}$, which may affect microvascular elements such as endothelial and smooth muscle cells and impinge on their function.[19,21]

ACKNOWLEDGMENT

This work was supported by grants from the MRC (UK) and NINDS (NIH), and a Zenith Award (RNK) from the National Alzheimer's Association, Chicago, USA.

REFERENCES

1. IWATSUBO, T., A. ODAKA, N. SUZUKI, H. MIZUSAWA, N. NUKINA & Y. IHARA. 1994. Visualization of A beta 42(43) and A beta 40 in senile plaques with end-specific A beta monoclonals: evidence that an initially deposited species is A beta 42(43). Neuron **13:** 45–53.
2. KALARIA, R.N., D.L. COHEN, B.D. GREENBERG, M.J. SAVAGE, N.E. BOGDANOVIC, B. WINBLAD, L. LANNFELT & A. ADEM. 1996. Abundance of the longer Aβ42 in neocortical and cerebrovascular amyloid deposits in Swedish familial Alzheimer's disease and Down's syndrome subjects. Neuroreport **7:** 1377–1381.
3. KALARIA, R.N. & P. HEDERA. 1995. Differential degeneration of the endothelium and basement membrane of capillaries in Alzheimer's disease. Neuroreport **6:** 477–480.
4. KAWAI, M., R.N. KALARIA, S.I. HARIK & G. PERRY. 1990. The relationship of amyloid plaques to cerebral capillaries in Alzheimer's disease. Am. J. Pathol. **137:** 1435–1446.
5. KALARIA, R.N. & P. HEDERA. 1996. β-Amyloid vasoactivity in Alzheimer's disease. Lancet **347:** 1492–1493.
6. KALARIA, R.N. 1997. Cerebrovascular degeneration is related to amyloid-β protein deposition in Alzheimer's disease. Ann. N.Y. Acad. Sci. **826:** 263–271.
7. MIYAKAWA, T., S. KATSURAGI, Y. HIGUCHI, K. YAMASHITA, T. KIMURA, K. TERAOKA, T. ONO & K. ISHIZUKA. 1997. Changes of microvessels in the brain with Alzheimer's disease. Ann. N.Y. Acad. Sci. **826:** 428–432.
8. MIYAKAWA, T. 1996. Electron microscopy of amyloid fibrils and microvessels. Ann. N.Y. Acad. Sci. **826:** 25–34.
9. THOMAS, T., G. THOMAS, C. MCLENDON, T. SUTTON & M. MULLAN. 1996. Beta-amyloid-mediated vasoactivity and vascular endothelial damage. Nature **380:** 168–171.
10. DAVIS, J., D.H. CRIBBS, C.W. COTMAN & W.E. VAN NOSTRAND. 1999. Pathogenic amyloid beta-protein induces apoptosis in cultured human cerebrovascular smooth muscle cells. Amyloid **6:** 157–164.
11. WISNIEWSKI, H.M., J. FRACKOWIAK & B. MAZUR-KOLECKA. 1995. *In vitro* production of beta-amyloid in smooth muscle cells isolated from amyloid angiopathy-affected vessels. Neurosci. Lett. **183:** 120–123.
12. KAWAI, M., R.N. KALARIA, P. CRAS, S.L. SIEDLAK, E.R. SHELTON, H.W. CHAN, B.D. GREENBERG & G. PERRY. 1993. Degeneration of amyloid precursor protein-containing smooth muscle cells in cerebral amyloid angiopathy. Brain Res. **623:** 142–146.
13. INCE, P.G., F.K. MCARTHUR, E. BJERTNESS, A. TROVIK, J.M. CANDY & J.A. EDWARDSON. 1996. Neuropathological diagnoses in elderly patients in Oslo: Alzheimer's disease, Lewy body disease, vascular lesions. Dementia **6:** 162–168.
14. MORRIS, C.M., R. BENJAMIN, A. LEAKE, F.K. MCARTHUR, J.M. CANDY, P.G. INCE, A. TORVIK, E. BJERTNESS & J.A. EDWARDSON. 1995. Effect of apolipoprotein E genotype on Alzheimer's disease neuropathology in a cohort of elderly Norwegians. Neurosci Lett. **201:** 45–47.
15. PREMKUMAR, D.L., D.L. COHEN, P. HEDERA, R.P. FRIEDLAND & R.N. KALARIA. 1996. Apolipoprotein E ε4 alleles in cerebral amyloid angiopathy and cerebrovascular pathology in Alzheimer's disease. Am. J. Pathol. **148:** 2083–2095.
16. WISNIEWSKI, H.M. & J. WEGIEL. 1994. Beta-amyloid formation by myocytes of leptomeningeal vessels. Acta Neuropathol. (Berl) **87:** 233–241.
17. DAVIS-SALINAS, J., S.M. SAPORITO-IRWIN, C.W. COTMAN & W.E. VAN NOSTRAND. 1995. Amyloid beta-protein induces its own production in cultured degenerating cerebrovascular smooth muscle cells. J. Neurochem. **65:** 931–934.
18. KALARIA, R.N., A.B. PAX, D.R.D. PREMKUMAR & I. LIEBERBURG. 1996. Production and increased detection of amyloid β-protein and amyloidogenic fragments in brain

microvessels, meningeal vessels and choroid plexus in Alzheimer disease. Mol. Brain Res. **35:** 58–68.

19. PRIOR, R., D. D'URSO, R. FRANK, I. PRIKULIS & G. PAVLAKOVIC. 1996. Loss of vessel wall viability in cerebral amyloid angiopathy. Neuroreport **7:** 562–564.

20. KALARIA, R.N. 1996. Cerebral vessels in ageing and Alzheimer's disease. Pharmacol. Ther. **72:** 193–214.

21. WELLER, R.O., A. MASSEY, T.A. NEWMAN, M. HUTCHINGS, Y.M. KUO & A.E. ROHER. 1998. Cerebral amyloid angiopathy: amyloid beta accumulates in putative interstitial fluid drainage pathways in Alzheimer's disease. Am. J. Pathol. **153:** 725–733.

Cerebrovascular Smooth Muscle Cell Surface Fibrillar Aβ

Alteration of the Proteolytic Environment in the Cerebral Vessel Wall

WILLIAM E. VAN NOSTRAND,[a] JERRY MELCHOR,
MATTHEW WAGNER, AND JUDIANNE DAVIS

*Departments of Medicine and Pathology, State University of New York,
Stony Brook, New York 11794-8153, USA*

ABSTRACT: Cerebrovascular deposition of the amyloid β-protein (Aβ) is a common pathologic event in patients with Alzheimer's disease (AD) and certain related disorders including hereditary cerebral hemorrhage with amyloidosis Dutch-type (HCHWA-D). Aβ deposition occurs primarily in the medial layer of the cerebral vessel wall in an assembled fibrillar state. These deposits are associated with several pathological responses including degeneration of the smooth muscle cells in the cerebral vessel wall. Severe cases of cerebrovascular Aβ deposition are also accompanied by loss of vessel wall integrity and hemorrhagic stroke. Although the reasons for this pathological consequence are unclear, altered proteolytic mechanisms within the cerebral vessel wall may be involved. Recent studies from our laboratory have shown that cell-surface assembly of Aβ into fibrillar structures causes cellular degeneration via an apoptotic pathway and creates an altered proteolytic microenvironment on the cell surface of human cerebrovascular smooth muscle cells (HCSM cells). For example, HCSM cell-surface Aβ fibrils serve as a site for tight binding of cell-secreted amyloid β-precursor protein (AβPP). Since AβPP is a potent inhibitor of key proteinases of coagulation cascade, its enhanced localization on the Aβ fibrils would provide an strong anticoagulant environment. In addition, HCSM cell-surface Aβ fibrils are potent stimulators of tissue plasminogen activator (tPA) creating a profibrinolytic milieu. Our findings indicate that Aβ fibril assembly on the HCSM cell surface causes cellular degeneration and results in both a strong anticoagulant and fibrinolytic environment. Together, these altered proteolytic events could create a setting that is conducive to loss of vessel wall integrity and hemorrhagic stroke.

INTRODUCTION

Cerebral amyloid angiopathy (CAA) is an age-associated condition that is pathologically characterized by deposition of amyloid in the medial layer of primarily small and medium-sized arteries and arterioles of the cerebral cortex and leptomeninges.[1–3] This condition accounts for up to 20% of the cases of primary in-

[a]Address for correspondence: Dr. William E. Van Nostrand, Departments of Medicine and Pathology, HSC T-15/081, State University of New York, Stony Brook, NY 11794-8153. Tel.: (631) 444-1661; fax: (631) 444-7518.
e-mail: wevn@mail.som.sunysb.edu

tracerebral hemorrhage and is a key pathologic lesion in most patients with Alzheimer's disease (AD) and certain related disorders including hereditary cerebral hemorrhage with amyloidosis Dutch-type (HCHWA-D).[4–6] In contrast to AD, the cerebrovascular amyloid deposition in HCHWA-D occurs earlier in life and is so severe that it leads to recurrent, and often fatal, intracerebral hemorrhages by a mean age of fifty years.[5,7] The CAA observed in patients with AD and patients with HCHWA-D share a common amyloid subunit known as the amyloid β-protein (Aβ).[8,9] In addition to the walls of the cerebral blood vessels, Aβ is also found deposited in plaques within the neuropil of patients with either of these disorders. Aβ is a 39–42 amino acid peptide that has the propensity to self-assemble into insoluble, β-pleated sheet fibrils. Aβ is proteolytically derived from a large transmembrane precursor protein, termed the amyloid β-precursor protein (AβPP), which can be translated from primarily three alternatively spliced mRNAs resulting in polypeptides of 695, 751, and 770 amino acids; the latter two species contain an additional insert, which is structurally similar to Kunitz-type serine protease inhibitors (KPI).[10,11] Individuals with HCHWA-D have a point mutation in their AβPP gene that results in a glutamine for glutamic acid substitution at position 22 in the Aβ domain.[12] It has been postulated that this mutation plays a role in Aβ formation and/or deposition in the cerebral vasculature of patients afflicted with this rare disorder. Although the mechanism as to how cerebrovascular Aβ is deleterious in CAA remains unresolved, it has been proposed that the amyloid deposition weakens the vessel wall, possibly through degeneration of the smooth muscle cells, leading toward a tendency for vessel rupture.[13,14]

A number of ultrastructural and immunohistochemical studies performed on autopsy brain tissue have shown that Aβ deposition in the walls of cerebral blood vessels is accompanied by degeneration and eventual disappearance of smooth muscle cells suggesting that the amyloid is toxic to these cells *in vivo*.[15–18] The degenerating smooth muscle cells in the amyloid-laden cerebral vessels have been implicated in the overproduction of AβPP.[16,19] In addition, recent ultrastructural and immunohistochemical studies have implicated cerebrovascular smooth muscle cells in the formation of Aβ.[20–22] Each of these studies points to smooth muscle cells in the cerebral blood vessel wall as active participants in the condition of CAA.

PATHOGENIC Aβ INDUCES DEGENERATION OF CULTURED HCSM CELLS

In light of the above findings we have established a number of primary cell cultures of human cerebrovascular smooth muscle (HCSM) cells.[23] Our recent studies suggest that these HCSM cells may provide a useful and valid cell culture paradigm to investigate some of the cellular processes involved with the cerebrovascular pathology of AD and related disorders. We have described that $A\beta_{1-42}$, a prominent isoform of Aβ found in CAA,[24,25] is toxic to these cultured HCSM cells supporting the findings that are observed *in vivo*.[26–28] However, in contrast to studies with cultured neurons,[29] the shorter $A\beta_{1-39}$ and $A\beta_{1-40}$ peptides failed to elicit degenerative responses in the cultured HCSM cells. In these studies we reported that the degeneration of cultured HCSM cells induced by $A\beta_{1-42}$ is accompanied by a striking increase in the levels of cell-associated AβPP and soluble Aβ peptide. These novel findings demonstrated that $A\beta_{1-42}$ can induce overproduction of its precursor and subsequent formation of additional $A\beta$ in the cultured HCSM cells. In addition, we now have shown that the HCHWA-D mutation converts the normally nonpathogenic $A\beta_{1-40}$ into a highly pathogenic form of the peptide for cultured HCSM cells. HCHWA-D $A\beta_{1-40}$ was even more robust than wild-type $A\beta_{1-42}$.[30] This finding suggests that the altered functional properties of HCHWA-D-mutated $A\beta$ may contribute to the early and often severe cerebrovascular pathology that is the hallmark of this disorder. It is noteworthy that the pathogenic effects of $A\beta_{1-42}$ or HCHWA-D $A\beta_{1-40}$ were not observed in cultured human fibroblasts nor glioblastoma cells suggesting that these particular pathogenic effects are somewhat specific for smooth muscle cells in the cerebral blood vessel wall.

There are several indications that our proposed mechanism and cell culture findings are consistent with the *in vivo* pathologic features of CAA. First, $A\beta$ is found deposited within the tunica media of the cerebral vessel wall.[1,2,6,7,15–19] Second, $A\beta$ deposition within the vessel wall leads to smooth muscle cell degeneration.[1,15–18] Third, the degenerating smooth muscle cells express increased amounts of $A\beta PP$[16,19] and produce more $A\beta$ peptide.[20–22] Lastly, in HCHWA-D each of these effects is enhanced, apparently due to the altered functional properties of the mutant $A\beta$ peptide.[5,7,19] These properties suggest that the HCSM cell culture paradigm is a valid and useful *in vitro* model for further elucidating the cellular mechanistic aspects of this condition.

PATHOGENIC Aβ ASSEMBLES INTO FIBRILS
ON THE SURFACE OF HCSM CELLS

We recently conducted studies to determine why HCHWA-D $A\beta_{1-40}$, but not wild-type $A\beta_{1-40}$, is highly pathogenic for cultured HCSM cells.[31] We showed by several quantitative criteria including thioflavin T fluorescence binding, circular dichroism spectroscopy, and transmission electron microscopic analysis, that at a concentration of 25 μM neither pathogenic HCHWA-D $A\beta_{1-40}$ nor nonpathogenic wild-type $A\beta_{1-40}$ appreciably assembled into β-pleated sheet-containing fibrils in solution over a six-day incubation period. In contrast, at the same concentrations HCHWA-D $A\beta_{1-40}$, but not wild-type $A\beta_{1-40}$, selectively bound and assembled into abundant fibrils on the surface of cultured HCSM cells. As shown in FIGURE 1, the HCHWA-D $A\beta_{1-40}$ peptide clearly assembled into a network of fibrils on the surface of the cultured HCSM cells. This demonstrates that initially unassembled HCHWA-D $A\beta_{1-40}$ in solution assembles into a fibrillar network on the surfaces of HCSM cells. This *in vitro* finding is consistent with electron microscopy studies which showed pathologic $A\beta$ deposition around smooth muscle cells in vessels *in vivo* in patients with CAA.[17,32] Assembly of HCSM cell surface fibrils was also observed with the pathogenic wild-type $A\beta_{1-42}$ peptide but, as stated above, not with the nonpathogenic wild-type $A\beta_{1-40}$. An equimolar concentration of the dye Congo red prevented the cell-surface fibril assembly of HCHWA-D $A\beta_{1-40}$. Moreover, Congo red effectively blocked the key pathologic responses induced by HCHWA-D $A\beta_{1-40}$ in cultured HCSM cells. This finding demonstrated that formation of these $A\beta$ fibrils coincides with the induction of pathologic responses in the HCSM cells. Importantly, this suggests that assembly of $A\beta$ fibrils on the surface of smooth muscle cells is required

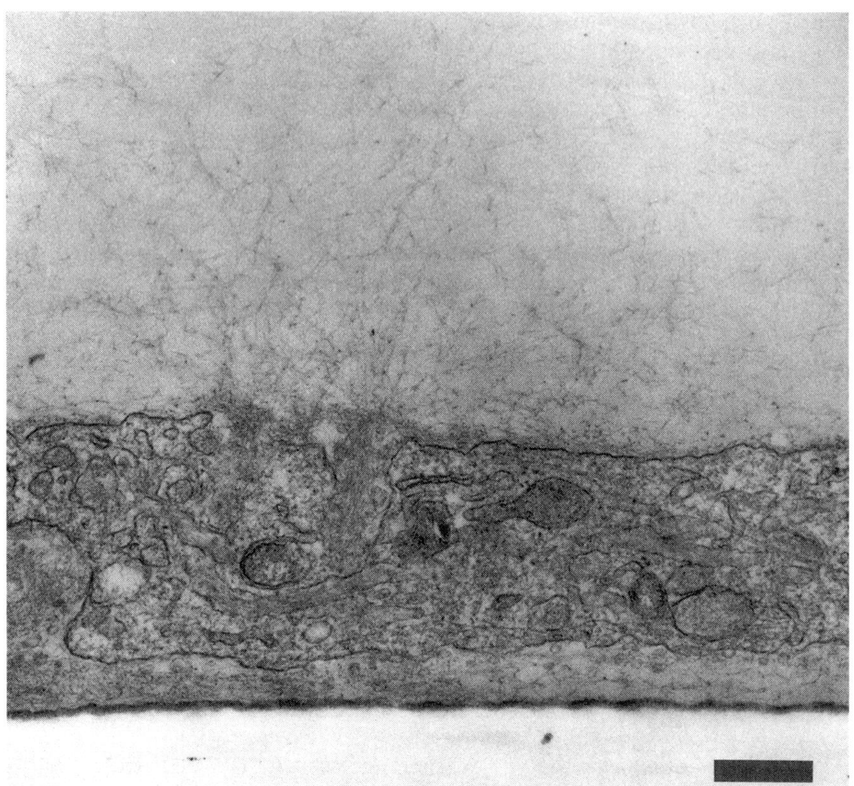

FIGURE 1. HCHWA-D $A\beta_{1-40}$ fibril formation on the surface of HCSM cells. HCSM cells were incubated in the presence of freshly solublized HCHWA-D $A\beta_{1-40}$ at a concentration of 25 µM for six days. The cells were then washed, fixed with a solution 2% paraformaldehyde and 2.5% glutaraldehyde, stained, embedded, thin sectioned, and placed on carbon formar-coated 200-mesh copper grids. The sections were viewed with a JEOL 1200 EX Transmission Electron Microscope at 60 kV. Note the extensive formation of fibrils on the cell surface. *Scale bar* = 0.4 µm.

for it to induce pathologic responses in these cells. As we described above, the assembly of $A\beta$ into fibrils in solution abolished its pathogenic properties to HCSM cells.[27] These present findings suggest that the surfaces of HCSM cells may selectively orchestrate the assembly of pathogenic HCHWA-D $A\beta_{1-40}$ fibrils and that cell-surface $A\beta$ fibril formation plays an important role in causing the pathologic responses in HCSM cells.

HCSM CELL SURFACE Aβ FIBRILS BIND SECRETED AβPP

We have recently further investigated the nature of the increased HCSM cell-associated $A\beta PP$ that results in response to treatment with pathogenic $A\beta$. HCSM cells were incubated in the presence or absence of HCHWA-D $A\beta_{1-40}$ for six days.

In one set of experiments the cell-surface proteins were removed by incubation with trypsin and the remaining AβPP was quantitated by immunoblotting. Incubation of the HCHWA-D $Aβ_{1-40}$-treated HCSM cells with trypsin erased the increased levels of cell-associated AβPP. In a second set of experiments the cell-surface proteins were biotinylated, then precipitated using streptavidin-agarose beads, and the AβPP that was precipitated was quantitated by immunoblotting. Both these techniques revealed that the increased cell-associated AβPP was present on the HCSM cell surface. To further determine the nature of the increased cell surface AβPP in the HCHWA-D $Aβ_{1-40}$-treated HCSM cells we used antibodies directed against the amino- and carboxyl-terminus of AβPP. Although the levels of full-length AβPP increased modestly ($≈2$ to 3-fold), the majority of the total AβPP increase was due to secreted AβPP (sAβPP). This result suggests that sAβPP may bind back to HCSM cells, possibly to the cell-surface fibrils formed by the pathogenic Aβ peptide. Binding of biotinylated-sAβPP to Aβ fibrils formed in solution was observed by transmission electron microscopy. Solid-phase binding assays showed that biotinylated-sAβPP binds to fibrillar Aβ in a dose-dependent manner with a K_d of $≈30$ nM. Subsequent domain mapping studies implicate the amino-terminal region of the AβPP molecule in this high-affinity interaction with fibrillar Aβ. These recent studies suggest that an interaction between fibrillar pathogenic Aβ peptide and its secreted parent molecule, sAβPP, occurs on the cell-surface of cultured HCSM cells. This interaction may contribute to the pathologic responses evoked by pathogenic Aβ in HCSM cells leading to their degeneration.

FIBRILLAR Aβ STIMULATES THE INHIBITION OF COAGULATION FACTOR XIA BY PN-2/AβPP

Severe cases of CAA, particularly in HCHWA-D, lead to recurrent and often fatal hemorrhagic strokes. Although the reasons for this pathological consequence remain unclear, alterations in proteolytic hemostasis mechanisms have been implicated. For example, protease nexin-2 (PN-2), the sAβPP forms that contain the Kunitz-type serine proteinase inhibitory domain, is elevated in cerebral vessels with Aβ deposits.[16,19] PN-2/AβPP is a potent inhibitor of several key enzymes in coagulation cascade.[33–36] As described above, we recently showed that fibrillar Aβ binds PN-2/AβPP in a dose-dependent manner with a K_d of $≈30$ nM. Subsequently, we found that PN-2/AβPP bound to fibrillar Aβ is active in inhibiting coagulation factor XIa (FXIa). Quantitative kinetic measurements revealed that fibrillar Aβ enhanced the inhibition of FXIa by PN-2/AβPP with an IC_{50} of $≈5$ μM. This effectively lowered the K_i of the reaction $≈10$-fold. These findings suggest that fibrillar Aβ deposits in cerebral vessels can serve to localize and enhance the anticoagulant properties of PN-2/AβPP thereby contributing to a microenvironment conducive to hemorrhaging.

FIBRILLAR Aβ STIMULATES THE ACTIVITY OF tPA

In addition to the potential increased anticoagulant activities described above, alterations in the fibrinolytic proteinases may also contribute to hemorrhaging in CAA. For example, previous studies by Kingston *et al.*[37] showed that fibrillar forms of Aβ can stimulate the enzymatic activity of tissue-type plasminogen activator (tPA) *in vitro*. Recently, we investigated the stimulation of tPA by freshly solubilized Aβ_{1-40}. The rate of tPA stimulation by Aβ_{1-40} increased dramatically over time suggesting that Aβ may be altered during the course of the reaction. SDS-PAGE analysis showed that Aβ_{1-40} was cleaved during the course of the reaction. Subsequent studies showed that it was plasmin, the product of tPA activation of plasminogen, that specifically cleaved Aβ_{1-40} in the amino terminal region between Arg[5] and His[6]. Plasmin effectively cleaved a chromogenic substrate corresponding to this cleavage site in Aβ. Circular dichroism spectral analysis showed that Aβ_{6-40} adopted a strong β-sheet secondary structure. This truncated Aβ_{6-40} peptide was a potent stimulator of tPA *in vitro*. These results indicate that β-sheet secondary structure of Aβ, which can be promoted by plasmin cleavage, stimulates tPA activity. These findings suggest that pathologic interactions between Aβ, tPA, and plasmin in the cerebral vessel walls of patients with CAA could result in excessive proteolysis contributing to intracerebral hemorrhages. Furthermore, HCHWA-D patients, with their exaggerated cerebrovascular Aβ deposition, would be even more inclined to suffer from excessive plasminogen activation.

SUMMARY

Our studies have shown that soluble pathogenic forms of Aβ assemble into fibrils on the surface of cultured HCSM cells, and this process is related to inducing an apoptotic mechanism of cell death. Secreted forms of AβPP extensively bind to this cell-surface assembly of Aβ fibrils and may contribute to the induction of Aβ-induced HCSM cell death. These Aβ fibrils may also serve as surface to localize and stimulate the anticoagulant properties of PN-2/AβPP as well as localize and stimulate the activity of tPA. The combined effects of HCSM cell death and altered proteolytic hemostatic mechanisms in the Aβ-laden cerebral vessel wall may significantly contribute to the development of hemorrhagic strokes in patients with severe CAA.

ACKNOWLEDGMENTS

This work was supported by NIH grants NS35781, AG16223, HL49566, and HL03229.

REFERENCES

1. VINTERS, H.V. 1987. Cerebral amyloid angiopathy: a critical review. Stroke **18:** 311–324.
2. IWAMOTO, N., T. ISHIHARA, H. ITO & F. UCHINO. 1993. Morphological evaluation of amyloid-laden arteries in leptomeninges, cortices, and subcortices in cerebral amyloid angiopathy with subcortical hemorrhage. Acta Neuropathol. **86:** 418–421.
3. CORIA, F. & I. RUBIO. 1996. Cerebral amyloid angiopathies. Neuropathol. Appl. Neurobiol. **22:** 216–227.
4. GLENNER, G.G., J.H. HENRY & S. FUJIHARA. 1981. Congophilic angiopathy in the pathogenesis of Alzheimer's degeneration. Ann. Pathol. **1:** 120–129.

5. LUYENDIJK, W., G.T.A.M. BOTS, M. VEGTER-VAN DER VLIS & L.N. WENT. 1988. Hereditary cerebral hemorrhage caused by cortical amyloid angiopathy. J. Neurol. Sci. **85:** 267–280.

6. HIRAI, S. & K. OKAMOTO. 1993. Amyloid beta/A4 peptide associated with Alzheimer's disease and cerebral amyloid angiopathy. Internal Med. **32:** 923–925.

7. WATTENDORFF, A.R., B. FRANGIONE, W. LUYENDIJK & G.T.A.M. BOTS. 1995. Hereditary cerebral haemorrhage with amyloidosis, Dutch type (HCHWA-D): clinicopathological studies. J. Neurol. Neurosurg. Psychiatry **59:** 699–705.

8. GLENNER, G.G. & C.W. WONG. 1984. Alzheimer's disease: initial report of the purification and characterization of a novel cerebrovascular amyloid protein. Biochem. Biophys. Res. Commun. **122:** 885–890.

9. PRELLI, F., E. CASTANO, G.G. GLENNER & B. FRANGIONE. 1988. Differences between vascular and plaque core amyloid in Alzheimer's disease. J. Neurochem. **51:** 648–651.

10. SELKOE, D.J. 1996. Amyloid β-protein and the genetics of Alzheimer's disease. J. Biol. Chem. **271:** 18295–18298.

11. YANKNER, B.A. 1996. Mechanisms of neuronal degenration in Alzheimer's disease. Neuron **16:** 921–932.

12. LEVY, E., M.D. CARMAN, I.J. FERNANDEZ-MADRID, M.D. POWER, I. LIEBERBURG, S.G. VAN DUINEN, G.T.A.M. BOTS, W. LUYENDIJK & B. FRANGIONE. 1990. Mutation of the Alzheimer's disease amyloid gene in hereditary cerebral hemorrhage, Dutch type. Science **248:** 1124–1126.

13. OKAZAKI, H., T.J. REAGEN & R.J. CAMPBELL. 1979. Clinicopathologic studies of primary cerebral amyloid angiopathy. Mayo Clin. Proc. **54:** 22–31.

14. MARUYAMA, K., S. IKEDA, T. ISHIHARA, D. ALLSOP & N. YANGISAWA. 1990. Immunohistochemical characterization of cerebrovascular amyloid in 46 autopsied cases using antibodies to β-protein and cystatin C. Stroke **21:** 397–403.

15. CORIA, F., M. LARRONDO-LILLO & B. FRANGIONE. 1989. Degeneration of smooth muscle cells in beta-amyloid angiopathies. J. Neuropathol. Exp. Neurol. **48:** 368–375.

16. KAWAI, M., R.N. KALARIA, P. CRAS, S.L. SIEDLAK, M.E. VELASCO, E.R. SHELTON, H.W. CHAN, B.D. GREENBERG & G. PERRY. 1993. Degeneration of vascular muscle cells in cerebral amyloid angiopathy of Alzheimer disease. Brain Res. **623:** 142–146.

17. VINTERS, H.V., D.L. SECOR, S.L. READ, J.G. FRAZEE, U. TOMIYASY, T.M. STANLEY, J.A. FERREIRO & M.-A. AKERS. 1994. Microvasculature in brain biopsy specimens from patients with Alzheimer's disease: an immunohistochemical and ultrastructural study. Ultrastruct. Pathol. **18:** 333–348.

18. PRIOR, R., D. D'URSO, R. FRANK, I. PRIKULIS & G. PAVLAKOVIC. 1996. Loss of vessel wall viability in cerebral amyloid angiopathy. Neuroreport **7:** 562–564.

19. ROZEMULLER, A.J.M., R.A.C. ROOS, G.T.A.M. BOTS, W. KAMPHORST, P. EIKELENBBOM & W.E. VAN NOSTRAND. 1993. Distribution of β/A4 and amyloid precursor protein in hereditary cerebral hemorrhage with amyloidosis-Dutch type and Alzheimer's disease. Am. J. Pathol. **142:** 1449–1457.

20. WISNIEWSKI, H.M. & J. WEIGEL. 1994. β-Amyloid formation by myocytes of leptomeningeal vessels. Acta Neuropathol. **87:** 233–241.

21. WISNIEWSKI, H.M., J. FRACKOWIAK, A. ZOLTOWSKA & K.S. KIM. 1994. Vascular β-amyloid in Alzheimer's disease angiopathy is produced by proliferating and degenerating smooth muscle cells. Amyloid **1:** 8–16.

22. WISNIEWSKI, H.M., J. FRACLOWIAK & B. MAZUR-KOLECKA. 1995. *In vitro* production of β-amyloid in smooth muscle cells isolated from amyloid angiopathy-affected vessels. Neurosci. Lett. **183:** 120–123.

23. VAN NOSTRAND, W.E, A.J.M. ROZEMULLER, R. CHUNG, C.W. COTMAN & S.M. SAPORITO-IRWIN. 1994. Amyloid β-protein precursor in cultured leptomeningeal smooth muscle cells. Amyloid **1:** 1–7.

24. ROHER, A.E., J.D. LOWENSON, S. CLARKE, A.S. WOODS, R.J. COTTER, E. GOWING & M.J. BALL. 1993. β-Amyloid-(1–42) is a major component of cerebrovascular amyloid deposits: implications for the pathology of Alzheimer's disease. Proc. Natl. Acad. Sci. USA **90:** 10836–10840.

25. SHINKAI, Y., M. YOSHIMURA, Y. ITO, A. ODAKA, N. SUZUKI, K. YANAGISAWA & Y. IHARA. 1995. Amyloid β-proteins 1–40 and 1–42(43) in the soluble fraction of extra- and intracranial blood vessels. Ann. Neurol. **38:** 421–428.

26. DAVIS-SALINAS, J., S.M. SAPORITO-IRWIN, C.W. COTMAN & W.E. VAN NOSTRAND. 1995. Alzheimer's amyloid β-protein induces its own production in cultured cerebrovascular smooth muscle cells. J. Neurochem. **65:** 931–934.

27. DAVIS-SALINAS, J. & W.E. VAN NOSTRAND. 1995. Aggregation of amyloid β-protein nullifies its pathologic properties in cultured cerebrovascular smooth muscle cells. J. Biol. Chem. **270:** 20887–20890.

28. VAN NOSTRAND, W.E., J. DAVIS-SALINAS & S.M. SAPORITO-IRWIN. 1996. Amyloid β-protein induces the cerebrovascular cellular pathology of Alzheimer's disease and related disorders. Ann. N.Y. Acad. Sci. **777:** 297–302.

29. PIKE, C.J., D. BURDICK, A.J. WALENCEWICZ, C.G. GLABE & C.W. COTMAN. 1993. Neurodegeneration induced by β-amyloid peptides *in vitro*: the role of peptide assembly state. J. Neurosci. **13:** 1676–1687.

30. DAVIS, J. & W.E. VAN NOSTRAND. 1996. Enhanced pathologic properties of Dutch-type mutant amyloid β-protein. Proc. Natl. Acad. Sci. USA **93:** 2996–3000.

31. VAN NOSTRAND, W.E., J.P. MELCHOR & L.D. RUFFINI. 1998. Pathologic amyloid β-protein cell-surface fibril assembly in cultured human cerebrovascular smooth muscle cells. J. Neurochem. **70:** 216–223.

32. YAMAGUCHI, H., T. YAMAZAKI, C.A. LEMERE, M.P. ROSCH & D.J. SELKOE. 1992. Beta amyloid is focally deposited within the outer basement membrane in the amyloid angiopathy of Alzheimer's disease. An immunoelectron microscopic study. Am. J. Pathol. **141:** 249–259.

33. VAN NOSTRAND, W.E., S.L. WAGNER, J.S. FARROW & D.D. CUNNINGHAM. 1990. Immunopurification and protease inhibitory properties of protease nexin-2/amyloid β-protein precursor. J. Biol. Chem. **265:** 9591–9594.

34. SCHMAIER, A.H., L.D. DAHL, A.J.M. ROZEMULLER, R.A.C. ROOS, S.L. WAGNER, R. CHUNG & W.E. VAN NOSTRAND. 1993. Protease nexin-2/amyloid β-protein precursor: a tight binding inhibitor of coagulation factor IXa. J. Clin. Invest. **92:** 2540–2545.

35. SCHMAIER, A.H., L.D. DAHL, A.A.K. HASAN, D.B. CINES & W.E. VAN NOSTRAND. 1995. Factor IXa inhibition by protease nexin-2/amyloid β-protein precursor on phospholipid vesicles and cell membranes. Biochemistry **34:** 1171–1178.

36. MAHDI, F., W.E. VAN NOSTRAND & A.H. SCHMAIER. 1995. Protease nexin-2/amyloid β-protein precursor inhibits Factor Xa in the prothrombinase complex. J. Biol. Chem. **270:** 23468–23474.

37. KINGSTON, I.B., M.J.M. CASTRO & S.A. ANDERSON. 1995. *In vitro* stimulation of tissue-type plasminogen activator by Alzheimer amyloid β-peptide analogues. Nat. Med. **1:** 138–142.

Aβ Vasoactivity: An Inflammatory Reaction

DANIEL PARIS, TERRENCE TOWN, TIMOTHY PARKER, JAMES HUMPHREY, AND MICHAEL MULLAN[a]

The Roskamp Institute, University of South Florida, Tampa, Florida 33613, USA

ABSTRACT: Mounting evidence from *in vitro* and *in vivo* studies in transgenic mice overproducing β-amyloid peptides (Aβ) suggests that Aβ can induce vasoconstriction and decrease cerebral blood flow. In this report, we describe the vasoactive properties of Aβ, in particular the enhancement of endothelin-1-induced vasoconstriction and Aβ's induction of a long-lasting vasoconstrictive event. Furthermore, we show that low doses (as low as 50 nM) of freshly solubilized Aβ similar to those observed in the plasma of patients suffering from Alzheimer's disease are vasoactive. By using various inhibitors and activators of the phospholipase A_2 (PLA_2)/arachidonic acid (AA) cascade, we demonstrate that Aβ vasoactivity is dependent on activation of this intracellular signaling pathway, resulting in stimulation of downstream cyclooxygenase-2 and 5-lipoxygenase, which mediate production of proinflammatory eicosanoids. Taken together, our data show that Aβ directly activates an intracellular proinflammatory pathway, which is responsible for its vasoactive properties.

BACKGROUND

Vascular pathology frequently co-occurs with Alzheimer's disease (AD), and, in particular, cerebral amyloid angiopathy (CAA) is one of the commonest abnormalities detected at autopsy in carefully standardized examination (83% of AD cases as assessed by the Consortium to Establish a Registry for Alzheimer's Disease (CERAD)[1]). It is becoming increasingly accepted that such vascular pathology may modify the risk of developing AD, may alter clinical presentation, and may modify the progression of the disease. However, we are concerned here not with the effects of gross anatomic pathological changes associated with AD, but, rather, with the hypothesis that β-amyloid peptides (Aβ) may induce functional abnormalities in the microvasculature of AD patients, and that these functional changes may contribute to the clinical picture, pathology, and progression of the disease. This hypothesis arises from mounting evidence that soluble forms of Aβ peptides have vasoactive effects in isolated mammalian vessels and in transgenic animal models where Aβ peptides are overexpressed.[2–4] At the clinical level, it is possible that these "physiologic" effects of soluble Aβ mediate hypoperfusion and perhaps ischemia in AD brains, thereby amplifying the AD pathological process. This hypothesis includes the tenet that Aβ peptides exert these effects in their soluble form, and that deposition of insoluble amyloid is not required to produce these effects. With regard

[a]Address for correspondence: Dr. Michael Mullan, The Roskamp Institute, University of South Florida, 3515 E. Fletcher Ave., Tampa, FL 33613. Tel.: (813) 974-3722; fax: (813) 974-3915.
e-mail: mmullan@com1.med.usf.edu

to hypoperfusion, both single photon emission computed tomography (SPECT) and positron emission tomography (PET) studies confirm reduction in cerebral blood flow in AD,[5–6] but the concomitant decrease in glucose metabolism has prompted the interpretation that the former observation is a consequence of reduced neuronal metabolic demand.[7]

Although the potential vasoactive effects of Aβ have not been demonstrated in humans, data from transgenic animal models of AD and CAA are highly supportive of the hypothesis that soluble Aβ peptides can induce vasoconstriction and oppose normal vasorelaxation. For instance, transgenic mice that overexpress Aβ peptides exhibit decreased cerebral blood flow in response to vasodilators[4] prior to the formation of amyloid plaques, suggesting that the isolated vessel bath system may be an accurate model of the preclinical effects of soluble Aβ levels on the microcerebrovasculature in AD. Other transgenic models of AD also overexpressing Aβ do not respond well after vascular insult compared to their nontransgenic littermates. In particular, after middle cerebral artery occlusion there is enlarged infarct size, reduced blood flow in the penumbra of the infarct, and reduced response to vasodilators in the same area.[8] Again, this is consistent with a vasoactive role for soluble Aβ peptides, as their levels reach supraphysiologic amounts around the microcerebrovasculature in the brain parenchyma.

However, in persons affected with AD, there has been no direct testing of the existence or clinical importance of any Aβ-induced vasoactive effects similar to those observed *in vitro* or in transgenic animals. Indeed, a primary role of hypoperfusion is not established and, as mentioned, thought to be largely consequent upon reduced metabolic demand of dysfunctional neurons. For instance, in a small study conducted by Jagust and colleagues,[9] it was suggested that there was no evidence to propose that the prominent perfusion changes seen in AD were primary and that AD cases had similar increases in perfusion compared to normals when challenged by hypocapnia. By contrast, Nagata and colleagues[10] observed increased oxygen extraction in AD cases compared to controls, suggesting a primary role for the vasculature in limiting perfusion to the brain. Interestingly, the same study suggested no change in vascular reactivity, at least in relation to changes in $PaCO_2$. Already, then, there are important differences in studies of blood flow in AD cases and transgenic models of AD. Some of these differences may be due to the different experimental paradigms between human and animal studies and, in particular, the restrictions inherent in human studies that preclude challenge of the appropriate vasoactive mechanisms triggered by Aβ. For instance, although vascular reactivity is maintained in AD in relation to hypercapnia, it may not be maintained in relation to compounds that directly relate to the proposed mechanism of Aβ vasoactivity. The experimental design of studies that would contribute such information is not obvious, but much needed. As a first step to elucidating the contribution of Aβ's vasoactive effects in transgenic models of AD and in AD itself, we must be clear on exactly how Aβ mediates its vasoactive effects, and this is the subject of this report.

MATERIALS AND METHODS

Freshly dissected aortae were prepared from normal male Sprague-Dawley rats (7–8 months old, purchased from Zivic Miller, Zelienople, PA) as previously de-

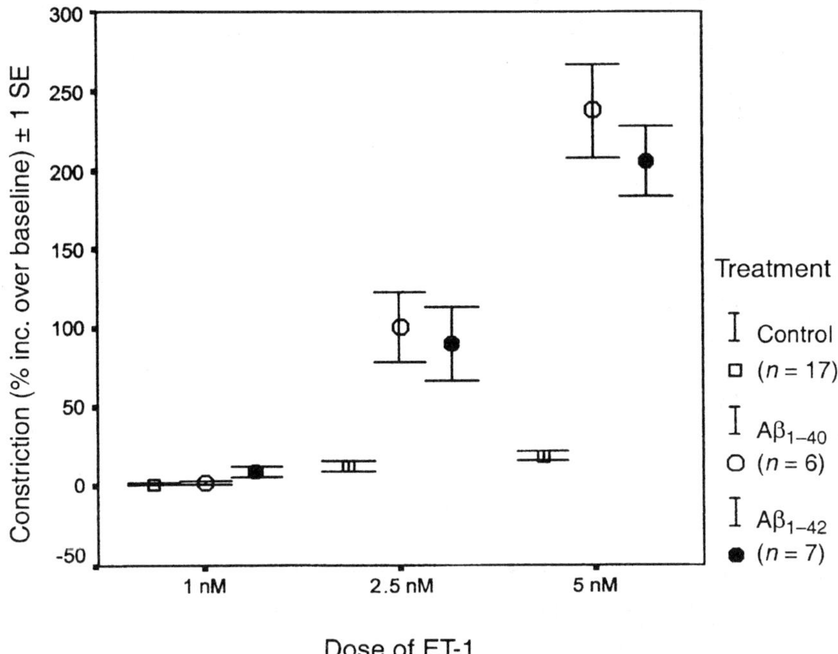

FIGURE 1. Freshly solubilized $A\beta_{1-40}$ or $A\beta_{1-42}$ enhance ET-1-induced vasoconstriction. Certain aortic rings were treated with $A\beta_{1-40}$ or $A\beta_{1-42}$ 5 min prior to the addition of a dose range of ET-1. Analysis of variance (ANOVA) showed significant main effects of ET-1 dose (p <0.001), $A\beta_{1-40}$ (p <0.001), and $A\beta_{1-42}$ (p <0.001). ANOVA also revealed significant interactive terms between ET-1 dose and either $A\beta_{1-40}$ (p <0.001) or $A\beta_{1-42}$ (p = 0.001), indicating ET-1 dose-dependent enhancement of vasoconstriction by $A\beta$.

scribed.[3] Rat aortae were segmented into rings and suspended in Kreb's buffer on hooks connected to a tensiometer linked to a MacLab system. Aortic rings were equilibrated for 2 h, in 7 ml tissue baths thermoregulated to 37°C containing Kreb's buffer oxygenated with 95% O_2 : 5% CO_2. A baseline tension of 2 g was applied to each ring, and the first set of aortic rings was pretreated with various inhibitors or activators of the phopholipase A_2 (PLA_2)/arachidonic acid (AA) cascade, either alone or in combination with $A\beta$ peptides. After 5 min of incubation in the presence or absence of $A\beta$, vessels were subjected to a dose range of endothelin-1 (ET-1, from 1 nM to 5 nM). The second set of vessels was treated with 1 μM of $A\beta$ peptides prior to the addition of ET-1. A third set received only ET-1 treatment (control). Each ET-1 dose was added only after the constriction response to the previous dose had reached a plateau. In all cases the means ± 1 standard error (SE) of the percentage vasoconstriction increase over baseline were determined for each dose of ET-1 used.

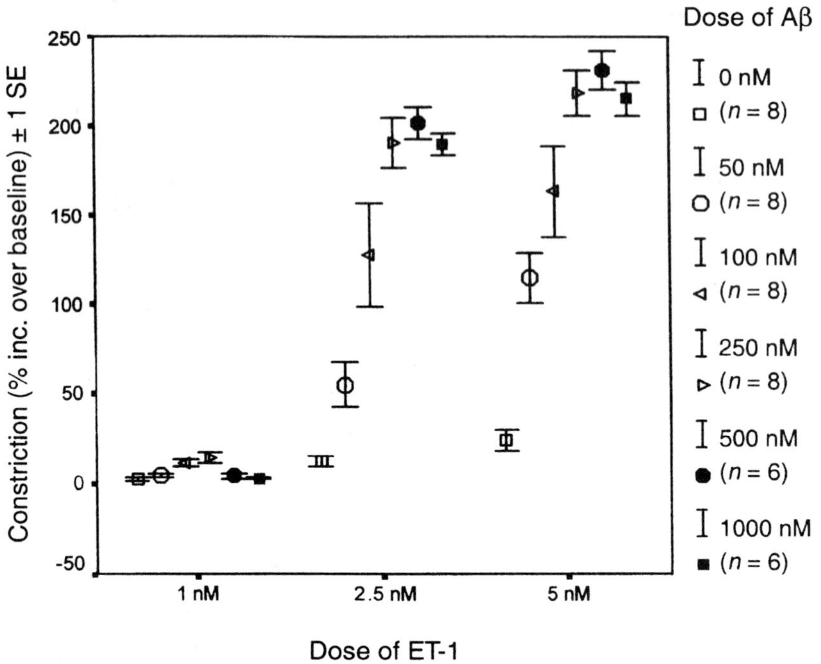

FIGURE 2. Dose-response curve showing $A\beta_{1-40}$ vasoactivity. Certain aortic rings were treated with a dose range of $A\beta_{1-40}$ 5 min prior to the addition of a dose range of ET-1. ANOVA revealed significant main effects of ET-1 dose ($p < 0.001$), $A\beta$ dose ($p < 0.001$), and an interactive term between them ($p < 0.001$). One-way ANOVA across ET-1 doses revealed significant between-groups differences ($p < 0.001$), and Bonferonni's post-hoc comparison across the 2.5 nM and 5 nM doses of ET-1 showed a significant difference between the 50 nM dose of $A\beta$ and the $A\beta$-free condition ($p = 0.001$).

RESULTS AND DISCUSSION

$A\beta_{1-40}$ has previously been shown to exhibit vasoactive properties, and it has been suggested that this effect is mediated by free radical production.[2] However, we have excluded the involvement of free radical and reactive oxygen species as possible contributors to the vasoactive properties of $A\beta$ peptides, since Mn(111)tetrakis(4-benzoic acid)porphyrin chloride (MnTBAP), a superoxide mimetic and peroxynitrite scavenger, catalase, and Trolox were unable to reduce or oppose the effect of $A\beta$ in rat aortae.[11] Interestingly, $A\beta$ vasoactivity appears to be related to the conformation adopted by the peptide in solution, and is observable with soluble, but not with aggregated forms of $A\beta$.[12] To determine the impact of $A\beta$ on endogenous vasoconstrictors, we examined the effect of ET-1 on vessels pretreated with $A\beta$. ET-1

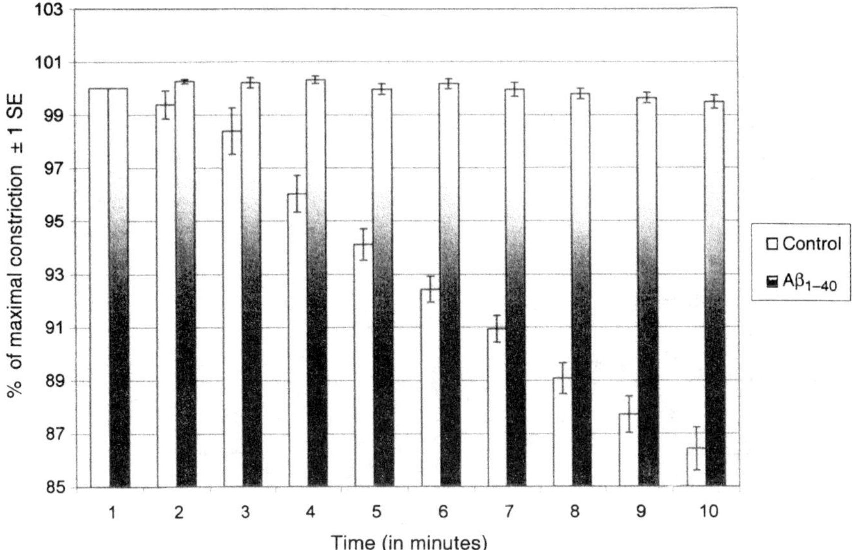

FIGURE 3. Aβ induces a long-lasting vasoconstriction. Certain aortic rings were treated with 1 µM Aβ$_{1-40}$ 5 min prior to the addition of a dose range of ET-1 (1, 2.5, and 5 nM). Following the 5 nM dose of ET-1, maximum tension was taken as the t = 0 time point (and standardized to 100% both in control and Aβ-treated vessels), with vasotension assessed for each following minute until t = 10 min. n = 8 for control and Aβ-treated vessels. ANOVA revealed significant main effects of Aβ (p <0.001), time (p <0.001), and an interaction between them (p <0.001). Post-hoc t test for independent samples across time points revealed a significant difference (p <0.001) between control and Aβ-treated rat aortae.

is one of the most potent cerebral vasoconstrictors known in the brain, and, together with NO, controls cerebral vasoregulation.[13] Our data show that Aβ peptides (1 µM, 1–40 or 1–42) synergistically enhance ET-1-induced vasoconstriction to a similar extent (FIG. 1). Furthermore, Aβ's response to ET-1 is much more potent than with phenylephrine (PE[2]), and is observable within minutes. This observation led us to focus on the ET-1 system as an assay for Aβ vasoactivity.

The initial experiments showing Aβ's vasoactive response employed relatively high doses of Aβ. However, it is entirely possible that such elevated doses of Aβ are not physiologically relevant. In order to approach physiologic levels of Aβ, we assessed the vasoconstrictive effect of low doses of Aβ. Furthermore, we employed freshly solubilized Aβ, as this form of the peptide may exert its bioactivity prior to clinical presentation of the disease. Data show that Aβ's vasoactivity is observable within minutes with nanomolar doses of freshly solubilized Aβ (as low as 50 nM, plateauing at 250 nM), which are physiologic (FIG. 2). Specifically, it has been shown that circulating levels of Aβ range between 30 and 150 nM in AD blood.[14] This dose-response curve shows that the vasculature is extremely sensitive to the effects of soluble Aβ, suggesting that, in AD and CAA where perivascular Aβ levels

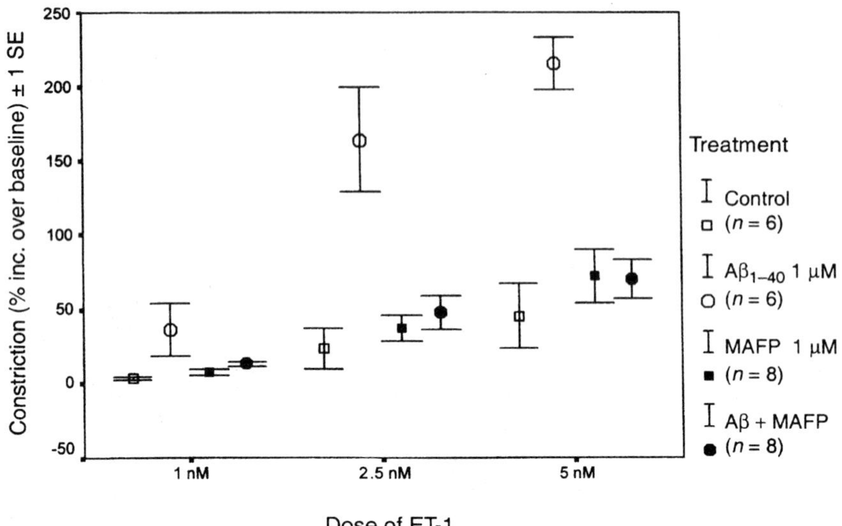

FIGURE 4. Effect of $cPLA_2$ inhibition on Aβ-induced vasoactivity. Certain aortic rings were treated with 1 µM freshly solubilized $Aβ_{1-40}$, 1 µM MAFP, or MAFP + Aβ 5 min prior to the addition of a dose range of ET-1. There were significant main effects by ANOVA of ET-1 dose ($p < 0.001$), Aβ ($p < 0.001$), but not MAFP ($p < 0.001$). There were also significant interactive terms between ET-1 dose and Aβ ($p < 0.01$), and among ET-1, Aβ, and MAFP ($p < 0.01$). One-way ANOVA across ET-1 doses revealed significant between-groups differences ($p < 0.001$), and post-hoc testing showed significant differences between control and Aβ ($p < 0.001$), and Aβ and Aβ + MAFP ($p = 0.001$).

are substantially increased, the cerebrovasculature may play an important role in the pathogenesis of the disease prior to the formation of Aβ aggregates.

Interestingly, Aβ not only increases the magnitude of contraction induced by ET-1, but also enhances the sustained phase of ET-1-induced vasoconstriction at doses as low as 20 nM of freshly solubilized Aβ (FIG. 3). Long-lasting vasoconstriction induced by Aβ is evident with other vasoconstrictors, such as phenylepherine or a thromboxane A_2 analogue (U-46619), indicating that long-lasting vasoconstriction is not specific to the vasoconstrictor used. However, Aβ's enhancement of maximum vasoconstriction was observable only with ET-1, and not with these other vasoconstrictors (named above).

Although considerable information is available regarding the mechanism by which vasoconstrictors mediate their effects, less is known about the intracellular events that lead to a sustained contraction. It has been suggested that activation of mitogen-activated protein kinase (MAPK) may be associated with sustained smooth muscle contraction.[15] Interestingly, activation of the MAPK module has been shown to be a critical player in mediating inflammatory reactions in various cell types, including smooth muscle cells.[16–18] Inflammation is becoming increasingly substantiated as a contributor to AD pathogenesis, and the possible involvement of Aβ in the induction of this inflammatory process has been suggested. For example, the oc-

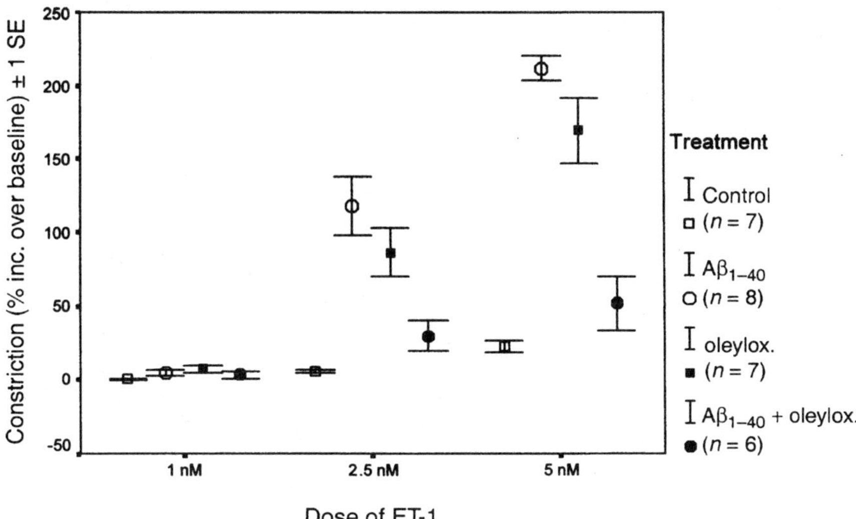

FIGURE 5. Interaction among oleyloxyethylphosphocholine (oleylox.), Aβ, and ET-1 on vasoconstriction. Certain aortic rings were treated with 1 μM freshly solubilized Aβ$_{1-40}$, 1 μM oleylox., or oleylox. + Aβ 5 min prior to the addition of a dose range of ET-1. There were significant main effects by ANOVA of ET-1 dose (p <0.001), Aβ (p <0.001), and oleylox. (p <0.001). There were also significant interactive terms between ET-1 dose and either Aβ (p <0.001) or oleylox. (p <0.001), and among ET-1, Aβ and oleylox. (p <0.001). One-way ANOVA across ET-1 doses revealed significant between-groups differences (p <0.001), and post-hoc testing showed significant differences between control and Aβ (p <0.001), and Aβ and Aβ + oleylox. (p = 0.001).

currence of immune system proteins, activated microglia, and astrocytes in perivascular senile plaques suggests that Aβ may play a substantial role in neuroinflammation.[19–22] Based on such circumstantial evidence for a proinflammatory role of Aβ peptides in AD brains, we asked whether Aβ might mediate vasoactivity through activation of an inflammatory response involving stimulation of the MAPK module. AA release and production of eicosanoids are prerequisites for inflammation, and PLA$_2$s are key enzymes that initiate the AA cascade, which leads to the generation of multiple eicosanoid products during both acute and chronic inflammation. Thus, we first investigated the effect of blocking PLA$_2$ on Aβ vasoactivity.

Data show that inhibition of either cytosolic PLA$_2$ (cPLA$_2$) by MAFP (a specific cPLA$_2$ inhibitor, FIG. 4) or secretory PLA$_2$ (sPLA$_2$) by oleyloxyphosphorylcholine (type I sPLA$_2$ inhibitor, FIG. 5) is sufficient to completely abolish Aβ vasoactivity, suggesting that Aβ mediates its effects via an activation of sPLA$_2$ and cPLA$_2$. Melittin and mastoparan, two small peptides known to stimulate cPLA$_2$, are able to mimic the effects of Aβ by enhancing ET-1-induced vasoconstriction to a similar extent as Aβ. Interestingly, when melittin or mastoparan are used in combination with Aβ, a statistical interaction is observed among ET-1, Aβ, and either peptide, further

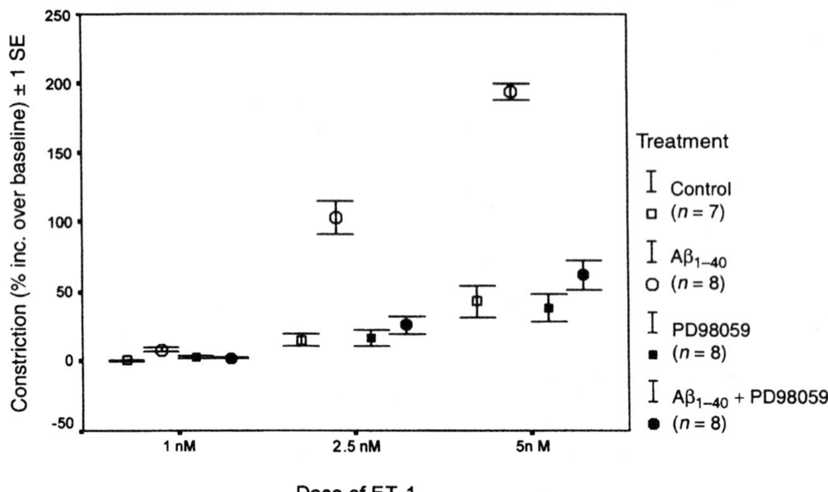

FIGURE 6. Effect of MEK1/2 inhibition on Aβ-enhancement of ET-1-induced vaso-constriction. Certain aortic rings were treated with 1 μM freshly solubilized $A\beta_{1-40}$, 25 μM PD98059, PD98059 + Aβ, or untreated (control) 5 min prior to the addition of a dose range of ET-1. ANOVA revealed significant main effects of ET-1 dose ($p < 0.001$), Aβ ($p < 0.001$), and PD98059 ($p < 0.001$). There were also significant interactive terms between ET-1 dose and either Aβ ($p < 0.001$) or PD98059 ($p < 0.001$), and among ET-1 dose, Aβ, and PD98059 ($p < 0.001$). One-way ANOVA across ET-1 doses revealed significant between-groups differences ($p < 0.001$), and post-hoc testing showed significant differences between control and Aβ ($p < 0.001$), Aβ and Aβ + PD98059 ($p < 0.001$), and control and Aβ + PD98059 ($p < 0.001$), but not between control and PD98059 ($p = 1.00$), or PD98059 and Aβ + PD98059 ($p = 0.880$).

confirming that Aβ vasoactivity is mediated via activation of $cPLA_2$ (data not shown). Low doses of purified type I $sPLA_2$ from porcine pancreas also mimic Aβ's vasoactive effect by enhancing ET-1-induced vasoconstriction to a similar extent as Aβ. Furthermore, as with Aβ, statistical interaction is observed among $sPLA_2$, Aβ, and ET-1 (data not shown). Interestingly, not all of the PLA_2 isoforms are involved in this process. In particular, inactivation of type II $sPLA_2$ with quercetin or inhibition of calcium-independent PLA_2 (type VI) with haloenol lactone suicide substrate (HELSS) does not inhibit Aβ vasoactivity. Moreover, we have confirmed that Aβ vasoactivity is selectively mediated by an activation of the PLA_2 cascade, but not by an activation of phospholipase C, phospholipase D, or protein kinase C. Thus, our data show that the vasoactive effects exerted by Aβ are specifically mediated by an activation of the PLA_2 pathway.

Taken together, our data show that both $sPLA_2$ and $cPLA_2$ are necessary to mediate Aβ vasoactivity, leaving the possibility open that $sPLA_2$ may activate $cPLA_2$. This effect has recently been shown, and involves a stimulation of p38 MAPK, as well as p44/42 MAPK, both of which result in the phosphorylation and concomitant activation of $cPLA_2$.[23-25] Thus, we investigated the effect of inhibition of the MAPK

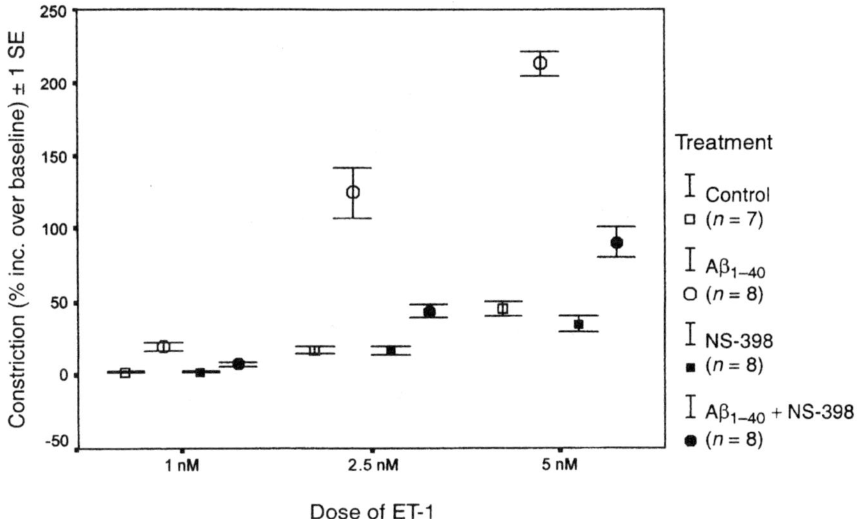

FIGURE 7. Effect of COX-2 inhibition on Aβ-enhancement of ET-1-induced vasoconstriction. Certain aortic rings were treated with 1 μM freshly solubilized Aβ$_{1-40}$, 5 μM NS-398, NS-398 + Aβ, or untreated (control) 5 min prior to the addition of a dose range of ET-1. ANOVA revealed significant main effects of ET-1 dose ($p < 0.001$), Aβ ($p < 0.001$), and NS-398 ($p < 0.001$). There were also significant interactive terms between ET-1 dose and either Aβ ($p < 0.001$) or NS-398 ($p < 0.001$), and among ET-1 dose, Aβ, and NS-398 ($p < 0.001$). One-way ANOVA across ET-1 doses revealed significant between-groups differences ($p < 0.001$), and post-hoc testing showed significant differences between control and Aβ ($p < 0.001$), and Aβ and Aβ + NS-398 ($p = 0.001$).

module in our vessel bath system. Vessels were pretreated with PD 98059, a highly specific MEK1/2 (MAPK kinase) inhibitor that has been shown to completely block the activation of p44/42 MAPK.[25] We observed complete blockade of Aβ vasoactivity by PD 98059, showing that MEK1/2 activity is necessary to mediate Aβ vasoactivity (Fig. 6). Interestingly, PD 98059 was also able to completely inhibit sPLA$_2$ enhancement of ET-1-induced vasoconstriction, showing that sPLA$_2$ induction of vasoconstriction, like Aβ, is essentially mediated via MEK1/2 (data not shown). Moreover, inhibition of p38 MAPK by SB 202190 resulted in complete blockade of Aβ vasoactivity (data not shown), further confirming that the MAPK module is necessary to ensure the activation of cPLA$_2$ via Aβ.

AA will give rise to various eicosanoids, via the cyclooxygenase (COX) and lipoxygenase (LOX) pathways, which are proinflammatory compounds. We show that both COX-2 (Fig. 7) and 5-LOX (data not shown) mediate Aβ vasoactivity, since specific inhibition of COX-2 with NS-398 or 5-LOX by MK-886 results in partial blockade of Aβ vasoactivity. Furthermore, when added in combination, NS-398 and MK-886 completely abolish Aβ's vasoconstrictive effect (data not shown). In the final analysis, we have dissected the intracellular signaling events which leads to the vasoactive properties induced by Aβ peptides. Specifically, our data show that

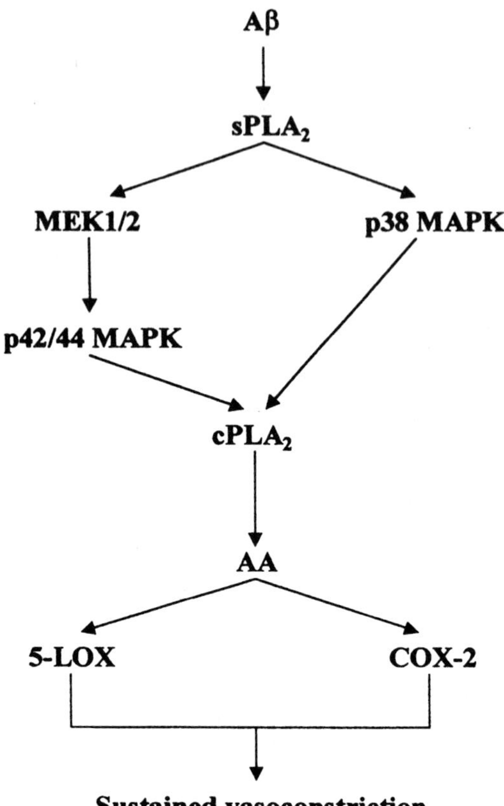

Sustained vasoconstriction

FIGURE 8. Aβ's signaling pathway.

freshly solubilized Aβ induces vasoconstriction by initially stimulating sPLA$_2$, which, in turn, results in activation of the MAPK module, which ensures the stimulation of cPLA$_2$, thus inducing the release of AA. COX-2 and 5-LOX then convert AA into various proinflammatory eicosanoids, which ultimately bring about Aβ's vasoconstrictive effect. These events are summarized in FIGURE 8.

We have previously shown that cyclic guanosine monophosphate (cGMP)-elevating agents, in particular the type V cGMP phosphodiesterase inhibitor dipyridamole, are able to block the Aβ-induced proinflammatory response in microglial cells.[11] Also, these agents are able to inhibit the release of tumor necrosis factor-α (TNF-α) from microglia which are activated by lipopolysaccharide (LPS, data not shown). Interestingly, we have also shown that dipyridamole can block Aβ vasoactivity.[11] We now suggest that dipyridamole and other cGMP-elevating compounds may influence the PLA$_2$ pathway described above, since it has been shown that cGMP can inhibit the MAPK module,[26,27] and, via this mechanism, cGMP-elevating agents may block the induction of cPLA$_2$, thereby inhibiting Aβ's vasoactive effect. Another effect of cGMP is to lower levels of intracellular calcium, by blocking the release of Ca^{++} from intracellular stores as well as the entry of extracellular calcium. Since Ca^{++} is necessary for $cPLA_2$ translocation to the nuclear membrane, where COX-2 and 5-LOX are located, cGMP-elevating agents may inhibit $cPLA_2$ translocation via decreasing intracellular Ca^{++}.

CONCLUSION

We have shown that low doses (in the nM range similar to the level of circulating Aβ found in AD) of freshly solubilized Aβ peptides are able to potentiate ET-1-induced vasoconstriction, and are also able to increase the duration of the constriction induced by various vasoconstrictors. We have dissected the signal transduction pathway that is responsible for the vasoactive properties of soluble Aβ peptides, and find that this effect is mediated via the activation of a proinflammatory pathway. Therefore, our data suggest that soluble Aβ peptides initiate an inflammatory cascade, and, at the clinical level, may be responsible for the initiation of AD-type neuroinflammation prior to Aβ deposition. Since we have shown that specific inhibitors of the PLA_2 pathway are efficient blockers of Aβ's proinflammatory vasoactivity, this provides a basis for novel therapies aimed at blocking Aβ's bioactivity.

ACKNOWLEDGMENTS

This work was supported by the generosity of Mr. and Mrs. Robert Roskamp. M. Mullan is the recipient of a Veteran's Administration Merit Award.

REFERENCES

1. ELLIS, R.J., J.M. OLICHNEY, L.J. THAL, S.S. MIRRA, J.C. MORRIS, D. BEEKLY & A. HEYMAN. 1996. Cerebral amyloid angiopathy in the brains of patients with Alzheimer's disease: the CERAD experience, Part XV. Neurology **46:** 1592–1596.
2. THOMAS, T., G. THOMAS, C. MCLENDON, T. SUTTON & M. MULLAN. 1996. β-Amyloid mediated vasoactivity and vascular endothelial damage. Nature **380:** 168–171.
3. PARIS, D., T.A. PARKER, T. TOWN, Z. SUO, C. FANG, J. HUMPHREY, F. CRAWFORD & M. MULLAN. 1998. Role of peroxynitrite in the vasoactive and cytotoxic effects of Alzheimer's β-amyloid peptide. Exp. Neurol. **152:** 116–122.
4. IADECOLA, C., F. ZHANG, K. NIWA, C. ECKMAN, S. TURNER, E. FISCHER, S. YOUNKIN, D. BORCHELT, K. HSAIO & G. CARLSON. 1999. SOD1 rescues cerebral endothelial dysfunction in mice overexpressing amyloid precursor protein. Nat. Neurosci. **2:** 157–161.
5. DUARA, R., C. GRADY, J. HAXBY, M. SUNDARAM, N.R. CUTLER, L. HESTON, A. MOORE, N. SCHLAGETER, S. LARSON & S.I. RAPOPORT. 1986. Positron emission tomography in Alzheimer's disease. Neurology **36:** 879–887.
6. JOHNSON, K.A., S.T. MUELLER, T.M. WALSHE, R.J. ENGLISH & B.L. HOLMAN. 1987. Cerebral perfusion imaging in Alzheimer's disease. Use of a single photon emission computed tomography and iofetamine hydrochloride I 123. Arch. Neurol. **44:** 165–168.
7. FRIEDLAN, R.P., T.F. BUDINGER, E. GANZ, Y. YANO, C.A. MATHIS, B. KOSS, B.A. OBER, R.H. HUESMAN & S.E. DERENZO. 1983. Regional cerebral metabolic alterations in dementia of the Alzheimer type: positron emission tomography with $[^{18}F]$fluorodeoxyglucose. J. Comput. Assist. Tomogr. **7:** 590–598.

8. ZHANG, F., C. ECKMAN, S. YOUNKIN, K. HSIAO & C. IADECOLA. 1997. Increased susceptibility to ischemic brain damage in mice overexpressing the amyloid precursor protein. J. Neurosci. **17:** 7655–7661.

9. JAGUST, W.J., J.L. EBERLING, B.R. REED, C.A. MATHIS & T.F. BUDINGER. 1997. Clinical studies of cerebral blood flow in Alzheimer's disease. Ann. N.Y. Acad. Sci. **826:** 254–262.

10. NAGATA, K., R.J. BUCHAN, E. YOKOYAMA, Y. KONDOH, M. SATO, H. TERASHI, Y. SATO, Y. WATAHIKI, M. SENOVA, Y. HIRATA & J. HATAZAWA. 1997. Misery perfusion with preserved vascular reactivity in Alzheimer's disease. Ann. N.Y. Acad. Sci. **826:** 272–281.

11. PARIS, D., T. TOWN, T.A. PARKER, J. HUMPHREY, J. TAN, F. CRAWFORD & M. MULLAN. 1999. Inhibition of Alzheimer's β-amyloid induced vasoactivity and pro-inflammatory response in microglia by a cGMP-dependent mechanism. Exp. Neurol. **157:** 211–221.

12. CRAWFORD, F., C. SOTO, Z. SUO, C. FANG, T. PARKER, A. SAWAR, B. FRANGIONE & M. MULLAN. 1998. Alzheimer's β-amyloid vasoactivity: identification of a novel β-amyloid conformational intermediate. FEBS Lett. **436:** 445–448.

13. DOUGLAS, S.A. & E.H. OHLSTEIN. 1997. Signal transduction mechanisms mediating the vascular actions of endothelin. J. Vasc. Res. **34:** 152–164.

14. KUO, Y.M., M.R. EMMERLING, H.R. LAMPERT, S.R. HEMPELMAN, T.A. KOKJOHN, A.S. WOODS, R.J. COTTER & A.E. ROHER. 1999. High levels of circulating Aβ42 are sequestered by plasma proteins in Alzheimer's disease. Biochem. Biophys. Res. Commun. **257:** 787–791.

15. EPSTEIN, A.M., D. THROCKMORTON & C.M. BROPHY. 1997. Mitogen-activated protein kinase activation: an alternate signaling pathway for sustained vascular smooth muscle contraction. J. Vasc. Surg. **26:** 327–332.

16. BALBOA, M.A., J. BALSINDE, D.A. DILLON, G.M. CARMAN & E.A. DENNIS. 1999. Proinflammatory macrophage-activating properties of the novel phospholipid diacylglycerol pyrophosphate. J. Biol. Chem. **274:** 522–526.

17. SAKLATVALA, J., J. DEAN & A. FINCH. 1999. Protein kinase cascades in intracellular signalling by interleukin-1 and tumor necrosis factor. Biochem. Soc. Symp. **64:** 63–77.

18. PARK, J., G.T. GORES & T. PATEL. 1999. Lipopolysaccharide induces cholangiocyte proliferation via an interleukin-6-mediated activation of p44/42 mitogen-activated protein kinase. Hepatology **29:** 1037–1043.

19. CORIA, F., A. MORENO, I. RUBIO, M.A. GARCIA, E. MORATO & F. MAYOR. 1993. The cellular pathology associated with Alzheimer β-amyloid deposits in non-demented aged individuals. Neuropathol. Appl. Neurobiol. **19:** 261–268.

20. GRIFFIN, W.S.T., J.G. SHENG, G.W. ROBERTS & R.E. MRAK. 1995. Interleukin-1 expression in different plaque types in Alzheimer's disease: significance in plaque evolution. J. Neuropathol. Exp. Neurol. **54:** 276–281.

21. ITAGAKI, S., P.L. MCGEER, H. AKIYAMA, S. ZHU & D. SELKOE. 1989. Relationship of microglia and astrocytes to amyloid deposits of Alzheimer's disease. J. Neuroimmunol. **24:** 173–182.

22. LUE, L.F., L. BRACHOVA, W.H. CIVIN & J. ROGERS. 1996. Inflammation, abeta deposition, and neurofibrillary tangle formation as correlates of Alzheimer's disease neurodegeneration. J. Neuropathol. Exp. Neurol. **55:** 1083–1088.

23. MURAKAMI, M., T. KAMBE, S. SHIMBARA & I. KUDO. 1999. Functional coupling between various phospholipase A_2s and cyclooxygenases in immediate and delayed prostanoid biosynthetic pathways. J. Biol. Chem. **274:** 3103–3115.

24. HERNANDEZ, M., S.L. BURILLO, M.S. CRESPO & M.L. NIETO. 1998. Secretory phospholipase A_2 activates the cascade of mitogen-activated protein kinases and cytosolic phospholipase A_2 in the human astrocytoma cell line 1321N1. J. Biol. Chem. **273:** 606–612.

25. HUWILLER, A., G. STAUDT, R.M. KRAMER & J. PFEILSCHIFTER. 1997. Cross-talk between secretory phospholipase A_2 and cytosolic phospholipase A_2 in rat mesangial cells. Biochem. Biophys. Acta **1348:** 257–272.

26. HANEDA, M., S. ARAKI, T. SUGIMOTO, M. TOGAWA, D. KOYA & R. KIKKAWA. 1996. Differential inhibition of mesangial MAP kinase cascade by cyclic nucleotides. Kidney Int. **50:** 384–391.
27. SUGIMOTO, T., R. KIKKAWA, M. HANEDA, S. ARAKI, D. KOYA, M. TOGAWA & Y. SHIGETA. 1995. Cyclic nucleotides attenuate endothelin-1-induced activation of mitogen-activated protein kinase in cultured rat mesangial cells. J. Diabetes Complications **9:** 249–251.

Cerebral Amyloid Angiopathy: Accumulation of Aβ in Interstitial Fluid Drainage Pathways in Alzheimer's Disease

ROY O. WELLER,[a,c] ADRIAN MASSEY,[a] YU-MIN KUO,[b] AND ALEX E. ROHER[b]

[a]*Department of Neuropathology, University of Southampton, Southampton, UK*

[b]*Haldeman Laboratory for Alzheimer Disease Research, Sun Health Research Institute, Sun City, Arizona 85151, USA*

ABSTRACT: Cerebral amyloid angiopathy (CAA) is characterized by the accumulation of β-amyloid (Aβ) peptides in the walls of arteries both in the cortex and meninges. Here, we test the hypothesis that CAA results from the progressive accumulation of Aβ in the perivascular interstitial fluid drainage pathways of the brain. Experimental studies have shown that interstitial fluid (ISF) from the rat brain flows along periarterial spaces to join the cerebrospinal fluid (CSF) to drain to cervical lymph nodes. Such lymphatic drainage plays a key role in B-cell and T-cell mediated immunity of the brain. Anatomical studies have defined periarterial ISF drainage pathways in the human brain that are homologous with the lymphatic pathways in the rat brain but are largely separate from the CSF. Periarterial channels in the brain in man are in continuity with those of leptomeningeal arteries and can be traced from the brain to the extracranial portions of the internal carotid arteries related to deep cervical lymph nodes. The pattern of deposition of Aβ in senile plaques and in CAA suggests that Aβ accumulates in pericapillary and periarterial ISF drainage pathways. Aβ could accumulate in CAA due to either (i) increased production of Aβ, (ii) reduced solubility of Aβ peptides, or (iii) impedance of drainage of Aβ along periarterial ISF drainage pathways within the brain and leptomeninges due to aging factors in cerebral arteries. Elucidation of factors that reduce elimination of Aβ via perivascular drainage pathways may lead to their rectification and to new strategies for treatment of Alzheimer's disease.

INTRODUCTION

Alzheimer's disease is characterized by the intracellular accumulation of neurofibrillary tangles containing ubiquitin and hyperphosphorylated tau, and by extracellular plaques of β-amyloid (Aβ) peptides. In addition to accumulation within senile plaques, Aβ also accumulates in the walls of capillaries and arteries within the brain and in leptomeningeal arteries as cerebral amyloid angiopathy (CAA). CAA may occur throughout the cerebral hemispheres and in the cerebellum but is most

[c]Address for correspondence: Professor R.O. Weller, M.D., Ph.D., FRCPath, Department of Pathology (Neuropathology), Mailpoint 813, Laboratory and Pathology Block, Southampton General Hospital, Southampton, SO16 6YD, UK. Tel.: +44(0)1703 796669; fax: +44(0)1703 796603.

e-mail: row@soton.ac.uk

prevalent in the occipital lobes.[1] In a number of types of familial Alzheimer's disease, excessive Aβ deposition appears to be due to overproduction of Aβ peptides associated with defects in the amyloid precursor protein gene on chromosome 21; similar overproduction of Aβ peptides occurs in Down's syndrome with Trisomy 21.[2] CAA is present in 62–95% of patients with Alzheimer's disease and consistently in Down's syndrome, but it also occurs in the brains of nondemented elderly individuals.[3] In some patients, CAA is very prominent and is associated with intracerebral hemorrhage, especially in the syndromes of hereditary cerebral hemorrhage with amyloidosis (HCHWA), of the Dutch, Flemish and British types.[4] It is not only Aβ peptides, however, that accumulate in the walls of cerebral arteries as CAA occurs in cystatin C amyloidosis and in familial prion diseases.[4,5] This suggests that there may be a common factor in the deposition of all these proteins within perivascular compartments and blood vessel walls, and that common factor is the focus of this paper.

A number of mechanisms have been proposed for the deposition of Aβ in blood vessel walls in CAA. The close association of plaques of amyloid with cerebral capillaries and the confluence of plaques with capillary basement membranes have led to the suggestion that Aβ is derived from the blood.[6] However, plaques of amyloid only occur in the brain and, although Aβ is described in other tissues such as in skeletal muscle in inclusion body myositis,[7] it rarely accumulates in the extracellular spaces of organs other than the brain. It has also been proposed that the Aβ deposited in blood vessel walls in CAA is due to its production by smooth muscle cells.[8] But, CAA predominantly affects small arteries and not the larger intracranial arteries which contain more smooth muscle cells; furthermore, CAA rarely, if ever, occurs in extracranial arteries.[9]

In the present study, we explore the concept that the accumulation of Aβ peptides within senile plaques and in the walls of blood vessels in CAA, reflects a failure of the elimination of Aβ peptides along the perivascular interstitial fluid (lymphatic) drainage pathways of the human brain.

PERIVASCULAR DRAINAGE OF INTERSTITIAL FLUID (ISF) AND PROTEINS FROM THE BRAIN

Extracellular fluid in the brain can be broadly divided into cerebrospinal fluid (CSF) in the ventricles and interstitial fluid (ISF) within the grey and white matter of the brain itself. Experiments in animals such as the rat have shown that some 50% of tracer injected into the ventricular or cisternal CSF drains to cervical lymph nodes.[10] Arachnoid villi are very small and primitive in the rat but may account for the other 50% of CSF drainage.[11] When tracers are injected into the grey matter of the rat brain, they pass along periarterial spaces within the brain and alongside arteries in the subarachnoid space to the cribriform plate, enter nasal lymphatics and drain to lymph nodes in the neck[11,12] (FIG. 1). Resident macrophages (perivascular cells) ingest proteins and particles within these periarterial fluid drainage pathways.[12]

The immunological significance of lymphatic drainage of ISF from the rat brain has been illustrated both for B-cell and for T-cell mediated immunity. Injection of

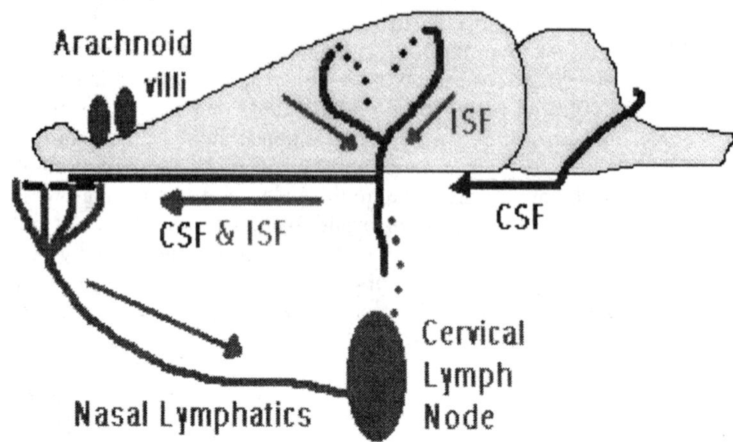

FIGURE 1. Lymphatic drainage of interstitial fluid (ISF) and cerebrospinal fluid (CSF) from the rat brain. ISF drains along perivascular pathways, both within the brain and alongside the middle cerebral artery. CSF enters the subarachnoid space from the ventricular system, and, together with ISF, drains alongside the ethmoidal artery to the cribriform plate and thence into nasal lymphatics to the cervical lymph nodes. Some drainage also occurs alongside the internal carotid artery. Primitive arachnoid villi account for some intracranial fluid drainage.

human serum albumin into the caudate-putamen of the rat brain results in antibody production predominantly in cervical lymph nodes; removal of these nodes results in a significant reduction in the antibody response.[10] Involvement of cervical lymph nodes in T-cell mediated immunity has been determined through a series of experiments with experimental autoimmune encephalomyelitis (EAE).[13–15] When active, acute EAE is induced by injection of antigen in complete Freund's adjuvant into the foot pads of Lewis rats, the initial inflammatory disease is predominantly in the spinal cord. A brain wound, in the form of a cryolesion to one cerebral hemisphere, results in a sixfold increase in inflammation in the brain,[13] but this enhancement of cerebral EAE is reduced by 50% if the cervical lymph nodes are removed at the time of the cryolesion.[14] The results of these experiments and of adoptive transfer studies[15] suggest that cervical lymph nodes play a very significant role in the development of T-cell mediated inflammatory reactions in the brain possibly as the major source of T lymphocytes that home to the brain.

DRAINAGE OF CSF AND ISF FROM THE HUMAN BRAIN

In man, it appears that the drainage pathways for the CSF have become largely separated from the ISF drainage pathways.[16] A large amount (some 350 µl/min) of CSF is produced by the choroid plexuses and flows through the ventricular system into the subarachnoid space. Numerous studies have shown that the major pathways for the drainage of CSF in man are via arachnoid granulations and villi associated with venous sinuses in the dura mater (FIG. 2a).[16] The extensive investigation of CSF

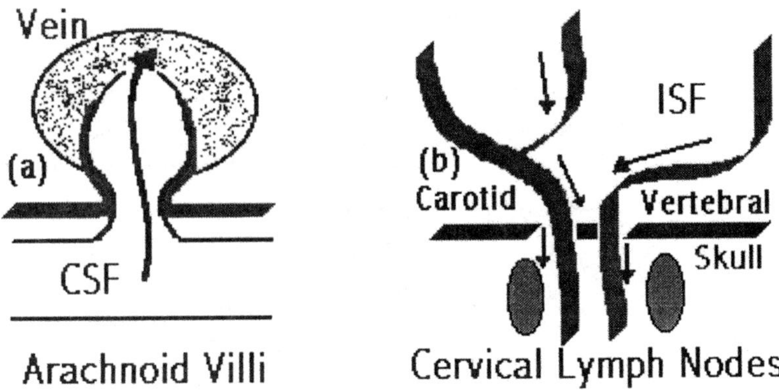

FIGURE 2. Separation of CSF and interstitial fluid (ISF) drainage from the human brain. **(a)** The classical pathway of drainage of CSF from the subarachnoid space through arachnoid granulations and villi into veins in the dura. **(b)** The putative lymphatic drainage pathways of ISF are along perivascular spaces of branches of the internal carotid and vertebral arteries, passing through the base of the skull to the region of cervical lymph nodes.

with its large daily volume and ease of access has overshadowed the investigation of ISF drainage from the human brain.[16]

Anatomical studies have shown that periarterial compartments, homologous with ISF drainage pathways in the rat, are present in the human brain.[17,18] Extracellular spaces in the brain are very narrow, and the pericapillary and periarterial channels appear to act as conduits for bulk drainage of ISF.[10] The basement membrane surrounding capillaries may act as the initial conduit for ISF draining from grey matter; this pericapillary compartment may enlarge under conditions of cerebral inflammation and cerebral edema by the separation of the endothelial and glial components of the basement membrane and the creation of a wider perivascular space. Arterioles within the cortex have a perivascular space surrounded not only by the glia limitans but also by a layer of leptomeningeal cells derived from the pia mater.[17] In normal brain, this space is largely occupied by basement membrane coating the smooth muscle cells. At the surface of the brain (FIG. 3), the periarterial compartments are continuous with those of leptomeningeal arteries and are separated from the subpial and subarachnoid spaces by a coating of leptomeninges. Perivascular compartments of leptomeningeal arteries are wider than those of cortical arteries, and they contain loosely packed collagen fibres; this compartment becomes widely dilated when there is edema of the underlying cortex. The perivascular compartment of leptomenigeal arteries can be followed to the middle cerebral artery to become continuous with the perivascular compartment of the internal carotid artery as it traverses the base of the skull (Kelsey, Djuanda & Weller, manuscript in preparation). Just below the carotid foramen are deep cervical lymph nodes that are closely associated with the internal carotid arteries. Thus, there is a continuous periarterial compartment that can be traced anatomically from capillaries and arteries within the brain to lymph nodes in the neck as the putative lymphatic drainage pathways for ISF from the human brain

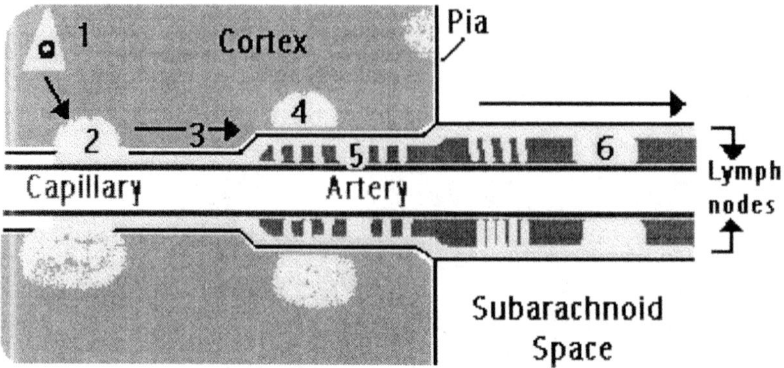

FIGURE 3. Elimination of β-amyloid peptides from the brain: a working hypothesis. The perivascular space is continuous from brain capillaries to the internal carotid artery in the neck. (1) β-Amyloid produced by cells within the CNS accumulates in the extracellular space. (2) Plaques related to the glia limitans and continuous with Aβ in capillary perivascular spaces. (3) It is proposed that amyloid moves in the direction of the *arrow* towards intracortical arteries. (4) Plaques of Aβ around arteries, in general, stop at the glia limitans and do not enter directly into the perivascular space. (5) Within arterial walls, Aβ is mainly in basement membrane on the surface of the artery and surrounding smooth muscle cells (shown here as *light bands* in the artery wall). (6) As Aβ flows along perivascular spaces (direction of *arrow*) in leptomeningeal arteries, it also accumulates between smooth muscle cells and as large deposits within the artery wall. It is suggested here that in this way Aβ may drain all the way to cervical lymph nodes.

(FIG. 2b). It is not feasible to perform, in man, the tracer experiments that are possible in the rat, but Aβ peptides appear to serve as as natural tracers to define the ISF drainage pathways from the human brain.

ACCUMULATION OF Aβ IN ISF DRAINAGE PATHWAYS IN CAA

Biochemical, histological and immunocytochemical studies of brains from patients with Alzheimer's disease and from nondemented elderly patients strongly suggest that Aβ accumulates in pericapillary and periarterial ISF drainage pathways in CAA.[5] Drawing upon data from this study[5] and from many other descriptions of Aβ deposition in the brain and blood vessel walls, it is possible to construct a working hypothesis for the elimination of Aβ peptides from the normal brain and to suggest how drainage of Aβ may be impeded due to age changes in cerebral arteries. FIGURE 3 sets out the proposed pathway by which the Aβ, produced by cells in the central nervous system (CNS), passes through interstitial spaces towards the low-resistant perivascular drainage channels. Plaques of Aβ form within the extracellular space, and many fibrillar Aβ plaques are associated with capillaries, both in the white matter and in the cortex.[6] Thus, when blood vessels are isolated, such plaques can be seen arranged as globules on the surface of small blood vessels, and there is linear deposition of Aβ in their walls.[5] Electron microscopy has shown that fibrillar plaques are confluent with the basement membrane and that Aβ is present in the perivascular spaces of very small blood vessels.[6] Elimination of Aβ could be blocked at the perivascular glia limitans, on its entry into pericapillary compartments or by impedance of flow along compartments in the walls of intracortical and leptomeningeal arteries.

Plaques of Aβ in the glia limitans around arteries tend not to be confluent with the walls of arteries in the same way that they are confluent with capillary basement membranes. This suggests that Aβ enters perivascular spaces mainly at the capillary level and then flows along vessel walls into periarterial compartments (FIG. 3). Aβ accumulation in leptomeningeal arteries is heaviest in the small arteries (<60 μm in diameter), often with replacement of smooth muscle in the artery wall by Aβ.[5] In the larger vessels, small deposits may be seen in the periarterial connective tissue suggesting that this peripheral compartment is the pathway for ISF and Aβ drainage from the brain and that only later does Aβ accumulate in the media.[5] Although the larger arteries, such as the middle cerebral and basilar arteries, rarely contain stainable deposits of amyloid, biochemical studies have revealed the presence of Aβ peptides, not only in the walls of these vessels in Alzheimer's disease but also in normal young adults;[9] in that study, no Aβ was detected in extracranial portions of the internal carotid artery. These observations, again, suggest that Aβ drains along perivascular compartments even of the larger vessels possibly en route to the cervical lymph nodes (FIG. 3).

CAUSES AND EFFECTS OF Aβ ACCUMULATION IN THE BRAIN AND IN ARTERY WALLS

If, as strongly suggested by the evidence,[5] Aβ accumulates in ISF drainage pathways, both within the brain and in leptomeningeal vessels, defining the reasons why elimination of Aβ fails would be important for devising therapeutic strategies for Alzheimer's disease. Although the more soluble $A\beta_{1-40}$ is detected in walls of large leptomeningeal arteries in younger people, the relative proportion of the more insoluble $A\beta_{1-42}$ to the more soluble $A\beta_{1-40}$ is higher in cortical vessels than in leptomeningeal vessels.[19] In CAA, some vascular amyloid deposits in vessels are solely composed of $A\beta_{1-42}$, but deposits consisting of $A\beta_{1-40}$ alone have not been recorded.[9] Such observations suggest that $A\beta_{1-42}$, derived from the brain, may be the initial amyloid to be deposited in vessel walls and that it entraps the more soluble $A\beta_{1-40}$, which would normally drain from the brain along perivascular spaces more easily than $A\beta_{1-42}$ due to its greater solubility.[5]

There may be a number of reasons why Aβ is deposited in artery walls: (a) Aβ may bind to collagen IV and to glycosaminoglycans present within the vessel wall;[20] (b) there could be a defect in a chaperon molecule that decreases the solubility of Aβ; the association of CAA with the apolipoprotein E_4 isotype[21] suggests that there may be a defect in apolipoprotein transport molecules; or (c) there may be a decrease in the normal motive force by which Aβ drains along periarterial pathways.

The close association of Aβ with smooth muscle cells in CAA suggests that the motive force for the drainage of ISF and Aβ could be the pulsation of the artery with its regular dilatation and recoil driving ISF and proteins in the opposite direction to the flow of blood through the lumen of the vessel. If this is the case, the changes in elasticity of cerebral arteries that occur in arteriosclerosis may impede the flow of ISF and $A\beta$ from the brain. Advancing age is not only a risk factor for the development of Alzheimer's disease but it is also a risk factor for development of arteriosclerosis with thickening of the intima, fibrosis of vessel walls, and increasing rigidity and ectasia of larger intracranial arteries such as the middle cerebral and basilar arteries. Whereas in infants and young adults, the internal elastic lamina is highly corrugated in the relaxed artery, in an arteriosclerotic artery, the wall may be held in a more distended state reflecting a lack of expansion and elastic recoil during systole and diastole. Such a reduction in expansion, recoil, and pulsation of aging arteries may be a factor in reducing the motive force for drainage of ISF and proteins, including $A\beta$, from the brain.

The consequences of $A\beta$ accumulation within vessel walls in CAA are more clearly defined. An increase in frequency of intracerebral hemorrhage in CAA is probably due to weakening of the vessel wall following replacement of smooth muscle cells by $A\beta$ with the consequent formation and rupture of aneurysms. Furthermore, $A\beta$ deposition may affect constriction of arteries and, therefore, perfusion and autoregulation. Such changes may play a significant role in the clinical symptomatology of Alzheimer's disease.

THERAPEUTIC IMPLICATIONS

The studies outlined above suggest that one important factor in the accumulation of $A\beta$ in the brains of demented and nondemented elderly individuals is reduced elimination of $A\beta$ due to impedence of ISF drainage from the brain. If this is due to defects in chaperon molecules, possibly apolipoprotein E (ApoE), therapeutic strategies to compensate for defective chaperon molecules may lead to the prevention of amyloid accumulation. Control of hypertension and cerebrovascular disease may also play a role in maintaining motive forces for the drainage of ISF and $A\beta$ peptides from the brain, through a reduction in arteriosclerosis.

REFERENCES

1. PREMKUMAR, D.R., D.L. COHEN, P. HEDERA, R.P. FRIEDLAND & R.N. KALARIA. 1996. Apolipoprotein E ε4 alleles in cerebral amyloid angiopathy and cerebrovascular pathology in Alzheimer's disease. Am. J. Pathol. **148:** 2083–2095.
2. STOREY, E. & R. CAPPAI. 1999. The amyloid precursor protein of Alzheimer's disease and the $A\beta$ peptide. Neuropathol. Appl. Neurobiol. **25:** 81–97.
3. VINTERS, H.V., Z.Z. WANG & D.L. SECOR. 1996. Brain parenchymal and microvascular amyloid in Alzheimer's disease. Brain Pathol. **6:** 179–195.
4. COHEN, D.L., P. HEDERA, D.R.D. PREMKUMAR, R.P. FRIEDLAND & R.N. KALARIA. 1997. Amyloid-β protein angiopathies masquerading as Alzheimer's disease? Ann. N.Y. Acad. Sci. **826:** 390–395.
5. WELLER, R.O., A. MASSEY, T.A. NEWMAN, M. HUTCHINGS, Y.-M. KUO & A.E. ROHER. 1998. Cerebral amyloid angiopathy: β-amyloid accumulates in putative interstitial fluid drainage pathways in Alzheimer's disease. Am. J. Pathol. **153:** 725–734.
6. MIYAKAWA, T. 1997. Electron microscopy of amyloid fibrils and microvessels. Ann. N.Y. Acad. Sci. **826:** 25–34.

7. ASKANAS, V., W.K. ENGEL, C.C. YANG, R.B. ALVAREZ, V.M. LEE & T. WISNIEWSKI. 1998. Light and electron microscopic immunolocalization of presenilin 1 in abnormal muscle fibers of patients with sporadic inclusion-body myositis and autosomal-recessive inclusion-body myopathy. Am. J. Pathol. **152:** 889–895.

8. WISNIEWSKI, H., J. WEGIEL & L. KOTULA. 1996. Some neuropathological aspects of Alzheimer disease and its relevance to other disciplines. Neuropathol. Appl. Neurobiol. **22:** 3–11.

9. SHINKAI, Y., M. YOSHIMURA, Y. ITO, A. ODAKA, N. SUZUKI, K. YANAGISAWA & Y. IHARA. 1995. Amyloid beta-proteins 1–40, and 1–42(43) in the soluble fraction of extra- and intracranial blood vessels. Ann. Neurol. **38:** 421–428.

10. CSERR, H.F., C.J. HARLING-BERG & P.M. KNOPF. 1992. Drainage of brain extracellular fluid into blood and deep cervical lymph and its immunological significance. Brain Pathol. **2:** 269–276.

11. KIDA, S., A. PANTAZIS & R.O. WELLER. 1993. CSF drains directly from the subarachnoid space into nasal lymphatics in the rat. Anatomy, histology and immunological significance. Neuropathol. Appl. Neurobiol. **19:** 480–488.

12. ZHANG, E.T., H.K. RICHARDS, S. KIDA & R.O. WELLER. 1992. Directional and compartmentalised drainage of interstitial fluid and cerebrospinal fluid from the rat brain. Acta Neuropathol. **83:** 233–239.

13. PHILLIPS, M.J., R.O. WELLER, S. KIDA & F. IANNOTTI. 1995 Focal brain damage enhances experimental allergic encephalomyelitis in brain and spinal cord. Neuropathol. Appl. Neurobiol. **21:** 189–200.

14. PHILLIPS, M.J., M. NEEDHAM & R.O. WELLER. 1997. Role of cervical lymph nodes in autoimmune encephalomyelitis in the Lewis rat. J. Pathol. **182:** 457–464.

15. LAKE , J., R.O. WELLER, M.J. PHILLIPS & M.J. NEEDHAM. 1999. Lymphocyte targeting of the brain in adoptive transfer cryolesion-EAE. J. Pathol. **187:** 259–265.

16. WELLER, R.O. 1998. Pathology of cerebrospinal fluid and interstitial fluid of the CNS: significance for Alzheimer disease, prion disorders and multiple sclerosis. J. Neuropathol. Exp. Neurol. **57:** 885–894.

17. ZHANG, E.T., C.B.E. INMAN & R.O. WELLER. 1990. Interrelationships of the pia mater and the perivascular (Virchow-Robin) spaces in the human cerebrum. J. Anat. **170:** 111–123.

18. POLLOCK, H., M. HUTCHINGS, R.O. WELLER & E.-T. ZHANG. 1997. Perivascular spaces in the basal ganglia of the human brain: their relationship to lacunes. J. Anat. **191:** 337–346.

19. ROHER. A.E. 1993. β-Amyloid (1–42) is a major component of cerebrovascular amyloid deposits: implications for the pathology of Alzheimer's disease. Proc. Natl. Acad. Sci. USA **90:** 10836–10840.

20. ZHANG, W.W., H. LEMPESSI & Y OLSSON. 1998. Amyloid angiopathy of the human brain: immunohistochemical studies using markers for components of extracellular matrix, smooth muscle actin and endothelial cells. Acta Neuropathol. **96:** 558–563.

21. ALONZO, N.C., B.T. HYMAN, G.W. REBECK & S.M. GREENBERG. 1998. Progression of cerebral amyloid angiopathy: accumulation of amyloid-beta40 in affected vessels. J. Neuropathol. Exp. Neurol. **57:** 353–359.

Traumatic Brain Injury Elevates the Alzheimer's Amyloid Peptide $A\beta_{42}$ in Human CSF

A Possible Role for Nerve Cell Injury

M.R. EMMERLING,[a,e] M.C. MORGANTI-KOSSMANN,[b] T. KOSSMANN,[b] P.F. STAHEL,[b] M.D. WATSON,[a] L.M. EVANS,[a] P.D. MEHTA,[c] K. SPIEGEL,[a] Y.-M. KUO,[d] A.E. ROHER,[d] AND C.A. RABY[a]

[a]*Neuroscience Therapeutics, Parke-Davis Pharmaceutical Research Division, Warner-Lambert Company, 2800 Plymouth Road., Ann Arbor, Michigan 48105, USA*

[b]*Department of Surgery, Division of Trauma Surgery, University Hospital, CH-8091 Zürich, Switzerland*

[c]*New York Institute for Basic Research, 1050 Forrest Hill Road, Staten Island, New York 10314, USA*

[d]*Haldeman Laboratory for Alzheimer's Disease Research, Sun Health Research Institute, Sun City, Arizona 85372, USA*

ABSTRACT: The increased risk for Alzheimer's Disease (AD) associated with traumatic brain injury (TBI) suggests that environmental insults may influence the development of this age-related dementia. Recently, we have shown that the levels of the β-amyloid peptide ($A\beta_{1-42}$) increase in the cerebrospinal fluid (CSF) of patients after severe brain injury and remain elevated for some time after the initial event. The relationships of elevated $A\beta$ with markers of blood-brain barrier (BBB) disruption, inflammation, and nerve cell or axonal injury were evaluated in CSF samples taken daily from TBI patients. This analysis reveals that the rise in $A\beta_{1-42}$ is best correlated with possible markers of neuronal or axonal injury, the cytoskeletal protein *tau*, neuron-specific enolase (NSE), and apolipoprotein E (ApoE). Similar or better correlations were observed between $A\beta_{1-40}$ and the three aforementioned markers. These results imply that the degree of brain injury may play a decisive role in determining the levels of $A\beta_{1-42}$ and $A\beta_{1-40}$ in the CSF of TBI patients. Inflammation and alterations in BBB may play lesser, but nonetheless significant, roles in determining the $A\beta$ level in CSF after brain injury.

INTRODUCTION

How does the β-amyloid peptide ($A\beta$) come to dominate the Alzheimer disease (AD) brain? In a handful of AD cases (less than 5%), genetic mutations in the genes coding for the β-amyloid precursor protein ($A\beta PP$) on chromosome 21, or for pres-

[e]Address for correspondence: Mark R. Emmerling, Ph.D., Parke-Davis, 2800 Plymouth Road, Ann Arbor, MI 48106. Tel.: (734) 622-5917; fax: (734) 622-1193.
  e-mail: mark.emmerling@wl.com

enilin protein 1 (PS1) or 2 (PS2), respectively on chromosomes 14 and 1, lead to increased $A\beta$ production by cells, especially the longer form with 42 amino acids.[1] However, we are still trying to grasp what factors lead to the accumulation of $A\beta$ in the vast majority of AD cases. Recently, more attention has been focused on the role of environmental factors in the development of AD. In particular, factors that chronically diminish cerebral perfusion or cause nerve cell damage like brain trauma, or cardiovascular and cerebral vascular diseases, have become suspects in this sabotage. It has been well documented since 1990 that severe traumatic brain injury (TBI) associated with accidents or boxing lead to amyloid deposition in brain and an increased risk for AD. The cascade of events suspected of being initiated by brain trauma[3] are not that dissimilar from those suggested for AD.[4] The increased immunocytochemical detection of $A\beta$ in brains after TBI indicates that some or all of the pathophysiological changes in the central nervous system (CNS) contribute to the formation and/or accumulation of this amyloid peptide. Recently, we found that the average level of $A\beta_{1-42}$ increases in the cerebrospinal fluid (CSF) from patients with severe brain injury. Presumably, this elevation of $A\beta$ in the CSF reflects changes in the CNS resulting from trauma or inflammation. In the present study, we performed correlation analyses on $A\beta_{1-40}$ and $A\beta_{1-42}$ in CSF from TBI patients with markers of blood-brain barrier (BBB) dysfunction, inflammation, the acute phase response, and axonal or neuronal damage. The results suggest that neuronal damage might be crucial to the observed elevation of $A\beta$ in the CSF of TBI patients.

METHODS

Samples of CSF were obtained daily from brain trauma patients through intraventricular catheters as described previously.[5] The cohort under study has already been described.[6] The CSF samples were collected on ice over 24-h periods from each patient, centrifuged, and thereafter stored at $-70°C$. A total of 113 CSF samples was obtained from the six TBI patients. Phenotyping of apolipoprotein E (ApoE) in these patients was also done.[7] All patients survived their accidents.

The measurement of $A\beta_{1-40}$, $A\beta_{1-42}$, and $A\beta PP$ has been described previously.[6] The quantitation of the cytokines tumor necrosis factor-α (TNF-α), interleukin 6 (IL-6), interleukin 8 (IL-8), and transforming growth factor-β (TGF-β) was measured by methods reported in previous publications,[8] as were the measurements of tau,[9] α-antichymotrypsin (α_1-ACT),[10] neuron-specific enolase (NSE),[11] and ApoE.[12]

Correlation analysis was done using a Spearman r, two-tailed test using commercially available statistical software (Prism; Graphpad Sorftware, San Diego). Comparisons were performed between the daily values of the various parameters measured by our biochemical assays.

RESULTS

On the average, the levels of $A\beta_{1-40}$ found in CSF from TBI patients were significantly different only from $A\beta_{1-40}$ levels in non-AD CSF.[6] Nonetheless, we found that the level of $A\beta_{1-40}$ correlated best with the amount of ApoE (r = 0.691,

TABLE 1. Spearman r correlations between Aβ levels and other markers in CSF from TBI patients

	$A\beta_{1-40}$	$A\beta_{1-42}$
Albumin	0.39 ($p = 0.0001$)	0.254 ($p = 0.01$)
Neuronal markers		
Tau	0.39 ($p = 0.0005$)	0.513 ($p < 0.0001$)
NSE	0.350 ($p = 0.0006$)	0.48 ($p < 0.0001$)
Acute phase proteins		
AβPP	NS[a]	NS
ApoE	0.691 ($p < 0.0001$)	0.514 ($p < 0.0001$)
α_1-ACT	0.239 ($p = 0.0240$)	NS
Cytokines		
IL-6	0.30 ($p = 0.0012$)	0.26 ($p = 0.005$)
IL-8	NS	NS
TGF-β	0.39 ($p < 0.0001$)	0.36 ($p = 0.0003$)
TNF-α	NS	NS

[a]NS = not significant.

$p < 0.0001$) present in the CSF of TBI patients. The "r value" accounted for almost 49% of the variability between the levels of ApoE and $A\beta_{1-40}$. Because the patients in this study were phenotyped as ApoE ε2 or ApoE ε3, it was not possible to determine if ApoE ε4 influenced the CSF levels of $A\beta_{1-40}$. The remaining calculated "r values" between $A\beta_{1-40}$ and the other CSF markers were 0.39 or less.

With regard to $A\beta_{1-42}$, the amount in CSF from TBI patients was significantly higher than that measured in CSF from control and AD subjects.[6] Correlations between $A\beta_{1-42}$ with ApoE ($p < 0.0001$), *tau* ($p < 0.0001$), or NSE ($p < 0.0001$) have had similar and statistically significant "r values" (0.48–0.51), each accounting for about 25% of the variability of $A\beta_{1-42}$. The remaining correlation coefficients were 0.36 or less. The tau levels measured in CSF from our TBI cohort (2308 ng/ml of CSF) were higher than those reported in CSF from normal and AD patients[13] and in good agreement with the results (1,519 ng/ml of CSF) recently published by Zemlan.[14]

DISCUSSION

NSE,[11] tau,[14] and ApoE[15] are all suggested to be markers of nerve cell damage. Based on the substantial correlations between $A\beta_{1-42}$ and tau, NSE, and ApoE, it is tempting to speculate that a major factor determining the levels of $A\beta_{1-42}$ in CSF from TBI patients is neuronal and axonal injury. Studies done in AβPP transgenic mice show a similar relationship in that neuronal death in the hippocampus after TBI in these animals relates to a transitory increase in brain levels of $A\beta_{1-42}$.[16] Smaller but significant correlations with $A\beta_{1-42}$ were determined with the cytokines IL-6 and TGF-β, but not TNF-α or IL-8 measured in the CSF from TBI patients. Again, this may suggest that damage rather than inflammation *per se* governs the increased expression of $A\beta_{1-42}$, since both IL-6 and TGF-β may be associated with an acute phase response.

Further study is needed to understand fully the implications of these associations and their relevance to AD. However, it is provocative that CSF samples taken from mildly cognitively impaired individuals show increased $A\beta_{1-42}$ levels preceding the development of AD dementia.[17] Taken literally, the above observations imply that the elevation of $A\beta_{1-42}$ in CSF from individuals possibly reflects underlying nerve cell injury. It follows that the decrease in $A\beta_{1-42}$ in CSF seen in late stages of AD might be a consequence of nerve cell loss, rather than a consequence of $A\beta$ sequestration in amyloid plaques. It will be of great interest to determine if volumetric changes seen in medial temporal lobes of individuals who go on to develop AD[18] also exhibit at the same time an elevation of $A\beta_{1-42}$ in their CSF.

REFERENCES

1. SELKOE, D.J. 1998. The cell biology of β-amyloid precursor protein and presenilin in Alzheimer's disease. Trends Cell Biol. **8:** 447–453.
2. NICOLL, J.A., G.W. ROBERTS & D.I. GRAHAM. 1996. Amyloid β-protein, APOE genotype and head injury. Ann. N.Y. Acad Sci. **777:** 271–275.
3. STAHEL, P.F., M.C. MORGANTI-KOSSMANN & T. KOSSMANN. 1998. The role of the complement system in traumatic brain injury. Brain Res. Brain Res. Rev. **27:** 243–256.
4. EMMERLING, M.R., S. GRACON & A.E. ROHER. 1999. Towards a Unifying Hypothesis of Alzheimer's Disease: Pathogenesis and Pathophysiology.: 33–53. Martin Dunitz Ltd. London.
5. KOSSMANN, T., V.H. HANS, H.G. IMHOF, R. STOCKER, P. GROB O. TRENTZ & C. MORGANTI-KOSSMANN. 1995. Intrathecal and serum interleukin-6 and the acute-phase response in patients with severe traumatic brain injuries. Shock **4:** 311–317.
6. RABY, C.A., M.C. MORGANTI-KOSSMANN, T. KOSSMANN, P.F. STAHEL, M.D. WATSON, L.M. EVANS, P.D. MEHTA, K. SPIEGEL, Y.M. KUO, A.E. ROHER & M.R. EMMERLING. 1998. Traumatic brain injury increases β-amyloid peptide 1–42 in cerebrospinal fluid. J. Neurochem. **71:** 2505–2509.
7. LEHTIMAKI, T., T. PIRTTILA, P.D. MEHTA, H.M. WISNIEWSKI, H. FREY & T. NIKKARI. 1995. Apolipoprotein E (ApoE) polymorphism and its influence on ApoE concentrations in the cerebrospinal fluid in Finnish patients with Alzheimer's disease. Hum. Genet. **95:** 39–42.
8. MORGANTI-KOSSMAN, M.C., P.M. LENZLINGER, V. HANS, P. STAHEL, E. CSUKA, E. AMMANN, R. STOCKER, O. TRENTZ & T. KOSSMANN. 1997. Production of cytokines following brain injury: beneficial and deleterious for the damaged tissue. Mol. Psychiatry **2:** 133–136.
9. VANDERMEEREN, M., M. MERCKEN, E. VANMECHELEN, J. SIX, A. VAN DE VOORDE, J.J. MARTIN & P. CRAS. 1993. Detection of tau proteins in normal and Alzheimer's disease cerebrospinal fluid with a sensitive sandwich enzyme-linked immunosorbent assay. J. Neurochem. **61:** 1828–1834.
10. PIRTTILA, T., P.D. MEHTA, H. FREY & H.M. WISNIEWSKI. 1994. α-1-Antichymotrypsin and IL-1β are not increased in CSF or serum in Alzheimer's disease. Neurobiol. Aging **15:** 313–317.
11. ROSS, S.A., R.T. CUNNINGHAM, C.F. JOHNSTON & B.J. ROWLANDS. 1996. Neuron-specific enolase as an aid to outcome prediction in head injury. Br. J. Neurosurg. **10:** 471–476.
12. PIRTTILA, T., H. SOININEN, O. HEINONEN, T. LEHTIMAKI, N. BOGDANOVIC, L. PALJARVI, O. KOSUNEN, B. WINBLAD, P. RIEKKINEN, SR., H.M. WISNIEWSKI & P.D. MEHTA. 1996. Apolipoprotein E (apoE) levels in brains from Alzheimer disease patients and controls. Brain Res. **722:** 71–77.
13. BLENNOW, K., A. WALLIN, H. AGREN, C. SPENGER, J. SIEGFRIED & E. VANMECHELEN. 1995. Tau protein in cerebrospinal fluid: a biochemical marker for axonal degeneration in Alzheimer disease? Mol. Chem. Neuropathol. **26:** 231–245.

14. ZEMLAN, F.P., W.S. ROSENBERG, P.A. LUEBBE, T.A. CAMPBELL, G.E. DEAN, N.E. WEINER, J.A. COHEN, R. RUDICK & D. WOO. 1999. Quantification of axonal damage in traumatic brain injury: affinity purification and characterization of cerebrospinal fluid tau proteins. J. Neurochem. **72:** 741–750.
15. POIRIER, J. 1994. Apolipoprotein E in animal models of CNS injury and in Alzheimer's disease. Trends Neurosci. **17:** 525–530.
16. SMITH, D.H., M. NAKAMURA, T.K. MCINTOSH, J. WANG, A. RODRIGUEZ, X.H. CHEN, R. RAGHUPATHI, K.E. SAATMAN, J. CLEMENS, M.L. SCHMIDT, V.M. LEE & J.Q. TROJANOWSKI. 1998. Brain trauma induces massive hippocampal neuron death linked to a surge in beta-amyloid levels in mice overexpressing mutant amyloid precursor protein. Am. J. Pathol. **153:** 1005–1010.
17. JENSEN, M., J. SCHRODER, M. BLOMBERG, B. ENGVALL, J. PANTEL, N. IDA, H. BASUN, L.O. WAHLUND, E. WERLE, M. JAUSS, K. BEYREUTHER, L. LANNFELT & T. HARTMANN. 1999. Cerebrospinal fluid A beta42 is increased early in sporadic Alzheimer's disease and declines with disease progression. Ann. Neurol. **45:** 504–511.
18. SMITH, A.D. & K.A. JOBST. 1996. Use of structural imaging to study the progression of Alzheimer's disease. Br. Med. Bull. **52:** 575–586.

Prospects for Noninvasive Imaging of Brain Amyloid β in Alzheimer's Disease

R.P. FRIEDLAND,[a,d] J. SHI,[a] J.C. LAMANNA,[b] M.A. SMITH,[c] AND G. PERRY[c]

Departments of [a]Neurology, [b]Anatomy and [c]Pathology, School of Medicine,
Case Western Reserve University, Cleveland, Ohio 44106, USA

ABSTRACT: The brain in patients with Alzheimer's disease (AD) contains large amounts of fibrillary amyloid β protein. Studies attempting to use levels of amyloid β protein in plasma, cerebrospinal fluid or skin as diagnostic tests for the disease have not been fruitful. A method for the noninvasive detection of cerebral amyloid β would be valuable for dementia differential diagnosis, pathophysiology and monitoring of anti-amyloid therapies. Anti-amyloid monoclonal antibody 10H3 has been evaluated as an amyloid-imaging ligand, without success. Important considerations in the development of amyloid-imaging ligands include choice of radiolabel and physical and biological half-lives, route of administration, protein binding, use of control molecules, and imaging techniques. It is important that imaging studies be designed to reflect the slow nature of the process of amyloid deposition. We used a transgenic mouse model overexpressing β protein precursor (βPP) to assess the binding of basic fibroblast growth factor (bFGF) and serum amyloid P component (SAP) to amyloid β (Aβ) plaques in mouse brain. Although the binding of these ligands is similar to AD, neither is found endogenously associated with Aβ deposits. Because SAP is a component of mouse serum, these findings suggest the blood-brain barrier in transgenic mice is not affected as it is in AD. These findings suggest that the transgenic mouse may be used as a model for evaluation of Aβ imaging methods.

INTRODUCTION

Brain imaging with pneumoencephalography first appeared at the beginning of this century and revealed *in vivo* the presence of cortical atrophy in patients with Alzheimer's disease (AD), Pick's disease and related disorders. Thanks to great advances in physics, a variety of brain imaging techniques were subsequently invented. We are now able to document both anatomical and metabolic features of the brain, *in vivo*. However, we have not yet found a way of noninvasively diagnosing or monitoring AD in living patients. The time lag between the onset of AD to the appearance of clinically noticeable symptoms and signs may be 20 years or more. The development of a novel noninvasive method to detect amyloid in AD brain will be helpful to diagnose AD and possibly treat AD in its early stages. Also there is currently no way to assess cerebral amyloid deposition *in vivo*. An amyloid imaging

[d]Address for correspondence: Robert P. Friedland, M.D., Department of Neurology, Case Western Reserve University, School of Medicine, Room TG2A, 10900 Euclid Avenue, Cleveland, OH 44106, USA. Tel.: (216) 368-1912; fax: (216) 368-1989.
e-mail: rpf2@po.cwru.edu

technique would aid our ability to study the pathophysiology of the disease and measure the effects of drugs altering amyloid β (Aβ) aggregation and deposition.

We now have considerable knowledge of the complicated pathological mechanisms and the chronic progression of AD. The Aβ protein which constitutes the core of neuritic plaques and deposits in cerebral vessels (congophilic angiopathy) is the main pathological feature of AD.[1] Other manifestations of AD include neurofibrillary tangles,[2] astrocytic activation,[3,4] decreased cerebral blood flow in temporal and parietal lobes, decreased cerebral metabolic rate of oxygen and glucose,[5,6] cortical atrophy, ventricular enlargement,[7,8] altered patterns of fMRI activation,[9] and altered receptor density and function. These features are not only observed in AD, but also in other neurodegenerative and psychiatric disorders.

POSSIBLE LIGANDS FOR AMYLOID IMAGING STUDIES

We evaluated the use of 10H3, a monoclonal antibody to Aβ protein 1–28, labeled with Tc-99m, and applied single photon emission computed tomography to six subjects with probable AD.[10] Images showed nonspecifically diffuse staining of 10H3 around the scalp and cranial bone marrow, but no evidence of cerebral uptake of the antibody.[10] Lovat *et al.* have used I-123 labeled serum amyloid P component (SAP) and successfully imaged amyloid deposits in peripheral tissues of subjects with systemic amyloidosis.[11] However, they were unable to show cerebral amyloid deposits in AD with SAP labeled either by I-123 or I-124 using single photon emission computerized tomography or positron emission tomography.[12] Congo red is a histologic dye that binds to many amyloid proteins because of their extensive β-sheet structure. Klunk and colleagues have evaluated Chrysamine G, an analogue of Congo red, as a candidate for imaging Aβ.[13] The disturbance of iron stores in AD brains may provide another candidate for imaging. Bartzokis *et al.* quantified brain tissue iron with MRI based on the fact that ferritin affects transverse relaxation time in a field-dependent manner. The iron content in AD was significantly higher in the caudate and globus pallidus than in age- and gender-matched controls.[14,15] Several lines of evidence implicate oxidative stress in the progression of AD.[16–19] The reduction of Cu (II) to Cu (I) by amyloid precursor protein involves an electron-transfer reaction and could lead to a production of hydroxyl radicals.[20] The oxidative by-products of this reaction could be paramagnetic and possibly imaged. All these agents have the potential to target Aβ or to be the target by itself for imaging AD brains. However, none has been developed sufficiently to provide diagnostic or *in vivo* information.

METHODOLOGICAL CONSIDERATIONS IN THE DEVELOPMENT OF AMYLOID IMAGING AGENTS

Various methodological issues require consideration. The effects of label on the binding, electric charge and pH of the ligand, routes of administration, the half-life of the ligand, and signal/noise ratio are all important. The difficulty in transporting labeled ligands into the brain is due in most part to the blood-brain barrier (BBB). Although Kalaria *et al.* suggested leakiness of the BBB from studies of postmortem

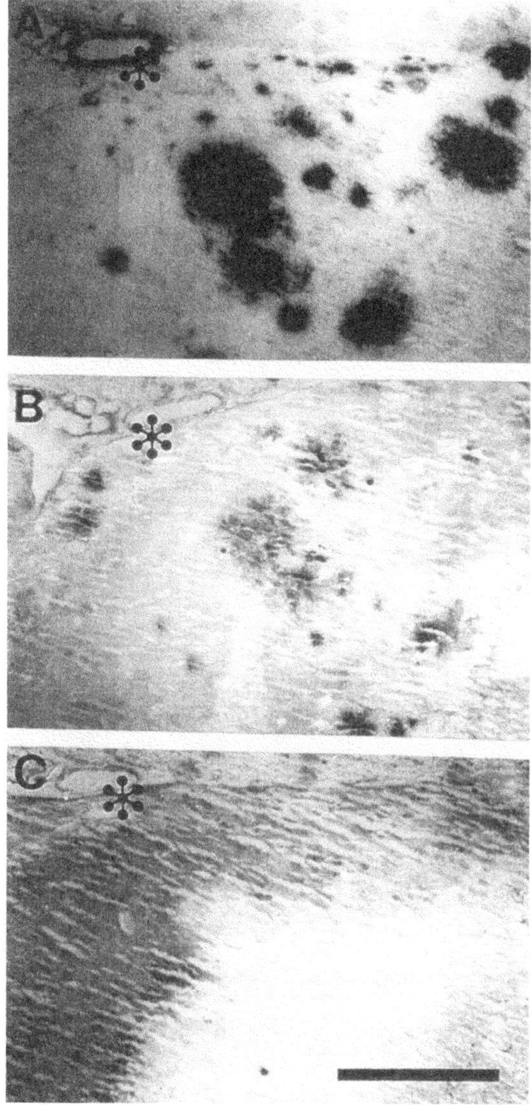

FIGURE 1. Adjacent sections of transgenic mouse brain were treated with (**A**) a rabbit antiserum to $A\beta_{1-42}$, (**B**) bFGF-binding, followed by 48.1, a monoclonal antibody to bFGF, and (**C**) rabbit antiserum to SAP. The core of $A\beta$ plaque and the basement membrane of cerebral microvessel walls (∗) are intensely $A\beta$-immunoreactive and bound to bFGF. There is no evidence of immunoreactivity of SAP in $A\beta$ plaques. Bar = 200 μm.

AD brains,[21] definitive evidence of abnormality of the BBB in living AD patients is lacking. There are several choices of animal models in amyloid imaging studies. Rhesus and squirrel monkeys develop neuritic plaques containing $A\beta$ at the age of

25 and 15 years, respectively.[22] Dogs older than 15 years may also develop neuritic plaques.[23] Due to the scarcity of resources and the expense of nonhuman primates, transgenic mice overexpressing the Aβ precursor protein[24] are a good surrogate that develop Aβ deposits with great predictability.

PRELIMINARY RESULTS OF bFGF AND SAP BINDING

We studied the C57B6/SJL transgenic mouse model overexpressing β protein precursor (βPP) to assess whether SAP and basic fibroblastic growth factor (bFGF) bound to cortical senile plaques. Our goal was to evaluate this mouse as a model for development of amyloid imaging agents. SAP and bFGF bind to neuritic plaques and NFT of AD by interacting with extracellular matrix molecules.[25–28] Because SAP is synthesized only by peripheral organs, its presence in the brain of AD suggests impairment of the BBB.

In the Tg mouse brain section, both SAP and bFGF (FIG. 1) bound to all the Aβ deposits defined by antibodies to Aβ. The binding in Aβ deposits was found in both cortical and hippocampal regions. Double staining of bFGF and Aβ in neuritic plaques showed the binding of bFGF to be at the center of the plaques (data not shown). For both bFGF and SAP, the binding to Aβ was dependent on heparinase-sensitive sites, because heparinase pretreatment diminished the binding intensity. This is consistent with the presence of HSPG within these sites. In contrast, there was little endogenous immunoreactivity of SAP (FIG. 1) and bFGF on the Tg mouse brain section as detected by antibodies. SAP is associated with amyloid plaques in human AD brains. Since SAP is associated with all Aβ deposits in amyloid A amyloidosis found in mice spleens, it clearly demonstrates that SAP can rapidly associate with amyloid in non-BBB areas. The absence of SAP binding in the Tg mouse suggests that the BBB may not be altered in these mice as it is in AD.

CONCLUSION

Our results suggest that the Tg mouse can be used to develop tracer molecules for amyloid imaging. Although most pathological features of Tg mouse are similar to those of AD, there are certain differences between them. The difficult issue of BBB entry needs to be addressed.

ACKNOWLEDGMENTS

This work is supported in part by the National Institute of Aging (AG08012-05), the Joseph and Florence Mandel Foundation, the Nickman Family, the Institute for the Study of Aging, NY, and Philip Morris, USA. The authors also thank K.H. Ashe for the use of transgenic mice that she developed.

REFERENCES

1. HARDY, J., K. DUFF, K.G. HARDY, J. PEREZ-TUR & M. HUTTON. 1998. Genetic dissection of Alzheimer's disease and related dementias: amyloid and its relationship to tau. Nat. Neurosci. **1:** 355–358.
2. TAKAHASHI, M., Y. TSUJIOKA, T. YAMADA, Y. TSUBOI, H. OKADA, T. YAMAMOTO & Z. LIPOSITS. 1999. Glycosylation of microtubule-associated protein tau in Alzheimer's disease brain [In Process Citation]. Acta Neuropathol. (Berl.) **97:** 635–641.
3. JOHNSTONE, M., A. J. GEARING & K.M. MILLER. 1999. A central role for astrocytes in the inflammatory response to beta- amyloid; chemokines, cytokines and reactive oxygen species are produced [In Process Citation]. J. Neuroimmunol. **93:** 182–193.
4. SCHUBERT, P., T. OGATA, H. MIYAZAKI, C. MARCHINI, S. FERRONI & K. RUDOLPHI. 1998. Pathological immuno-reactions of glial cells in Alzheimer's disease and possible sites of interference. J. Neural Transm. Suppl. **54:** 167–174.
5. SIMPSON, I.A., K.R. CHUNDU, T. DAVIES-HILL, W.G. HONER & P. DAVIES. 1994. Decreased concentrations of GLUT1 and GLUT3 glucose transporters in the brains of patients with Alzheimer's disease [see comments]. Ann. Neurol. **35:** 546–551.
6. HARIK, S.I. & J.C. LaMANNA. 1991. Altered glucose metabolism in microvessels from patients with Alzheimer's disease [letter; comment]. Ann. Neurol. **29:** 573.
7. FOX, N.C., E.K. WARRINGTON & M.N. ROSSOR. 1999. Serial magnetic resonance imaging of cerebral atrophy in preclinical Alzheimer's disease [letter] [In Process Citation]. Lancet **353:** 2125.
8. STOUT, J.C., M.W. BONDI, T.L. JERNIGAN, S.L. ARCHIBALD, D.C. DELIS & D.P. SALMON. 1999. Regional cerebral volume loss associated with verbal learning and memory in dementia of the Alzheimer type [In Process Citation]. Neuropsychology **13:** 188–197.
9. ICHIMIYA, A. 1998. Functional and structural brain imagings in dementia. Psychiatry Clin. Neurosci. **52**(Suppl.): S223–S225.
10. FRIEDLAND, R.P., R. KALARIA, M. BERRIDGE, F. MIRALDI, P. HEDERA, J. RENO, L. LYLE & C.A. MAROTTA.1997. Neuroimaging of vessel amyloid in Alzheimer's disease. Ann. N. Y. Acad. Sci. **826:** 242–247.
11. LOVAT, L.B., M.R. PERSEY, S. MADHOO, M.B. PEPYS & P.N. HAWKINS. 1998. The liver in systemic amyloidosis: insights from ^{123}I serum amyloid P component scintigraphy in 484 patients. Gut **42:** 727–734.
12. LOVAT, L.B., A.A. O'BRIEN, S.F. ARMSTRONG, S. MADHOO, C.J. BULPITT, M.N. ROSSOR, M.B. PEPYS & P.N. HAWKINS. 1998. Scintigraphy with ^{123}I-serum amyloid P component in Alzheimer disease. Alzheimer Dis. Assoc. Disord. **12:** 208–210.
13. KLUNK, W.E., R.F. JACOB & R.P. MASON. 1999. Quantifying amyloid beta-peptide (Abeta) aggregation using the Congo red-Abeta (CR-abeta) spectrophotometric assay. Anal. Biochem. **266:** 66–76.
14. BARTZOKIS, G., J. MINTZ, D. SULTZER, P. MARX, J.S. HERZBERG, C.K. PHELAN & S.R. MARDER. 1994. In vivo MR evaluation of age-related increases in brain iron. Am. J. Neuroradiol. **15:** 1129–1138.
15. BARTZOKIS, G., D. SULTZER, J. MINTZ, L.E. HOLT, P. MARX, C.K. PHELAN & S.R. MARDER. 1994. In vivo evaluation of brain iron in Alzheimer's disease and normal subjects using MRI. Biol. Psychiatry **35:** 480–487.
16. GONZALEZ-FRAGUELA, M.E., O. CASTELLANO-BENITEZ & M. GONZALEZ-HOYUELA. 1999. Estres oxidativo en las neurodegeneraciones. [Oxidative stress in neurodegeneration]. Rev. Neurol. **28:** 504–511.
17. PERRY, G. & M.A. SMITH. 1999. Es la lesion producida por oxidacion una parte central en la patogenia de la enfermedad de Alzheimer? [Is the lesion produced by oxidation a central part in the pathogenesis of Alzheimer's disease?] Neurologia **14:** 78–84.
18. BEHL, C. 1999. Alzheimer's disease and oxidative stress: implications for novel therapeutic approaches. Prog. Neurobiol. **57:** 301–323.
19. RETZ, W., W. GSELL, G. MUNCH, M. ROSLER & P. RIEDERER. 1998. Free radicals in Alzheimer's disease. J. Neural Transm. Suppl. **54:** 221–236.
20. MULTHAUP, G. 1997. Amyloid precursor protein, copper and Alzheimer's disease. Biomed. Pharmacother. **51:** 105–111.

21. KALARIA, R.N. & I. GRAHOVAC. 1990. Serum amyloid P immunoreactivity in hippocampal tangles, plaques and vessels: implications for leakage across the blood-brain barrier in Alzheimer's disease. Brain Res. **516:** 349–353.
22. WALKER, L.C. 1997. Animal models of cerebral beta-amyloid angiopathy. Brain Res. Brain Res. Rev. **25:** 70–84.
23. CUMMINGS, B.J., E. HEAD, W. RUEHL, N.W. MILGRAM & C.W. COTMAN. 1996. The canine as an animal model of human aging and dementia. Neurobiol. Aging **17:** 259–268.
24. HSIAO, K., P. CHAPMAN, S. NILSEN, C. ECKMAN, Y. HARIGAYA, S. YOUNKIN, F. YANG & G. COLE. 1996. Correlative memory deficits, Abeta elevation, and amyloid plaques in transgenic mice [see comments]. Science **274:** 99–102.
25. PERRY, G., S.L. SIEDLAK , P. RICHEY, M. KAWAI, P. CRAS, R.N. KALARIA, P.G. GALLOWAY, J.M. SCARDINA, B. CORDELL & B.D. GREENBERG. 1991. Association of heparan sulfate proteoglycan with the neurofibrillary tangles of Alzheimer's disease. J. Neurosci. **11:** 3679–3683.
26. SNOW, A.D., H. MAR, D. NOCHLIN, R.T. SEKIGUCHI, K. KIMATA, Y. KOIKE & T.N. WIGHT. 1990. Early accumulation of heparan sulfate in neurons and in the beta-amyloid protein-containing lesions of Alzheimer's disease and Down's syndrome. Am. J. Pathol. **137:** 1253–1270.
27. SCHUBERT, D., M. LaCORBIERE, T. SAITOH & G. COLE. 1989. Characterization of an amyloid beta precursor protein that binds heparin and contains tyrosine sulfate. Proc. Natl. Acad. Sci. USA **86:** 2066–2069.
28. KATO, T., H. SASAKI, T. KATAGIRI, K. KOIWAI, H. YOUKI, S. TOTSUKA & T. ISHII. 1991. The binding of basic fibroblast growth factor to Alzheimer's neurofibrillary tangles and senile plaques. Neurosci. Lett. **122:** 33–36.

A Newly Formed Amyloidogenic Fragment due to a Stop Codon Mutation Causes Familial British Dementia

J. GHISO,[a,d] R. VIDAL,[a] A. ROSTAGNO,[a] S. MEAD,[b] T. RÉVÉSZ,[c] G. PLANT,[c] AND B. FRANGIONE[a]

[a]Department of Pathology, New York University School of Medicine, New York, New York, USA

[b]The National Hospital for Neurology and Neurosurgery, London, United Kingdom

[c]Department of Neuropathology, Institute of Neurology, London, United Kingdom

ABSTRACT: Familial British dementia (FBD) is an early-onset autosomal dominant disorder characterized by progressive cognitive impairment, spasticity, and cerebellar ataxia. Hippocampal neurofibrillar degeneration and widespread parenchymal and vascular amyloid deposits are the main neuropathological lesions. Amyloid fibrils are composed of a novel 34 amino acid subunit (ABri) with no sequence identity to any known amyloid molecule. The peptide derives from a larger precursor protein codified by a single gene *BRI* on chromosome 13. Affected family members have a single base substitution at the stop codon of the *BRI* gene that generates a longer open-reading frame resulting in a larger precursor protein. The release of the 34 C-terminal amino acids from the mutated precursor originates the ABri amyloid subunit. Our discovery of a new amyloid associated with the development of dementia supports the concept that amyloid peptides may be of primary importance in the initiation of neurodegeneration.

Cerebral amyloid angiopathy (CAA) is a disorder most commonly associated with normal aging, Alzheimer's disease (AD), Down's syndrome (DS), and cerebral hemorrhage. Familial conditions in which amyloid is deposited as CAA include hereditary cerebral hemorrhage with amyloidosis of Icelandic (HCHWA-I)[1] and Dutch (HCHWA-D)[2] types, and the Hungarian and Ohio kindreds of meningocerebrovascular amyloidosis.[3,4] In most of the cases, the biochemical identification of the amyloid subunit responsible for the deposits have led to the discovery of a genetic defect associated with the disease. As summarized in FIGURE 1, the constituent protein of the cerebrovascular amyloid in HCHWA-I is a variant of cystatin C (ACys-Q68) codified by a single gene located on chromosome 20. The 110-residue-long ACys-Q68 amyloid subunit is a degradation product of the cysteine protease inhibitor cystatin C, starting at position 11 and bearing an amino acid substitution (glutamine for leu-

[d]Corresponding author: Jorge Ghiso, Ph.D., NYU School of Medicine, 550 First Avenue, Room TH-432, New York, NY 10016, USA. Tel.: (212) 263-7997; fax (212) 263-6751.
e-mail: ghisoj01@popmail.med.nyu.edu

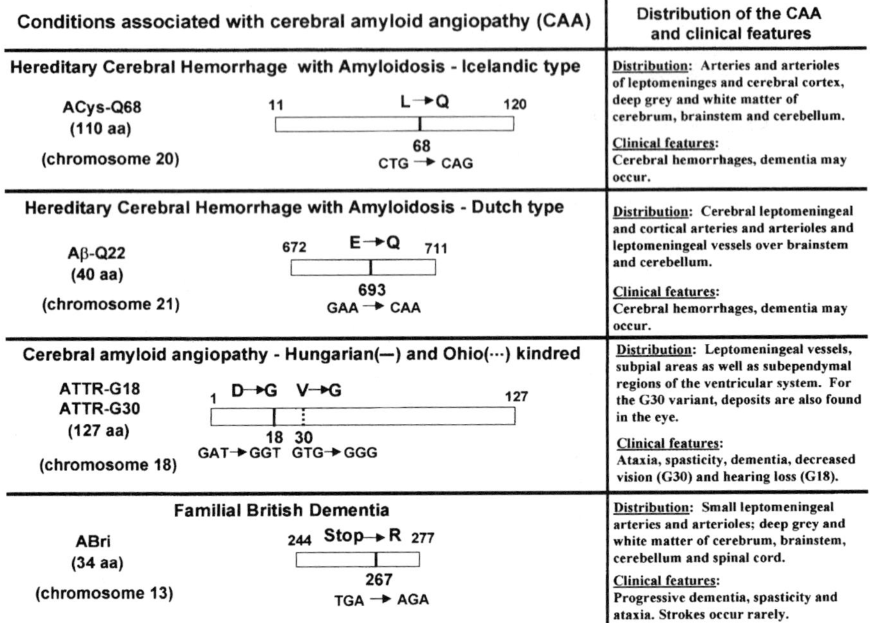

FIGURE 1. Conditions associated with cerebral amyloid angiopathy: amyloid molecules, clinical features, and tissue distribution.

cine)[5] as a result of a single nucleotide change, A for T at codon 68.[6] In HCHWA-D, amyloid deposits are formed by a mixture of wild-type Aβ peptide and the Aβ-Q22 variant.[7,8] The Aβ peptide is a fragment of the larger precursor APP codified by a single gene on chromosome 21. The Aβ-Q22 variant is due to a single nucleotide change, G for C, at codon 693 of APP.[9] Cerebral amyloid deposits consisting of transthyretin (TTR) variants ATTR-G18[3] and ATTR-G30[4] have been reported in two families carrying different point mutations in the TTR gene mapped to chromosome 18. Familial TTR amyloidosis is usually associated with peripheral neuropathy and involvement of visceral organs, whereas signs of central nervous system involvement are exceptional. In the Hungarian kindred, a single nucleotide change (A for G) at codon 18 results in the presence of glycine instead of aspartic acid whereas in the Ohio family, a T for G substitution at codon 30 results in the change of valine for glycine (FIG. 1).

FAMILIAL BRITISH DEMENTIA

Familial British dementia (FBD) is an autosomal dominant form of CAA clinically characterized by progressive dementia, spastic tetraparesis and cerebellar ataxia, with an age of onset in the fourth to fifth decade and full penetrance by age 60. Neuropathologically, many areas of the central nervous system are affected. The

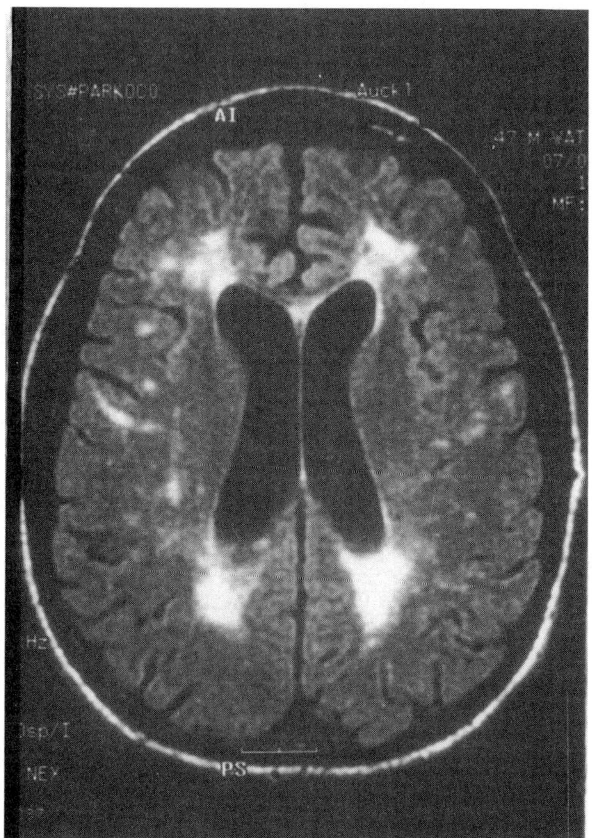

FIGURE 2. MRI scan of a patient affected with FBD. Axial FLAIR image in one of the early affected family members shows the typical confluent patches of high signal around the frontal and occipital poles of the lateral ventricles.

findings consist of (1) severe and widespread amyloid angiopathy of the brain and spinal cord with perivascular amyloid plaque formation, (2) periventricular white matter changes resembling Binswanger's leukoencephalopathy, (3) nonneuritic amyloid plaques affecting cerebellum, hippocampus, amygdala and occasionally cerebral cortex, and (4) neurofibrillary degeneration of hippocampal neurons.[10] Large intracerebral hemorrhage is a rare feature of the disease. Because of the extensive cerebrovascular involvement, the disorder has been previously designated as familial cerebral amyloid angiopathy–British type[10] and cerebrovascular amyloidosis–British type.[11]

FBD was first reported in 1933 by Worster-Drought *et al.*[12] in two siblings. The pedigree has been followed and expanded since then,[10] and common ancestors have been identified with separate family case reports by Griffiths *et al.*[13] and Love and Duchen.[14] At present, the Worster-Drought pedigree comprises 343 individuals over nine generations dating back to ~1780. Although this pedigree is large, it is not complete because the descendants of 22 individuals from early generations who were at risk of the disease could not be traced. The family originally lived in South London, but branches have now emigrated around the world. It is likely that the disease has gone unrecognized. Only one other family with two affected siblings is known, but no common ancestor can be found with the larger pedigree.[15]

Fifty-six members of the family have been identified as at-risk of inheriting FBD. Five affected members of this group, ages between 45 and 50 years, showed early signs of the disease on the basis of a neurological examination, neuropsychological assessment, and MRI brain scan. All five patients had abnormal imaging; a typical example is shown in FIGURE 2. The most consistent finding was patchy or confluent high signal on T2-weighted scans in the deep white matter. This abnormality was located around the frontal and occipital poles of the lateral ventricles and probably represents white matter ischemic changes. Other abnormalities included circumscribed corpus callosum lesions, corpus callosum atrophy, and lacunar infarcts. The neuropsychology was abnormal in four of the five patients. Three had impaired recognition and recall memory, and another had a mild impairment of delayed visual recall. The memory loss is probably related to neuronal loss in the hippocampus. Tests of general intelligence, frontal lobe function, naming, and perception were normal. Neurological signs were found in three of the five individuals with abnormal imaging consisting of gait ataxia and lower-limb spasticity. This could be accounted for by cerebellum and spinal cord pathology.

FBD AMYLOID SUBUNIT

Since the original description by Worster-Drought, the identity of the amyloid protein subunit has remained elusive. Immunohistochemical attempts to classify the disease using a number of antibodies against known amyloidogenic molecules (Cystatin C, Aβ, Gelsolin, TTR, Amyloid A, PrP, κ and λ light chains, ApoA-I, ApoA-II, calcitonin, and β2-microglobulin) failed to identify the nature of the amyloid subunit.[16] We carried out biochemical studies on amyloid fibrils extracted from leptomeningeal amyloid deposits of a patient with FBD, solubilized in 99% formic acid and further purified by gel filtration chromatography. The main component (M_r ~4 kDa on SDS-PAGE) featured pyroglutamate at the N-terminus, which precluded direct sequence analysis. The final amino acid sequence was obtained by combining partial sequence data retrieved from internal peptides generated via trypsin digestion and purified by reverse-phase HPLC, mass spectrometry analysis of the isolated 4 kDa subunit, and homology search in expressed sequence-tagged (EST) data banks. The novel amyloid subunit, named ABri, is composed of 34 amino acids (EASNCFAIRHFENKFAVETLICSRTVKKNIIEEN) with no sequence identity to any known amyloid protein.[17] The peptide is devoid of glycine, methionine, proline, aspartic acid, tryptophane, tyrosine, and glutamine. ABri features two cysteine residues at positions 5 and 22 that may be of importance for polymerization and fibrillization. Mass spectrometry analysis revealed a mass of $3,937.5 \pm 1.0$ Da. The predicted pI (7.0) suggests low-solubility properties at physiologic pH. Synthetic peptides homologous to the full-length ABri spontaneously polymerize in solution and form amyloid-like fibrils *in vitro*.

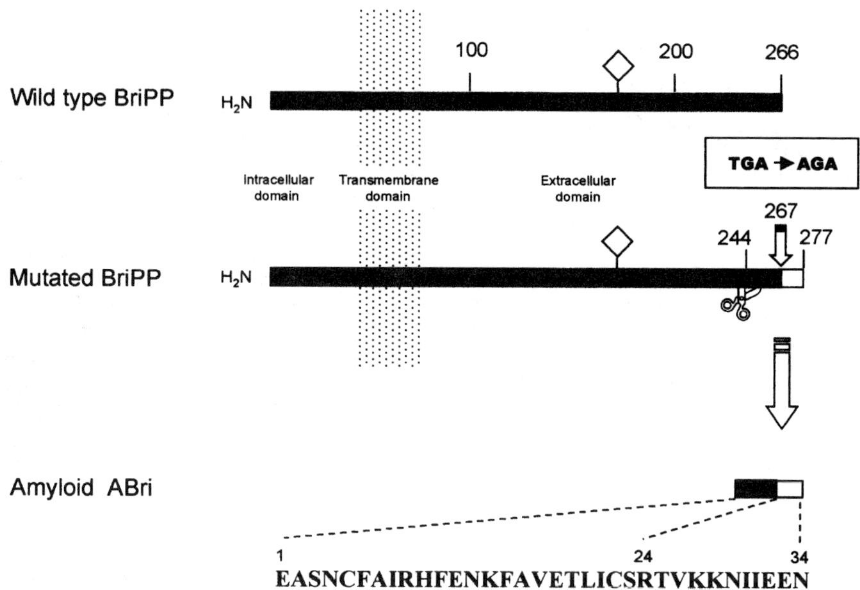

FIGURE 3. Schematic representation of the wild-type and mutated Bri precursor molecules. A single nucleotide change T for A at codon 267 abolishes the normally occurring stop codon resulting in a longer 277 residues Bri precursor protein. The ABri amyloid is generated by proteolytic cleavage of the 34 C-terminal amino acids of the mutated precursor protein (peptide bond 243-244).

ABri PRECURSOR PROTEIN

Because the ABri peptide was not homologous to any known protein and the EST databanks indicated the presence of a larger precursor, the gene codifying the precursor molecule of ABri was cloned and sequenced.[17] The novel gene BRI was located on the long arm of chromosome 13 (13q14) by FISH analysis. It codifies for a 266 amino acid protein with a calculated M_r of 30,329 Da and a theoretical pI of 4.86. Hydropathy analysis[18,19] indicated the presence of a putative single transmembrane spanning domain at positions 52–74, suggesting that the ABri precursor molecule is a type II integral transmembrane protein with the C-terminal part being extracellular (FIG. 3). A putative single N-glycosylation site was located at asparagine 170. The complete nucleotide sequence of the human transcript[17] was highly homologous to sequences obtained from other EST clones of chicken, rat, mouse, rabbit, and pig origin that had been deposited in the data banks. In fact, the mouse and rat amino acid sequences were 95.5 and 96.2% identical to the human homologue, whereas the chicken sequence exhibited 75.9% homology to the human counterpart.

Nucleotide sequence analysis of the precursor protein from a number of available affected members of FBD revealed a single nucleotide substitution in the stop codon, TGA to AGA at codon 267[17] resulting in the presence of an arginine residue and an open-reading frame of 277 amino acids instead of 266. The nucleotide substitution

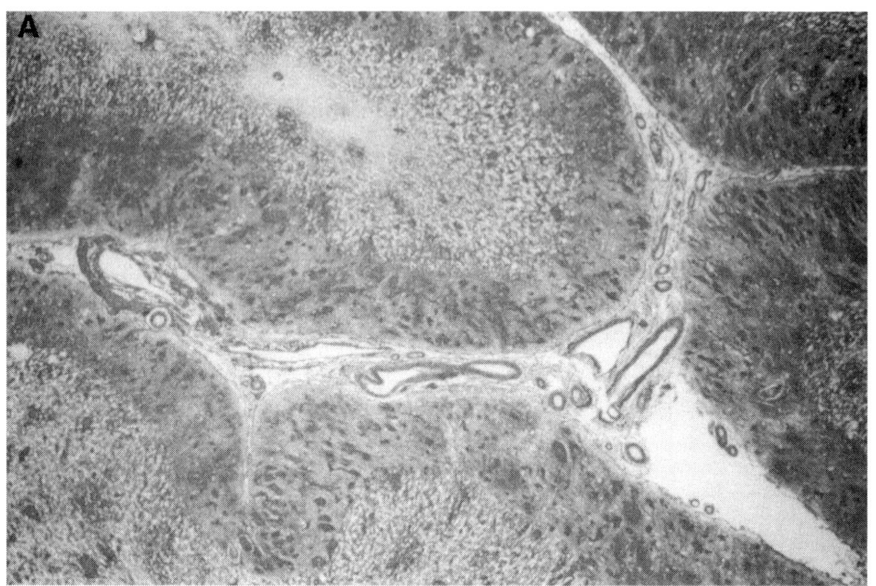

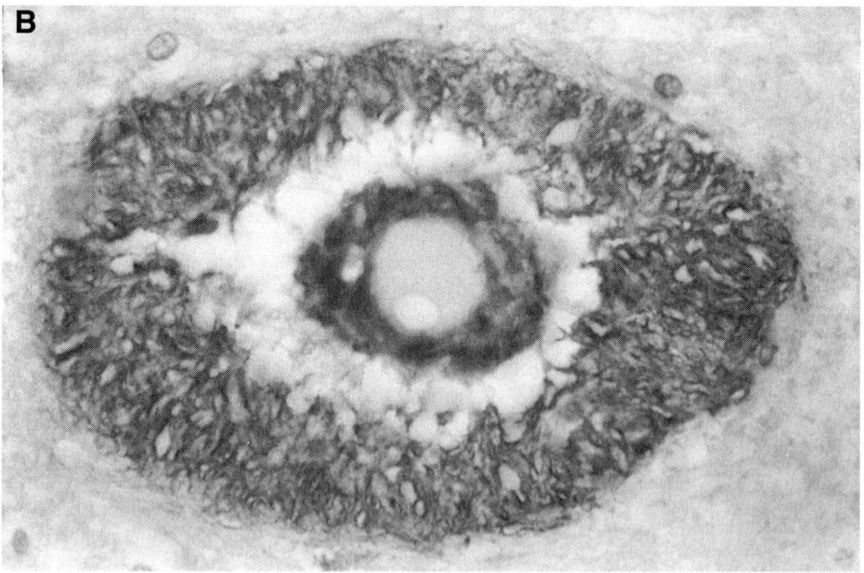

FIGURE 4. Immunohistochemical analysis. (**A**) Parenchymal (nonneuritic and peri-vascular) plaques and vascular amyloid in cerebellum (×120); (**B**) details of a perivascular plaque (×1,200). Staining was carried out with antibody 338, specific for the 10 C-terminal residues of the ABri molecule. Paraffin sections, hematoxylin counterstain.

creates a *XbaI* restriction site useful to detect asymptomatic carriers. The ABri amyloid peptide is formed by the last 34 amino acids of the mutated precursor protein (FIG. 3). Mass spectrometry analysis of the isolated amyloid showed N- and C-terminal heterogeneity. This feature is a common finding in almost every type of amyloidosis, regardless of the protein composing the amyloid subunit.[20]

The mechanism that generates the ABri deposits in patients with FBD remains unknown. Since there is a classical motif for subtilisin-like proprotein convertases (PCs)[21] immediately before the glutamic acid (peptide bond 243–244 of the ABri precursor sequence), it is possible that the ABri peptide is generated by a PC-like cleavage and that further degradation by local amino- or carboxyl- peptidases may take place *in situ*, producing the N- and C-terminal heterogeneity observed in the mass spectrometry. The experimental molecular mass of the main component was 18 Da lower than the expected mass deduced from the cDNA sequence, corroborating a blocked N-terminus. It is interesting to note that pyroglutamate is usually formed by deamination of glutamine; in the case of the ABri amyloid, the nucleotide sequence clearly indicated the presence of glutamic acid at the N-terminus. This finding suggests dehydration as the possible mechanism that results in a blocked ABri. Similar data have been previously published for other amyloids, i.e., the peptides derived from the Alzheimer's Aβ.[22–24]

A synthetic peptide comprising the last 10 residues of the ABri sequence was used to raise polyclonal antibodies in rabbits. As indicated in FIGURE 4, antibody 338 specifically recognized parenchymal and perivascular plaques, as well as vascular amyloid deposits. Specificity of the immunostaining was corroborated by absorption of the antibody with a synthetic peptide homologous to the 34-amino acid full-length ABri amyloid. The immunoreactivity co-localized with yellow-green birefringent material observed under polarized light after Congo red staining (not shown). No immunoreactivity using antibody 338 was observed in brain sections of sporadic CAA, sporadic AD, Down's syndrome, HCHWA-D, HCHWA-I, Hungarian transthyretin cerebral amyloidosis, and systemic cases of light-chain amyloidosis (kidney), light-chain deposition disease (kidney), and amyloid A (heart).

In summary, our data indicate that FBD is not related to any of the known cerebral or systemic forms of human amyloidosis. Since the stop codon at position 267 was always present in asymptomatic family members ($n = 7$) and normal controls from comparable ethnic origins ($n = 113$) and is conserved in the murine homologues, the nucleotide substitution found in patients with FBD is a pathogenic mutation rather than innocent polymorphism. ABri is structurally unrelated to all known amyloids, including those deposited in the brain; however, immunohistochemical and electron microscopical studies on three cases of FBD demonstrated that the cytoskeletal pathology in these patients is almost identical to that seen in patients with other neurodegenerative conditions, including Alzheimer's disease, Prion disorders, brain trauma, or mutations in chromosome 17.[11,25–28] Therefore, different amyloid peptides could trigger similar neuropathological changes leading to the same scenario: neuronal loss and dementia. All these data support the concept that amyloid peptides may be of primary importance in the initiation of neurodegeneration.

[NOTE ADDED IN PROOF: K. Pittois *et al.*[29] independently reported the cloning and identification of the *BRI* gene under the name of *Itm2b* (EMBL/GenBank Data Libraries accession number U76253).]

REFERENCES

1. GUDMUNDSSON, G., J. HALLGRIMSSON, T. JONASSON & O. BUGIANI. 1972. Hereditary cerebral haemorrhage with amyloidosis. Brain **95:** 387–404.
2. LUYENDIJK, W. & J. SCHOEN. 1964. Intracerebral haematomas. A clinical study of 40 surgical cases. Psychiat. Neurol. Neurochir. **67:** 445–468.
3. VIDAL, R., F. GARZULY, H. BUDKA, M. LALOWSKI, R. LINKE, F. BRITTIG, B. FRANGIONE & T. WISNIEWSKI. 1996. Meningocerebrovascular amyloidosis associated with a novel transthyretin mis-sense mutation at codon 18 (TTRD18G). Am. J. Pathol. **148:** 361–366.
4. PETERSEN, R., H. GOREN, M. COHEN, S. RICHARDSON, N. TRESSER, A. LYNN, M. GALI, M. ESTES & P. GAMBETTI. 1997. Transthyretin amyloidosis: a new mutation associated with dementia. Ann. Neurol. **41:** 307–313.
5. GHISO, J., O. JENSSON & B. FRANGIONE. 1986. Amyloid fibrils in hereditary cerebral haemorrhage with amyloidosis of Icelandic type is a variant of g-trace basic protein (cystatin-C). Proc. Natl. Acad. Sci. USA **83:** 2974–2978.
6. LEVY, E., C. LOPEZ-OTIN, J. GHISO, D. GELTNER & B. FRANGIONE. 1989. Stroke in Icelandic patients with hereditary amyloid angiopathy is related to a mutation in the cystatin-C gene, an inhibitor of cysteine proteases. J. Exp. Med. **169:** 1771–1778.
7. VAN DUINEN, S., E. CASTAÑO, F. PRELLI, G. BOTS, W. LUYENDIJK & B. FRANGIONE. 1987. Hereditary cerebral haemorrhage with amyloidosis in patients of Dutch origin is related to Alzheimer's disease. Proc. Natl. Acad. Sci. USA **84:** 5991–5994.
8. PRELLI, F., E. LEVY, S. VAN DUINEN, G. BOTS, W. LUYENDIJK & B. FRANGIONE. 1990. Expression of a normal and variant Alzheimer's β-protein gene in amyloid of hereditary cerebral hemorrhage, Dutch type: DNA and protein diagnostic assays. Biochem. Biophys. Res. Commun. **170:** 301–307.
9. LEVY, E., M. CARMAN, I. FERNANDEZ-MADRID, M. POWER, I. LIEBERBURG, S. VAN DUINEN, G. BOTS, W. LUYENDIJK & B. FRANGIONE. 1990. Mutation of the Alzheimer's disease amyloid gene in hereditary cerebral hemorhage, Dutch type. Science **248:** 1124–1126.
10. PLANT, G., T. RÉVÉSZ, R. BARNARD, A. HARDING & P. GAUTIER-SMITH. 1990. Familial cerebral amyloid angiopathy with nonneuritic plaque formation. Brain **113:** 721–747.
11. RÉVÉSZ, T., J. HOLTON, B. DOSHI, B. ANDERTON, F. SCARAVILLI & G. PLANT. 1999. Cytoskeletal pathology in familial cerebral amyloid angiopathy (British type) with non-neuritic plaque formation. Acta Neuropathol. **97:** 170–176.
12. WORSTER-DROUGHT, C., T. HILL & W. MCMENEMEY. 1933. Familial presenile dementia with spastic paralysis. J. Neurol. Psychopathol. 27–34.
13. GRIFFITHS, R., T. MORTIMER, D. OPPENHEIMER & J. SPALDING. 1982. Congophilic angiopathy of the brain: a clinical and pathological report on two siblings. J. Neurol. Neurosurg. Psychiatry **45:** 396–408.
14. LOVE, S. & L. DUCHEN. 1982. Familial cerebellar ataxia with cerebrovascular amyloid. J. Neurol. Neurosurg. Psychol. **45:** 271–273.
15. DOSHI, B., T. RÉVÉSZ, G. HARWOOD & G. PLANT. 1996. Familial cerebral amyloid angiopathy (British type) with non-neuritic plaque formation is not restricted to a single family. J. Neuropathol. Appl. Neurobiol. **22:** 163.
16. GHISO, J., G. PLANT, T. RÉVÉSZ, T. WISNIEWSKI & B. FRANGIONE. 1995. Familial cerebral amyloid angiopathy (British type) with nonneuritic amyloid plaque formation may be due to a novel amyloid protein. J. Neurol. Sci. **129:** 74–75.
17. VIDAL, R., B. FRANGIONE, A. ROSTAGNO, S. MEAD, T. RÉVÉSZ, G. PLANT & J. GHISO. 1999. A stop codon in the BRI gene associated with familial British dementia. Nature **399:** 776–781.
18. KYTE, J. & R. DOOLITTLE. 1982. A simple method for displaying the hydropathic character of a protein. J. Mol. Biol. **157:** 105–132.
19. SONNHAMMER, E., G. VON HEIJNE & A. KROGH. 1998. A hidden Markov model for predicting transmembrane helices in protein sequences. I.S.M.B. 175–182.
20. GHISO, J., T. WISNIEWSKI & B. FRANGIONE. 1994. Unifying features of systemic and cerebral amyloidosis. Mol. Neurobiol. **8:** 49–64.

21. ZHOU, A., G. WEBB, X. ZHU & D.F. STEINER. 1999. Proteolytic processing in the secretory pathway. J. Biol. Chem. **274:** 20745–20748.

22. MORI, H., K. TAKIO, M. OGAWARA & D. SELKOE. 1992. Mass spectrometry of purified amyloid beta protein in Alzheimer's disease. J. Biol. Chem. **267:** 17082–17086.

23. SAIDO, T., W. YAMAO-HARIGAYA, T. IWATSUBO & S. KAWASHIMA. 1996. Amino- and carboxyl-terminal heterogeneity of beta-amyloid peptides deposited in human brain. Neurosci. Lett. **13:** 173–176.

24. TEKIRIAN, T., T. SAIDO, W. MARKESBERY, M. RUSSELL, D. WEKSTEIN, E. PATEL & J. GEDDES. 1998. N-terminal heterogeneity of parenchymal and cerebrovascular Aβ deposits. J. Neuropathol. Exp. Neurol. **57:** 76–94.

25. DICKSON, D. 1997. Neurodegenerative diseases with cytoskeletal pathology: a biochemical classification. Ann. Neurol. **42:** 541–544.

26. GIACCONE, G., F. TAGLIAVINI, L. VERGA, B. FRANGIONE, M. FARLOW, O. BUGIANI & B. GHETTI. 1990. Neurofibrillary tangles in the Indiana kindred of Gerstmann-Straussler-Scheinker disease share antigenic determinants with those of Alzheimer's disease. Brain Res. **530:** 325–329.

27. TOKUDA, T., S. IKEDA, N. YANAGISAWA, Y. IHARA & G. GLENNER. 1991. Re-examination of ex-boxers' brains using immunohistochemistry with antibodies to amyloid beta-protein and tau protein. Acta Neuropathol. **82:** 280–285.

28. CLARK, L., P. POORKAJ, Z. WSZOLEK, D. GESCHWIND, Z. NASREDDINE, B. MILLER, D. LI, H. PAYAMI, F. AWERT, K. MARKOPOULOU, A. ANDREADIS, I. D'SOUZA, V.-Y. LEE, J. TROJANOWSKI, V. ZHUKAREVA, T. BIRD, G. SCHELLENBERG & K. WILHELMSEN. 1998. Pathogenic implications of mutations in the tau gene in pallido-ponto-nigral degeneration and related neurodegenerative disorders linked to chromosome 17. Proc. Natl. Acad. Sci. USA **95:** 13103–13107.

29. PITTOIS, K., W. DELEERSNIJDER & J. MERREGAERT. 1998. cDNA sequence analysis, chromosomal assignment and expression pattern of the gene coding for integral membrane protein 2B. Gene **217:** 141–149.

Relationship between Severe Amyloid Angiopathy, Apolipoprotein E Genotype, and Vascular Lesions in Alzheimer's Disease

J.M. OLICHNEY,[a,b,e] L.A. HANSEN,[a] J.H. LEE,[c] C.R. HOFSTETTER,[d] R. KATZMAN,[a] AND L.J. THAL[a,b]

[a]*Alzheimer's Disease Research Center and Department of Neurosciences, University of California, San Diego, La Jolla, California 92093-0948, USA*

[b]*Neurology Service, Veteran's Affairs Medical Center, San Diego, California 92161, USA*

[c]*Department of Neurology, University of Ulsan, Asan Medical Center, Seoul, South Korea*

[d]*Alzheimer's Disease Research Center, University of California, San Diego, La Jolla, California 92093-0948, USA*

ABSTRACT: In this brief review, we aim to describe the complex relationship between cerebral amyloid angiopathy (CAA), apolipoprotein E (ApoE), and cerebrovascular lesions in Alzheimer's disease (AD). First, we review the evidence that CAA is associated with, and may cause, specific types of vascular lesions (VLs). In addition to being a leading cause of lobar hemorrhages in the elderly, CAA has been implicated as a likely cause of small infarcts, microinfarcts, and incomplete infarctions in the deep white matter. We also review the role that ApoE4 (the major genetic risk factor for AD) has in predisposing toward CAA, coronary artery disease, and possibly toward cerebrovascular disease. Last, we provide evidence that the association between CAA and VLs is *not* a spurious one due to an increase in the ApoE4 genotype. Even within patient groups with the same ApoE genotype (specifically, E4/4 homozygotes and E3/3 homozygotes), our recent analyses have found significant increases in VLs in association with severe CAA. We discuss the implications of this finding as advancing a pathogenic role for severe CAA in producing many of the VLs commonly found in AD cases.

INTRODUCTION

In this brief review article, we aim to describe the complex relationship between cerebral amyloid angiopathy (CAA), apolipoprotein E (ApoE), and cerebrovascular lesions in Alzheimer's disease (AD). First, we review the evidence that CAA is associated with, and may be the cause of, specific types of vascular lesions (VLs).

[e]Address for correspondence: John Olichney, M.D., Neurology Service (127), V.A. Medical Center, 3350 La Jolla Village Drive, San Diego, CA 92161. Tel.: (619) 552-8585, ext. 3685; fax: (619) 552-7513.
e-mail: olichney@cogsci.ucsd.edu

Next, we review the role ApoE4 has in predisposing toward CAA, coronary artery disease, and possibly toward cerebrovascular disease. Last, we show how the association between CAA and VLs is *not* a spurious one due to an increase in the ApoE4 genotype. We discuss the implications of this finding as advancing a pathogenic role for severe CAA in producing the VLs commonly found in AD cases.

ASSOCIATION OF CAA WITH HEMORRHAGES AND INFARCTIONS

While cerebral amyloid angiopathy (CAA) is best known as a leading cause of lobar hemorrhages in the elderly and as a very common finding in AD, it has also been implicated in the production of other types of cerebrovascular lesions. In 1978, Okazaki and colleagues[1] reported a strikingly high prevalence of small infarcts in their series of 23 cases with "primary cerebrovascular amyloidosis" (only two of whom had advanced AD pathology, but nearly all of whom had some senile plaques). Ferriero *et al.*,[2] like Okazaki, found cerebral infarcts to be even more common than hemorrhages in a series of 25 AD cases with CAA. CAA has also been suggested to be a neuropathological correlate of leukoaraiosis. Gray *et al.*[3] hypothesized that amyloid deposits in the meningocortical segments of the long-perforating arterioles, where CAA is typically prominent, may induce stenosis of these vessels with consequent chronic hypoperfusion of the deep white matter. Incomplete infarctions of the deep white matter, which have been shown in approximately 60% of autopsied AD cases,[4] are frequently associated with CAA.

In 1995, we reported on the relationship between the severity of CAA and cerebral infarctions in what was then the largest pathological AD series ($n = 188$) ever studied in this manner.[5] We found a strong relationship between severe CAA (SAA) and infarction (overall odds-ratio (OR) of 3.5; 95% CI = 1.4–8.9), which was particularly strong within the AD patients who had a history of hypertension. The risk of infarction was most dramatically increased (OR = 14.2; 95% CI = 3.2–63.4) in hypertensive SAA cases relative to nonhypertensive cases with mild or absent amyloid angiopathy (MAA). In a later study,[6] we analyzed an even larger autopsy series (combining the University of California, San Diego and the Consortium to Establish a Registry for Alzheimer's Disease brain autopsy series) in order to better define the types of infarcts to which AD patients with SAA are prone. This analysis showed that SAA cases were at particularly high risk for cortical microinfarcts, intracerebral hemorrhages, and multiple lesion types. There were also trends for increases in small/lacunar infarctions and large (volume >10 cc) infarcts, which did not reach statistical significance. These results were generally consistent with the past neuropathological literature which has strongly implicated, albeit in smaller samples, CAA as a cause of cerebral infarction and hemorrhage.[7] The predilection for specific types of vascular lesions in CAA, which are biologically plausible given the abundant vascular amyloid usually found in the small superficial cortical arterioles, suggests that CAA is directly involved in the pathogenesis of these lesions. CAA does not appear to be a nonspecific marker for cerebrovascular disease, atherosclerosis, or end-stage AD.

ASSOCIATION OF CAA WITH APOE4

Apolipoprotein E4 (ApoE4) has received a great deal of attention since being established as the major genetic risk factor for typical "late-onset" (i.e., after age 60) AD.[8] In 1993, two groups of investigators[9,10] demonstrated that AD cases with the ApoE4 allele have even more severe intraparenchymal β-amyloid than cases without an E4 allele. Greenberg *et al.*[11] extended this finding to the cerebral blood vessels, both within the AD and non-AD series. We, like several other groups, have since replicated this association of ApoE4 with more severe amyloid angiopathy, but have been impressed with how little of the variance ApoE genotype explains within AD. For example, we reported that only when large groups of AD and LBV cases were combined did the ApoE4 effect on CAA severity even reach statistical significance.[12] Therefore, it is clear that other unidentified features are operative in determining the genetic and/or environmental susceptibility for developing CAA. While advanced age is clearly associated with a greater prevalence of CAA, this statement does not necessarily hold within AD cohorts. This may be because ApoE4 carriers tend to present fairly early (especially the E4/4 homozygotes), both with respect to the onset of cognitive/AD symptoms[8] and age of cerebral hemorrhage.[13]

ASSOCIATION OF APOE4 WITH CORONARY ARTERY DISEASE AND ATHEROSCLEROSIS

Prior to its discovery as a risk factor for AD, ApoE was primarily known for its role in cholesterol metabolism. Premature coronary artery disease and atherosclerosis had been well described in ApoE4 carriers, although the relative risks are generally more modest than those now described for AD.[14] This association of ApoE4 with both coronary artery disease and AD may help explain a report from Sparks *et al.*,[15] which was surprising at the time, that patients with high-grade stenoses of coronary vessels had an greatly increased prevalence of AD pathology (mainly diffuse plaques) at autopsy. Alternatively, the poor cardiac function of this group may have increased AD pathology through mechanisms related to ischemia/hypoperfusion, independent of ApoE status. However, one recent autopsy study has found no relationship between cardiovascular status and severity of AD neuropathological changes[16] in a nondemented sample.

POSSIBLE ASSOCIATION OF APOE4 WITH CEREBROVASCULAR DISEASE

In contrast to being clearly implicated in the risk of ischemic heart disease, the role ApoE4 may play in stroke and vascular dementia is much less established. In the stroke literature, some studies have found a modest increase in ApoE4. For example, Pedro-Botet and colleagues[17] found an increased prevalence of ApoE3/4 heterozygotes in their sample of patients with prior stroke. However, other studies have found no increased representation of ApoE4,[18] with one study finding an increase in the uncommon ApoE2/3 genotype.[19] ApoE2 has also been found to be associated with CAA and CAA-related hemorrhages,[20] but no consistent increase in overall stroke risk has been demonstrated.

In studies of clinically defined vascular dementia, the results are again mixed with many,[21,22] but not all,[23,24] finding an increase in ApoE4. However, it should be emphasized that these studies lacked neuropathological verification and therefore superimposed AD pathology (i.e., the common entity of "mixed" AD/vascular dementia) is not excluded. Interestingly, one neuropathological study[25] found a striking overrepresentation of ApoE4 (51% allele frequency) in "mixed" dementia, but no increase in pure vascular dementia (8% ApoE4). This suggests that ApoE4 carriers with stroke are very likely to also develop intraparenchymal amyloid deposits and meet neuropathologic criteria for AD. What remains unclear is how often the cerebrovascular pathology is the primary cause of dementia, and to what extent CAA may contribute to the early cerebrovascular disease and/or subsequent strokes. Also, ApoE may be important in neuronal repair and regeneration,[26] with ApoE4 carriers having less resistance to the cognitive impact of cerebral ischemia. Along these lines, Isoe *et al.*[27] found increased ApoE4 among subjects with clinically defined "vascular dementia," but no increase of ApoE4 in subjects with cerebrovascular disease but without dementia.

SEVERE CAA IS ASSOCIATED WITH VASCULAR LESIONS INDEPENDENT OF APOE STATUS

With these multiple roles of ApoE4, it is certainly plausible that the association between severe CAA and vascular lesions is a spurious one, mediated by ApoE4 and/or atherosclerosis. Therefore, we recently re-examined our brain autopsy series at the University of California, San Diego to test whether severe CAA is an independent risk factor for vascular lesions in AD.[28] We did this by stratifying the 247 autopsy-confirmed AD dementia cases that had been ApoE genotyped by the number of E4 alleles. Within two of the three strata (i.e., the E4/4 homozygotes and the E3/3 group), significant increases were found in VLs in association with SAA. Within E4/4 homozygotes, 47% of the SAA cases had one or more VL compared to 9.5% of MAA cases (chi-square, $p = 0.01$). Within the E3/3 group, 56% of SAA versus 21% of MAA had VLs ($p = 0.02$). We also performed logistic regression models to see which factors best predicted VLs in our AD cases. This showed that while the presence of SAA (OR = 3.53; $p = 0.0016$) and advanced age of death (OR = 1.07; $p = 0.013$) were significantly associated with VLs, the number of ApoE4 alleles had no significant independent effect. In fact, when we looked at the prevalence of VLs, we found no significant difference between cases with 0, 1 or 2 ApoE4 alleles.

CONCLUSIONS

In summary, severe CAA appears to be etiologically related to the production of VLs in AD. Our recent analyses have shown that the association between severe amyloid angiopathy and vascular lesions in Alzheimer's disease is not a spurious one due to ApoE4. Further, the associated VLs show some specificity in their lesion type with particularly high risks for small cortical infarcts and hemorrhages.[6] Because CAA predominantly affects leptomeningeal and small cortical arterioles and the associated VLs are commonly small infarcts in the neocortical ribbon,[5] a causal relationship is suggested. Recent research has provided additional insights into the possible mechanisms by which amyloid in the vessel may produce VLs. Thomas *et al.*[29] have shown β-amyloid to be a vasoactive substance which can induce vasospasm *in vitro* at low concentrations. Platelets have been shown capable of producing β-amyloid,[30] which could make platelet-endothelial interactions particularly important in patients with CAA. Also, an agonist effect of aggregated amyloid upon tPA has been described,[31] which could account for the excess in intracerebral hemorrhages (with or without microaneurysms). Although ApoE4 is a well-established risk factor for CAA, it does not appear to be in itself a strong predictor of stroke in the general population, or of cerebral infarction in AD.

ACKNOWLEDGMENT

This work was supported by NIH Grant No. AG-05131.

REFERENCES

1. OKAZAKI, H. *et al.* 1979. Clinicopathologic studies of primary cerebral amyloid angiopathy. Mayo Clin. Proc. **54:** 22–31.
2. FERREIRO, J.A. *et al.* 1989. Stroke related to cerebral amyloid angiopathy: the significance of systemic vascular disease. J. Neurol. **236:** 267–272.
3. GRAY, F. *et al.* 1985. Leukoencephalopathy in diffuse hemorrhagic cerebral amyloid angiopathy. Ann. Neurol. **18:** 54–59.
4. BRUN, A. *et al.* 1986. A white matter disorder in dementia of the Alzheimer type: a pathoanatomical study. Ann. Neurol. **19:** 253–262.
5. OLICHNEY, J.M. *et al.* 1995. Cerebral infarction in Alzheimer's disease is associated with severe amyloid angiopathy and hypertension. Arch. Neurol. **52:** 702–708.
6. OLICHNEY, J.M. *et al.* 1997. Types of cerebrovascular lesions associated with severe cerebral amyloid angiopathy in Alzheimer's disease. Ann. N.Y. Acad. Sci. **826:** 493–497.
7. MANDYBUR, T.I. 1986. Cerebral amyloid angiopathy: the vascular pathology and complications. J. Neuropathol. Exp. Neurol. **45:** 79–90.
8. SAUNDERS, A.M. *et al.* 1993. Association of apolipoprotein E allele ε4 with late-onset familial and sporadic Alzheimer's disease. Neurology **43:** 1467–1472.
9. SCHMECHEL, D.E. *et al.* 1993. Increased amyloid β-peptide deposition in cerebral cortex as a consequence of apolipoprotein E genotype in late-onset Alzheimer's disease. Proc. Natl. Acad. Sci. USA **90:** 9649–9653.
10. REBECK, G.W. *et al.* 1993. Apolipoprotein E in sporadic Alzheimer's disease: allelic variation and receptor interactions. Neuron **11:** 575–580.
11. GREENBERG, S.M. *et al.* 1995. Apolipoprotein E4 and cerebral hemorrhage associated with amyloid angiopathy. Ann. Neurol. **38:** 254–259.
12. OLICHNEY, J.M. *et al.* 1996. The apolipoprotein E ε4 allele is associated with increased neuritic plaques and cerebral amyloid angiopathy in Alzheimer's disease and Lewy body variant. Neurology **47:** 190–196.
13. GREENBERG, S.M. *et al.* 1996. Apolipoprotein E ε4 is associated with the presence and earlier onset of hemorrhage in cerebral amyloid angiopathy. Stroke **27:** 1333–1337.
14. WILSON, P.W.F. *et al.* 1994. Apolipoprotein E alleles, dyslipidemia, and coronary heart disease: the Framingham Offspring Study. JAMA **272:** 1666–1671.
15. SPARKS, D.L. *et al.* 1990. Cortical senile plaques in coronary artery disease, aging and Alzheimer's disease. Neurobiol. Aging **11:** 601–607.

16. ALAFUZOFF, I. *et al.* 1999. β-Amyloid load is not influenced by the severity of cardiovascular disease in aged and demented patients. Stroke **30**: 613–618.
17. PEDRO-BOTET, J. *et al.* 1992. Lipoprotein and apolipoprotein profile in men with ischemic stroke. Roles of lipoprotein(a), triglyceride-rich lipoproteins, and lipoprotein E polymorphism. Stroke **23**: 1556–1562.
18. BASUN, H. *et al.* 1996. Apolipoprotein E polymorphism and stroke in a population sample aged 75 years or more. Stroke **27**: 1310–1315.
19. COUDERC, R. *et al.* 1993. Prevalence of apolipoprotein E phenotypes in ischemic cerebrovascular disease. A case-control study. Stroke **24**: 661–664.
20. NICOLL, J.A.R. *et al.* 1997. High frequency of apolipoprotein E2 allele in hemorrhage due to cerebral amyloid angiopathy. Ann. Neurol. **41**: 716–721.
21. SHIMANO, H. *et al.* 1989. Plasma apolipoproteins in patients with multi-infarct dementia. Atherosclerosis **79**: 257–260.
22. FRISONI, G.B. *et al.* 1994. Apolipoprotein E ε4 allele in Alzheimer's disease and vascular dementia. Dementia **5**: 240–242.
23. KAWAMATA, J. *et al.* 1994. Apolipoprotein E polymorphism in Japanese patients with Alzheimer's disease and vascular dementia. J. Neurol. Neurosurg. Psychiatry **57**: 1414–1416.
24. PALUMBO, B. *et al.* 1997. Apolipoprotein E genotype in normal aging, age-associated memory impairment, Alzheimer's disease, and vascular dementia patients. Neurosci. Lett. **231**: 59–61.
25. BERTARD, C. *et al.* 1994. Apo E allele frequencies in Alzheimer's disease, Lewy body dementia, Alzheimer's disease with cerebrovascular disease and vascular dementia. Neuroreport **5**: 1893–1896.
26. POIRIER, J. *et al.* 1991. Astrocytic apolipoprotein E mRNA and GFAP mRNA in hippocampus after entorhinal cortex lesioning. Mol. Brain Res. **11**: 97–106.
27. ISOE, K. *et al.* 1996. Apolipoprotein E in patients with dementia of the Alzheimer type and vascular dementia. Acta Neurol. Scand. **93**: 133–137.
28. OLICHNEY, J.M. *et al.* The association between severe cerebral amyloid angiopathy and cerebrovascular lesions in Alzheimer's disease is not a spurious one due to apolipoprotein E4. Arch. Neurol. In press.
29. THOMAS, T. *et al.* 1996. β-Amyloid-mediated vasoactivity and vascular endothelial damage. Nature **380**: 168–171.
30. LI, Q.X. *et al.* 1998. Secretion of Alzheimer's disease Abeta amyloid peptide by activated human platelets. Lab. Invest. **78**: 461–469.
31. KINGSTON, I.B. *et al.* 1995. In vitro stimulation of tissue-type plasminogen activator by Alzheimer amyloid β-peptide analogues. Nature Med. **1**: 138–142.

Plasma β-Amyloid Peptide, Transforming Growth Factor-β1, and Risk for Cerebral Amyloid Angiopathy

STEVEN M. GREENBERG,[a,c] HYUN-SOON CHO,[a] HEATHER C. O'DONNELL,[a] JONATHAN ROSAND,[a] ALAN Z. SEGAL,[a] LINDA H. YOUNKIN,[b] STEVEN G. YOUNKIN,[b] AND G. WILLIAM REBECK[a]

[a]*Massachusetts General Hospital and Harvard Medical School, Boston, Massachusetts 02114, USA*

[b]*Mayo Clinic, Jacksonville, Florida 32224, USA*

ABSTRACT: Despite the documented association between apolipoprotein E genotype and cerebral amyloid angiopathy (CAA), a substantial proportion of CAA-related hemorrhages occur in patients without known risks for this disorder. Two other factors implicated in the pathogenesis of CAA are the amyloid-β peptide (preferentially deposited in vessels as a 40-amino acid species) and the multifunctional cytokine transforming growth factor-β1 (a specific promoter of vascular amyloid deposition in transgenic models). We measured plasma concentrations of these factors in a series of 25 patients diagnosed with probable or definite CAA-related hemorrhage and compared them with 21 patients with hemorrhage due to probable hypertensive vasculopathy and 42 elderly control subjects without hemorrhage. We found no differences among the groups in concentrations of the 40- or 42-amino acid species of β-amyloid or either the active or latent form of transforming growth factor-β1. While the data do not exclude important roles for these molecules as risks for CAA, they indicate that plasma measurements are not useful in its diagnosis.

Despite the close molecular relationship between cerebral amyloid angiopathy (CAA) and Alzheimer's disease (AD), the diseases do not entirely overlap. Indeed, clinical dementia precedes only about 25–40% of CAA-related hemorrhages,[1] while only 5% of patients with AD demonstrate CAA-related hemorrhages.[2] These observations suggest the existence of factors that specifically favor one of these processes over the other.

Previous studies of apolipoprotein E (APOE) genotype have highlighted some of the similarities and differences between CAA and AD. Whereas APOE ε4 associates with increased amyloid deposition in both plaques and vessels,[3-5] APOE ε2, a protective factor in AD,[6] appears to promote rather than prevent CAA.[7,8] CAA-related

[c]Address correspondence to Steven M. Greenberg, M.D., Ph.D., Massachusetts General Hospital, Wang ACC 836, Boston, MA 02114, USA. Tel.: (617) 724-1874; fax: (617) 726-5346. e-mail: greenberg@helix.mgh.harvard.edu

hemorrhages nonetheless occur commonly in the absence of either allele,[7,8] indicating a high likelihood of further specific risk factors.

The current study examined plasma concentrations of two molecules implicated in the pathogenesis of CAA: the amyloid-β peptide (Aβ) and the multifunctional cytokine transforming growth factor-β1 (TGF-β1). Aβ, the primary constituent of both cerebrovascular and plaque amyloid, exists primarily as a 39–40 amino acid peptide (Aβ_{40}) in vascular deposits as opposed to the 42–43 amino acid species (Aβ_{42}) that predominates in plaques.[9,10] Alterations in cerebrospinal (though not plasma) concentrations of Aβ_{42} have been suggested as a potential diagnostic marker for AD.[11,12] The evidence for the role of TGF-β1 in CAA comes from its ability to promote largely vascular amyloid deposition in a transgenic mouse model.[13] Human brains demonstrate TGF-β1 in plaques[14,15] and an association between TGF-β1 mRNA levels and the severity of CAA.[13]

We therefore sought to determine whether patients with CAA-related hemorrhage might be distinguished by specific alterations in plasma Aβ—particularly Aβ_{40}—and TGF-β1. We compared CAA patients to those diagnosed with a different type of primary intracerebral hemorrhage (i.e., one related to hypertensive vasculopathy) and to elderly volunteers. The results did not demonstrate significant differences among the groups.

METHODS

Patient Selection

Hemorrhage patients and control subjects were recruited and evaluated as described previously.[16,17] Study subjects included 25 patients diagnosed with definite or probable CAA-related hemorrhage (5 with CAA on postmortem exam or hematoma specimen, 20 diagnosed clinically by the presence of multiple, strictly lobar, hemorrhages[4]), 21 with probable hypertensive (HTN) hemorrhage (hemorrhagic focus in putamen, thalamus, or pons), and 42 consecutive elderly (age $\geq$55) volunteers undergoing annual physical examination at a primary care practice. Hemorrhage patients underwent routine clinical, radiographic, and laboratory evaluation to exclude other specific causes of hemorrhage such as trauma, metastatic neoplasm, vascular malformation, hemorrhagic transformation of ischemic infarction, vasculitis, coagulopathy, or blood dyscrasia. Control subjects were excluded if they had previous intracerebral hemorrhage.

Analysis of Plasma Samples

Nonfasting blood samples were obtained at least one month following the most recent hemorrhage (or, for controls, at the time of the annual physical examination). Samples were drawn into EDTA-containing tubes, placed on ice, and centrifuged within one hour. Clear plasma was removed without disturbing the buffy coat, aliquoted, and stored at $-80°$ until time of assay.

Plasma Aβ_{40} and Aβ_{42} were measured by sandwich ELISA as described in Reference 18. (One individual with probable CAA included in the TGF-β1 analysis was not assayed for Aβ.)

TABLE 1. Plasma Aβ and TGF-β1 concentrations in hemorrhage cases and controls

	CAA (n = 25)	HTN (n = 21)	Control (n = 42)
Gender, male/female	12/13	13/8	18/24
Age, mean ± SD	74.5 ± 7.8*	66.8 ± 11.9	68.6 ± 9.3
Plasma Aβ, pM, median (25th/75th percentile)			
Aβ$_{40}$	133.6 (97.5/178.2)	167.3 (109.6/196.9)	144.5 (112.7/192.0)
Aβ$_{42}$	16.7 (13.1/26.0)	18.0 (14.4/19.9)	16.6 (13.9/22.4)
Total TGF-β1, ng/ml, median (25th/75th percentile)			
Males†	6.5 (3.9/9.2)	5.5 (2.8/6.2)	6.5 (4.1/8.7)
Females	6.9 (5.4/11.1)	8.8 (5.5/10.9)	8.5 (4.8/10.4)

*$p < 0.02$ vs. either other group; †$p < 0.02$ vs. females.
ABBREVIATIONS: CAA, probable cerebral amyloid angiopathy-related hemorrhage; HTN, probable hypertensive hemorrhage.

TGF-β1 was measured by the Promega ELISA system specific for this cytokine according to the manufacturer's instructions (see Ref. 19). All measurements were performed in duplicate, and all samples assayed in a single batch. Total TGF-β1 (naturally active + latent) was measured at final dilution of 1:100 following activation with HCl; naturally active TGF-β1 was assayed at 1:5 dilution. Samples with active TGF-β1 concentrations of less than 78 pg/ml fell below the linear range of the standard curve after dilution and were recorded as nondetectable. A control series was used to establish that blood samples drawn under our routine conditions (with use of tourniquets) yielded similar TGF-β1 levels to those drawn from the same individuals without use of tourniquet or vacuum containers. All biochemical analyses were performed without knowledge of the patient's diagnosis.

Aβ and TGF-β1 concentrations were compared among groups by nonparametric methods (Wilcoxon rank-sum test or Kruskal-Wallis test) because of nonnormal distributions. Potential covariates examined included gender, age at time of sample collection (categorized as <70 or ≥70 years old), and history of hypertension, determined as described previously.[16,17]

RESULTS

Individuals diagnosed with probable CAA-related hemorrhage were older than patients with HTN hemorrhage or control subjects without hemorrhage (TABLE 1). Plasma concentrations of Aβ$_{40}$, Aβ$_{42}$, and the ratio of Aβ$_{40}$ to Aβ$_{42}$ did not differ among the groups ($p > 0.4$). Aβ levels also did not significantly vary with gender, age, or history of hypertension (data not shown).

Total TGF-β1 levels (naturally active plus latent activity released by acid treatment) were greater in women than in men; naturally active TGF-β1 and the ratio of active to total enzyme did not differ between the sexes. Similar concentrations of total TGF-β1 were detected among patients with CAA-related hemorrhages, HTN hemorrhages, and elderly controls (TABLE 1). On assay of naturally active TGF-β1, most (53/88) of the samples fell below the lower level of detection of the assay

(78 pg/ml). There were no apparent differences among the groups in proportion with detectable active TGF-β1 (12/25, or 48%, of CAA samples were above limit of detection compared with 18/42, or 43%, of controls, 5/21, or 24%, of HTN hemorrhages) or mean concentration (data not shown). Similar results were obtained in comparisons stratified for gender, age, or history of hypertension.

DISCUSSION

Altered plasma concentrations of Aβ and TGF-β have been noted in association with several specific disease states. Aβ_{40} and Aβ_{42} are elevated in patients with Down's syndrome or the β-amyloid precursor protein (βAPP)-670/671 mutation,[18,20] whereas the ßAPP-717 and pathogenic presenilin mutations (including those in the presymptomatic carrier state) are associated with selective increases in plasma Aβ_{42}.[18,21] Sporadic AD patients demonstrate normal plasma concentrations of Aβ.[18,22] The latter observation suggests that circulating Aβ, while a marker of altered βAPP processing in familial AD, is probably not a direct cause of brain pathology.

Altered plasma concentrations of active TGF-β1 have been reported in coronary artery disease.[19,23,24] TGF-β exerts numerous effects on vessels that might underlie these observations, including protection of endothelium,[25] maintenance of smooth muscle differentiation,[26] and deposition of vascular extracellular matrix proteins.[27,28] TGF-β1 levels have not been reported in cerebrovascular disease or most other human neurologic diseases. One small study found elevated serum levels of TGF-β in six patients who died with AD.[29]

We found that plasma Aβ and TGF-β1 concentrations are not altered in patients with CAA-related hemorrhage and thus have no role in the detection of this disorder. Although the data do not offer support for a specific role for Aβ or TGF-β as either diagnostic markers or risk factors for CAA, there are several potential pitfalls in this interpretation. From a technical standpoint, the fact that a majority of naturally active TGF-β1 samples fell below the assay's limit of detection (and were generally lower than previously reported values[19,23]) leaves open the possibility that significant differences exist in the very low range of active cytokine. A larger issue is whether significant differences in Aβ or TGF-β might exist in cerebrospinal fluid rather than plasma, as has been noted for Aβ_{42} in AD.[11,12] Another possibility in the case of Aβ is that its role as a risk factor might be confounded by the progression of the disease, as potentially high initial levels of circulating peptide are converted into intracranial Aβ deposits. Finally, it is possible that elevated Aβ or TGF-β1 might have a pathogenic role in only a subgroup of CAA patients, a possibility to be addressed in future studies of disease progression and hemorrhage recurrence in this cohort.

The APOE genotype remains the strongest identified risk factor for sporadic CAA. Cumulative evidence has pointed to roles for both APOE ϵ2 and ϵ4 in promoting the presence,[5,7,16] early onset,[7,8] and recurrence[30] of CAA-related hemorrhage. Such genetically based studies offer substantial practical advantages over the nongenetic studies reported here, obviating many of the pitfalls in interpretation such as location of sampling (blood versus cerebrospinal fluid) or confounding by disease progression. Further identification of the genes regulating β-amyloid deposition and toxicity thus offers perhaps the most promising approach to finding new candidate risk factors for CAA.

ACKNOWLEDGMENTS

This work was supported by grants from the National Institute of Health (AG00725), the American Heart Association, and the Edward Mallinckrodt, Jr. Foundation.

REFERENCES

1. GREENBERG, S.M. 2000. Clinical aspects and diagnostic criteria of sporadic CAA-related hemorrhage. *In* Cerebrovascular Amyloidosis in Alzheimer's Disease and Related Disorders. M.M. Verbeek, H.V. Vinters & R.M.W. de Waal, Eds. Wolters Kluwer Academic Publishers. Dordrecht, the Netherlands.
2. ELLIS, R.J., J.M. OLICHNEY, L.J. THAL, S.S. MIRRA, J.C. MORRIS, D. BEEKLY & A. HEYMAN. 1996. Cerebral amyloid angiopathy in the brains of patients with Alzheimer's disease: the CERAD experience, Part 15. Neurology **46:** 1592–1596.
3. SCHMECHEL, D.E., A.M. SAUNDERS, W.J. STRITTMATTER, B.J. CRAIN, C.M. HULETTE, S.H. JOO, M.A. PERICAK-VANCE, D. GOLDGABER & A.D. ROSES. 1993. Increased amyloid beta-peptide deposition in cerebral cortex as a consequence of apolipoprotein E genotype in late-onset Alzheimer disease. Proc. Natl. Acad. Sci. USA **90:** 9649–9653.
4. GREENBERG, S.M., G.W. REBECK, J.P.V. VONSATTEL, T. GOMEZ-ISLA & B.T. HYMAN. 1995. Apolipoprotein E e4 and cerebral hemorrhage associated with amyloid angiopathy. Ann. Neurol. **38:** 254–259.
5. PREMKUMAR, D.R., D.L. COHEN, P. HEDERA, R.P. FRIEDLAND & R.N. KALARIA. 1996. Apolipoprotein E-epsilon4 alleles in cerebral amyloid angiopathy and cerebrovascular pathology associated with Alzheimer's disease. Am. J. Pathol. **148:** 2083–2095.
6. CORDER, E.H., A.M. SAUNDERS, N.J. RISCH, W.J. STRITTMATTER, D.E. SCHMECHEL, P.C.J. GASKELL, J.B. RIMMLER, P.A. LOCKE, P.M. CONNEALLY, K.E. SCHMADER, G.W. SMALL, A.D. ROSES, J.L. HAINES & M.A. PERICAK-VANCE. 1994. Protective effect of apolipoprotein E type 2 allele for late onset Alzheimer disease. Nat. Genet. **7:** 180–184.
7. NICOLL, J.A., C. BURNETT, S. LOVE, D.I. GRAHAM, D. DEWAR, J.W. IRONSIDE, J. STEWART & H.V. VINTERS. 1997. High frequency of apolipoprotein E epsilon 2 allele in hemorrhage due to cerebral amyloid angiopathy. Ann. Neurol. **41:** 716–721.
8. GREENBERG, S.M., J.P. VONSATTEL, A.Z. SEGAL, R.I. CHIU, A.E. CLATWORTHY, A. LIAO, B.T. HYMAN & G.W. REBECK. 1998. Association of apolipoprotein E epsilon2 and vasculopathy in cerebral amyloid angiopathy. Neurology **50:** 961–965.
9. MANN, D.M., T. IWATSUBO, Y. IHARA, N.J. CAIRNS, P.L. LANTOS, N. BOGDANOVIC, L. LANNFELT, B. WINBLAD, M.L. MAAT-SCHIEMAN & M.N. ROSSOR. 1996. Predominant deposition of amyloid-beta 42(43) in plaques in cases of Alzheimer's disease and hereditary cerebral hemorrhage associated with mutations in the amyloid precursor protein gene. Am. J. Pathol. **148:** 1257–1266.
10. ALONZO, N.C., B.T. HYMAN, G.W. REBECK & S.M. GREENBERG. 1998. Progression of cerebral amyloid angiopathy. Accumulation of amyloid-β40 in already affected vessels. J. Neuropathol. Exp. Neurol. **57:** 353–359.
11. MOTTER, R., C. VIGO-PELFREY, D. KHOLODENKO, R. BARBOUR, K. JOHNSON-WOOD, D. GALASKO, L. CHANG, B. MILLER, C. CLARK, R. GREEN, D. OLSON, P. SOUTHWICK, R. WOLFERT, B. MUNROE, I. LIEBERBURG, P. SEUBERT & D. SCHENK. 1995. Reduction of beta-amyloid peptide42 in the cerebrospinal fluid of patients with Alzheimer's disease. Ann. Neurol. **38:** 643–648.
12. ANDREASEN, N., C. HESSE, P. DAVIDSSON, L. MINTHON, A. WALLIN, B. WINBLAD, H. VANDERSTICHELE, E. VANMECHELEN & K. BLENNOW. 1999. Cerebrospinal fluid β-amyloid(1–42) in Alzheimer disease and stability during the course of the disease. Arch. Neurol. **56:** 673–680.

13. WYSS-CORAY, T., E. MASLIAH, M. MALLORY, L. MCCONLOGUE, K. JOHNSON-WOOD, C. LIN & C. MUCKE. 1997. Amyloidogenic role of cytokine TGF-ß1 in transgenic mice and in Alzheimer's disease. Nature **389:** 603–606.

14. VAN DER WAL, E.A., F. GOMEZ-PINILLA & C.W. COTMAN. 1993. Transforming growth factor-beta 1 is in plaques in Alzheimer and Down pathologies. Neuroreport **4:** 69–72.

15. PERESS, N.S. & E. PERILLO. 1995. Differential expression of TGF-beta 1, 2 and 3 isotypes in Alzheimer's disease: a comparative immunohistochemical study with cerebral infarction, aged human and mouse control brains. J. Neuropathol. Exp. Neurol. **54:** 802–811.

16. GREENBERG, S.M., M.E. BRIGGS, B.T. HYMAN, G.J. KOKORIS, C. TAKIS, D. S. KANTER, C.S. KASE & M.S. PESSIN. 1996. Apolipoprotein E e4 is associated with the presence and earlier onset of hemorrhage in cerebral amyloid angiopathy. Stroke **27:** 1333–1337.

17. SEGAL, A.Z., R.I. CHIU, P.M. EGGLESTON-SEXTON, A. BEISER & S.M. GREENBERG. 1999. Low cholesterol as a risk factor for primary intracerebral hemorrhage. A case-control study. Neuroepidemiology **18:** 185–193.

18. SCHEUNER, D., C. ECKMAN, M. JENSEN, X. SONG, M. CITRON, N. SUZUKI, T.D. BIRD, J. HARDY, M. HUTTON, W. KUKULL, E. LARSON, L.E. LEVY, M. VIITANEN, E. PESKIND, P. POORKAJ, G. SCHELLENBERG, R. TANZI, W. WASCO, L. LANNFELT, D. SELKOE & S. YOUNKIN. 1996. Secreted amyloid beta-protein similar to that in the senile plaques of Alzheimer's disease is increased in vivo by the presenilin 1 and 2 and APP mutations linked to familial Alzheimer's disease. Nat. Med. **2:** 864–870.

19. WANG, X.L., S.X. LIU & D.E. WILCKEN. 1997. Circulating transforming growth factor beta 1 and coronary artery disease. Cardiovasc. Res. **34:** 404–410.

20. TOKUDA, T., T. FUKUSHIMA, S. IKEDA, Y. SEKIJIMA, S. SHOJI, N. YANAGISAWA & A. TAMAOKA. 1997. Plasma levels of amyloid beta proteins Abeta1-40 and Abeta1-42(43) are elevated in Down's syndrome. Ann. Neurol. **41:** 271–273.

21. KOSAKA, T., M. IMAGAWA, K. SEKI, H. ARAI, H. SASAKI, S. TSUJI, A. ASAMI ODAKA, T. FUKUSHIMA, K. IMAI & T. IWATSUBO. 1997. The beta APP717 Alzheimer mutation increases the percentage of plasma amyloid-beta protein ending at A beta42(43). Neurology **48:** 741–745.

22. TAMAOKA, A., T. FUKUSHIMA, N. SAWAMURA, K. ISHIKAWA, E. OGUNI, Y. KOMATSUZAKI & S. SHOJI. 1996. Amyloid beta protein in plasma from patients with sporadic Alzheimer's disease. J. Neurol. Sci. **141:** 65–68.

23. GRAINGER, D.J., P.R. KEMP, J.C. METCALFE, A.C. LIU, R.M. LAWN, N.R. WILLIAMS, A.A. GRACE, P.M. SCHOFIELD & A. CHAUHAN. 1995. The serum concentration of active transforming growth factor-beta is severely depressed in advanced atherosclerosis. Nat. Med. **1:** 74–79.

24. TASHIRO, H., H. SHIMOKAWA, K. YAMAMOTO, M. MOMOHARA, H. TADA & A. TAKESHITA. 1997. Altered plasma levels of cytokines in patients with ischemic heart disease. Coronary Artery Dis. **8:** 141–147.

25. KENNY, D., M.G. COUGHLAN, P.S. PAGEL, J.P. KAMPINE & D.C. WARLTIER. 1994. Transforming growth factor beta 1 preserves endothelial function after multiple brief coronary artery occlusions and reperfusion. Am. Heart J. **127:** 1456–1461.

26. GRAINGER, D.J., J.C. METCALFE, A.A. GRACE & D.E. MOSEDALE. 1998. Transforming growth factor-beta dynamically regulates vascular smooth muscle differentiation in vivo. J. Cell Sci. **111:** 2977–2988.

27. BORDER, W.A. & E. RUOSLAHTI. 1992. Transforming growth factor-beta in disease: the dark side of tissue repair. J. Clin. Invest. **90:** 1–7.

28. WYSS-CORAY, T., L. FENG, E. MASLIAH, M.D. RUPPE, H.S. LEE, S.M. TOGGAS, E.M. ROCKENSTEIN & L. MUCKE. 1995. Increased central nervous system production of extracellular matrix components and development of hydrocephalus in transgenic mice overexpressing transforming growth factor-beta 1. Am. J. Pathol. **147:** 53–67.

29. CHAO, C.C., S. HU, W.H. FREY II, T.A. ALA, W.W. TOURTELLOTTE & P.K. PETERSON. 1994. Transforming growth factor beta in Alzheimer's disease. Clin. Diagn. Lab. Immunol. **1:** 109–110.

30. O'DONNELL, H.C., J. ROSAND, K.A. KNUDSEN, K.L. FURIE, A.Z. SEGAL, R.I. CHIU, D. IKEDA & S.M. GREENBERG. 2000. Apolipoprotein E and risk of recurrent lobar intracerebral hemorrhage. N. Engl. J. Med. In press.

The Effect of Iron and Aluminum on Transferrin and Other Serum Proteins as Revealed by Isoelectric Focusing Gel Electrophoresis

S.J. VAN RENSBURG,[a,c] M.E. CARSTENS,[a] F.C.V. POTOCNIK,[b]
AND J.J.F. TALJAARD[a]

*Departments of [a]Chemical Pathology and [b]Psychiatry, Tygerberg Hospital and
University of Stellenbosch Medical School, 7505 Tygerberg, South Africa*

INTRODUCTION

Transferrin (Tf) is a carrier protein which binds metals such as iron (Fe) and aluminum (Al) in the blood. Although it has been demonstrated that Al binds to Tf,[1] very little is known about the absorption, transport, or tissue distribution of Al, since there is no suitable radioisotope of Al which could be used in such studies.[2] Conflicting reports on the binding of Al to serum proteins are found in the literature, for example, Rahman *et al.*[3] found that Al bound exclusively to Tf, in contrast to King *et al.*,[4] who demonstrated that Al was associated with five (unidentified) serum proteins. In the present study, we used isoelectric focusing (IEF) to determine the binding of Fe and Al to serum proteins.

MATERIALS AND METHODS

Isolated Tf was obtained from Dr. G. Johnson, Department of Chemical Pathology, University of Cape Town. Serum was obtained from healthy volunteers. Fe and Al were added to the Tf and serum as ferrous ammonium sulphate (FAS), $FeCl_3$, and $AlCl_3$ to produce Fe- and Al-saturated Tf. The serum solutions were left overnight at 4°C to allow the metals to bind to the proteins. These concentrations were higher than normal values, since Tf is normally only 30% saturated. (Normal iron concentrations: 50–160 mg/L. Al values in serum of healthy individuals: 6.4–11.6 µg/L and patients on hemodialysis: 21–235 µg/L;[3] in patients with Alzheimer's disease, after ingestion of Al citrate: 104.5 µg/L.[2])

For IEF, the method of Kühnl and Spielmann[5] was used, with certain modifications. Composition of the gel: 2.91 g acrylamide (Merck), 0.09 g N,N'-methylene-bisacrylamide (Merck), 8.01 g sucrose; 3 ml Pharmalytes pH 5–8 and 30 µl TEMED (N,N,N',N'-tetramethylethylenediamine; Merck) were added together and made up

[c]Address for correspondence: Dr. S.J. van Rensburg, Department of Chemical Pathology, Tygerberg Hospital and University of Stellenbosch Medical School, P.O. Box 19113, 7505 Tygerberg, South Africa. Tel.: +21 938 4611; fax: +21 938 4640.
e-mail: sjvr@gerga.sun.ac.za

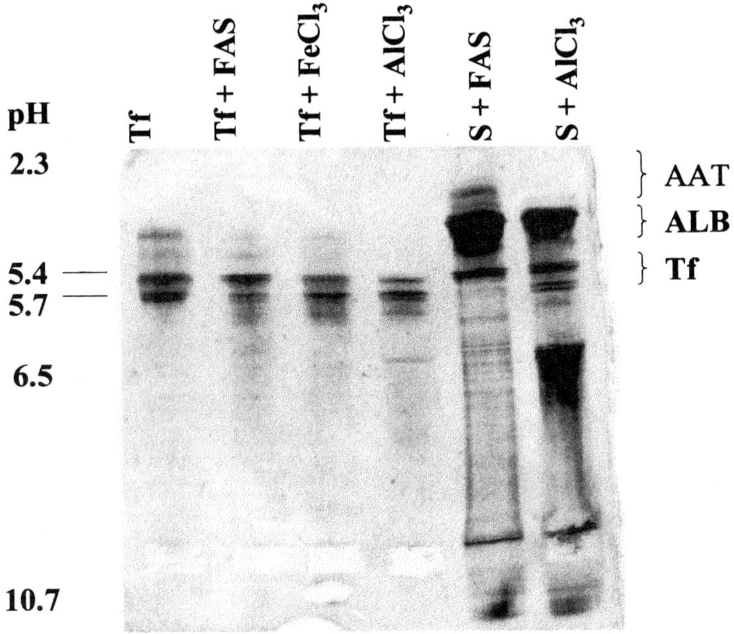

FIGURE 1. Isoelectric focusing gel electrophoresis of isolated transferrin and serum proteins. S, serum; Tf, transferrin; AAT, α1-antitrypsyn; ALB, albumin.

to 60 ml with distilled water. The solution was degassed for a few minutes, after which 1.5 ml of a 20 mg/ml ammonium persulphate solution was added to the gel solution. After mixing gently, the gel solution was poured into a mould using a 50-ml syringe to which a 19-gauge intravenous infusion tube had been attached. The dimensions of the gel were $245 \times 115 \times 2$ mm. Anode and cathode solutions: 0.5 M H_3PO_4 and 0.5 M NaOH, respectively. After prefocusing the gel for 30 minutes at 300 V, sample papers were applied to the gel 0.5 cm from the cathode. Power settings: 1000 V, 18 mA, and 8 Watts. Staining procedure: The gel was stained for 10 minutes in 1 g Coomassie Brilliant Blue R250 (Merck) dissolved in a 1:5:5 mixture of glacial acetic acid:methanol:water (destaining solution) at 37°C, and destained in destaining solution for 1 hour at 37°C. This procedure renders the bands visible for reading the genetic pattern. However, to destain completely, the following destaining solution was used additionally: 500 ml ethanol and 160 ml acetic acid, made up to 2 liters with water.

Gels were dried and preserved using the method of Popescu *et al.*[6]

RESULTS

The effect of Fe and Al on Tf and other serum proteins is illustrated in FIGURES 1–4. On the gels, the following serum proteins are visible from the cathode to the anode:

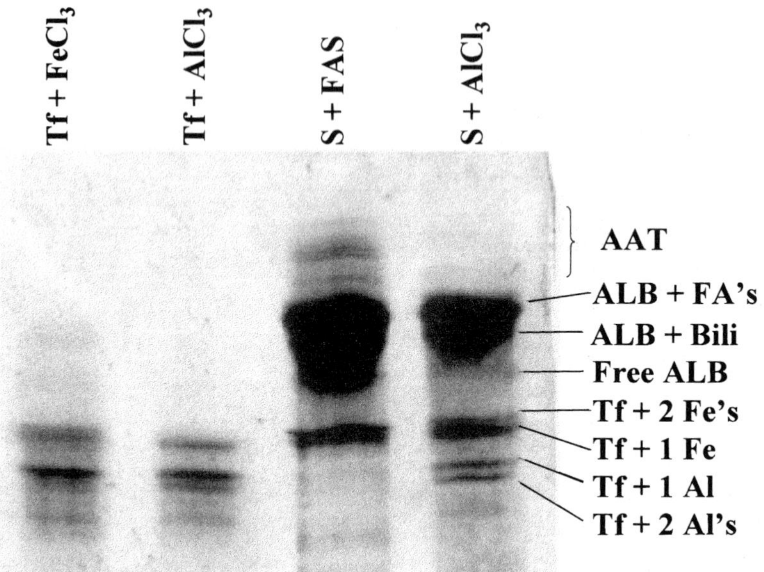

FIGURE 2. Detail of FIGURE 1. S, serum; Tf, transferrin; FAS, ferrous ammonium sulphate; AAT, α1-antitrypsyn; ALB, albumin; FA's, fatty acids; Bili, bilirubin.

(1) Several alpha-1 antitrypsin (AAT) bands,
(2) Three prominent albumin (ALB) bands (corresponding to ALB bound to fatty acids, ALB bound to bilirubin, and free ALB), and
(3) Two groups of Tf bands.

Transferrin

Untreated Tf demonstrated two groups of bands (FIG. 1), seeming to correspond to iron-Tf (3 bands; pH 5.4–5.5) and aluminum-Tf (2 bands; pH 5.7–5.8). These bands were also visible in untreated serum (FIG. 3).

Upon addition of FAS to Tf, the aluminum-Tf bands became less intense, while the iron-Tf bands became darker, especially the more cathodal band, which presumably corresponded to iron-saturated Tf (pH 5.4, FIG. 1). $FeCl_3$ similarly increased the prominence of the iron-Tf bands, although one of the $AlCl_3$ bands also became darker. Addition of $AlCl_3$ increased both the aluminum-Tf bands, and removed the iron-saturated Tf band, but did not remove the other two iron Tf bands, corresponding to the two "one iron-TF" molecules (FIGS. 1–4).

Transferrin in Serum

In untreated serum, bands corresponding to iron-Tf as well as aluminum-Tf were visible, although the latter bands were less prominent than the former (FIG. 3). Upon addition of FAS or $FeCl_3$, the aluminum-Tf bands disappeared, and the iron-Tf

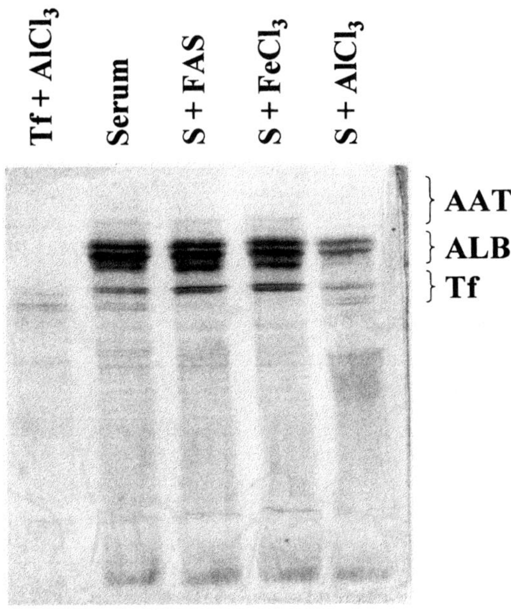

FIGURE 3. Isoelectric focusing gel electrophoresis of isolated transferrin and serum proteins. S, serum; Tf, transferrin; FAS, ferrous ammonium sulphate; AAT, α1-antitrypsyn; ALB, albumin.

bands became more prominent, especially the iron-saturated Tf band (FIGS. 1–4). Upon addition of AlCl₃, the aluminum-Tf bands became more prominent, but all three iron-Tf bands were present as well.

Other Proteins in Serum

The electrophoretic patterns of some other serum proteins were also affected by AlCl₃, but not FeCl₃ (FIGS. 1–4): ALB: the anodal band of ALB which represents the unbound ALB decreased (FIG. 2) or disappeared from the electrophoretic pattern (FIG. 4).

(1) AAT: these bands also disappeared completely from their normal position in the serum treated with AlCl₃ (Figs. 1–4).

(2) A diffuse band appeared at pH 6.5–7 in the Al-treated serum (FIGS. 1 and 3).

DISCUSSION

On the IEF gels, Tf gave bands corresponding to iron-Tf as well as aluminum-Tf, indicating that commercially available Tf contains aluminum as well as iron, as was found by Roskams and Connor.[1] The aluminum-Tf bands occurred in serum as well, indicating that IEF can be used to detect the presence of Al in serum, although this would not be a quantitative measure of the amount of Al present.

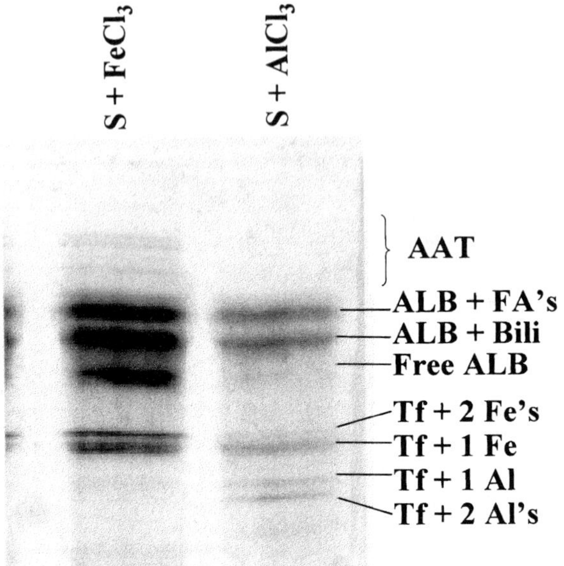

FIGURE 4. Detail of FIGURE 3. S, serum; Tf, transferrin; AAT, α1-antitrypsyn; ALB, albumin; FA's: fatty acids; Bili, bilirubin.

It is clear that adding Al to serum affects some serum proteins in such a way that their electrophoretic mobility is altered. From the results it may be inferred that:

    (1) Fe can displace Al from Tf in serum, but Al does not completely displace Fe, since the aluminum-Tf bands disappeared when Fe was added, but not vice versa. This is in accordance with the belief that Tf binds Fe with approximately 200 times greater stability than Al.[8]

    (2) Al binds to the fraction of ALB which is not bound to its ligands bilirubin or fatty acids. The concentrations of Al in the present study was higher than normal, but serum Al has been demonstrated to be higher in patients on renal dialysis,[3] and in patients with Alzheimer's disease.[2]

    (3) Al binds to AAT and alters its electrophoretic mobility. A low serum level of AAT is associated with lung disease.[9] In AD patients lung infections are frequently found; in fact such patients often die of pneumonia. It is interesting that in 20 patients with AD and 20 nondemented controls, significantly lower ALB and AAT concentrations (39 g/L vs 43 g/L, $p < 0.02$ and 1.57 vs 2.14 g/L, $p < 0.02$, respectively) were found.[10]

    (4) Since ALB is involved with fatty acid transport, any decrease in ALB concentration could jeopardize the availability of fatty acids for incorporation into cell membranes. Lipid peroxidation of cell membranes may play an important role in the etiology of AD.[11]

CONCLUSION

In this study it was confirmed that Tf binds both Fe and Al. Since it has previously been demonstrated that Al exacerbates iron-induced damage to cell membranes at low pH,[12] Tf may be acting as a Trojan Horse, carrying metal ions into the cells in such a way that they are capable of causing oxidative damage.[13] In addition, it was found that increased concentrations of aluminum had an effect on several other serum proteins, confirming that Al as environmental factor may interact with Tf as genetic factor in the etiology of diseases such as AD.

ACKNOWLEDGMENTS

The authors would like to thank Dr. G. Johnson, Department of Chemical Pathology, University of Cape Town, for supplying the transferrin, and Mr. David Dunn, of the South African Institute of Medical Research, Johannesburg, for technical help. We also gratefully acknowledge the financial support given by the Cape Provincial Administration, the Medical Research Council of South Africa and ARDA Western Cape.

REFERENCES

1. ROSKAMS, A.J. & J.R. CONNOR. 1990. Aluminium access to the brain: a role for transferrin and its receptor. Proc. Natl. Acad. Sci. USA **87:** 9024–9027.
2. TAYLOR, G.A., I.N. FERRIER, I.J. MCLOUGHLIN, A.F. FAIRBAIRN, I.G. MCKEITH, D. LETT & J.A. EDWARDSON. 1992. Gastrointestinal absorption of aluminium in Alzheimer's disease: response to aluminium citrate. Age Ageing **21:** 81–90.
3. RAHMAN, H., A.W. SKILLEN, S.M. CHANNON, M.K. WARD & D.N.S. KERR. 1985. Methods for studying the binding of aluminium by serum protein. Clin. Chem. **31:** 1969–1973.
4. KING, S.W., J. SAVORY & M.R. WILLS. 1982. Aluminum distribution in serum following hemodialysis. Ann. Clin. Lab. Sci. **12:** 143–149.
5. KÜNHL, P. & W. SPIELMANN. 1979. A third common allele in the transferrin system, TFC3, detected by isoelectric focussing. Hum. Genet. **50:** 193–198.
6. POPESCU, O. 1983. A simple method for drying polyacrylamide slab gels using glycerol and gelatin. Electrophoresis **4:** 432–433.
7. GIANAZZA, E., A. FRIGERIO, S. ASTRUA-TESTORI & P.G. RIGHETTI. 1984. The behavior of serum albumin upon isoelectric focusing on immobilized pH gradients. Electrophoresis **5:** 310–312.
8. BIRCHALL, J.D. & J.S. CHAPPELL. 1988. Aluminium, chemical physiology, and Alzheimer's disease. Lancet **ii:** 1008–1010.
9. CARRELL, R.W. 1988. The molecular pathology of α-1 antitrypsin. Ann. Clin. Biochem. **25:** 11s–13s.
10. VAN RENSBURG, S.J. 1993. The relationship between some genetic and environmental factors in the etiology of Alzheimer's disease. Ph.D thesis. Stellenbosch University, Stellenbosch.
11. VAN RENSBURG, S.J., W.M.U. DANIELS, J. VAN ZYL, F.C.V. POTOCNIK, B.J. VAN DER WALT & J.J.F. TALJAARD. 1994. Lipid peroxidation and platelet membrane fluidity—implications for Alzheimer's disease? NeuroReport **5:** 2221–2224.
12. GUTTERIDGE, J.M.C., G.J. QUINLAN, I. CLARK & B. HALLIWELL. 1985. Aluminium salts accelerate peroxidation of membrane lipids stimulated by iron salts. Biochim. Biophys. Acta **835:** 441–447.
13. VAN RENSBURG, S.J., M.E. CARSTENS, F.C.V. POTOCNIK, G.D. VAN DER SPUY, B.J. VAN DER WALT & J.J.F. TALJAARD. 1995. Transferrin C2 and Alzheimer's disease: another piece of the puzzle found? Med. Hypotheses **44:** 229–306.

Aβ Vasoactivity *in Vivo*

ZHIMING SUO,[a] GEORGE SU, ANDON PLACZEK, AMY KUNDTZ,
JAMES HUMPHREY, FIONA CRAWFORD, AND MIKE MULLAN

Roskamp Institute, Tampa, Florida 33613, USA

ABSTRACT: Bilateral temporoparietal hypoperfusion has been frequently observed early in the Alzheimer's disease (AD) process. The β-amyloid (Aβ) peptide is believed to play a central role in the pathogenesis of AD. *In vitro* experiments have shown that freshly solubilized Aβ enhances constriction of cerebral and peripheral vessels. We proposed that *in vivo*, Aβ would also have vasoactive properties. To test this hypothesis, we intraarterially infused freshly solubilized $A\beta_{1-40}$ in rats and observed changes in peripheral blood pressure, cerebral blood flow, and cerebrovascular resistance. We found that infusion of Aβ *in vivo* significantly increased the blood pressure in hypotensive rats but not in normotensive and hypertensive rats. Moreover, Aβ infusion also resulted in a decreased blood flow and increased vascular resistance specifically in cerebral cortex but not in heart or kidneys. These data suggest that Aβ has a direct and specific constrictive effect on cerebral vessels *in vivo*, which may contribute to the cerebral hypoperfusion observed early in the AD process.

INTRODUCTION

Bilateral temporoparietal hypoperfusion is one of the major clinical features evident in the early phases of Alzheimer's disease (AD),[1,2] and regional reduction in cerebral blood flow (CBF) is closely associated with the severity of dementia.[2,3] In addition, hypertension is recognized as a risk factor for AD,[4,5] and both hypertension and hypotension have been associated with the disease.[6,7] Although hypertension may be an independent risk factor for the disease, it is feasible that the disease process itself induces hypertension well before the onset of clinically observable symptoms.

Increased β-amyloid (Aβ) production is one of the pathological features of AD and is believed to play a central role in its pathogenesis. Aβ is deposited in the brain parenchyma of Alzheimer patients as senile plaques, and also in the walls of cerebral vessels in cerebral amyloid angiopathy (CAA). In addition to the fibrillar Aβ deposition that occurs during the formation of senile plaques, levels of nonfibrillar $A\beta_{1-40}$ are also increased in the leptomeningeal vessels of AD cases compared to those of age-matched controls.[8,9] Since deposition of Aβ fibrils also derives from the accumulation of the nonfibrillar form of Aβ, nonfibrillar Aβ may have early pathogenic consequences in the AD process prior to extensive Aβ deposition in the brain parenchyma and cerebral vessels.

[a]Address for correspondence: Dr. Zhiming Suo, Roskamp Institute, 3515 E. Fletcher Avenue, Tampa, FL 33613. Tel.: (813) 974-3722; fax: (813) 974-3915.
e-mail: zsuo@com1.med.usf.edu

We have previously shown Aβ, added to isolated peripheral arteries, results in enhancement of vasoconstriction.[10,11] Recent data from transgenic mice overexpressing mutant human amyloid precursor protein show a significant impairment of cerebral vasoregulation.[12] These data suggest that Aβ may be vasoactive *in vivo*, and that this may contribute to the vascular abnormalities observed in AD patients. To test this hypothesis, we infused rats with Aβ in order to directly observe its effects on both peripheral and cerebral blood circulation.

METHODS

Animal Surgery

Male Sprague-Dawley rats (7–11 months old) were anesthetized (sodium pentobarbital 55 mg/kg, i.p.), and cannulated (P-50) at the right common carotid artery, positioned at the aortic arch for intraarterial infusions and arterial blood pressure (BP) measurements with a digital blood pressure analyzer (Micro-Med). For blood flow (BF) measurements, animals were also cannulated at the left femoral artery to obtain a reference blood sample. After a short stabilization period, animals received an infusion of 0.5 ml peptide solution [40 nmol/kg of freshly solubilized human $A\beta_{1-40}$ (QCB), rat $A\beta_{1-40}$ (QCB), and rat amylin (RBI), respectively] or vehicle (0.9% NaCl) over one minute. Four minutes later, 1 mL of fluorescent microsphere (100,000 spheres/ml, 15 μm diameter, Molecular Probes) suspension in 0.9% NaCl solution was infused at the carotid cannula at a rate of 1 ml/min, while simultaneously withdrawing reference blood from the femoral artery at the same rate. After another ten minutes animals were sacrificed by decapitation, and the target tissues (kidney, heart, and cerebral cortex) were dissected and then followed by digestion and fluorometric quantification as described.[13] BF and vascular resistance (VR) for specific organs were calculated using previously established equations.[14–16] For cerebral cortices and kidneys, the BF and VR were determined separately for either left or right side. Since statistical analyses did not reveal any significant differences between left and right sides for these organs, data from both sides were combined for the final analysis.

Experimental Groups

Two independent experiments were performed to evaluate the Aβ vasoactive effects *in vivo* in the intraarterial Aβ infusion rat model:

BP Experiment

The effects of freshly solubilized human $A\beta_{1-40}$ on mean arterial blood pressure (MAP) were observed in the following groups: (1) spontaneous hypotension (MAP <100 mm Hg, $n = 4$); (2) normotension (MAP = 100–129 mm Hg, $n = 8$); and (3) spontaneous hypertension (MAP >130 mm Hg, $n = 7$). Peak MAP within the 15-minute postinfusion period was analyzed.

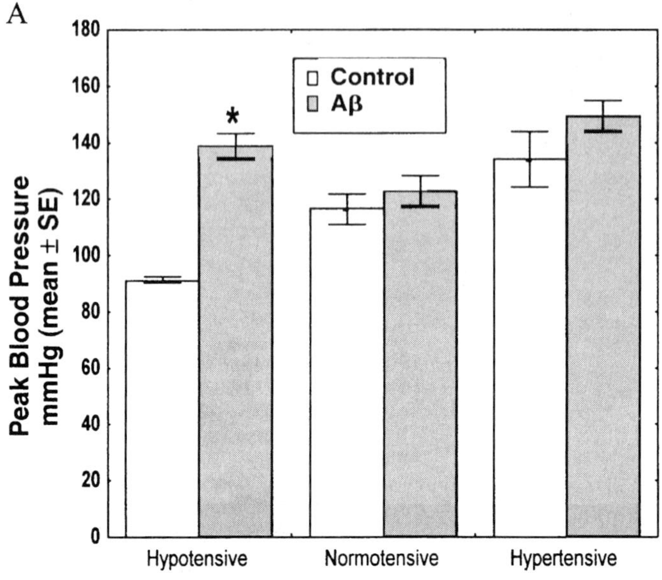
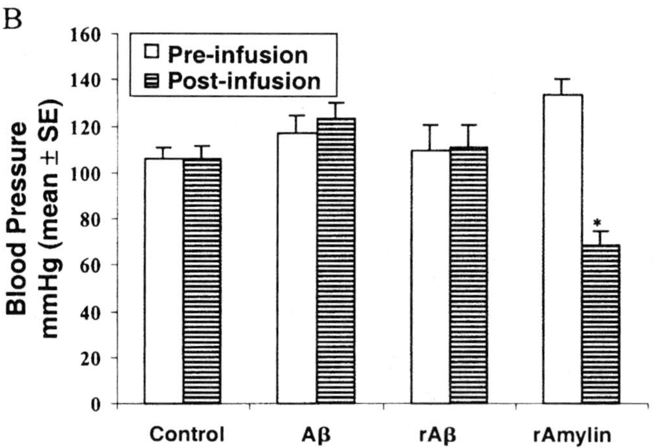

FIGURE 1. Changes in arterial blood pressure in Aβ-infused rats. **(A)** Peak mean arterial blood pressure in normotensive, hypotensive, and hypertensive rats after Aβ infusion. *p <0.01. **(B)** Effects of human Aβ, rat Aβ, and rat amylin on blood pressure. *p <0.001.

BF Experiment

Changes in BF and VR as well as BP were determined as grouped: (1) control, $n = 4$; (2) human $A\beta_{1-40}$ (AB), $n = 5$; (3) rat $A\beta_{1-40}$ (rAB), $n = 4$ and (4) rat amylin (rAmylin), $n = 4$.

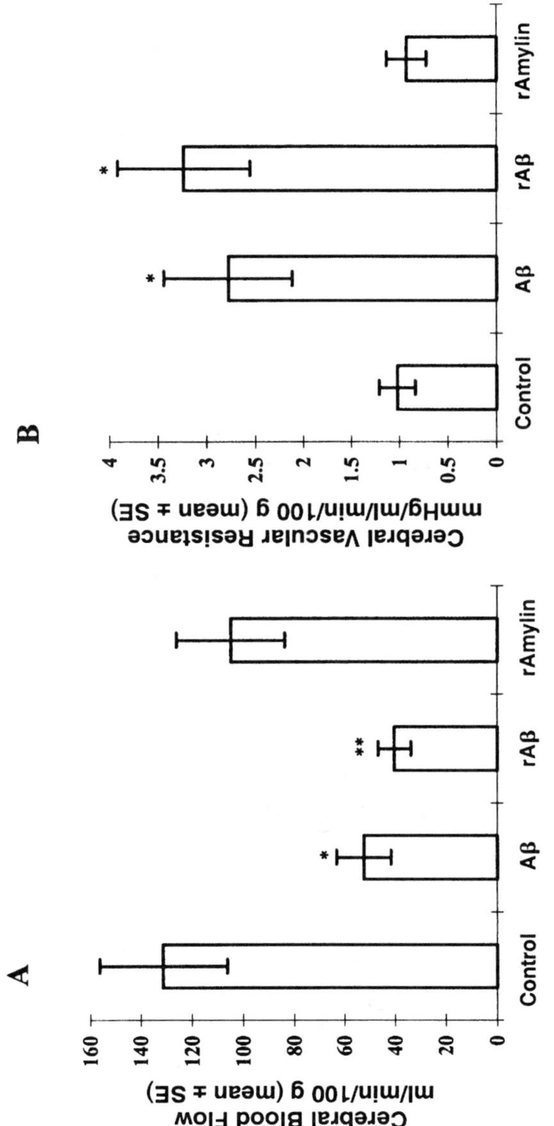
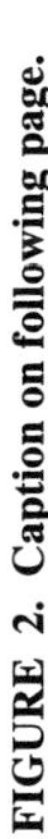

FIGURE 2. Caption on following page.

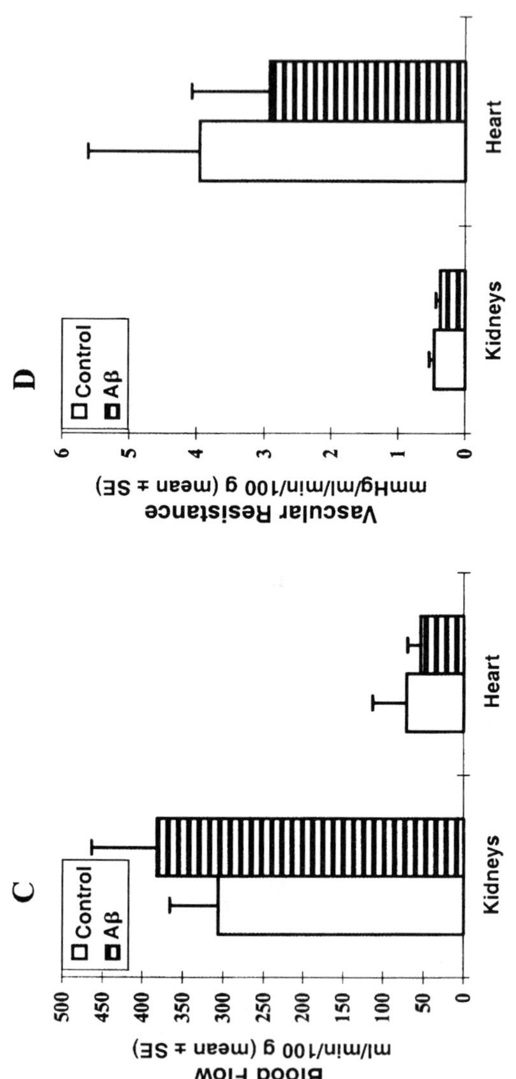

FIGURE 2. BF and VR changes in cerebral cortex (**A,B**) and in kidneys and heart (**C,D**) in Aβ-infused rats. (A) Cerebral blood flow; *p <0.05, **p = 0.01 compared to control. (B) Cerebral vascular resistance; *p <0.05 compared to control.

Statistical Analysis

Data were expressed as means ± SE. Analysis of variance (ANOVA) followed by post-hoc testing (Sheffé) was used to reveal any significant differences.

RESULTS

In the BP experiment, infusion of $A\beta_{1-40}$ into hypotensive rats induced an immediate increase (p <0.01) in MAP (FIG. 1A). However, neither normotensive nor hypertensive rats displayed this increase after Aβ infusion. These data suggested that Aβ *in vivo* can be vasoactive, especially in hypotension.

In an independent experiment on the purpose of BF measurements, the changes in BP were also monitored throughout the experiment. As shown in FIGURE 1B, infusion of human $A\beta_{1-40}$ or rat $A\beta_{1-40}$ did not result in significant changes to BP in these normotensive rats, but infusion of rat amylin, a vasodilatory peptide[17] of similar size to $A\beta_{1-40}$ used as a methodological control, significantly decreased the BP in these animals (p <0.001). By contrast, measurement of CBF during 14 minutes of treatment with either human or rat $A\beta_{1-40}$ revealed a significant (p <0.05) decrease compared to controls, but no such decrease occurred with rat amylin (FIG. 2A). Consequently, a calculation of cerebral vascular resistance (CVR) revealed significant (p <0.05) increases for the $A\beta_{1-40}$ treatments (FIG. 2B). By way of comparison, BF and VR in the heart and kidneys in animals treated with human $A\beta_{1-40}$ were not significantly different from controls (FIG. 2C & D). These results are in agreement with the BP experiment, that Aβ had no significant influence in peripheral BP in normotensive rats. The major effect of Aβ *in vivo* was cerebral microvascular constriction, which was evident by an increased CVR. It should be noted that both rat and human $A\beta_{1-40}$ exhibited similar potency on cerebral vessels, suggesting that *in vivo* Aβ vasoactivity did not reflect an acute species-specific immune response. Taken together, these data indicate that relatively low doses of freshly solubilized $A\beta_{1-40}$ have a direct and specific effect on cerebral vessel constriction *in vivo*.

DISCUSSION

AD is a multifactorial disease. Accumulating evidence suggests that vascular factors contribute to AD pathogenesis by modifying the risk of developing AD, altering clinical presentation, and changing the progression of the disease.[18,19] Of the pathological changes observed in AD cases, regional-specific reduction of CBF and disturbance of BP are the earliest preclinical symptoms associated with this disease process.[1,2,8,9] Meanwhile, a large body of evidence suggests that Aβ may be the central pathological molecule in the AD pathogenesis. Therefore, the relationship between Aβ and cerebral vascular change is of high interest.

It has been demonstrated repeatedly that Aβ is vasoconstrictive *in vitro*, with the effective concentration as low as 50 nM (Paris, unpublished data). Taken together with the recent finding that normal human plasma Aβ level is approximately 10 nM and elevated at least 5 times in AD cases,[20] it is entirely plausible that the elevated plasma Aβ level in AD cases can be effectively vasoconstrictive in the presence of proper mediators.

In this study, we demonstrated that intraarterial infusion of Aβ significantly increases MAP only in hypotensive animals. More importantly, Aβ does not significantly change peripheral BP but it does significantly constrict cerebral microvessels in normotensive animals. Therefore, our results suggest that Aβ is vasoactive *in vivo*, and preferentially influences cerebral microvessels. This phenomenon may explain why, despite the fact that there are increased levels of circulating Aβ in AD patients, there appear to be predominantly cerebral rather than systemic vascular consequences.

As none of the variables that were measured in the present experimental paradigm reflect activity of large vessels, the current study does not preclude the possibility that circulating Aβ also affects large and medium sized arteries, and perhaps veins. Since peripheral blood pressure is mainly determined by changes in resistance vessels, the absence of change in peripheral blood pressure in normotensive rats does not necessarily reflect an absence of vasoconstriction in large vessels.

The cerebral specificity of the observed *in vivo* vasoconstrictive effects can be explained in several ways; there may be phenotypic differences in response to Aβ stimulation between the peripheral and cerebral vessels. For instance, it is known that endothelin is the major vasoconstrictor controlling cerebral vascular tension, whereas epinephrine and norepinephrine are major regulators of vasoconstriction in the periphery. We have previously shown that the same dose of Aβ enhances endothelin vasoconstriction much more (5–10-fold) than an epinephrine analogue (phenylephrine)-mediated vasoconstriction.[10,11] Therefore, it may be that the selective cerebral effects are due to the potentiation of endothelin vasoconstriction. Although the specificity of our findings may suggest a receptor-mediated event, it is also possible that distribution of the infused Aβ *in vivo* differs in cerebral and peripheral vessels. Additional investigation, including the examination of the kinetics of an Aβ dose-dependent response, will be necessary to further characterize the mechanism of *in vivo* Aβ vasoactivity, and clarify the differences observed between cerebral and peripheral tissues.

ACKOWLEDGMENT

The authors would like to thank Mr. and Mrs. R. Roskamp for their generous support to this work. This research was supported, in part, by a Zenith award from the Alzheimer's Association to M.M.

REFERENCES

1. WALDEMAR, G., P. HOGH & O.B. PAULSON. 1997. Functional brain imaging with single-photon emission computed tomography in the diagnosis of Alzheimer's disease. Int. Psychogeriatr. **9**(Suppl. 1): 223–227.
2. HIRSCH, C., P. BARTENSTEIN, S. MINOSHIMA, D. MOSCH, F. WILLOCH, K. BUCH, D. SCHAD, M. SCHWAIGER & A. KURZ. 1997. Reduction of regional cerebral blood flow and cognitive impairment inpatients with Alzheimer's disease: evaluation of an observer-independent analytic approach. Dement. Geriatr. Cogn. Disord. **8**(2): 98–104.

3. BROWN, D.R., R. HUNTER, D.J. WYPER, J. PATTERSON, R.C. KELLY, D. MONTALDI & J. MCCULLOUCH. 1996. Longitudinal changes in cognitive function and regional cerebral function in Alzheimer's disease: a SPECT blood flow study. J. Psychiatr. Res. **30**(2): 109–126.

4. HARRIS, Y., P.B. GORELICK, S. FREELS, M. BILLINGSLEY, N. BROWN & D. ROBINSON. 1995. Neuroepidemiology of vascular and Alzheimer's dementia among African-American women. J. Natl. Med. Assoc. **87**: 741–745.

5. KOKMEN, E., C.M. BEARD, V. CHANDRA, K.P. OFFORD, B.S. SCHOENBERG & D.J. BALLARD. 1991. Clinical risk factors for Alzheimer's disease: a population-based case-control study. Neurology **41**: 1393–1397.

6. SKOOG, I., B. LERNFELT, S. LANDAHL, B. PALMERTZ, A. ANDREASSON, L. NILSSON, G. PERSSON, A. ODEN & A. SVANBORG. 1996. 15-year longitudinal study of blood pressure and dementia. Lancet **347**: 1141–1145.

7. PASSANT, U., S. WARKENTIN & L. GUSTAFSON. 1997. Orthostatic hypotension and low blood pressure in organic dementia: a study of prevalence and related clinical characteristics. Int. J. Geriatr. Psychiatry **12**: 395–403.

8. HAMANO, T., M. YOSHIMURA, T. YAMAZAKI, Y. SHINKAI, K. YANAGISAWA, M. KURIYAMA & Y. IHARA. 1997. Amyloid beta-protein (A beta) accumulation in the leptomeninges during aging and in Alzheimer disease. J. Neuropathol. Exp. Neurol. **56**(8): 922–932.

9. SHINKAI, Y., M. YOSHIMURA, Y. ITO, A. ODAKA, N. SUZUKI, K. YANAGISAWA & Y. IHARA. 1995. Amyloid beta-proteins 1–40 and 1–42(43) in the soluble fraction of extra- and intracranial blood vessels. Ann. Neurol. **38**(3): 421–428.

10. THOMAS, T., G. THOMAS, C. MCCLENDON, T. SUTTON & M. MULLAN. 1996. β-Amyloid-mediated vasoactivity and vascular endothelial damage. Nature **380**: 168–171.

11. CRAWFORD, F., Z. SUO, C. FANG & M. MULLAN. 1998. Characteristics of the *in vitro* vasoactivity of β-amyloid peptides. Exp. Neurol. **150**: 159–168.

12. IADECOLA, C., F. ZHANG, K. NIWA, C. ECKMAN, S.K. TURNER, E. FISCHER, S. YOUNKIN, D.R. BORCHELT, K.K. HSIAO & G.A. CARLSON. 1999. SOD1 rescues cerebral endothelial dysfunction in mice overexpressing amyloid precursor protein. Nat. Neurosci. **2**(2): 157–161.

13. MARCUS, M.L., D.D. HEISTAD, J.C. EHRHARDT & F.M. ABBOUD. 1976. Total and regional cerebral blood flow measurement with 7-, 10-, 15-, 25-, and 50-mum microspheres. J. Appl. Physiol. **40**(4): 501–507.

14. NAKIA, M., K. TAMAKI, J. YAMAMOTO, A. SHIMOUCHI & M. MAEDA. 1990. A minimally invasive technique for multiple measurement of regional blood flow of the rat brain using radiolabeled microspheres. Brain Res. **507**(1): 168–171.

15. SUO, Z., J. HUMPHREY, A. KUNDTZ, F. SETHI, A. PLACZEK, F. CRAWFORD & M. MULLAN. 1998. Soluble Alzheimer's β-amyloid constricts the cerebral vasculature *in vivo*. Neurosci. Lett. **257**: 77–80.

16. ARENDASH, G.W., G.C. SU, F.C. CRAWFORD, K.B. BJUGSTAD & M. MULLAN. 1999. Intravascular β-amyloid infusion increases blood pressure: implications for a vasoactive role of β-amyloid in the pathogenesis of Alzheimer's disease. Neurosci. Lett. **268**: 17–20.

17. WESTFALL, T.C. & M. CURFMAN-FALVEY. 1995. Amylin-induced relaxation of the perfused mesenteric arterial bed:meditatin by calcitonin gene-related peptide receptors. J. Cardiovasc. Pharmacol. **26**(6): 932–936.

18. SLOOTER, A., M.X. TANG, C. VAN DUIJN, Y. STERN, A. OTT, K. BELL, M. BRETELER, C. VAN BROECKHOVEN, T. TATEMICHI, B. TYCKO, A. HOFMAN & R. MAYEUX. 1997. Apolipoprotein E ε4 and the risk of dementia with stroke. A population-based investigation. JAMA **277**: 818–821.

19. SNOWDON, D.A., L.H. GREINER, J.A. MORTIMER, K.P. RILEY, P.A. GREINER & W.R. MARKESBERY. 1997. Brain infarction and the clinical expression of Alzheimer disease. The nun study. JAMA **277**: 813–817.

20. KUO, Y.M., M.R. EMMERLING, H.C. LAMPERT, S.R. HEMPELMAN, T.A. KOKJOHN, A.S. WOODS, R.J. COTTER & A.E. ROHER. 1999. High levels of circulating abeta42 are sequestered by plasma proteins in Alzheimer's disease. Biochem. Biophys. Res. Commun. **257**: 787–791.

Cytochemistry of Intraplatelet Ca^{++} Spots as a Peripheral Marker of Age-related Brain Impairment

CARLO BERTONI-FREDDARI,[a,c] TIZIANA CASOLI,[a] PATRIZIA FATTORETTI,[a] LUCIANO GALEAZZI,[a] GIUSEPPINA DI STEFANO,[a] NATASCIA BELARDINELLI,[b] EUGENIO PUCCI,[b] AND MARIO SIGNORINO[b]

[a]*Neurobiology of Aging Laboratory, "N. Masera" Research Department, INRCA, Ancona, Italy*

[b]*Neurology Clinic, University of Ancona, Torrette, Ancona, Italy*

The etiology and/or the causative events leading to dementing illnesses typical of the third age are still poorly understood. However, an early diagnosis may offer a good opportunity to tackle the problem in due time and, hopefully, to retard the progressive and relentless decline of the senile demented brain. Precocious changes in peripheral cells have been hypothesized to mirror alterations occurring in neurons.[1,2] Conceivably these alterations may constitute potential markers of the risk to develop an age-related dementing pathology. In agreement with this rationale, a consistent proliferation of internal membranes has been reported within the platelets of patients affected by Alzheimer's disease.[1,2] These newly synthesized membranes are supposed to be involved in sequestering the free calcium ions escaping impaired homeostatic mechanisms.[2,3] With the aim of assessing the calcium content in human platelets, we set up a morphometric procedure to verify whether cytochemically evidenced intraplatelet calcium aggregates can be considered as a predictive risk factor of a dementing pathology of the senile brain.

Human platelets were isolated from 10 ml of blood samples obtained from 6 adult healthy volunteers (mean age: 45.3 years). Intraplatelet calcium ions were cytochemically evidenced by the oxalate pyroantimonate (OPA) preferential staining.[4,5] Embedding, sectioning, and contrasting were carried out according to conventional electron microscopic procedures. The number and the area of the OPA aggregates/μm^2 of the total sampled area, the area of the OPA deposits/μm^2 of platelet surface, and the percentage of OPA-positive platelets were measured by random sampling and point counting methods adapted to our image analysis system. Collection of data was terminated when 100 OPA-positive platelets were analyzed. The OPA-Ca^{++} reaction sites can be easily identified within platelets as discrete dark spots with a sharp membrane (FIG. 1). The histograms reported in FIGURE 2 show

[c]Address for correspondence: Dr. Carlo Bertoni-Freddari, Neurobiology of Aging Laboratory, "N. Masera" Research Department, INRCA, Via Birarelli 8, 60121 Ancona, Italy. Tel.: +39 71 8004153; fax: +39 71 206791.

e-mail: c.bertoni@inrca.it

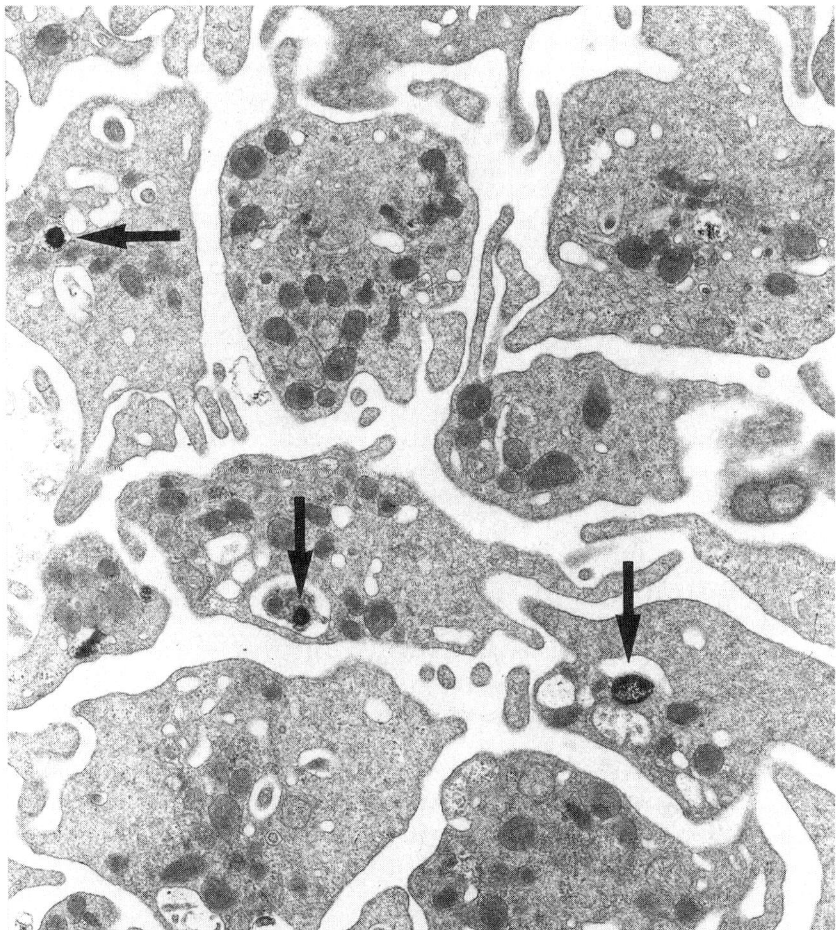

FIGURE 1. Electron microscopic picture of human platelets stained by the OPA procedure. The dark spots (*arrows*) are due to Ca^{++} ions stored within vesicles. Enlargement: 20,800×.

that the standard error of the mean of our measured parameters is rather high (24–27%), with the exception of the spot area/platelet surface where it accounts for 12%.

Our studies document that the intraplatelet calcium aggregates due to OPA reaction can be semiautomatically quantified by computer-assisted morphometry. Since the OPA procedure allows the identification of millimolar quantities of calcium ions,[4] only the sites where these ions are concentrated can be evidenced as sharp deposits and possibly indicate an increased Ca^{++} sequestering activity by platelets. Conceivably, the amount of ions represents a critical determinant in the cytochemistry of intraplatelet calcium aggregates evidenced by the OPA reaction. Previous studies have reported that only a discrete population (15%) of platelets is altered in senile demented patients.[2] Thus, despite the limiting step of Ca^{++} ions concentration, mor-

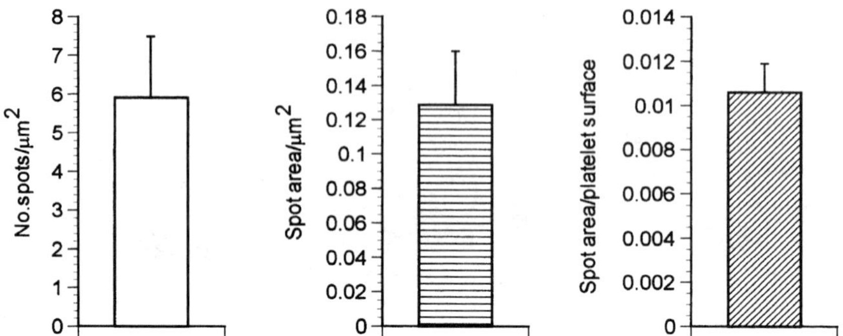

FIGURE 2. Morphometric parameters of theintraplatelet OPA-Ca^{++} deposits. Number of spots/μm^2 of the total sampled area, spot area/μm^2 of total sampled area, and spot area/platelet surface. The high value of the standard error of the mean (SEM) for each parameter is due to the still reduced number of subjects (6) investigated. The OPA-positive platelets accounted for 1% of the total thrombocytes screened.

phometric investigations appear to be very useful, since they enable one to select the fraction of thrombocytes where changes have occurred and to carry out quantitative analyses on the specific ultrastructural features of the OPA-Ca^{++} spots. Ca^{++} ions concentration within discrete cellular compartments has physiological significance, since it is closely coupled with specific functional activities;[4,5] in turn, alteration of intracellular calcium homeostasis is documented to constitute an early detrimental event in physiological brain aging and, to a higher extent, in age-related pathologies, e.g., Alzheimer's disease.[6] If changes in peripheral cells mirror neuronal alterations,[1,2] the assessment of an increased Ca^{++} sequestering activity by platelets of normal elderly subjects may represent an early and quantifiable marker of the risk to develop a dementing syndrome and may help to set up strategies to prevent or at least retard the steep progression of the demented state.

REFERENCES

1. PILETZ, J.E., M. SARASUA, P. WHITEHOUSE *et al.* 1991. Intracellular membranes are more fluid in platelets of Alzheimer's disease patients. Neurobiol. Aging **12:** 401–406.
2. ZUBENKO, G.S., I. MALINAKOVA & B. CHOJNACKI. 1987. Proliferation of internal membranes in platelets from patients with Alzheimer's disease. J. Neuropathol. Exp. Neurol. **46:** 407–418.
3. HAJIMOHAMMADREZA, I., M.J. BRAMMER, S. EAGGER *et al.* 1990. Platelet and erythrocyte membrane changes in Alzheimer's disease. Biochim. Biophys. Acta **1025:** 208–214.
4. HOROYAN, M., M. SOLER, A.M. BENOLIEL *et al.* 1992. Localization of calcium changes in stimulated mast cells. J. Histochem. Cytochem. **40:** 51–63.
5. MATA, M., J. STAPLE & D.J. FINK. 1987. Ultrastructural distribution of Ca^{++} within neurons: an oxalate pyroantimonate study. Histochemistry **87:** 339–349.
6. KHACHATURIAN, Z.S. 1989. The role of calcium regulation in brain aging: re-examination of a hypothesis. Aging **1:** 17–34.

Lipoproteins in the Central Nervous System

MARY JO LADU,[a,b] CATHERINE REARDON,[b] LINDA VAN ELDIK,[c]
ANNE M. FAGAN,[d] GUOJUN BU,[e] DAVID HOLTZMAN,[d] AND
GODFREY S. GETZ[b]

[b]Department of Pathology, University of Chicago, Chicago, Illinois, USA

[c]Department of Cell and Molecular Biology, Northwestern University Medical School,
Chicago, Illinois, USA

Departments of [d]Neurology and [e]Pediatrics, Washington University School of Medicine,
St. Louis, Missouri, USA

ABSTRACT: Although the synthesis and metabolism of plasma lipoproteins are
well characterized, little is known about lipid delivery and clearance within the
central nervous system (CNS). Our work has focused on characterizing the lipoprotein particles present in the cerebrospinal fluid (CSF) and the nascent
particles secreted by astrocytes. In addition to carrying lipids, we have found
that β-amyloid (Aβ) associates with lipoproteins, including the discoidal particles secreted by cultured astrocytes and the spherical lipoproteins found in
CSF. We believe that association with lipoproteins provides a means of transport and clearance for Aβ. This process may be further influenced by an interaction between Aβ and apoprotein E (apoE), the primary protein component
of CNS lipoproteins. Specifically, we have investigated the formation and physiologic relevance of a SDS-stable complex between apoE and Aβ. In biochemical assays, native apoE2 and E3 (associated with lipid particles) form an SDS-
stable complex with Aβ that is 20-fold more abundant than the apoE4:Aβ complex. In cell culture, native apoE3 but not E4 prevents Aβ-induced neurotoxicity by a mechanism dependent on cell surface apoE receptors. In addition,
apoE and the inhibition of apoE receptors prevent Aβ-induced astrocyte activation. Therefore, we hypothesize that the protection from Aβ-induced neurotoxicity afforded by apoE3 may result from clearance of the peptide by SDS-
stable apoE3:Aβ complex formation and uptake by apoE receptors.

Apoprotein E (apoE), a component of several classes of lipoproteins, regulates plasma lipid transport and clearance by acting as a ligand for cell surface lipoprotein
receptors. Recent genetic, immunohistochemical, and biochemical evidence suggesting a correlation between apoE allelic variation and Alzheimer's disease (AD)
has produced interest in the general function of apoproteins and lipoproteins in the
brain. This chapter summarizes our current understanding of the composition of
CNS lipoproteins, and discusses possible functions for these particles in neurobiology and the pathogenesis of AD.

[a]Address for correspondence: Mary Jo LaDu, Evanston Northwestern Healthcare Research Institute, 1801 Maple Ave., Suite 6240, Evanston, IL 60201. Tel.: (847) 467-5975; fax: (240) 352-4077.
e-mail: mjladu@enhri.birl.nwu.edu

LIPOPROTEINS AND PLASMA LIPID METABOLISM

In the aqueous environment of the blood, neutral lipids circulate packaged as lipoproteins. Lipoproteins are composed of a phospholipid (PL) and free cholesterol shell surrounding a triglyceride (TG) and cholesteryl-ester (CE) core. Lipoproteins are stabilized by surface apoproteins. Apoproteins also serve as cofactors for enzymatic reactions and ligands for lipoprotein receptors. Plasma lipoproteins can be separated by size and density into four major classes that vary in their core TG/CE content and apoprotein composition: chylomicrons, very low-density lipoproteins (VLDL), low-density lipoproteins (LDL), and high-density lipoproteins (HDL). The soluble apoprotein gene family, which includes apoE and apoJ, encodes proteins with amphipathic α-helical structures in the C-terminus that allow the proteins to exist at the water-lipid interface.[1]

ApoE

ApoE is a 35-kDa glycoprotein that circulates in the plasma associated with several classes of lipoproteins including chylomicron remnants, VLDL, and a subset of HDL. ApoE-containing lipoproteins are bound and internalized via receptor-mediated endocytosis by a number of receptors in the LDL receptor (LDLR) family including LDLR, LDL receptor-related protein (LRP), VLDL receptor (VLDLR), LR8/apoE receptor-2, and megalin/glycoprotein 330.[2,3] ApoE plays a major role in the transport of lipoproteins in the bloodstream, where it participates in the delivery and clearance of plasma lipid and cholesterol. For example, in reverse cholesterol transport, cholesterol from peripheral tissues is transported to the liver either directly by apoE-containing HDL or via transfer of the cholesteryl esters to larger particles by cholesteryl ester transfer protein (CETP).

In humans, apoE has 299 amino acids and three major isoforms that differ at two residues: E2 (Cys^{112}, Cys^{158}), E3 (Cys^{112}, Arg^{158}), and E4 (Arg^{112}, Arg^{158}). These single amino acid changes result in functional differences between the apoE isoforms including their relative affinities for both apoE receptors and lipoproteins subtypes.[4]

ApoJ

One of the more recently identified apoproteins is apoJ, or clusterin. In regard to its potential role as an apoprotein, apoJ was first identified by immunoaffinity chromatography localized to a specific subclass of dense plasma HDL, specifically HDL-3.[5] ApoJ has several similarities to apoE. The concentration of both proteins in human plasma is similar (~50 μg/ml), and both apoE and apoJ are highly expressed in liver and brain. However, although there is a clear requirement for apoE in normal plasma cholesterol and TG homeostasis, a specific role for apoJ in plasma lipoprotein metabolism has not yet been defined.

LIPOPROTEINS AND LIPID TRANSPORT IN THE BRAIN

CSF Lipoproteins

In addition to the plasma, lipoproteins are also present in other body fluids such as the CSF. CSF is produced by the choroid plexus and also contains non-resorbed products derived from the interstitial space of the brain and, to a lesser degree, the plasma. As determined by lipid and apoprotein profiles, gel electrophoresis and electron microscopy (EM), CSF lipoproteins are the size (7–15 nM) and density of plasma HDL, contain the core lipid CE, and are spherical.[6–8] CSF lipoproteins appear to be heterogeneous in apoprotein content with apoE, the most abundant apoprotein, localized to the largest particles, apoAI and apoAII localized to progressively smaller particles, and apoJ distributed across the particle size range.

Astrocyte Lipoproteins

While the small apoAI and AII containing CSF lipoproteins may originate from the plasma, evidence suggests that apoE and apoJ are made within the blood-brain barrier (BBB). Following liver transplantation, while the plasma apoE phenotype of the recipient changes to that of the liver donor, the apoE phenotype in CSF does not change, evidence that the apoE component of CSF lipoproteins is synthesized locally.[9] In the CNS, apoE is expressed predominantly by astrocytes and microglia (for review, see Ref. 10). ApoJ mRNA is present in astrocytes, neurons, and the ependymal cells lining the ventricles. We have characterized the lipoproteins secreted by astrocytes cultured from wild-type (WT), apoE (–/–), apoJ (–/–), and apoE transgenic mice expressing human apoE3 or E4 under the control of the GFAP promoter in a mouse apoE (–/–).[11] Non-denaturing size exclusion chromatography demonstrates that WT, apoJ(–/–), apoE3, and E4 astrocytes secrete a population of particles the size of HDL, composed of PL, FC, and primarily apoE and apoJ. The lack of core lipids (CE or TG) suggests that at least a portion of these particles are discoidal in shape, an observation confirmed by EM analysis. ApoE localizes across a range of particle sizes, whereas apoJ localizes only to the smaller particles. Non-denaturing immunoprecipitation and gel electrophoresis of astrocyte particles from WT mice confirm that apoE and apoJ reside predominantly on distinct particles. ApoE (–/–) astrocytes secrete little detectable PL or FC despite comparable apoJ expression whereas apoJ (–/–) astrocytes secrete particles comparable to WT. In addition, particles were not detected in apoE (–/–) samples analyzed by EM. These data suggest that apoE is both necessary and sufficient for normal secretion of astrocyte lipoproteins. The apoJ secreted by cultured astrocytes appears to be in small lipid-poor particles or protein aggregates.

Function of CNS Lipoproteins in Lipid Transport

Unlike the peripheral pathways, little is known about cholesterol and lipid transport and metabolism in the CNS. The fact that both apoE and apoJ are expressed within the brain, isolated from the circulation by the BBB, suggests that in addition to their role in plasma lipid transport, apoE and apoJ may also have a paracrine-like function, delivering and clearing lipid in the brain. ApoE-containing particles generated within neural tissue may deliver their contents to the surrounding cells via uptake by apoE receptors. Brain cells express a variety of receptors in the LDLR family, with glia expressing primarily the LDLR and neurons expressing LRP,[12] apoE receptor 2,[13] and the VLDLR.[14] Cells expressing apoE receptors that have a need for cholesterol or lipid could acquire these lipids following receptor-mediated endocytosis. For example, *in vitro*, astrocyte-secreted apoE-containing particles interact with the LRP on neurons to facilitate neurite outgrowth processes.[15,16] These particles may also participate in the transfer of lipids from particles in the CSF to neural cells within the CNS.

While apoE-containing astrocyte particles may serve as ligands for neural apoE receptors, such a function for apoJ is less obvious because megalin (gp330, also known as LRP-2) is the only receptor identified for mammalian apoJ[17] and is not expressed by neurons or glia. Instead, cells of the choroid plexus and ependyma, as well as brain capillary endothelial cells at the BBB, express megalin.[18] This receptor distribution suggests that apoJ-containing particles may acquire lipid after secretion from astrocytes and may be involved in the transport of lipids and associated components between the brain, blood, and CSF.

ApoE-containing astrocyte lipoproteins may also play a role in lipid clearance. Because spherical CSF lipoproteins are in part derived from the brain parenchyma, it seems likely that nascent astrocyte lipoproteins secreted as discs acquire a CE core and become spherical before reaching the CSF. For example, small discoidal plasma HDL and CSF particles are efficient acceptors of cholesterol.[19] Thus, nascent astrocyte-secreted lipoproteins may participate in the efflux of cholesterol from neural cells, particularly under circumstances of cellular degeneration. Enzymes that participate in cholesterol esterification and transfer in the periphery (lecithin: cholesterol acyltransferase and CETP) are present in the brain[20,21] and may facilitate the incorporation of lipid into particles in the brain parenchyma. Further studies will be required to determine whether astrocyte-secreted lipoproteins can promote cholesterol delivery and clearance, and the role of apoE and apoJ in these processes.

POTENTIAL ROLES FOR APOE AND APOJ IN CNS DISEASE

Clearance and delivery of lipid components could be of particular importance following neural injury. Following a hippocampal denervating lesion, apoE −/− mice cleared lipid-laden axonal debris much more slowly than wild-type.[10] If there are differences in the ability of the apoE isoforms or apoJ to clear cholesterol and lipid following CNS injury, this could have an impact on neurologic outcome. Indeed, both apoE and apoJ increase in response to different brain insults.[22,23] Genetic epidemiological studies have shown that the ε4 allele of apoE is a major risk factor for AD.[24] In addition, recent data suggest that apoE4 is also associated with poor outcome after head trauma,[25] cerebral hemorrhage,[26] cardiac bypass,[27] and possibly stroke.[28] ApoE4 may also influence the age of onset of Parkinson's disease.[29]

Alzheimer's Disease

In regard to AD, one hypothesis is that CNS lipoproteins containing apoE and/or apoJ may provide a vehicle for clearing amyloid-β (Aβ) via lipoprotein receptors.[12,30,31] *In vivo*, apoE and apoJ immunoreactivity is localized to senile plaques.[32,33] *In vitro*, apoE and apoJ interact with Aβ to form a stable complex,[24,30,34–37] alter the aggregation of the Aβ peptide,[38–40] and affect Aβ-induced neurotoxicity.[41–43] In addition, soluble Aβ is found complexed to apoE- and apoJ-containing lipoproteins in plasma and CSF.[34,44] With regard to apoE, reports are conflicting as to whether differences exist between the apoE isoforms in terms of their interactions with Aβ. At least a portion of the apparent discrepancy between published accounts can be attributed to the apoE source. For example, in biochemical assays, native apoE2 and apoE3 (associated with lipid particles) form an SDS-stable complex with Aβ that is more abundant than apoE4:Aβ complex.[30,36,37,45,46] However, purified apoE3 and apoE4 exhibit a comparable affinity for Aβ.[24,37] These results are consistent with the general observation that functional activity of apoE is affected by its conformation, and the conformation of apoE is largely determined by the size, composition, and type (disc versus sphere) of particle with which it is associated. For example, the type of particle and ratio of apoE to lipid further determine the affinity of apoE for specific receptors.[47,48] To the extent that Aβ forms complexes to either the lipid or protein components of astrocyte lipoproteins within brain parenchyma, lipoprotein trafficking would affect the metabolism (deposition and/or clearance) of this pathologic peptide, thus perhaps directly influencing AD pathogenesis itself.

Several lines of evidence support the involvement of apoE receptors in neural homeostasis in general and particularly in processes that may relate to the pathogenesis of AD. First, as discussed above, a variety of receptors in the LDLR family are expressed in the brain. Second, apoE3 enhances neurite outgrowth in vitro by a mechanism requiring LRP.[15,49,50] Third, LRP may play a role in the metabolism of amyloid precursor protein (APP) as LRP has been shown to mediate the endocytosis of a secreted form of APP.[51] Fourth, immunoreactivity for LRP and a number of its ligands including apoE and α2-macroglobulin (α2M) is found associated with senile plaques.[52] Finally, genetic evidence suggests that polymorphism's in either LRP or α2M increase the risk of late-onset familial AD.[53,54] In vitro evidence further supports the hypothesis that apoE receptors are involved in modulating the activity of Aβ. Several studies have shown that the addition of exogenous apoE prevents Aβ-induced toxicity in neuronal cell cultures, as well as Aβ-induced activation of primary rat astrocytes.[42,43,55] Using primary rat hippocampal neurons, we have previously shown that apoE3, but not apoE4, protects against Aβ-induced neurotoxicity, a process inhibited by receptor associated protein (RAP), an antagonist to apoE receptors.[42] We have recently reported that Aβ-induced activation of primary rat astrocytes is also inhibited by the addition of RAP (LaDu and Van Eldik, unpublished observations), suggesting that apoE receptors are cell surface proteins that can translate the presence of extracellular Aβ into cellular responses in both neurons and glial cells.

In addition to clearance, apoE and/or apoJ may effect the trafficking of Aβ by altering deposition of the peptide. Recent studies suggest apoE may specifically influence the deposition of Aβ in vivo. Transgenic mice overexpressing a mutant form of the human amyloid precursor protein (APP^{V717F}), when crossed with apoE (−/−) mice, had less Aβ deposition and no thioflavine-S-positive (fibrillar) Aβ as is normally seen in the presence of mouse apoE.[56] However, recent work by Holtzman, Bales and colleagues demonstrated that when APP^{V717F}/apoE (−/−) mice were crossed with transgenic mice expressing human apoE by astrocytes within the brain, both apoE3 and E4 suppressed early Aβ deposition even when compared to APP^{V717F}/apoE (−/−) mice.[57] These and other recent data from human brain[58] further support the possibility that human apoE can influence Aβ clearance in vivo. For future studies, it will be important to characterize the interaction between apoE, apoJ, and Aβ, utilizing lipoprotein particles likely to be found in the brain, such as those secreted by astrocytes.

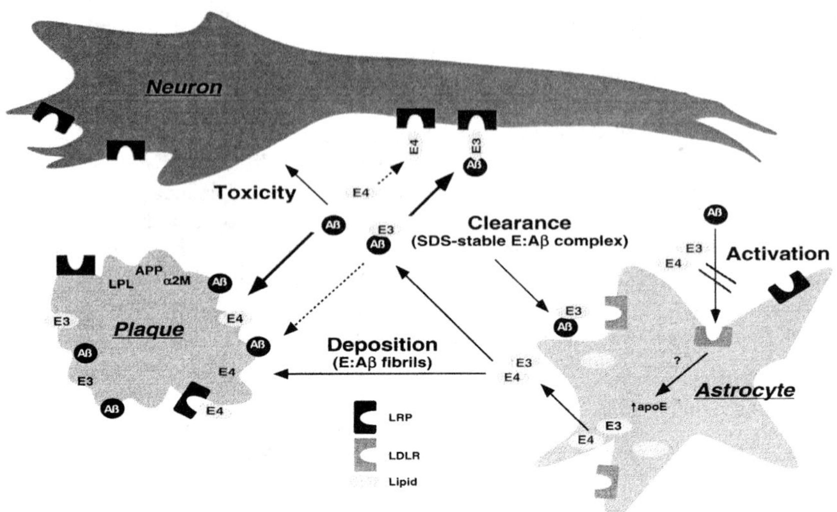

FIGURE 1. Effects of apoE/lipoproteins on the fate of β-amyloid in the CNS: Astrocytes secrete nascent lipoproteins primarily containing apoE. Although not illustrated here, these particles undoubtedly participate in intercellular lipid transport in the CNS. These lipoproteins may also interact with Aβ to (1) effect fibril formation and eventually amyloid deposition; (2) bind a soluble, active form of the peptide facilitating its cellular clearance either by neurons, via LRP, or LDLR on astrocytes and LRP on activated astrocytes. ApoE3 may be more efficient than apoE4 in this clearance pathway as *in vitro* assays demonstrate that apoE3 has a greater affinity for Aβ than apoE4. Aβ not associated with lipoproteins may induce neurotoxicity or astrocyte activation, processes blocked *in vitro* by the addition of apoE via a mechanism dependent on apoE receptors.

SUMMARY

ApoE and apoJ are apoproteins found in plasma in distinct subpopulations of lipoproteins. While an important role for apoE has been found in plasma cholesterol/lipid homeostasis, the role of apoJ remains to be defined. ApoE and apoJ appear to be the principal apoproteins produced in brain. Current research is focusing on characterizing the lipoprotein particles produced by neural cells, as well as determining the function of these particles in cerebral lipid transport both in normal and injured brains. Both genetic, biochemical, and cell biological studies suggest potential roles for apoE, apoJ and their receptors in AD and other CNS diseases.

ACKNOWLEDGMENTS

This work was supported by NIH AG13939 (L.V.E.), NS37525 (G.B.), AG13956 (D.M.H.), AG00861-01, AG05681-16 (A.M.F.); Alzheimer's Association RG3-96-026 (D.M.H.), L0I-96-508 (G.S.G.); American Health Assistance Foundation ADR-97006 (GSG); University of Missouri Alzheimer's Disease and Related Disorders

Program (A.M.F.); the Ruth K. Broad Biomedical Research Foundation (D.M.H.); a Paul Beeson Physician Faculty Scholar's Award from the American Federation from Aging Research (D.M.H.).

REFERENCES

1. LI, W-H. *et al.* 1988. The apolipoprotein multigene family: biosynthesis, structure, structure-function relationships, and evolution. J. Lipid Res. **29:** 245–271.
2. CHRISTIE, R.H. *et al.* 1996. Expression of the very low-density lipoprotein receptor (VLDL-r), an apoprotein-E receptor, in the central nervous system and in Alzheimer's disease. J. Neuropathol. Exp. Neurol. **55:** 491–498.
3. KIM, D.H. *et al.* 1996. Human apoprotein E receptor 2. A novel lipoprotein receptor of the low density lipoprotein receptor family predominantly expressed in brain. J. Biol. Chem. **271:** 8373–8380.
4. WEISGRABER, K.H. *et al.* 1994. Apolipoprotein E: structure-function relationships. Adv. Protein Chem. **45:** 249–302.
5. DE SILVA, H.V. *et al.* 1990. A 70-kDa apoprotein designated apoJ is a marker for subclasses of human plasma high density lipoproteins. J. Biol. Chem. **265:** 13240–13247.
6. ROHEIM, P.S. *et al.* 1979. Apoproteins in human cerebrospinal fluid. Proc. Natl. Acad. Sci. USA **76:** 4646–4649.
7. PITAS, R.E. *et al.* 1987. Lipoproteins and their receptors in the central nervous system. J. Biol. Chem. **262:** 14352—14360.
8. LADU, M.J. *et al.* 1998. Nascent astroctye particles differ from lipoproteins in CSF. J. Neurochem. **70:** 2070–2081.
9. LINTON, M.F. *et al.* 1991. Phenotypes of apoB and apoE after liver transplantation. J. Clin. Invest. **88:** 270–281.
10. HOLTZMAN, D.M. *et al.* 1999. Clusterin-apoE lipoprotein particles. *In* Clusterin in Normal Brain Functions and during Neurodegeneration. C.E. Finch, Ed.: 61–69. R.G. Landes. Georgetown, Texas.
11. FAGAN, A.M. *et al.* 1999. Unique lipoproteins secreted by primary astrocytes from wild type, apoE(–/–), and human apoE transgenic mice. J. Biol. Chem. **274:** 30001–30007.
12. REBECK, G.W. *et al.* 1993. Apolipoprotein E in sporadic Alzheimer's disease: allelic variation and receptor interactions. Neuron **11:** 575–580.
13. KIM, D.H. *et al.* 1996. Human apolipoprotein E receptor 2: a novel lipoprotein receptor of the low density lipoprotein receptor family predominantly expressed in brain. J. Biol. Chem. **271:** 8373–8380.
14. CHRISTIE, R.H. *et al.* 1996. Expression of the very low-density lipoprotein receptor (VLDL-r), an apolipoprotein E receptor, in the central nervous system and in Alzheimer's disease. J. Neuropathol. Exp. Neurol. **55:** 491–498.
15. SUN, Y. *et al.* 1998. GFAP-apoE transgenic mice: astrocyte specific expression and differing biological effects of astrocyte-secreted apoE3 and apoE4 lipoproteins. J. Neurosci. **18:** 3261–3272.
16. NARITA, M. *et al.* 1997. The low density lipoprotein receptor-related protein (LRP), a multifunctional apoE receptor, modulates hippocampal neurite development. J. Neurochem. **68:** 587–595.
17. KOUNNAS, M.Z. *et al.* 1995. Identification of glycoprotein 330 as an endocytic receptor for apolipoprotein J/clusterin. J. Biol. Chem. **270:** 13070–13075.
18. ZLOKOVIC, B.V. *et al.* 1996. Glycoprotein 330/megalin: probable role in receptor-mediated transport of apolipoprotein J alone and in a complex with Alzheimer's disease amyloid β at the blood-brain and blood-cerebrospinal fluid barriers. Proc. Natl. Acad. Sci. USA **93:** 4229–4234.
19. REBECK, G.W. *et al.* 1998. Structure and functions of human cerebrospinal fluid lipoproteins from individuals of different APOE genotypes. Exp. Neurol. **149:** 175–182.
20. ALBERS, J.J. *et al.* 1992. Cholesteryl ester transfer protein in human brain. Int. J. Clin. Lab. Res. **21:** 264–266.

21. SMITH, K.M. *et al.* 1990. Cellular localization of apolipoprotein D and lecithin:choles-terol acyltransferase mRNA in rhesus monkey tissues by in situ hybridization. J. Lipid Res. **31:** 995–1004.
22. MAY, P.C. *et al.* 1992. Sulfated glycoprotein 2: new relationships of this multifunctional protein to neurodegeneration. Trends Neurol. Sci. **15:** 391–396.
23. POIRER, J. 1994. Apolipoprotein E in animal models of CNS injury and Alzheimer's disease. Trends Neurol. Sci. **17:** 525–530.
24. STRITTMATTER, W.J. *et al.* 1993. Apolipoprotein E: high-avidity binding to β-amyloid and increased frequency of type 4 allele in late-onset familial Alzheimer disease. Proc. Natl. Acad. Sci. USA **90:** 1977–1981.
25. NICOLL, J.A.R. *et al.* 1996. Amyloid β-protein, APOE genotype and head injury. Ann. N.Y. Acad. Sci. **777:** 271–275.
26. ALBERTS, M.J. *et al.* 1995. ApoE genotype and survival from intracerebral hemor-rhage. Lancet **346:** 575.
27. TARDIFF, B.E. *et al.* 1997. Preliminary report of a genetic basis for cognitive decline after cardiac operations. The neurologic Outcome Research Group of the Duke Heart Center. Ann. Thorac. Surg. **64:** 715–720.
28. SLOOTER, A.J.C. *et al.* 1997. Apolipoprotein E epsilon-4 and the risk of dementia with stroke—a population based investigation. J. Am. Med. Assoc. **277:** 818–821.
29. ZAREPESI, S. *et al.* 1997. Modulation of the age at onset of Parkinson's disease by apoprotein E genotype. Ann. Neurol. **42:** 655–658.
30. LADU, M.J. *et al.* 1994. Isoform-specific binding of apolipoprotein E to β-amyloid. J. Biol. Chem. **269:** 23403–23406.
31. HAMMAD, S.M. *et al.* 1997. Interaction of apolipoprotein J-amyloid beta-peptide com-plex with low density lipoprotein receptor-related protein-2/megalin. A mechanism to prevent pathological accumulation of amyloid beta peptide. J. Biol. Chem. **272:** 18644–18649.
32. NAMBA, Y. *et al.* 1991. Apolipoprotein E immunoreactivity in cerebral amyloid deposits and neurofibrillary tangles in Alzheimer's disease and kuru plaque amyloid in Creutzfeldt-Jakob disease. Brain Res. **541:** 163–166.
33. CHOI-MIURA, N.H. *et al.* 1992. SP-40,40 is a constituent of Alzheimer's amyloid. Acta Neuropathol. **83:** 260–264.
34. GHISO, J. *et al.* 1993. The cerebral spinal-fluid soluble form of Alzheimer's amyloid beta is complexed to SP-40,40 (apolipoprotein J), an inhibitor of the complement membrane-attack complex. Biochem. J. **293:** 27–30.
35. MATSUBARA, E. *et al.* 1995. Characterization of apolipoprotein J–Alzheimer's Aβ inter-action. J. Biol. Chem. **270:** 7563–7567.
36. ALESHKOV, S. *et al.* 1997. Interaction of nascent apoE2, apoE3, and apoE4 isoforms expressed in mammalian cells with amyloid peptide β(1–40). Biochemistry **36:** 10571–10580.
37. LADU, M.J. *et al.* 1995. Purification of apolipoprotein E attenuates isoform-specific binding to β-amyloid. J. Biol. Chem. **270:** 9039–9042.
38. MA, J. *et al.* 1994. Amyloid-associated proteins α1-antichymotrypsin and apolipopro-tein E promote assembly of Alzheimer β-protein into filaments. Nature **372:** 92–94.
39. SANAN, D.A. *et al.* 1994. Apolipoprotein E associates with β amyloid peptide of Alzheimer's disease to form novel monofibrils. Isoform apoE4 associates more effi-ciently than apoE3. J. Clin. Invest. **94:** 860-869.
40. EVANS, K.C. *et al.* 1995. Apolipoprotein E is a kinetic but not a thermodynamic inhibi-tor of amyloid formation: implications for the pathogenesis and treatment of Alzheimer disease. Proc. Natl. Acad. Sci. USA **92:** 763–767.
41. MIYATA, M. *et al.* 1996. Apolipoprotein E allele-specific antioxidant activity and effects on cytotoxicity by oxidative insults and β-amyloid peptides. Nature Genet. **14:** 55–61.
42. JORDAN, J. *et al.* 1998. Isoform-specific effect of apolipoprotein E on cell survival and β-amyloid-induced toxicity in rat hippocampal pyramidal neuronal cultures. J. Neurosci. **18:** 195–204.
43. LAMBERT, M.P. *et al.* 1998. Diffusible, nonfibrillar ligands derived from Aβ1–42 are potent central nervous system toxins. Proc. Natl. Acad. Sci. USA **95:** 6448–6453.

44. KOUDINOV, A.R. *et al.* 1996. Biochemical characterization of Alzheimer's soluble beta protein in human cerebrospinal fluid-association with high density lipoprotein. Biochem. Biophys. Res. Commun. **223:** 592–597.
45. LaDu, M.J. *et al.* 1997. Association of human, rat, and rabbit apolipoprotein E with β-amyloid. J. Neurosci. Res. **49:** 9–18.
46. YANG, D.-S. *et al.* 1997. Characterization of the binding of amyloid-β peptide to cell culture-derived native apolipoprotein E2, E3, and E4 isoforms and to isoforms from human plasma. J. Neurochem. **68:** 721–725.
47. KOWAL, R. *et al.* 1990. Opposing effects of apolipoproteins E and C on lipoprotein binding to low density lipoprotein receptor-related protein. J. Biol. Chem. **265:** 10771–10779.
48. INNERARITY, T.L. *et al.* 1986. Type III hyperlipoproteinemia: a focus on lipoprotein receptor-apolipoprotein E2 interactions. *In* Advances in Experimental Medicine and Biology. A. Angel & J. Frohlich, Eds.: 273–288. Plenum Press. New York.
49. HOLTZMAN, D.M. *et al.* 1995. Low density lipoprotein receptor-related protein mediates apolipoprotein E-dependent neurite outgrowth in a central nervous system-derived neuronal cell line. Proc. Natl. Acad. Sci. USA **92:** 9480–9484.
50. BELLOSTA, S. *et al.* 1995. Stable expression and secretion of apolipoproteins E3 and E4 in mouse neuroblastoma cells produces differential effects on neurite outgrowth. J. Biol. Chem. **270:** 27063–27071.
51. KOUNNAS, M.Z. *et al.* 1995. LDL-receptor-related protein, a multifunctional apoE receptor, secreted β-amyloid precursor protein and mediates its degradation. Cell **82:** 331–340.
52. REBECK, G.W. *et al.* 1995. Multiple, diverse senile plaque-associated proteins are ligands of an apolipoprotein E receptor, the α-macroglobulin receptor/low-density-lipoprotein receptor-related protein. Ann. Neurol. **37:** 211–217.
53. KANG, D.E. *et al.* 1997. Genetic association of the low-density lipoprotein receptor-related protein gene (LRP), an apolipoprotein E receptor, with late-onset Alzheimer's disease. Neurology **49:** 56–61.
54. BLACKER, D. *et al.* 1998. Alpha-2 macroglobulin is genetically associated with Alzheimer-disease. Nature Genet. **19:** 357–360.
55. HU, J. *et al.* 1998. Apolipoprotein E attenuates β-amyloid-induced astrocyte activation. J. Neurochem. **71:** 1626–1634.
56. BALES, K.R. *et al.* 1997. Lack of apolipoprotein E dramatically reduces amyloid β-peptide deposition. Nature Genet. **17:** 263–264.
57. HOLTZMAN, D.M. *et al.* 1999. In vivo expression of apolipoprotein E reduces amyloid-β deposition in a mouse model of Alzheimer's disease. J. Clin. Invest. **103:** R15–R21.
58. RUSSO, C. *et al.* 1998. Opposite roles of apolipoprotein E in normal brains and in Alzheimer's disease. Proc. Natl. Acad. Sci. USA **95:** 15598–15602.

Apolipoprotein E Genotype and Cerebral Amyloid Angiopathy-related Hemorrhage

MARK O. McCARRON[a] AND JAMES A.R. NICOLL

Department of Neuropathology, University of Glasgow, Institute of Neurological Sciences, Southern General Hospital NHS Trust, Glasgow G51 4TF, United Kingdom

ABSTRACT: Following the identification of the role of the apolipoprotein E (*APOE*) gene polymorphism in Alzheimer's disease (AD), this gene was examined in cerebral amyloid angiopathy (CAA). As in AD, the *APOE* ε4 allele was found to be associated with CAA. Lobar intracerebral hemorrhage is the major clinical manifestation of CAA. Initial studies on a small number of patients with CAA-related hemorrhage (CAAH) identified overrepresentation of *APOE* ε4. However, it became clear that confounding bias from concomitant AD and the need for pathologically confirmed cases of CAAH would also have to be considered. A larger series of pathologically confirmed cases of CAAH, also assessed for AD pathology, found a surprising overrepresentation of the *APOE* ε2 allele. Because of the association between CAA and AD, it might have been predicted that patients with CAAH would have a low, rather than a high, ε2 frequency. The overrepresentation of *APOE* ε2 was present both in patients with and without AD, whereas a high ε4 frequency correlated with concomitant AD.

Further studies found that overrepresentation of *APOE* ε2 is specific for CAAH and is not found in intracranial hemorrhages due to other causes. In CAAH, *APOE* ε2 may interact with putative risk factors for hemorrhage, including antiplatelet/anticoagulant medication, minor head trauma, and hypertension. Several microvascular abnormalities in amyloid-laden blood vessels have been assumed to antedate CAAH and increase its likelihood. *APOE* ε2 has now been found to be associated with some of these vascular abnormalities, specifically a "double-barrel" appearance and fibrinoid necrosis.

The currently favored interpretation is that *APOE* ε4 enhances deposition of amyloid-β protein in the walls of cerebral blood vessels, whereas ε2 is a risk factor for hemorrhage from amyloid-laden blood vessels by promoting specific "CAA-associated vasculopathies."

Cerebral amyloid angiopathy (CAA) is characterized by the deposition of congophilic material, usually amyloid-β protein (Aβ), in the walls of cerebral cortical and leptomeningeal blood vessels. Until 1993, advancing age and Alzheimer's disease were the only recognized risk factors for sporadic CAA, which usually remains clinically silent. The identification of the apolipoprotein E (*APOE* for gene; apoE for protein) ε4 allele as a dose-dependent risk factor for late-onset familial and sporadic Alzheimer's disease,[1,2] as well as co-localization of apoE with Aβ in CAA,[3] has re-

[a]Corresponding author: Tel.: +44 141 201 2046; fax:+44 141 201 2998.
e-mail: mmc18f@clinmed.gla.ac.uk

cently prompted further study of CAA and its major clinical manifestation, CAA-related hemorrhage (CAAH) in patients with and without AD.

CAA increases with age so that nearly 50% of all individuals over 80 years of age have affected cortical and leptomeningeal blood vessels.[4] In addition, 90% of AD patients have evidence of CAA. In an autopsy study of AD brains, Schmechel *et al.*[5] found a strong dose-dependent association of the *APOE* ε4 allele with increased vascular Aβ deposition. Subsequent studies confirmed this association in AD patients[6,7] and in aged patients without AD.[8] A Japanese report has, however, failed to demonstrate this association in patients with and without AD.[9] Although CAA is a common finding in Japan,[10] the discrepancy may reflect the rather low frequency of the ε4 allele in the Japanese population.

Studies on the *APOE* allele distribution in CAAH followed.[8,11–14] The first report by Greenberg *et al.*[8] found in 15 patients with CAAH a statistically significant excess of the ε4 allele compared to a control population. However, only 8 of these patients had pathological evidence of CAA. Another study[14] that examined 13 patients with CAAH and AD also reported an excess of the *APOE* ε4 allele. A larger series followed consisting of 36 patients all of whom had pathologically confirmed diagnoses of CAAH.[11,12] The group was also assessed for neuropathological evidence of AD.[12] This revealed a surprising threefold excess of the ε2 allele (0.25), which had previously been documented to protect an individual from AD.[15] The elevated ε2 frequency in CAAH was present in patients both with and without pathological evidence of AD. One-third of the patients had evidence of multiple hematomas, and these had an even higher ε2 frequency (0.35 versus 0.20). The patients with CAAH and AD had an ε4 frequency similar to patients with AD alone. Patients with CAAH but not AD had an ε4 frequency similar to controls with neither AD nor CAAH. This was interpreted as indicating that the excess of ε4 in this population was due to the association of AD with CAA. The excess of the ε2 allele in CAAH appears to be specific for this pathological process and is not seen in patients with deep, hypertensive intracerebral hemorrhage or subarachnoid hemorrhage due to saccular aneurysms.[16]

Following this report, both clinical and pathological observations in CAAH patients were reviewed to determine the mechanism by which *APOE* ε2 might predispose an individual with CAA to hemorrhage. The larger pathological study[12] established that the ε2 allele was associated with hemorrhage at a younger age, a finding that has been subsequently confirmed,[17] but may also apply to ε4 carriers.[13,17] Clinical risk factors for CAAH have not been consistently established,[18–20] although hypertension,[18] minor head trauma,[21] antiplatelet or anticoagulant medication,[20,22,23] and thrombolytic therapy[24,25] have all been described as potential precipitants of CAAH. Intriguingly, the presence of any one of three of these features (antiplatelet/anticoagulant medication, minor head trauma or hypertension) has recently been shown to segregate with ε2 possession among 36 cases of pathologically confirmed CAAH; of particular prominence is the group taking antiplatelet or anticoagulant medication.[26] There has been some support for this finding in patients consuming warfarin, who appear to be at a higher risk of a lobar hemorrhage if they possess an ε2 allele.[27] These results suggest that in CAA an interaction between putative clinical risk factors and possession of ε2 may play an important role in leading to the rupture of amyloid-laden blood vessels.

It has been suspected for some time that CAA-associated vasculopathic complications precede vessel rupture and cerebral hemorrhage.[4,20,28,29] Two studies have demonstrated that the ε2 allele may be associated with some of these vascular complications. Among 75 brains with CAA, Greenberg *et al.*[17] found an elevated ε2 frequency (0.09) in brains that demonstrated both vessel wall cracking (i.e., "double-barrel" appearance) and evidence of paravascular blood leak compared to brains without this combination of vasculopathies (0.01). We have recently assessed each of six CAA-associated vasculopathic complications individually among 62 CAA patients with and without macroscopic evidence of lobar hemorrhage.[30] Apparently, stenosed blood vessels (i.e., with an increased ratio of wall thickness to lumen diameter), dilated/microaneurysmal vessels and, to a lesser extent, fibrinoid necrosis were more common in patients with CAAH than in patients with CAA but without macroscopic lobar hemorrhage. The former group of patients also demonstrated more immunoreactivity for cystatin C and perivascular-activated microglia. Of the CAA-associated vasculopathic complications only fibrinoid necrosis was associated with possession of the *APOE* ε2 allele. We have suggested that this structural change in the vessel wall may underpin the association of *APOE* ε2 with CAAH.[30] Indeed, it is plausible that the same association explains how an ε2-carrying individual may be more susceptible to CAAH when exposed to antiplatelet/anticoagulant medication, minor head trauma, and hypertension than patients without the ε2 allele.[26]

All of these findings have strengthened the current hypothesis that possession of the *APOE* ε4 allele is a risk factor for the deposition of Aβ in the walls of cortical and leptomeningeal blood vessels, whereas the *APOE* ε2 allele predisposes to rupture of Aβ-laden blood vessels by promoting one or more CAA-associated vasculopathic complications.

REFERENCES

1. STRITTMATTER, W. *et al.* 1993. Apolipoprotein E: high-avidity binding to beta-amyloid and increased frequency of type 4 allele in late-onset familial Alzheimer disease. Proc. Natl. Acad. Sci. USA **90:** 1977–1981.
2. SAUNDERS, A.M. *et al.* 1993. Association of apolipoprotein E allele ε4 with late-onset familial and sporadic Alzheimer's disease. Neurology **43:**1467–1472.
3. NAMBA ,Y. *et al.* 1991. Apolipoprotein E immunoreactivity in cerebral amyloid deposits and neurofibrillary tangles in Alzheimer's disease and kuru plaque amyloid in Creutzfeldt-Jakob disease. Brain Res. **541:** 163–166.
4. VONSATTEL, J.P. *et al.* 1991. Cerebral amyloid angiopathy without and with cerebral hemorrhages: a comparative histological study. Ann. Neurol. **30:** 637–649.
5. SCHMECHEL, D.E. *et al.* 1993. Increased amyloid beta-peptide deposition in cerebral cortex as a consequence of apolipoprotein E genotype in late-onset Alzheimer disease. Proc. Natl. Acad. Sci. USA **90:** 9649–9653.
6. PREMKUMAR, D.R. *et al.* 1996. Apolipoprotein E-ε4 alleles in cerebral amyloid angiopathy and cerebrovascular pathology associated with Alzheimer's disease. Am. J. Pathol. **148:** 2083–2095.
7. OLICHNEY, J.M. *et al.* 1996. The apolipoprotein E epsilon 4 allele is associated with increased neuritic plaques and cerebral amyloid angiopathy in Alzheimer's disease and Lewy body variant. Neurology **47:**190–196.
8. GREENBERG, S.M. *et al.* 1995. Apolipoprotein E ε4 and cerebral hemorrhage associated with amyloid angiopathy. Ann. Neurol. **38:** 254–259.
9. ITOH, Y. *et al.* 1996. Influence of apolipoprotein E genotype on cerebral amyloid angiopathy in the elderly. Stroke **27:** 216–218.
10. YAMADA, A.M. *et al.* 1987. Cerebral amyloid angiopathy in the aged. J. Neurol. **234:** 371–376.
11. NICOLL, J.A.R. *et al.* 1996. High frequency of apolipoprotein E ε2 in patients with cerebral hemorrhage due to cerebral amyloid angiopathy. Ann. Neurol. **39:** 682–683.2.

12. NICOLL, J.A.R. *et al.* 1997. High frequency of apolipoprotein E ε2 allele in hemorrhage due to cerebral amyloid angiopathy. Ann. Neurol. **41:** 716–721.
13. GREENBERG, S.M. *et al.* 1996. Apolipoprotein E ε4 is associated with the presence and earlier onset of hemorrhage in cerebral amyloid angiopathy. Stroke **27:** 1333–1337.
14. KALARIA, R.N. *et al.* 1995. Apolipoprotein E genotype and cerebral amyloid angiopathy. Lancet **346:** 1424.
15. CORDER, E.H. *et al.* 1994. Protective effect of apolipoprotein E type 2 allele for late onset Alzheimer disease. Nat.Genet. **7:** 180–184.
16. McCARRON, M.O. *et al.* 1998. High frequency of apolipoprotein E ε2 allele is specific for patients with cerebral amyloid angiopathy-related haemorrhage. Neurosci. Lett. **247:** 45–48.
17. GREENBERG, S.M. *et al.* 1998. Association of apolipoprotein E ε2 and vasculopathy in cerebral amyloid angiopathy. Neurology **50:** 961–965.
18. JELLINGER, K. 1977. Cerebrovascular amyloidosis with cerebral hemorrhage. J. Neurol. **214:** 195–206.
19. FERREIRO, J.A. *et al.* 1989. Stroke related to cerebral amyloid angiopathy: the significance of systemic vascular disease. J. Neurol. **236:** 267–272.
20. OKAZAKI, H. *et al.* 1979. Clinicopathologic studies of primary cerebral amyloid angiopathy. Mayo Clin. Proc. **54:** 22–31.
21. GREENE, G.M. *et al.* 1990. Surgical experience with cerebral amyloid angiopathy. Stroke 21:1545–1549.
22. SMITH, D.B. *et al.* 1985. Cerebral amyloid angiopathy presenting as transient ischemic attacks. Case report. J. Neurosurg. **63:** 963–964.
23. ANONYMOUS. 1996. Case records of the Massachusetts General Hospital. Weekly clinicopathological exercises. Case 22-1996. Cerebral hemorrhage in a 69-year-old woman receiving warfarin. N. Engl. J. Med. **335:**189–196.
24. LEBLANC, R. *et al.* 1992. Cerebral hemorrhage from amyloid angiopathy and coronary thrombolysis. Neurosurgery **31:** 586–590.
25. SLOAN, M.A. *et al.* 1995. Clinical features and pathogenesis of intracerebral hemorrhage after rt-PA and heparin therapy for acute myocardial infarction: the thrombolysis in myocardial infarction (TIMI) II pilot and randomized clinical trial combined experience. Neurology **45:** 649–658.
26. McCARRON, M.O. *et al.* 1999. Cerebral amyloid angiopathy-related hemorrhage: interaction of apolipoprotein E ε2 with putative clinical risk factors. Stroke **30:** 1643–1646.
27. ROSAND, J. *et al.* 1999. Cerebral amyloid angiopathy and warfarin-associated hemorrhage: a genetic and neuropathologic study [Abstr.]. Neurology 52(Suppl 2): A503.
28. MANDYBUR, T.I. 1986. Cerebral amyloid angiopathy: the vascular pathology and complications. J. Neuropathol. Exp. Neurol. **45:** 79–90.
29. VINTERS, H.V. 1987. Cerebral amyloid angiopathy. A critical review. Stroke **18:** 311–324.
30. McCARRON, M.O. *et al.* 1999. The apolipoprotein E ε2 allele and the pathological features in cerebral amyloid angiopathy-related hemorrhage. J. Neuropathol. Exp. Neurol. **58:** 711–718.

Apolipoprotein E, Smooth Muscle Cells and the Pathogenesis of Cerebral Amyloid Angiopathy: the Potential Role of Impaired Cerebrovascular Aβ Clearance

REINHARD PRIOR,[a] GÜNTHER WIHL, AND BRITTA URMONEIT

Department of Neurology, University of Duesseldorf, Moorenstrasse 5, D-40225 Duesseldorf, Germany

ABSTRACT: Cerebral amyloid angiopathy (CAA) is caused by the deposition of β-amyloid (Aβ) in Alzheimer disease brains. It also occurs isolated, representing a major cause for cerebral hemorrhage in the elderly. The E4 genotype of apolipoprotein E (ApoE) is a risk factor for CAA; however, the molecular mechanism underlying this genetic association is unknown. Various findings suggest that cerebrovascular Aβ is derived from the soluble Aβ contained in the cortical extracellular space or the cerebrospinal fluid (CSF) that communicates and surrounds small cortical or leptomeningeal vessels. CAA deposits are always intimately associated with smooth muscle cells (SMCs) or SMC-derived pericytes. As we have previously reported, SMCs internalize Aβ *in vitro* via a lipoprotein pathway involving ApoE and the low-density lipoprotein receptor family. Internalized Aβ is subsequently located to lysosomes, suggesting its intracellular degradation. We show that Aβ is internalized via multiple pathways, because class A and class B scavenger receptors are also colocalized to Aβ-containing endosomes in SMCs, and Aβ uptake is inhibited by various scavenger receptor antagonists. It has been recently shown for different cell types that the cellular uptake of ApoE is more efficient for the ApoE3 isoform when compared to ApoE4 and that this isoform-specific difference depends on the presence of heparan sulfate proteoglycan (HSPG). HSPG is produced by SMCs and promotes Aβ fibrillogenesis. We propose a pathogenetic model of CAA, in which the ApoE- and HSPG-mediated clearance of CSF-derived Aβ peptides by SMCs protects the vascular extracellular matrix against critical Aβ concentrations. Impairment of this pathway or its reduced efficiency in carriers of the ApoE4 genotype may increase the risk of developing CAA.

The occurrence of cerebral amyloid angiopathy (CAA) with the cerebrovascular deposition of β-amyloid (Aβ) as a feature of Alzheimer's disease or as a cause of cerebral hemorrhage is strictly associated with the presence of cerebrovascular smooth muscle cells (SMCs) or with pericytes around cortical capillaries that show many similarities to SMCs. SMCs therefore possess critical properties to facilitate the development of CAA. Such properties are likely to be related to SMC differen-

[a]Corresponding author.
e-mail: prior@uni-duesseldorf.de

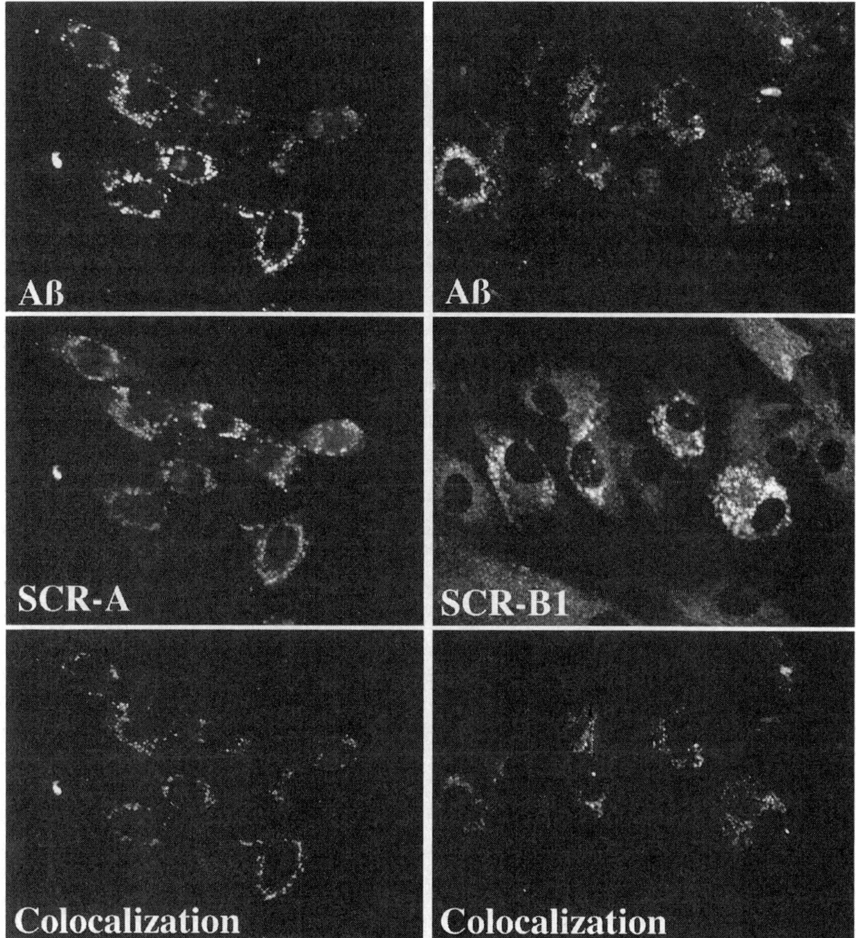

FIGURE 1. Confocal laser scanning micrographs demonstrating colocalization of fluorescein-conjugated $A\beta_{1-40}$ in endosomes of canine leptomeningeal SMCs after 2-h incubation with 1 μM $A\beta_{1-40}$. $A\beta_{1-40}$ is colocalized to class A scavenger receptors (visualized with a polyclonal antiserum against human type I and type II receptors, kindly provided by Dr. Ylä-Herttuala) and to class B scavenger receptors (visualized with a polyclonal antiserum against murine SR BI, kindly provided by Dr. Kozarsky).

tiation and biology. We describe our results with primary human and canine SMCs that were incubated with fluorescein-conjugated Aβ-peptides ($A\beta_{1-42}$ and $A\beta_{1-40}$) and analyzed by fluorescence and confocal laser scanning microscopy. In our opinion, this experimental setup reflects the situation *in vivo*, where vascular SMCs are surrounded by cerebrospinal fluid (CSF), which contains brain-derived Aβ peptides of extravascular, mostly of neuronal origin. An extravascular origin of cerebrovascular Aβ is supported by (1) the abluminal localization of early Aβ deposits in CAA,

(2) the almost exclusive distribution of CAA to cortical and leptomeningeal vessels and its absence in white matter where neurons are myelinated and do not secrete Aβ to the extracellular space, (3) the total absence of vascular Aβ deposition in systemic vessels, and (4) by recent findings in transgenic mice where prominent CAA develops in the absence of vascular amyloid precursor protein expression.[1] Our findings show that exogenous Aβ is bound to the extracellular matrix of SMCs but is also internalized by SMCs via different lipoprotein pathways, suggesting a central role of altered SMC lipoprotein metabolism in the pathogenesis of CAA. Based on these findings and on recent results obtained by others concerning the differential behavior of specific isoforms of apolipoprotein E (ApoE),[2–5] we propose a pathogenetic model of CAA in which a reduced or insufficient Aβ clearance by ApoE-containing lipoproteins contributes to the development of CAA. This model also suggests that reduced Aβ clearance by ApoE4 may determine the increased risk associated with this genotype, and finally considers a central role of SMC-derived extracellular matrix components such as heparan sulfate proteoglycan (HSPG) during the development of CAA.

We have previously shown that N-terminally fluorescein-conjugated Aβ_{1-40} and Aβ_{1-42} peptides bind selectively to senile plaques of Alzheimer brains[6] and to cerebrovascular Aβ deposits in organ cultures of canine leptomeninges,[7] and therefore reflect the behavior of Aβ *in vivo*. When primary cultures of SMCs were prepared from canine or human leptomeninges, we observed that Aβ bound first to the cell surface and was then internalized by receptor-mediated endocytosis.[8] The endocytosis appeared to be mediated via a lipoprotein pathway. In particular, Aβ was colocalized to ApoE and its receptor, the low-density lipoprotein receptor-related protein LRP on the cell surface and within SMC endosomes. The internalization of Aβ was partially inhibited by co-incubation with the 39-kDa receptor-associated protein (RAP), further indicating that Aβ is internalized via a receptor of the low-density lipoprotein receptor family. We show that the uptake of Aβ is also mediated by scavenger receptors, which represent another type of lipoprotein receptors expressed by SMCs. Confocal laser scanning microscopy of canine SMCs incubated for 2 h with 1 μM of fluorescein-conjugated Aβ_{1-40} demonstrates the presence of both class A and class B (SR-BI) scavenger receptors within Aβ containing endosomes (FIG.1). Moreover, the uptake of Aβ from the medium could be partially blocked by co-incubation with scavenger receptor antagonists (FIG.2). Therefore, multiple lipoprotein receptor pathways appear to contribute to the internalization of exogeneous Aβ into SMCs *in vitro*. After internalization, Aβ accumulated within SMC lysosomes as demonstrated by the colocalization of the lysosome-associated membrane protein LAMP1 and by enhanced intracellular accumulation after treatment with chloroquine.[8] The lysosomal localization of Aβ indicates that intracellular degradation is the ultimate fate of Aβ internalized by SMCs. To confirm the degradation of Aβ by cerebral vessels, small arterioles isolated from canine leptomeninges were kept in organ culture and incubated with 1 μM of Aβ_{1-40}. Analysis of the culture media showed a progressive reduction of Aβ contained in the medium when living vessels were incubated with Aβ, whereas no reduction was found when vessels had been previously inactivated (FIG. 3).

Because CSF contains high concentrations of ApoE and CSF-derived ApoE binds Aβ,[9,10] it appears likely that CSF-Aβ is actively internalized by the SMCs of cere-

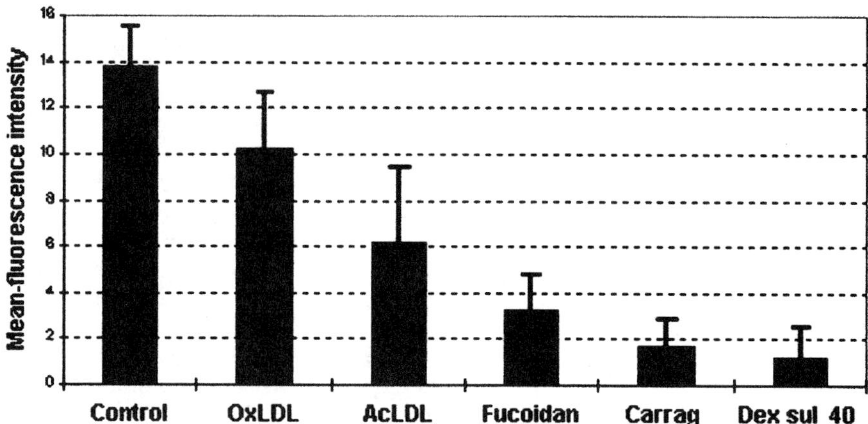

FIGURE 2. Inhibition of SMC internalization of $A\beta_{1-40}$ by different scavenger receptor antagonists. Bars represent the mean fluorescence intensity and standard deviations obtained by flow cytometry of trypsinized cells after a 2-h incubation with 1 μM fluorescein-conjugated $A\beta_{1-40}$ in five independent experiments (3,000 cells per experiment). Experiments were performed by co-incubation with oxidized LDL (100 μg/ml), acetylated LDL (25 μg/ml), carrageenan (2 mg/ml), fucoidan (200 μg/ml), and 40 kDa dextran sulfate (2 mg/ml).

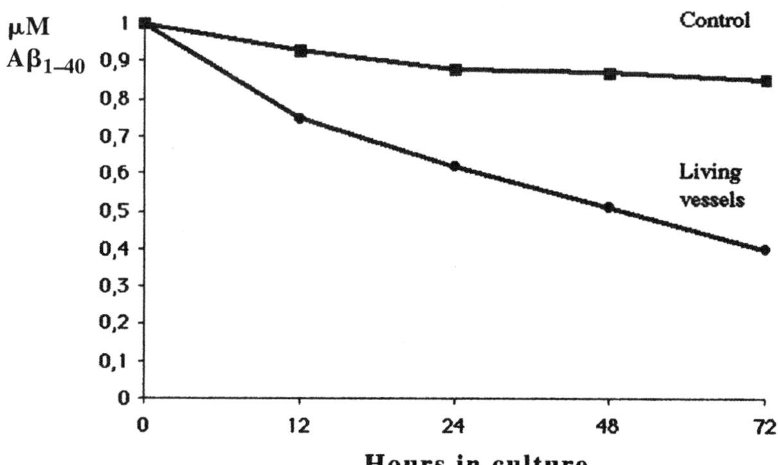

FIGURE 3. Removal of $A\beta_{1-40}$ by organ cultures of vessels isolated from canine meninges. Vessels were cultured in 200 μl of CSF and 1 μM $A\beta_{1-40}$. The concentration of $A\beta_{1-40}$ at different time points was measured by ELISA. Cultures of living vessels show a progressive decrease of the Aβ concentrations when compared to vessels that were inactivated by treatment with 1 M KCN.

bral vessels via ApoE-mediated lipoprotein pathways *in vivo*. The cerebrovascular accumulation of CSF-derived Aβ is further supported by the following data: CSF contains a heterogeneous set of Aβ peptides with the more soluble Aβ_{1-40} isoform being a major Aβ species within the CSF.[11] Accordingly, the presence of consistent amounts of Aβ_{1-40} was selectively found in brains with prominent CAA by various studies.[12–15] Interestingly, another study found a sharp peak of vessel-contained soluble Aβ between ages 50 and 70, even in the absence of CAA pathology.[16] The potential role of ApoE for cerebral Aβ clearance is also emphasized by recent results with transgenic mice in which cerebral Aβ deposition is reduced in the presence of human ApoE.[17] The internalization of soluble CSF-derived and lipoprotein-bound Aβ by brain vessel SMCs may be physiological and may represent a protective mechanism of Aβ clearance. However, such a physiological mechanism may become saturated leading to vascular Aβ concentrations above the solubility limit of Aβ with the result of Aβ precipitation and the formation of local extracellular Aβ seeds that would be at the origin of further amyloid deposition according to the current kinetic model of nucleation-dependent amyloid growth.[18] As we have previously reported in analyzing canine leptomeningeal organ cultures, physiological nanomolar CSF concentrations of Aβ are sufficient to sustain the further growth of preformed Aβ deposits.[7]

When cerebrovascular Aβ deposition is viewed as a consequence of reduced or insufficient Aβ clearance by SMCs, recently published findings by other groups may explain why CAA deposits form in the vascular extracellular space and why the ApoE4 genotype is a risk factor for CAA: (1) Binding of Aβ to ApoE was shown to be least efficient for ApoE4 with respect to ApoE3 when ApoE was produced by mammalian cells in two independent studies, suggesting a less efficient ApoE-

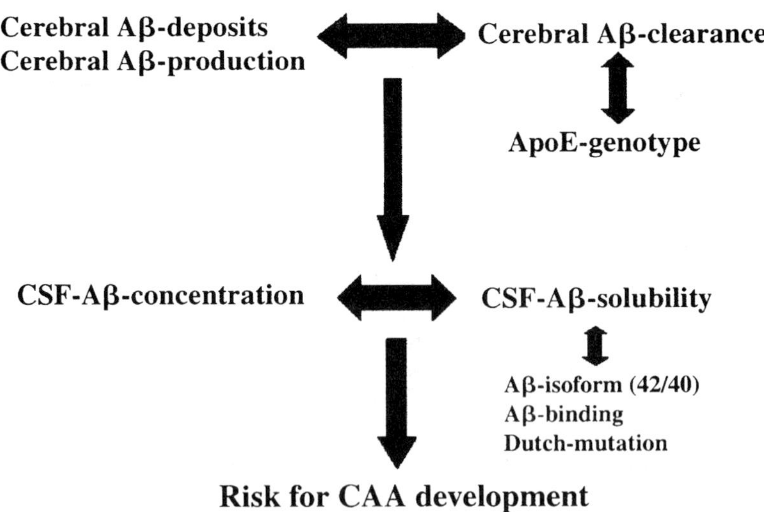

FIGURE 4. Model for the pathogenesis of CAA (see text).

mediated Aβ clearance in carriers of the E4 genotype.[2,19] (2) Intracellular accumulation or clearance of ApoE in fibroblasts[4] (a cell type that is mesenchymally derived and similar to SMCs), hepatocytes,[4] and neuronal cells[3–5] was significantly lower for ApoE4 when compared to ApoE3. Most importantly, the latter effect was only observed in the presence of cell surface HSPG,[4] which is abundantly expressed also by SMCs and has been convincingly implicated as an important cofactor in the development of cerebral and vascular Aβ-amyloid deposits.[20–23] We therefore propose that ApoE-mediated Aβ clearance by cerebrovascular SMCs may be a physiological and protective mechanism within a complex balance between Aβ production, Aβ clearance and Aβ solubility, the latter being also affected by Aβ binding to other CSF proteins or by changes in Aβ-peptide structure as in the case of hereditary cerebral hemorrhage with amyloidosis–Dutch type[24] (FIG. 4). Absolute or relative deficiency of Aβ clearance may lead to increased Aβ concentrations within the vascular extracellular matrix, where specific components such as HSPG ultimately promote deposition and growth of CAA deposits.

ACKNOWLEDGMENTS

This work was supported by DFG (Pr 299/3-1; Forschergruppe Molekularbiologie neurodegenerativer Erkrankungen, Teilprojekt 5).

REFERENCES

1. CALHOUN, M.E. *et al.* 1999. Neuronal overexpression of mutant amyloid precursor protein results in prominent deposition of cerebrovascular amyloid. Proc. Natl. Acad. Sci. USA **96:** 14088–14093.
2. LADU, M.J. *et al.* 1994. Isoform-specific binding of apolipoprotein E to beta-amyloid. J. Biol. Chem. **269:** 23403–23406.
3. JORDAN, J. *et al.* 1998. Isoform-specific effect of apolipoprotein E on cell survival and beta-amyloid-induced toxicity in rat hippocampal pyramidal neuronal cultures. J. Neurosci. **18:** 195–204.
4. JI, Z.S. *et al.* 1998. Differential cellular accumulation/retention of apolipoprotein E mediated by cell surface heparan sulfate proteoglycans. Apolipoproteins E3 and E2 greater than E4. J. Biol. Chem. **273:** 13452–13460.
5. BEFFERT, U. *et al.* 1999. Apolipoprotein E isoform-specific reduction of extracellular amyloid in neuronal cultures. Brain Res. Mol. Brain Res. **68:** 181–185.
6. PRIOR, R. *et al.* 1996. Selective binding of soluble Abeta1-40 and Abeta1-42 to a subset of senile plaques. Am. J. Pathol. **148:** 1749–1756.
7. PRIOR, R. *et al.* 1995. Experimental deposition of Alzheimer amyloid beta-protein in canine leptomeningeal vessels. Neuroreport **6:** 1747–1751.
8. URMONEIT, B. *et al.* 1997. Cerebrovascular smooth muscle cells internalize Alzheimer amyloid beta protein via a lipoprotein pathway: implications for cerebral amyloid angiopathy. Lab. Invest. **77:** 157–166.
9. STRITTMATTER, W.J. *et al.* 1993. Apolipoprotein E: high-avidity binding to beta-amyloid and increased frequency of type 4 allele in late-onset familial Alzheimer disease. Proc. Natl. Acad. Sci. USA **90:** 1977–1981.
10. WISNIEWSKI, T. *et al.* 1993. Apolipoprotein E: binding to soluble Alzheimer's beta-amyloid. Biochem. Biophys. Res. Commun. **192:** 359–365.
11. VIGO-PELFREY, C. *et al.* 1993. Characterization of beta-amyloid peptide from human cerebrospinal fluid. J. Neurochem. **61:** 1965–1968.

12. ALONZO, N.C. *et al.* 1998. Progression of cerebral amyloid angiopathy: accumulation of amyloid-beta40 in affected vessels. J. Neuropathol. Exp. Neurol. **57:** 353–359.

13. GRAVINA, S.A. *et al.* 1995. Amyloid beta protein (A beta) in Alzheimer's disease brain. Biochemical and immunocytochemical analysis with antibodies specific for forms ending at A beta 40 or A beta 42(43). J. Biol. Chem. **270:** 7013–7016.

14. SHINKAI, Y. *et al.* 1997. Amyloid beta-protein deposition in the leptomeninges and cerebral cortex. Ann. Neurol. **42:** 899–908.

15. SUZUKI, N. *et al.* 1994. High tissue content of soluble beta 1–40 is linked to cerebral amyloid angiopathy. Am. J. Pathol. **145:** 452–460.

16. SHINKAI, Y. *et al.* 1995. Amyloid beta-proteins 1–40 and 1–42(43) in the soluble fraction of extra- and intracranial blood vessels. Ann. Neurol. **38:** 421–428.

17. HOLTZMAN, D.M. *et al.* 1999. Expression of human apolipoprotein E reduces amyloid-beta deposition in a mouse model of Alzheimer's disease. J. Clin. Invest. **103:** R15–R21.

18. HARPER, J.D. & P.T. LANSBURY, JR. 1997. Models of amyloid seeding in Alzheimer's disease and scrapie: mechanistic truths and physiological consequences of the time-dependent solubility of amyloid proteins. Annu. Rev. Biochem. **66:** 385–407.

19. ALESHKOV, S. *et al.* 1997. Interaction of nascent ApoE2, ApoE3, and ApoE4 isoforms expressed in mammalian cells with amyloid peptide beta (1–40). Relevance to Alzheimer's disease. Biochemistry **36:** 10571–10580.

20. SNOW, A.D. *et al.* 1988. The presence of heparan sulfate proteoglycans in the neuritic plaques and congophilic angiopathy in Alzheimer's disease. Am. J. Pathol. **133:** 456-463P.

21. SNOW, A.D. *et al.* 1994. An important role of heparan sulfate proteoglycan (Perlecan) in a model system for the deposition and persistence of fibrillar A beta-amyloid in rat brain. Neuron **12:** 219–234.

22. SNOW, A.D. *et al.* 1995. Differential binding of vascular cell-derived proteoglycans (perlecan, biglycan, decorin, and versican) to the beta-amyloid protein of Alzheimer's disease. Arch. Biochem. Biophys. **320:** 84–95.

23. CASTILLO, G.M. *et al.* 1997. Perlecan binds to the beta-amyloid proteins (A beta) of Alzheimer's disease, accelerates A beta fibril formation, and maintains A beta fibril stability. J. Neurochem. **69:** 2452–2465.

24. VAN NOSTRAND, W.E. *et al.* 1998. Pathologic amyloid beta-protein cell surface fibril assembly on cultured human cerebrovascular smooth muscle cells. J. Neurochem. **70:** 216–223.

Amyloid-β-induced Degeneration of Human Brain Pericytes Is Dependent on the Apolipoprotein E Genotype

MARCEL M. VERBEEK,[a,c,d] WILLIAM E. VAN NOSTRAND,[b]
IRENE OTTE-HÖLLER,[a] PIETER WESSELING,[a,c] AND ROBERT M.W. DE WAAL[a]

*Departments of [a]Pathology and [c]Neurology, University Hospital Nijmegen,
P.O. Box 9101, 6500 HB Nijmegen, the Netherlands*

*[b]Departments of Medicine and Pathology, Health Sciences Center, State University of
New York, Stony Brook, New York, USA*

ABSTRACT: Amyloid-β (Aβ) deposition in cerebral vessels (cerebral amyloid angiopathy, CAA) is accompanied by degeneration of vascular cells, including pericytes and smooth muscle cells. Previous studies indicated that specific Aβ protein isoforms are toxic for cultured human brain pericytes and smooth muscle cells. In particular, $A\beta_{1-40}$ carrying the E22Q mutation, as in hereditary cerebral hemorrhage with amyloidosis of the Dutch type (HCHWA-D), is toxic. We investigated the effects of the Aβ-binding protein apolipoprotein E (ApoE) on the toxicity of Aβ for cultured human brain pericytes. We compared the toxicity of HCHWA-D $A\beta_{1-40}$ for pericyte cultures with different ApoE genotypes, studied the accumulation of Aβ and ApoE in these different cell cultures, and investigated the effects of exogenous ApoE. Pericyte cultures with an ApoE ε2/ε3 genotype were more resistant to HCHWA-D $A\beta_{1-40}$ treatment than cultures with a ε3/ε3 or ε3/ε4 genotype. Cell death was highest in cultures homozygous for ApoE ε4. The extent to which both Aβ and ApoE accumulated at the cell surface was parallel to the degree of toxicity. The addition of purified ApoE resulted in a decrease in cell death. These data suggest that ApoE4 may direct Aβ more efficiently than other ApoE isoforms into a pathological interaction with the HBP cell surface. The results of this study are in line with the observations that inheritance of the ApoE ε4 allele increases the risk of developing Alzheimer's disease, and that the ApoE ε2 allele has a relatively protective effect.

INTRODUCTION

The brains of patients with Alzheimer's disease (AD) are characterized by the presence of senile plaques, neurofibrillary tangles, and amyloid angiopathy of the vessels. The amyloid-β protein (Aβ), which consists of 40–42 amino acids, is the major constituent of both senile plaques and of cerebral amyloid angiopathy (CAA). The incidence of CAA in brains from patients over 60 years of age is 36%,[1] but in

[d]Address for correspondence: Dr. M. M. Verbeek, 319 Lab Pediatrics & Neurology, University Hospital Nijmegen, P.O. Box 9101, 6500 HB Nijmegen, the Netherlands. Tel.: 31-24-3615192; fax: 31-24-3540297.
e-mail: m.verbeek@CKSLKN.AZN.NL

association with AD this incidence is much higher, approximately 85%.[2,3] Aβ may assemble into aggregates, both *in vivo* and *in vitro*, resulting in the formation of insoluble amyloid.

Although both senile plaques and CAA primarily consist of Aβ, a number of differences in the pathogenesis of either lesion can be identified, among which are striking differences in the toxic properties of Aβ for either cultured neurons or vascular cells.[4] Aβ is toxic for cultured neurons,[5] and its neurotoxic properties are positively correlated with its degree of aggregation.[6] In contrast to fibrillar Aβ-induced neuronal toxicity, cultured smooth muscle cells and pericytes were completely unresponsive to preassembled, fibrillar forms of Aβ.[7] These cells have to be exposed to soluble, non β-sheet conformation of Aβ in order to induce cellular degeneration.[8–10]

Some years ago, apolipoprotein E (ApoE) was identified as a major risk factor for the sporadic late-onset form of AD. Three alleles are known of the *ApoE* gene, ε2, ε3 and ε4, the most frequent of which is the ε3 allele. Inheritance of one or two copies of the ε4 allele is associated with a dose-dependent increased risk for AD, and an earlier age of onset of AD,[11,12] although even subjects homozygous for ε4 may reach a high age without cognitive impairment.[13] On the contrary, the ε2 allele seems to have a protective effect against AD.[14] Surprisingly, however, both the ε2 and ε4 alleles are associated with an increased risk for CAA.[15–17]

ApoE may play an important role in the formation of the lesions of AD brains. It was found that an increase in the number of ε4 alleles corresponds to a high number of senile plaques and of vessels affected by CAA.[16,18] Furthermore, ApoE is present in senile plaques, neurofibrillary tangles, and CAA in AD brains.[19–21] ApoE is able to bind to Aβ, and may accelerate the formation of Aβ fibrils.[22–24] Finally, the deposition of Aβ in mice transgenic for a human mutant APP gene was strongly reduced when these mice were crossbred with ApoE knockout mice in comparison with ApoE[+/+] mice,[25] suggesting an important role for ApoE in mediating Aβ deposition in the brain.

Despite intensive research, the mechanism by which ApoE modifies the risk for development of AD has not yet been unraveled. In this study we investigated the influence of ApoE on Aβ-mediated cytotoxicity toward human vascular cells. We performed a comparative analysis of the cytotoxic effect of Aβ on cultures of pericytes with different ApoE genotypes, in order to study the role of endogenously produced ApoE. Additionally, to further investigate the role of ApoE in Aβ-mediated toxicity, purified protein was added to Aβ-treated cultures of human brain pericytes.

MATERIALS AND METHODS

Cells

Pericytes were isolated from human brain tissue, obtained after autopsy,[26] from a number of Alzheimer patients and neurologically unaffected individuals (TABLE 1). Pieces of frontal cortex were homogenized in a Dounce tissue grinder to release the capillaries from the remaining brain tissue. After several washing and centrifugation steps, the capillaries were treated with collagenase (1 mg/ml, 37°C, for approximately 1 h), and seeded on fibronectin-coated culture plates. Within a few days, endothelial cells started to grow from the digested capillary clumps, but their growth was

TABLE 1. Overview of patients from whom pericyte cultures were established after rapid autopsy

Number	Diagnosis	ApoE Genotype	Age	Sex
1	Control	2/3	84	F
2	AD	3/3	94	F
3	Control	3/3	48	M
4	Control	3/3	85	F
5	Control	3/3	81	M
6	AD	3/3	81	F
7	AD/MID	3/3	75	M
8	Control	3/3	84	F
9	AD	3/4	84	M
10	Control	3/4	83	F
11	AD	3/4	89	F
12	AD	4/4	83	F
13	AD	4/4	69	M

ABBREVIATIONS: AD, Alzheimer's disease; MID, multiinfarct dementia.

arrested by the appearance of pericytes that started to grow after approximately seven days in culture and which entirely replaced the endothelial cells. The cells were characterized using a panel of antibodies with which it was possible to distinguish them from endothelial cells, smooth muscle cells, and fibroblasts.[26,27]

Pericytes were maintained in Eagle's modification of essential medium (EMEM), supplemented with 10% human serum (Red Cross Blood Bank, Nijmegen, the Netherlands), 20% newborn calf serum (Gibco, Paisley, Scotland), recombinant basic fibroblast growth factor (1 ng/ml), heparin (5 U/ml, Organon, Boxtel, the Netherlands), and antibiotics.

Immunostaining

For staining experiments, cells were grown on gelatin-coated glass slides, which were cross-linked with glutaraldehyde prior to seeding of the cells. Cell cultures were washed with EMEM at confluency, and subsequently fixed in acetone. For double-staining experiments, primary antibodies were incubated simultaneously overnight at 4°C, followed by simultaneous incubation with fluorescein-isothiocyanate (FITC)-conjugated swine anti-rabbit antibodies (Cappel, Boxtel, the Netherlands) and biotinylated horse anti-mouse antibodies (Vector, Burlingame, CA) for 1 h. Cross-reactivity of these polyclonal antibodies with the primary antibodies was excluded. Finally, sections were incubated with Texas red-conjugated avidin (Vector). To both the FITC- and Texas red-conjugated antibodies, 4% human serum was added to eliminate a specific binding of the antibodies. All dilutions were made in PBS supplemented with 0.1% BSA, which also served as a negative control. Each incubation was followed by extensive washing with PBS.

Antibodies

Affinity-purified polyclonal anti-Aβ antibodies had been prepared previously by Dr. Van Nostrand. Monoclonal anti-ApoE antibody was purchased from Innogenetics (Antwerpen, Belgium).

Degeneration Experiments

Triplicate wells with cultured cells were preincubated with serum-free medium for 4 h. Subsequently, cells were incubated with fresh serum-free medium, supplemented with synthetic Aβ peptides at 25 µM, for six days. The Aβ peptides used in this study were synthesized and characterized as described previously.[9] Cells were routinely inspected and photographed using an Olympus phase-contrast microscope. Cell viability was quantitated using a fluorescence live/dead cell assay according to the manufacturer's description (Molecular Probes, Leiden, the Netherlands). The cultures were examined using an Olympus fluorescence microscope, and the percentage of dead cells was determined from at least five counts per well. Based on previous studies,[8,10] $Aβ_{1-40}$ containing the mutation found in patients with hereditary cerebral hemorrhage with amyloidosis of the Dutch type (HCHWA-D) was used in this study, because this peptide induced a robust degeneration of both pericytes and smooth muscle cells. This peptide contains a glutamine at amino acid 22 of Aβ instead of a glutamic acid. Lyophilized peptides were dissolved in sterile water at 250 µM. Purified ApoE peptides were obtained from PanVera (Madison, WI).

Western Blotting Analysis

For Western blotting analysis of cell lysates and culture supernatants, cells were grown in EMEM containing 0.1% bovine serum albumin and antibiotics (serum-free medium) for the indicated period of time. Both culture supernatant and cell lysates were collected to examine secreted or cell-bound expression of proteins, respectively. After incubation of the cells, culture supernatant was collected and diluted 1:1 with reducing sample buffer. Cells were washed twice with phosphate-buffered saline (PBS) and then solubilized in the wells with lysis buffer (50 mM Tris-HCl, 150 mM NaCl, pH 7.5, 1% sodium dodecyl sulfate (SDS), 5 mM EDTA, 500 µM 4-(2-aminoethyl)benzenesulfonyl fluoride, 10 µg/ml leupeptine and 10 µg/ml chymostatin) for 15 min. The protein content of diluted samples of the cell lysates was determined using the BCA method (Pierce, Rockford, IL). Equal protein amounts were loaded and fractionated on SDS-polyacrylamide gels and subsequently transferred electrophoretically to nitrocellulose membranes (Schleicher & Schuell, 's-Hertogenbosch, the Netherlands) in blotting buffer (25 mM Tris-HCl (pH 8.6), 192 mM glycine, 20% methanol). Blots were washed for 15 min in PBS containing 0.05% Tween-20 (PBST), preincubated with blocking solution (5% low-fat milk powder in PBST), washed three times with PBST, and subsequently incubated with primary antibodies and peroxidase-labeled secondary rabbit anti-mouse antibodies (Dako, Glostrup, Denmark). Detection was performed by chemiluminescence according to the manufacturer's description (Boehringer Mannheim, Almere, the Netherlands) and exposure to Kodak X-OMAT-R films.

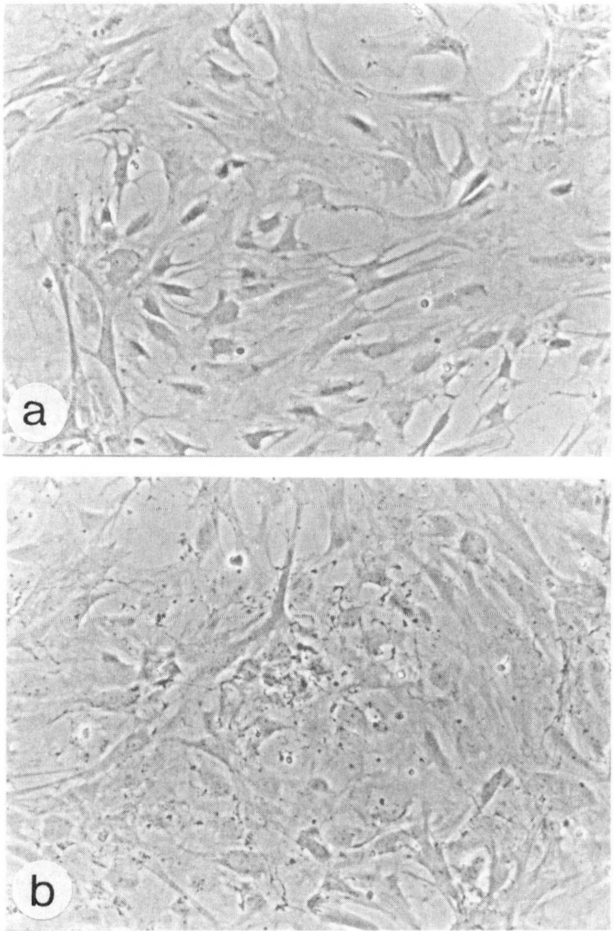

FIGURE 1. Phase contrast micrographs of cultured human brain pericytes treated for six days either in the absence (**A**) or presence of 25 μM HCHWA-D Aβ$_{1-40}$ (**B**). Note the degenerative changes in **B**. (Magnification: 300 ×.)

ApoE Genotyping

DNA was isolated from small pieces of brain tissue from which also cell cultures were derived, using a DNA isolation kit (Biozym, Landgraaf, the Netherlands). ApoE genotype was determined using PCR and HhaI restriction analysis according to previously described methods.[28,29]

RESULTS

Human brain pericytes (HBPs) were successfully isolated from 13 different donor brains, respectively. Cultured HBPs had a typical spindle-shaped or polygonal appearance with overlapping processes indicating the absence of contact inhibition. Only a subset of HBPs expressed smooth muscle cell α-actin. Both cell types expressed the high molecular weight melanoma-associated antigen and vascular cell adhesion molecule-1, which are neither expressed by cultured endothelial cells nor by fibroblasts, and lacked expression of endothelial markers. The cultured cells could be divided into four different groups according to their ApoE genotype: $\varepsilon2/\varepsilon3$, $\varepsilon3/\varepsilon3$, $\varepsilon3/\varepsilon4$, and $\varepsilon4/\varepsilon4$.

Cultured HBPs that were incubated with 25 μM HCHWA-D $A\beta_{1-40}$ clearly demonstrated signs of cellular degeneration after prolonged incubation periods, that is, after six or more days (FIG. 1). The cells lost their characteristic polygonal shape, individual cell contours became less evident, and signs of cellular atrophy were observed. Remarkable differences in the response to HCHWA-D $A\beta_{1-40}$ were observed between cell cultures with a different ApoE phenotype. Cultured HBPs homozygotic for ApoE $\varepsilon4$ exhibited widespread changes in the morphology of the cells, whereas cells with an ApoE $\varepsilon2/\varepsilon3$ genotype were much less vulnerable to HCHWA-D $A\beta_{1-40}$ treatment. These morphological observations were confirmed in a quantitative assay in which the proportion of dead cells after incubation with HCHWA-D $A\beta_{1-40}$ was determined in each cell culture. The highest number of dead cells was observed within $\varepsilon4/\varepsilon4$ cultures, whereas a relatively low number of dead cells was observed in $\varepsilon2/\varepsilon3$ cultures (FIG. 2). Cultures of HBPs either homozygous for $\varepsilon3$ or with an $\varepsilon3/\varepsilon4$ genotype demonstrated an intermediate loss of cell viability.

By use of Western blot analysis, it was demonstrated that cultured HBPs produced ApoE which, after a period of six days of incubation, predominantly accumulated in the supernatant and to a lesser extent was recovered from cell lysates (FIG. 3). After six days of incubation with HCHWA-D $A\beta_{1-40}$, the distribution of ApoE

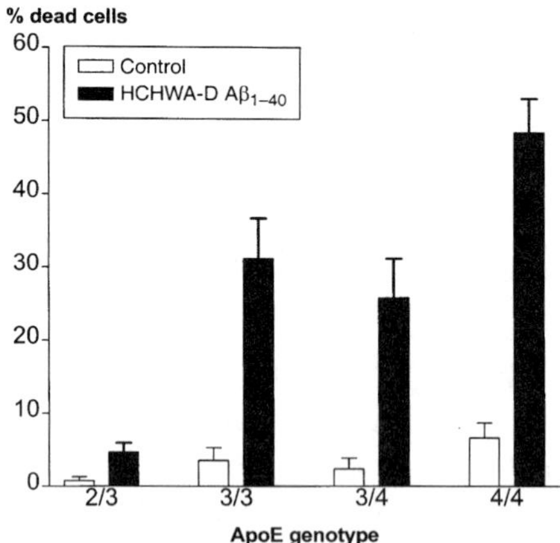

FIGURE 2. Comparison of the effect of treatment with 25 μM HCHWA-D $A\beta_{1-40}$ for six days of human brain pericytes cultures with different ApoE genotypes. An increasing number of dead cells was observed in the following order: $\varepsilon4/\varepsilon4 > \varepsilon3/\varepsilon4$, $\varepsilon3/\varepsilon3 >> \varepsilon2/\varepsilon3$. Significance of the observed differences (Student's t test): $\varepsilon2/\varepsilon3$ versus all others: $p < 0.001$; $\varepsilon4/\varepsilon4$ versus all others: $p < 0.001$.

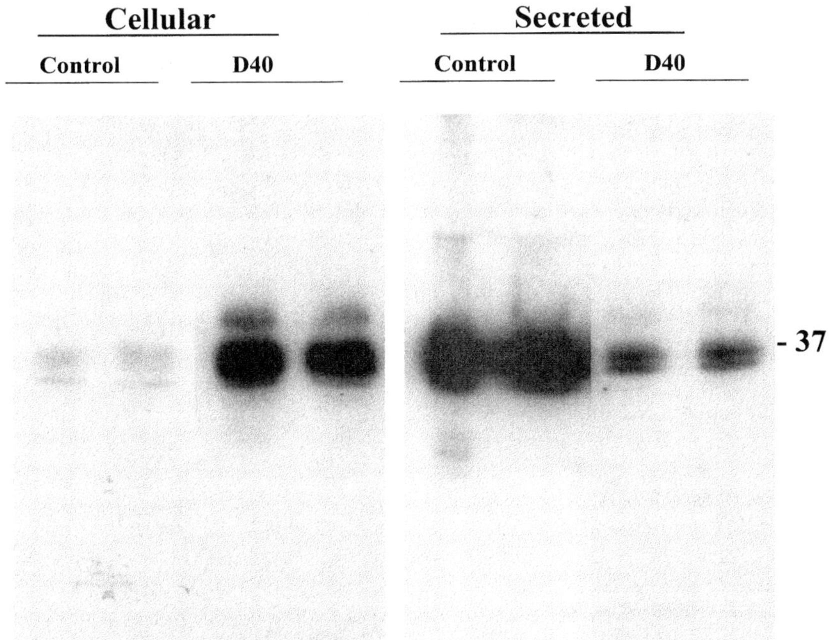

FIGURE 3. Western blotting analysis of cell-associated (*left panel*) and secreted ApoE (*right panel*) in cultured human brain pericytes treated for six days with 25 µM HCHWA-D $A\beta_{1-40}$. In untreated cultures, most ApoE (molecular weight approximately 37 kDa) was recovered from the supernatant, whereas in HCHWA-D $A\beta_{1-40}$ treated cells, ApoE was predominantly associated with the cellular fraction. Duplicate incubations are shown.

produced by the cultured HBPs over the supernatant and cell lysates was inverted (FIG. 3). The majority of ApoE was now recovered from the cell lysates and only small amounts were found in the supernatant, suggesting an increased association of ApoE with the cell. By applying double-immunofluorescence staining of cultured cells incubated with HCHWA-D $A\beta_{1-40}$, it was demonstrated that both $A\beta$ and ApoE were present in the cell or at the cell surface. The amounts of both $A\beta$ and ApoE that were associated with the cells were strongly dependent on the ApoE genotype of the cells: the strongest immunofluorescence signal of both $A\beta$ and ApoE was observed in cells with the ε4/ε4 genotype. Somewhat lower amounts of both $A\beta$ and ApoE were associated with cells of the ε3/ε4 or ε3/ε3 genotype, whereas both molecules could only occasionally be detected associated with ε2/ε3 cells (FIG. 4). In all cultures the area occupied by $A\beta$ deposition exceeded that of ApoE accumulation. In control cells, only sporadically present punctate staining for ApoE was observed, whereas staining for $A\beta$ was entirely absent (not shown).

Addition of purified ApoE to HBP cultures simultaneously with HCHWA-D $A\beta_{1-40}$ resulted in a decrease in the number of dead cells in the cultures, independent of the specific ApoE isoform applied (FIG. 5).

DISCUSSION

CAA is one of the neuropathological hallmarks of AD, together with senile plaques and neurofibrillary tangles. In vessels affected by CAA, smooth muscle cells, pericytes, and endothelial cells show a variable degree of degeneration.[30–33] Several *in vitro* studies have shown that specific Aβ isoforms, in particular, Aβ$_{1-42}$ and HCHWA-D Aβ$_{1-40}$ are toxic for cultures of HBPs and smooth muscle cells.[8–10]

It has been suggested that both ApoE ε2 and ε4 increase the risk of developing CAA, but by separate mechanisms. ApoE4 may enhance the deposition of Aβ in the vasculature, whereas ApoE2 may cause rupture of amyloid-laden vessels, possibly by interfering with smooth muscle cell integrity.[34] Given the association of ApoE genotypes with CAA and the co-occurrence of degenerating cells with the presence of both Aβ and ApoE in CAA,[19] ApoE might modulate the Aβ-induced cytotoxicity of cerebral vascular cells. According to the above-cited hypothesis,[34] it might be anticipated that ApoE2 enhances pericyte death. However, our *in vitro* data indicated an opposite relationship between the specific ApoE isoforms and Aβ-mediated cell death: cells with an ApoE ε2/ε3 genotype are significantly more resistant to incubation with HCHWA-D Aβ$_{1-40}$ than cells lacking the ApoE ε2 allele. Our data suggest that the absence of the ε2 allele renders cells more vulnerable to cell death initiated by Aβ. Extrapolation of these *in vitro* data would imply that the risk for rupture of cerebral vessels affected by CAA is increased in the absence of an ApoE ε2 allele. In this study we used the HCHWA-D Aβ$_{1-40}$ as a model peptide to study the effects of Aβ on cultured HBPs. Although previous studies indicated that both HCHWA-D Aβ$_{1-40}$ and wild-type Aβ$_{1-42}$ exerted similar, but quantitatively different, effects on cultured HBPs,[8,10] it remains to be investigated whether the effects of ApoE described in this report also apply to wild-type Aβ. This is particularly relevant because the vascular pathology in HCHWA-D is more severe than in AD.[35] Therefore, further studies with wild-type Aβ$_{1-42}$ are needed to investigate whether the cytotoxic properties of this peptide are modulated by ApoE in a way similar to HCHWA-D Aβ$_{1-40}$. Our data were obtained with a limited number of cell cultures only, which were derived from different patients. These limitations might interfere with our results. The ε2/ε3 cell culture was derived from a nondemented patient, and the ε4/ε4 cell cultures were established from AD patients (see TABLE 1). Although it is likely that cerebral factors, for example, the presence of Aβ, may have affected the viability of pericytes *in vivo*, it can be argued that such factors are no longer relevant after a few passages *in vitro*.

ApoE binds to Aβ in an isoform-dependent way. ApoE4 purified from plasma binds faster to Aβ than ApoE3,[22] and ApoE4 may promote Aβ fibril formation more efficiently than the other isoforms.[23,36] However, when different ApoE isoforms

---

FIGURE 4. Confluent monolayers of cultured human brain pericytes were treated with 25 μM HCHWA-D Aβ$_{1-40}$ and were double-stained using immunofluorescence for Aβ (**panels A,C,E, and G**) and ApoE (**panels B,D,F, and H**). Cells with the following ApoE genotypes were compared for the staining of Aβ and ApoE: ε2/ε3 (**A,B**); ε3/ε3 (**C,D**); ε3/ε4 (**E,F**); ε4/ε4 (**G,H**). In cultures with the ε2/ε3 genotype only a small area of the culture was stained for both Aβ and ApoE. An increasing amount of both Aβ and ApoE could be detected in the following order: ε4/ε4 > ε3/ε4, ε3/ε3 >> ε2/ε3. (Magnification: 330×.)

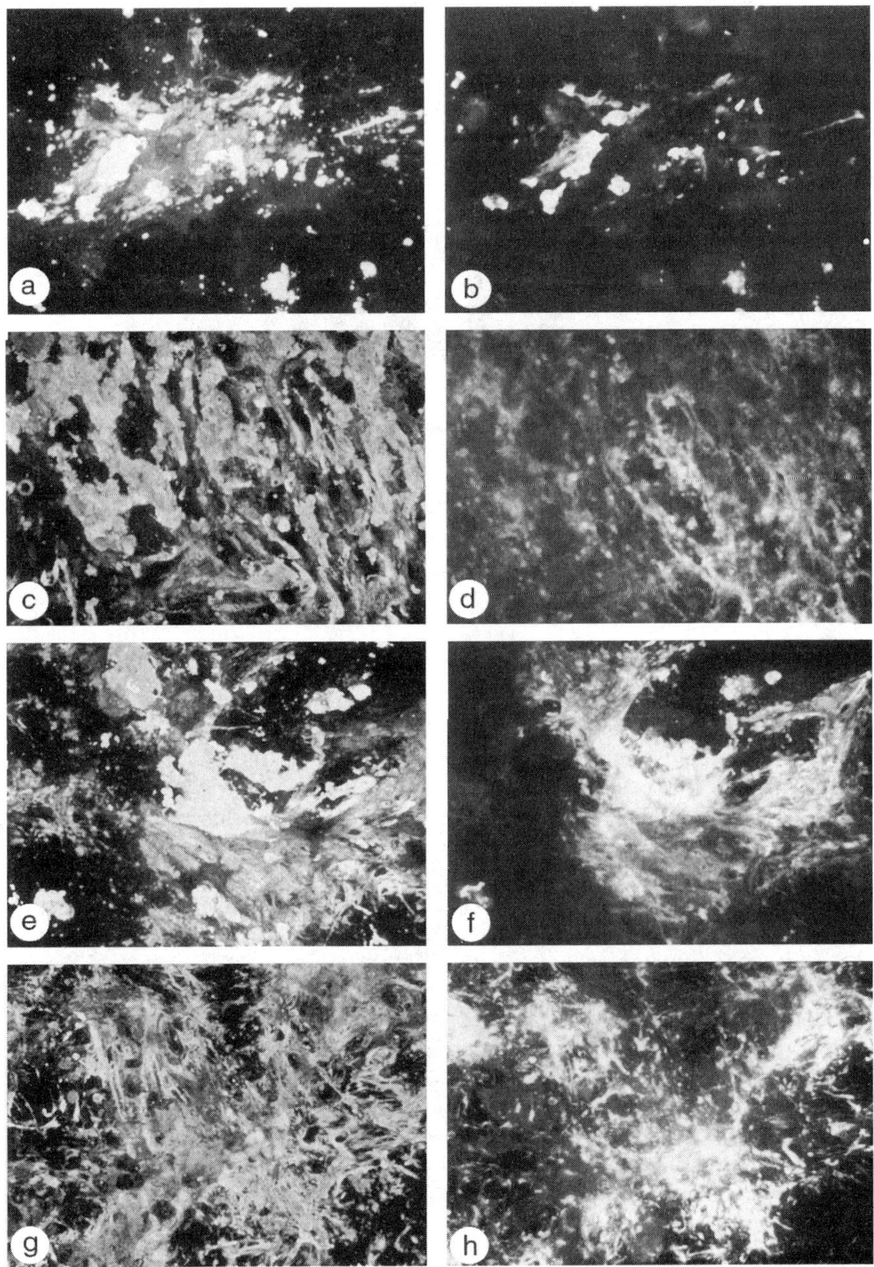

FIGURE 4. *Caption on previous page.*

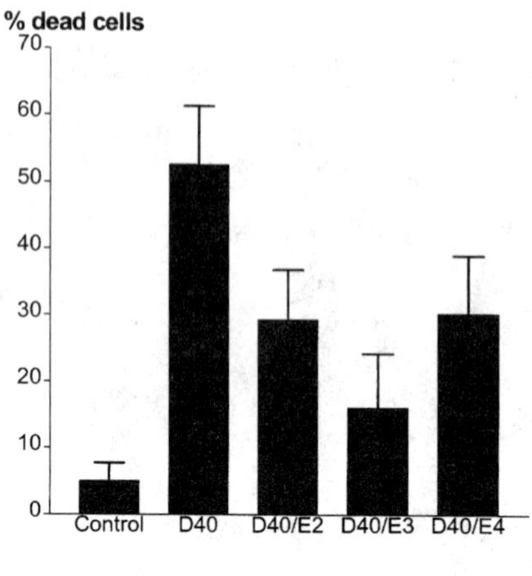

FIGURE 5. The effect of the addition of ApoE (100 ng) on the number of dead cells in cultures of human brain pericytes treated with 25 μM HCHWA-D Aβ_{1-40}. All ApoE isoforms decrease the number of dead cells induced by the addition of HCHWA-D Aβ_{1-40}. ABBREVIATIONS: D40: HCHWA-D Aβ_{1-40}; E2, E3, E4: ApoE2, 3, and 4, respectively.

produced by transfected cell cultures were compared in their capacity to bind to Aβ, it appeared that the binding capacity decreased in the following order: ApoE2 > ApoE3 >> ApoE4.[37,38] In line with previous reports,[39] our immunofluorescence data suggest that Aβ accumulates at the cell surface of cultured HBPs and aggregates into fibrils, thereby inducing a pathological cascade of events leading to cell death. Although we were not yet able to demonstrate this unequivocally, the ApoE secreted by cultured HBPs may bind to Aβ and form complexes. We did demonstrate, however, that ApoE colocalized with Aβ at the cell surface, suggesting that the endogeneously produced ApoE may bind to the HCHWA-D Aβ_{1-40} that was added to the cells, and that these complexes successively bind to the cell surface, which eventually will lead to the observed cell death. Our experiments suggest that—in line with the results of Strittmatter *et al.*[22]—ApoE4 either binds more efficiently to HCHWA-D Aβ_{1-40} than the other ApoE isoforms or specifically alters its conformation in such a way that it accelerates the interaction of HCHWA-D Aβ_{1-40} with the HBP cell surface. Probably, after binding Aβ, ApoE4 may direct Aβ more efficiently into a pathological interaction with the HBP cell surface, eventually leading to cell death. In this respect, it remains puzzling why the addition of ApoE to HCHWA-D Aβ_{1-40} treated cultured HBPs results in diminished cell death, irrespective of the specific ApoE isoform applied.

An alternative explanation for our observations might be the following. By means of interaction with specific cell-surface receptors, ApoE may block the interaction of Aβ with the cell surface. In this scenario, ApoE2 would be most efficient in blocking the interaction of Aβ with the cell surface. This latter possibility, however, seems less likely because in control incubations binding of ApoE to the cell surface was absent.

Our data reflect the general observations that inheritance of the ApoE ε4 allele increases the risk of developing Alzheimer's disease, and decreases the age of onset of the disease;[11–13] we demonstrated that cultured HBPs carrying the ApoE ε4 allele are more vulnerable to Aβ-mediated cell death than are cells with a different ApoE genotype. In addition, we found an even stronger effect of the ApoE ε2 allele, which renders cultured HBPs relatively resistant to Aβ-mediated cell death, in line with a protective effect of this allele in the development of Alzheimer's disease.[14]

ACKNOWLEDGMENTS

This work was supported by the Internationale Stichting Alzheimer Onderzoek.
We thank Dr. M. Mulder for performing the ApoE genotyping, and Dr. R. Koopmans, Dr. J.H.M. Cox-Claessens, and Dr. G. Woestenburg (Psychogeriatric Centers "Joachim en Anna" and "Margriet," Nijmegen, the Netherlands) for their cooperation in the rapid autopsy protocol.

REFERENCES

1. VINTERS, H.V. & J.J. GILBERT. 1983. Cerebral amyloid angiopathy: incidence and complications in the aging brain. II. The distribution of amyloid vascular changes. Stroke **14:** 924–928.
2. GLENNER, G.G., J.H. HENRY & S. FUJIHARA. 1981. Congophilic angiopathy in the pathogenesis of Alzheimer's degeneration. Ann. Pathol. **1:** 120–129.
3. ELLIS, R.J., J.M. OLICHNEY, L.J. THAL, S.S. MIRRA, J.C. MORRIS, D. BEEKLY & A. HEYMAN. 1996. Cerebral amyloid angiopathy in the brains of patients with Alzheimer's disease: the CERAD experience, Part 15. Neurology **46:** 1592–1596.
4. VERBEEK, M.M., P. EIKELENBOOM & R.M.W. DE WAAL. 1997. Differences in the pathogenesis between senile plaques and congophilic angiopathy in Alzheimer's disease. J. Neuropathol. Exp. Neurol. **56:** 751–761.
5. LORENZO, A. & B.A. YANKNER. 1994. β-Amyloid neurotoxicity requires fibril formation and is inhibited by Congo red. Proc. Natl. Acad. Sci. USA **91:** 12243–12247.
6. PIKE, C.J., D. BURDICK, A.J. WALENCEWICZ, C.G. GLABE & C.W. COTMAN. 1993. Neurodegeneration induced by β-amyloid peptides in vitro: the role of peptide assembly state. J. Neurosci. **13:** 1676–1687.
7. DAVIS-SALINAS, J. & W.E. VAN NOSTRAND. 1995. Amyloid beta-protein aggregation nullifies its pathologic properties in cultured cerebrovascular smooth muscle cells. J. Biol. Chem. **270:** 20887–20890.
8. VERBEEK, M.M., R.M.W. DE WAAL, J.J. SCHIPPER & W.E. VAN NOSTRAND. 1997. Rapid degeneration of cultured human brain pericytes by amyloid β protein. J. Neurochem. **68:** 1135–1141.
9. DAVIS-SALINAS, J., S.M. SAPORITO-IRWIN, C.W. COTMAN & W.E. VAN NOSTRAND. 1995. Amyloid β-protein induces its own production in cultured degenerating cerbrovascular smooth muscle cells. J. Neurochem. **65:** 931–934.
10. DAVIS, J. & W.E. VAN NOSTRAND. 1996. Enhanced pathologic properties of Dutch-type mutant amyloid β-protein. Proc. Natl. Acad. Sci. USA **93:** 2996–3000.
11. CORDER, E.H., A.M. SAUNDERS, W.J. STRITTMATTER, D.E. SCHMECHEL, P.C. GASKELL, G.W. SMALL, A.D. ROSES, J.L. HAINES & M.A. PERICAK-VANCE. 1993. Gene dose of apolipoprotein E type 4 allele and the risk of Alzheimer's disease in late onset families. Science **261:** 921–923.
12. SAUNDERS, A.M., W.J. STRITTMATTER, D. SCHMECHEL, P.H. ST. GEORGE-HYSLOP, M.A. PERICAK-VANCE, S.H. JOO, B.L. ROSI, J.F. GUSELLA, D.R. CRAPPER-MACLACHLAN, M.J. ALBERTS, C. HULETTE, B. CRAIN, D. GOLDGABER & A.D. ROSES. 1993. Associa-

tion of apolipoprotein E allele ε4 with late-onset familial and sporadic Alzheimer's disease. Neurology **43:** 1467–1472.

13. HENDERSON, A.S., S. EASTEAL, A.F. JORM, A.J. MACKINNON, A.E. KORTEN, H. CHRISTENSEN, L. CROFT & P.A. JACOMB. 1995. Apolipoprotein E allele epsilon 4, dementia, and cognitive decline in a population sample. Lancet **346:** 1387–1390.

14. CORDER, E.H., A.M. SAUNDERS, N.J. RISCH, W.J. STRITTMATTER, D.E. SCHMECHEL, J.P.C. GASKELL, J.B. RIMMLER, P.A. LOCKE, P.M. CONNEALLY, K.E. SCHMADER, G.W. SMALL, A.D. ROSES, J.L. HAINES & M.A. PERICAK-VANCE. 1994. Protective effect of apolipoprotein E type 2 allele for late onset Alzheimer disease. Nat. Genet. **7:** 180–183.

15. GREENBERG, S.M., M.E. BRIGGS, B.T. HYMAN, G.J. KOKORIS, C. TAKIS, D.S. KANTER, C.S. KASE & M.S. PESSIN. 1996. Apolipoprotein E ε4 is associated with the presence and earlier onset of hemorrhage in cerebral amyloid angiopathy. Stroke **27:** 1333–1337.

16. PREMKUMAR, D.R.D., D.L. COHEN, P. HEDERA, R.P. FRIEDLAND & R.N. KALARIA. 1996. Apolipoprotein E-ε4 alleles in cerebral amyloid angiopathy and cerebrovascular pathology associated with Alzheimer's disease. Am. J. Pathol. **148:** 2083–2095.

17. NICOLL, J.A.R., C. BURNETT, S. LOVE, D.I. GRAHAM, J.W. IRONSIDE & H.V. VINTERS. 1996. High frequency of apolipoprotein E ε2 in patients with cerebral hemorrhage due to cerebral amyloid angiopathy. Ann. Neurol. **39:** 682.

18. SCHMECHEL, D.E., A.M. SAUNDERS, W.J. STRITTMATTER, B.J. CRAIN, C.M. HULETTE, S.H. JOO, M.A. PERICAK-VANCE, D. GOLDGABER & A.D. ROSES. 1993. Increased amyloid β-peptide deposition in cerebral cortex as a consequence of apolipoprotein E genotype in late-onset Alzheimer disease. Proc. Natl. Acad. Sci. USA **90:** 9649–9653.

19. VERBEEK, M.M., I. OTTE-HÖLLER, R. VEERHUIS, D.J. RUITER & R.M.W. DE WAAL. 1998. Distribution of Aβ-associated proteins in cerebrovascular amyloid of Alzheimer's disease. Acta Neuropathol. **96:** 628–636.

20. NAMBA, Y., M. TOMONAGA, H. KAWASAKI, E. OTOMO & K. IKEDA. 1991. Apolipoprotein E immunoreactivity in cerebral amyloid deposits and neurofibrillary tangles in Alzheimer's disease and kuru plaque amyloid in Creutzfeld-Jakob disease. Brain Res. **541:** 163–166.

21. YAMAGUCHI, H., K. ISHIGURO, S. SUGIHARA, Y. NAKAZATO, T. KAWARABAYASHI, X. SUN & S. HIRAI. 1994. Presence of apolipoprotein E on extracellular neurofibrillary tangles and on meningeal blood vessels precedes the Alzheimer β-amyloid deposition. Acta Neuropathol. **88:** 413–419.

22. STRITTMATTER, W.J., K.H. WEISGRABER, D.Y. HUANG, L.-M. DONG, G.S. SALVESEN, M. PERICAK-VANCE, D. SCHMECHEL, A.M. SAUNDERS, D. GOLDGABER & A.D. ROSES. 1993. Binding of human apolipoprotein E to synthetic amyloid β peptide: isoform-specific effects and implications for late-onset Alzheimer disease. Proc. Natl. Acad. Sci. USA **90:** 8098–8102.

23. SANAN, D.A., K.H. WEISGRABER, S.J. RUSSELL, R.W. MAHLEY, D. HUANG, A. SAUNDERS, D. SCHEMEL, T. WISNIEWSKI, B. FRANGIONE, A.D. ROSES & W.J. STRITTMATTER. 1994. Apolipoprotein E associates with β-amyloid peptide of Alzheimer's disease to form novel monofibrils. J. Clin. Invest. **94:** 860–869.

24. WISNIEWSKI, T., E.M. CASTAÑO, A. GOLABEK, T. VOGEL & B. FRANGIONE. 1994. Acceleration of Alzheimer's fibril formation by apolipoprotein E in vitro. Am. J. Pathol. **145:** 1030–1035.

25. BALES, K.R., T. VERINA, R.C. DODEL, Y. DU, L. ALTSTIEL, M. BENDER, P. HYSLOP, E.M. JOHNSTONE, S.P. LITTLE, D.J. CUMMINS, P. PICCARDO, B. GHETTI & S.M. PAUL. 1997. Lack of apolipoprotein E dramatically reduces amyloid beta-peptide deposition [letter] [see comments]. Nat. Genet. **17:** 263–264.

26. VERBEEK, M.M., I. OTTE-HÖLLER, P. WESSELING, D.J. RUITER & R.M.W. DE WAAL. 1994. Induction of α-smooth muscle actin expression in cultured human brain pericytes by TGFβ1. Am. J. Pathol. **144:** 372–382.

27. VERBEEK, M.M., J.R. WESTPHAL, D.J. RUITER & R.M.W. DE WAAL. 1995. T lymphocyte adhesion to human brain pericytes is mediated via VLA-4/VCAM-1 interactions. J. Immunol. **154:** 5876–5884.

28. HIXSON, J.E. & D.T. VERNIER. 1990. Restriction isotyping of human apolipoprotein E by gene amplification and cleavage with HhaI. J. Lipid Res. **31:** 545–548.

29. WENHAM, P.R., W.H. PRICE & G. BLANDELL. 1991. Apolipoprotein E genotyping by one-stage PCR [letter]. Lancet **337:** 1158–1159.
30. WISNIEWSKI, H.M., J. WEGIEL, K.C. WANG & B. LACH. 1992. Ultrastructural studies of the cells forming amyloid in the cortical vessel wall in Alzheimer's disease. Acta Neuropathol. **84:** 117–127.
31. KIMURA, T., T. HASHIMURA & T. MIYAKAWA. 1991. Observations of microvessels in the brain with Alzheimer's disease by the scanning electron microscope. Jpn. J. Psychiatr. Neurol. **45:** 671–676.
32. KAWAI, M., R.N. KALARIA, P. CRAS, S.L. SIEDLAK, M.E. VELASCO, E.R. SHELTON, H.W. CHAN, B. GREENBERG & G. PERRY. 1993. Degeneration of vascular muscle cells in cerebral amyloid angiopathy of Alzheimer disease. Brain Res. **623:** 142–146.
33. PERRY, G., M.A. SMITH, C.E. McCANN, S.L. SIEDLAK, P.K. JONES & R.P. FRIEDLAND. 1998. Cerebrovascular muscle atrophy is a feature of Alzheimer's disease. Brain Res. **791:** 63–66.
34. GREENBERG, S.M., J.P. VONSATTEL, A.Z. SEGAL, R.I. CHIU, A.E. CLATWORTHY, A. LIAO, B.T. HYMAN & G.W. REBECK. 1998. Association of apolipoprotein E epsilon2 and vasculopathy in cerebral amyloid angiopathy. Neurology **50:** 961–965.
35. LUYENDIJK, W., G.T.A.M. BOTS, M. VEGTER-VAN DER VLIS, L.N. WENT & B. FRANGIONE. 1988. Hereditary cerebral haemorrhage caused by cortical amyloid angiopathy. J. Neurol. Sci. **85:** 267–280.
36. MA, J., A. YEE, H.B. BREWER, JR., S. DAS & H. POTTER. 1994. Amyloid associated proteins α1-antichymotrypsin and apolipoprotein E promote assembly of Alzheimer β-protein into filaments. Nature **372:** 92–94.
37. LADU, M.J., M.T. FALDUTO, A.M. MANELLI, C.A. REARDON, G.S. GETZ & D.E. FRAIL. 1994. Isoform-specific binding of apolipoprotein E to β-amyloid. J. Biol. Chem. **269:** 23403–23406.
38. ALESHKOV, S., C.R. ABRAHAM & V.I. ZANNIS. 1997. Interaction of nascent ApoE2, ApoE3, and ApoE4 isoforms expressed in mammalian cells with amyloid peptide beta (1–40). Relevance to Alzheimer's disease. Biochemistry **36:** 10571–10580.
39. VAN NOSTRAND, W.E., J.P. MELCHOR & L. RUFFINI. 1998. Pathologic amyloid β-protein cell surface assembly on cultured human cerebrovascular smooth muscle cells. J. Neurochem. **70:** 216–223.

Earlier Age of Onset of Alzheimer's Disease in Patients with Both the Transferrin C2 and Apolipoprotein E-ε4 Alleles

S.J. VAN RENSBURG,[a,d] F.C.V. POTOCNIK,[b] J.N.P. DE VILLIERS,[c] M.J. KOTZE,[c] AND J.J.F. TALJAARD[a]

Departments of [a]Chemical Pathology and [b]Psychiatry and [c]Division of Human Genetics, Tygerberg Hospital and University of Stellenbosch Medical School, 7505 Tygerberg, South Africa

ABSTRACT: The etiology of Alzheimer's disease is now known to be multifactorial. The genetic factors transferrin C2 (TfC2) and apolipoprotein E ε4 (ApoE-ε4) have both been associated with Alzheimer's disease (AD). Transferrin is the carrier protein for iron in the blood, while ApoE is involved with the transport and redistribution of lipids. In the present study, the polymerase chain reaction (PCR) method was used to determine the frequency of both TfC2 and ApoE-ε4 in 27 AD patients, 9 vascular dementia (VaD) patients, and 27 controls. Patients were diagnosed according to the criteria as set out in the 4th edition of the Diagnostic and Statistical Manual of the American Psychiatric Association (DSM-IV).

The frequency of the TfC2 allele for the AD patients was 24%, while for the VaD patients it was 12.5%, which was not significantly different from the controls at 13%. The frequency of ApoE-ε4 for the AD patients was 44%, for the VaD patients 22%, and controls 17%. Of the 27 AD patients, 8 had both TfC2 and ApoE-ε4. The age of onset of the disease in these 8 patients (51–67 years, mean 60.25) was significantly earlier ($p < 0.02$) than in the remaining AD patients (49–76 years, mean 66.9). None of the VaD patients had both the TfC2 and the ApoE-ε4 alleles.

INTRODUCTION

While there was once hope that a single cause for Alzheimer's disease (AD) would be found, permitting expedient testing and treatment, it has become increasingly clear that the cause of the disease is most likely multifactorial. Several mutational genetic factors have now been associated with AD, accounting for less than 5% of all cases (chromosomes 1, 14 and 21). Additionally, up to 60% of all AD patients are linked to a susceptibility gene, apolipoprotein E, situated on chromosome 19. However, studies with monozygotic twins have revealed a relatively low concordance for AD,[1] indicating that environmental factors interact with genetic factors to

[d]Address for correspondence: Dr. S.J. van Rensburg, Department of Chemical Pathology, Tygerberg Hospital and University of Stellenbosch Medical School, P.O. Box 19113, 7505 Tygerberg, South Africa. Tel.: +21 938 4611; fax: +21 938 4640.
e-mail: sjvr@gerga.sun.ac.za

cause the disease. Elucidating the interaction between the genetic and enviromental factors could thus enhance present knowledge as to the etiology of AD.

One of the genetic factors recently implicated in AD is a genetic variant of transferrin (Tf), an increased frequency of the TfC2 allele being found in patients with AD.[2–4] The principal function of Tf in the body is to carry iron in the blood. An additional function of Tf is to inhibit free radical reactions by removing iron from the Fenton reaction, thereby inhibiting the production of hydroxyl radicals, which are in turn responsible for damage to cell membranes by lipid peroxidation.[5] It was previously demonstrated that an increased frequency of TfC2 may be involved in other diseases thought to be caused by free radical damage, such as rheumatoid arthritis and phototoxic eczema.[6] This led to the hypothesis that AD may result from free radical-induced lipid peroxidation of neuronal membranes.[5] The iron binding capacity of TfC2 *in vitro* was found to be decreased in one study[7] and unchanged in another.[4]

Apolipoprotein E (ApoE), on the other hand, is involved in the transport and redistribution of membrane lipids, and may thus play a part in the regeneration of damaged membranes. Lipids are very important components of cell membranes, the unsaturated omega-6 and omega-3 fatty acids being indispensible for membrane regeneration. If the latter should be in short supply, however, cholesterol is utilized for this purpose. It has been demonstrated that cholesterol is required for rapid membrane biogenesis during axon regeneration, and that it is transferred to damaged sciatic nerve axonal membranes by low-density lipoprotein (LDL) containing ApoE.[8]

In the present study we determined the allele frequencies of TfC2 and ApoE-ε4 in patients with AD and vascular dementia (VaD).

MATERIALS AND METHODS

Twenty-seven AD patients and 9 VaD patients were diagnosed according to the criteria as set out in the *4th* edition of the Diagnostic and Statistical Manual of the American Psychiatric Association (DSM-IV). Twenty-seven nondemented subjects were used as controls.

Genomic DNA was extracted from 5 ml whole blood preserved in ethylenediaminetetraacetic acid (EDTA), using a standard lysis method.[9] ApoE and Tf genotyping was determined by polymerase chain reaction (PCR) amplification followed by *Hha* I/*Cfo* I and B*st*EII restriction enzyme digestion, respectively.[10,3] Amplification reaction for each amplication contained 50 ng DNA, 15 pmol of each primer (ApoE: forward F4 5′-ACAGAATTCGCCCCGGCCTGGTACAC-3′, reverse F6 5′-TAAGCTTGGCACGGCTGTCCAAGGA-3′; Tf: forward 5′-GCTGTGCCT-TGATGGTACCAGGTAA-3′, reverse primer 5′-GGACGCAAGCTTCCTTATCT-3′), 100 µM dNTP's, 0.5 units of Taq DNA polymerase and 1 × reaction buffer (Roche Diagnostics) in a total volume of 50 µl. The amplification profile was 2 min at 95°C, followed by 35 cycles at 95°C for 30 s, 60°C for 45 s and 72°C for 30 s, on a Perkin Elmer 9600 thermal cycler. The gel consisted of 12% polyacrylamide, with a 3.4% crosslink.

Statistics used: χ^2 test, Mann-Whitney U test.

RESULTS

In this study, 27 AD patients, 9 VaD patients, and 27 controls were tested at the DNA level. The allele frequency of TfC2 in the AD patients was 24%, in the VaD patients 12.5%, and in the controls 13%. The frequency of ApoE-ε4 for the AD patients was 44%, for the VaD patients 22%, and controls 17%.

Of the 27 AD patients, 8 had both the TfC2 and APOE-ε4 alleles. The age of onset of the disease in these 8 patients (51–67 years, mean 60.25) was significantly earlier (p <0.02; Mann-Whitney U test) than in the remaining AD patients (49–76 years, mean 66.9). None of the VaD patients had both the TfC2 and the ApoE-ε4 alleles, while two of the controls had both.

DISCUSSION

In these patients, the presence of both the TfC2 and the ApoE-ε4 alleles in combination appears to have been a predisposing factor for the earlier onset of AD, which may signal the importance of these two alleles in the etiology of AD. Although there is no direct proof as yet, TfC2 by virtue of its role in iron metabolism, suggests a link with free radical damage of neuronal membranes.[11] This may explain the efficacy of vitamin E, an antioxidant, in treating AD[12] and of nonsteroidal anti-inflammatory drugs, which have been found to decrease the incidence of AD.[1] These drugs lower the amount of free radicals by suppressing the immune response. Other studies using antioxidants, unsaturated fatty acids, and other nutrients have also been beneficial.[13,14]

An interesting observation is the low prevalence of AD in black Africans, including black South Africans. Kalaria *et al.*[15] showed in a comparison of several studies, that the allele frequency of ApoE-ε4 is surprisingly high in Tanzanians (21%), Kenyans (37%), Nigerians (29.6%), and South African Bushmen (37%). One would thus expect a higher incidence of AD in the black African, and must therefore assume that other susceptibility factors that would contribute towards AD are not yet in place. Although the frequency of TfC2 has not yet been determined in these population groups, this frequency has been found to be lower in black South Africans (8.2%) than in white South Africans (13.6%) 2, possibly offering a degree of protection in the former group. Determining the TfC2 in other population groups in Africa could possibly in part help explain a lower prevalence of AD in black Africans.

In summary, if the combination of TfC2 and ApoE-ε4 should be verified to be a predisposing factor for an earlier onset of AD, serious consideration should be given to including lipids, antioxidants, and free radical scavengers in the treatment regimen for AD.

ACKNOWLEDGMENTS

We gratefully acknowledge the financial support given by the Cape Provincial Administration, the Medical Research Council of South Africa, and ARDA Western Cape.

REFERENCES

1. PLASSMAN, B.L. & J.C.S. BREITNER. 1996. Recent advances in the genetics of Alzheimer's disease and vascular dementia with an emphasis on gene-environment interactions. J. Am. Geriatr. Soc. **44:** 1242–1250.
2. VAN RENSBURG, S.J., M.E. CARSTENS, F.C.V. POTOCNIK *et al.* 1993. Increased frequency of the transferrin C2 subtype in Alzheimer's disease. NeuroReport **4:** 1269–1271.
3. NAMEKATA, K., M. IMAGAWA, A. TERASHI *et al.* 1997. Association of transferrin C2 allele with late-onset Alzheimer's disease. Hum. Genet. **101:** 126–129.
4. VAN LANDEGHEM, G.F., C. SIKSTRÖM, L.E. BECKMAN *et al.* 1998. Transferrin C2, metal binding and Alzheimer's disease. NeuroReport **9:** 177–179.
5. VAN RENSBURG, S.J., W.M.U. DANIELS, J. VAN ZYL *et al.* 1994. Lipid peroxidation and platelet membrane fluidity—implications for Alzheimer's disease? NeuroReport **5:** 2221–2224.
6. BECKMAN, L. & G. BECKMAN. 1986. Transferrin C2 as an enhancer of cyto- and genotoxic damage. Prog. Clin. Biol. Res. **209B:** 221–224.
7. WONG, C.T. & N. SAHA. 1986. Effects of transferrin genetic phenotypes on total iron-binding capacity. Acta Haematol. **75:** 215–218.
8. BOYLES, J.K., C.D. ZOELLNER, L.J. ANDERSON *et al.* 1989. A role for apolipoprotein E, apolipoprotein A-I, and low density lipoprotein receptors in cholesterol transport during regeneration and remyelination of the rat sciatic nerve. J. Clin. Invest. **83:** 1015–1031.
9. MILLER, SA., D.D. DYKES & H.F. POLESKY. 1988. A simple salting out procedure for extracting DNA from human nucleated cells. Nucleic Acids Res. **16:** 1215.
10. HIXSON, J.E. & D.T. VERNIER. 1990. Restriction isotyping of human apolipoprotein E by gene amplification and cleavage with Hha I. J. Lipid Res. **31:** 545–548.
11. VAN RENSBURG, S.J., M.E. CARSTENS, F.C.V. POTOCNIK *et al.*1995. Transferrin C2 and Alzheimer's disease: another piece of the puzzle found? Med. Hypotheses **44:** 229–306.
12. SANO, M., C. ERNESTO, R.G. THOMAS *et al.* 1997. A controlled trial of selegiline, alpha-tocopherol, or both as treatment for Alzheimer's disease. The Alzheimer's Disease Cooperative Study. N. Engl. J. Med. **336:** 1216–1222.
13. CORRIGAN, F.M., A. VAN RHIJN & D.F. HORROBIN. 1991. Essential fatty acids in Alzheimer's disease. Ann. N.Y. Acad. Sci. **640:** 250–252.
14. ABALAN, F., G. MANCIER, J.-F. DARTIGUES *et al.*1992. Nutrition and SDAT. Biol. Psychiatry **31:** 99–105.
15. KALARIA, R.N., J.A. OGENG'O, N.B. PATEL *et al.* 1997. Evaluation of risk factors for Alzheimer's disease in elderly East Africans. Brain Res. Bull. **44:** 573–577.

Inherent Abnormalities in Energy Metabolism in Alzheimer Disease

Interaction with Cerebrovascular Compromise

JOHN P. BLASS,[a] REX KWAN-FU SHEU,[b] AND GARY E. GIBSON

Dementia Research Service, Burke Medical Research Institute, Weill Medical College of Cornell University, 785 Mamaroneck Avenue, White Plains, New York 10605, USA

ABSTRACT: Alzheimer disease (AD) is a form of the dementia syndrome. AD appears to have a variety of fundamental etiologies that lead to the neuropathological manifestations which define the disease. Patients who are at high risk to develop AD typically show impairments of cerebral metabolic rate *in vivo* even before they show any evidence of the clinical disease on neuropsychological, electrophysiological, and neuroimaging examinations. Therefore, impairment in energy metabolism in AD can not be attributed to loss of brain substance or to electrophysiological abnormalities. Among the characteristic abnormalities in the AD brain are deficiencies in several enzyme complexes which participate in the mitochondrial oxidation of substrates to yield energy. These include the pyruvate dehydrogenase complex (PDHC), the α-ketoglutarate dehydrogenase complex (KGDHC), and Complex IV of the electron transport chain (COX). The deficiency of KGDHC may be due to a mixture of causes including damage by free radicals and perhaps to genetic variation in the *DLST* gene encoding the core protein of this complex. Inherent impairment of glucose oxidation *by* the AD brain may reasonably be expected to interact synergistically with an impaired supply of oxygen and glucose *to* the AD brain, in causing brain damage. These considerations lead to the hypothesis that cerebrovascular compromise and inherent abnormalities in the brain's ability to oxidize substrates can interact to favor the development of AD, in individuals who are genetically predisposed to develop neuritic plaques.

INTRODUCTION

Dementia is a syndrome which can have many causes.[1] By definition, the characteristic abnormality in dementia is global cognitive impairment including impairment of memory.[2] Alzheimer disease (AD) is the most common cause of dementia. AD is found in more than 80% of patients in the United States who present clinically with dementia and come to autopsy.[3] As discussed elsewhere in this volume, cerebrovascular disease may contribute to the development of AD. Strokes can cause cognitive impairments, but the impairments caused by strokes alone do not tend to fit the syndrome of dementia as it is currently defined (see Hachinski & Munoz, this volume).

A consensus is emerging that AD is usefully thought of as a syndrome to which multiple factors contribute.[4–8] Rare patients have specific forms of familial early on-

[a]Corresponding author: Tel.: (914) 597-2356, (914) 597-2359; fax: (914) 597-2757.
e-mail: jpblass@mail.med.cornell.edu
[b]Deceased.

set AD associated with mutations in one of several specific genes (*APP*, *PS1*, or *PS2*). Even in these families, age of clinical onset varies. In some of these families penetrance is variable. These observations suggest that modifying factors play a role even in these putatively "monogenetic" forms of early-onset AD.[7,8] The common forms of later-onset AD appear to arise from the interactions of a variety of genetic and environmental risk factors.[4,6,9] The best established genetic risk factor in these later-onset forms of AD is the ε-4 allele of the *APOE* gene,[9] but many other genes have been proposed to contribute to the Alzheimer syndrome, at least in specific populations. Over 25 such genes are listed on the Alzheimer Association web site, <htpp://www.alzforum.org/members/research/gene/index.html>. By far the most important "nongenetic" risk factor for AD is age.[9] The various genetic and environmental risk factors converge to lead to the type of neuropathological brain damage that distinguishes Alzheimer disease from other dementias.[4] The common later-onset form of AD can usefully be thought of as a *convergence syndrome*, the Alzheimer syndrome.[4]

A number of abnormalities in AD have been proposed to play a role in causing the brain damage and the resulting clinical signs and symptoms.[4–11] They include loss of brain substance, particularly of synapses; accumulation of abnormal materials, particularly amyloid plaques and neurofibrillary tangles; inflammation; and impairments in energy/oxidative metabolism. The impairments in energy/oxidative metabolism have been linked to impairment in cerebral circulation (both macrovascular and microvascular), to damage due to reactive oxygen species (ROS) or other free radicals, and to inherent deficiencies in the major pathways of energy/oxidative metabolism. Those pathways include the Krebs tricarboxylic acid cycle and electron transport.[4,5,11] Evidence for and against the importance of each of these abnormalities is discussed in more detail elsewhere.[4,10] These different abnormalities may interact with each other. One may speculate that specific abnormalities may be more or less important in specific patients and in specific subgroups of patients. If biologically distinct subgroups of AD patients are combined in a "large study," then a factor that is a dominant cause in one of the subgroups may appear less important in the larger, mixed group.[5,6] This effect may account for some of the controversy about the relative importance of different causes of AD.

This discussion focuses on the abnormalities in energy/oxidative metabolism in AD. It focuses specifically on the potential interactions between deficiencies in cerebral circulation and inherent defeciencies in energy/oxidative metabolism in AD brain. This article discusses the potential effects on AD brain, which already has inherent weaknesses in its ability to utilise the oxygen and glucose supplied by the blood, of the additional stresses of compromises in cerebral circulation. This focused discussion is *not*, however, meant to imply that other mechanisms are not also important in the causation of AD.

ABNORMALITIES IN ENERGY/OXIDATIVE METABOLISM IN AD *IN VIVO*

The existence of metabolic abnormalities in the AD brain was implied in the original papers describing this condition.[12] In the late 1940s and 1950s, invasive methods demonstrated that the AD brain utilized glucose and oxygen more slowly than did the normal brain and also had lower blood flow.[13] Cerebral metabolic rate for glucose (CMR_{glu}) and for oxygen (CMR_{O2}) and in cerebral blood flow (CBF) were all reduced. These reductions have been extensively confirmed by studies of regional cerebral blood flow (rCBF) and by PET, SPECT, and fMRI.[14–17] The reductions in brain metabolism tend to be most marked in the brain regions that are most affected pathologically, but brain metabolism is also low in areas that are spared neuropathologically, such as caudate nucleus and cerebellum.[14–18] The reductions in brain metabolism are not accounted for quantitatively by atrophy.[19] The reductions become more profound as the disease progresses, but they cannot be accounted for by electrophysiologically demonstrable reductions of brain activity.[18]

Recent studies indicate that brain metabolism is reduced in patients who are going to develop AD *even before* abnormalities are detectable by detailed neuropsychological testing or by sophisticated brain imaging.[20–22] It was possible to make these observations by use of genetic markers which identify individuals who have a very high probability of developing clinical AD. For instance, individuals who are homozygous for the ε4 allele of the *APOE* gene can be studied while they are still well.[20] Because the diminutions in brain metabolism in AD are now known to occur before mental function is slowed and before atrophy is detectable, the reductions in brain metabolism in AD cannot now be attributed to slowing of mental function or brain atrophy. These highly replicable observations suggest that the cerebrometabolic impairment in AD contributes to the brain damage, rather than simply being a result of it.[4,5,18]

In addition to the direct evidence of abnormalities in energy/oxidative metabolism in AD brain *in vivo*, indirect evidence also suggests that energy/oxidative metabolism is also altered *in vivo* in other tissues of patients with this disease. AD patients tend to loss weight, even when they are monitored to be ingesting a diet that would normally be adequate calorically.[23,24] AD patients have been reported to have a lower incidence of diabetes than would be expected in their age group.[25–27] They have also been reported to have subtle abnormalities in regulation of blood glucose and insulin.[26,27] The resting metabolic rate of AD patients has, however, been reported to be normal.[28] As of yet, studies of overall body metabolism in AD have not taken into account the possibility of biological subgroups with the Alzheimer syndrome.

ABNORMALITIES IN ENERGY/OXIDATIVE METABOLISM IN AUTOPSIED AD BRAIN

Studies over the last 20 years in a number of laboratories have demonstrated abnormalities in the capacity of the AD brain to carry out carbohydrate catabolism. These findings have been extensively reviewed.[11,18,29] Deficiencies have been robustly demonstrated[29] in three mitochondrial components (FIG. 1): the pyruvate dehydrogenase complex (PDHC), which catalyzes the entry of carbons derived from glucose into the Krebs tricarboxylic acid cycle; the α-ketoglutarate dehydrogenase complex (KGDHC), which catalyzes a key step in the Krebs cycle and is also an enzyme of glutamate metabolism; and cytochrome oxidase (COX), the component of the electron transport chain which uses molecular oxygen as one of its substrates. COX is also known as Complex IV. The activities of other enzymes of energy me-

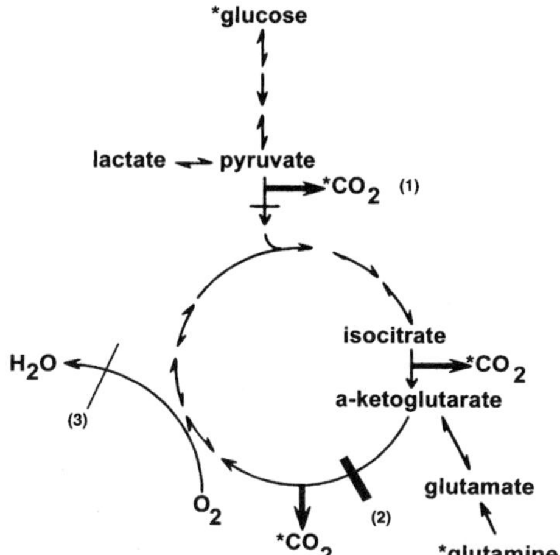

FIGURE 1. Sites of documented abnormalities in energy metabolism in AD. Major pathways of metabolism are diagrammed, with lines indicating where deficiencies in AD brain have been robustly demonstrated. 1, pyruvate dehydrogenase complex (PDHC); 2, α-ketoglutarate dehydrogenase complex (KGDHC); 3, Complex IV (cytochrome oxidase; COX).

tabolism may also be reduced, such as hexokinase which catalyzes the phosphorylation step by which glucose enters the pathway of glycolysis,[30] or phosphofructokinase which appears to be the major control step for glycolysis.[31,32] However, studies of the other enzymes in AD are less extensive.

PDHC was reported to be deficient in the AD brain in 1980.[33] That finding has subsequently been confirmed in at least three other laboratories,[34–36] with no contravening reports. Sheu and co-workers[34] reported that the deficiency is due to a reduction in the amount of immunochemically normal PDHC. Deficiency of PDHC activity occurs not only in regions of brain that are neuropathologically damaged in AD, but also in regions that are histopathologically normal.[33–36] However, no evidence has been reported for abnormalities in the genes encoding the components of PDHC in AD.

Deficient activity of KGDHC in the AD brain was reported in 1988.[37] This finding has been replicated in at least three other laboratories,[35,38,39] again with no contravening reports. The KGDHC deficiency cannot be explained by agonal or postmortem changes.[37,39] The deficiency of KGDHC also occurs both in histopathologically affected and in histopathologically normal regions of the AD brain,[37–39] and is discussed in more detail below, including the results of molecular genetic studies.

COX deficiency has been reported in the AD brain in most[40–44] but not all[45,46] studies. In most studies, the deficiency of COX is limited to regions of the brain which also show histopathological damage.[40,41,44] The expression of COX varies as a function of brain cell activity.[47] This effect is so prominent that immunohistochemical staining for COX has been used as an indicator of the extent of activity of specific neurons.[48,49] The close relationship between the activity of neurons and the amount of COX detected complicates the interpretation of the reduction in COX in histologically abnormal neurons.[48,49] The same considerations apply to the interpretation of the reported reduction in COX mRNA in histopathologically damaged neurons.[48,49] Abnormalities in the mtDNA genes encoding part of COX have been reported,[50] but were subsequently shown to be due to co-amplification of nuclear pseudogenes.[51–53] Decreases in COX activity have been reported in AD "cybrid" cells.[54,55] Cybrids are cells whose endogenous mtDNA has been replaced by exogenous "donor" mtDNA; in AD cybrid cells, the donor mtDNA comes from patients with AD. Defects that persist in cybrid cells are assumed to be due to mutations in the donor (e.g., AD) mtDNA. Studies of Alzheimer disease cybrids have, however, been criticized on technical grounds[56] and were not replicated in another laboratory.[57] By comparison, studies of cybrids implicating mtDNA mutations in a proportion of patients with Parkinson's disease have been replicable across laboratories.[58,59]

Immunohistochemical studies have also shown deficiencies in KGDHC[60] and COX[48,49] in affected areas of AD brain. These data suggest that cells that are normally rich in these mitochondrial components may be relatively vulnerable in AD.[60,61]

ABNORMALITIES IN ENERGY/OXIDATIVE METABOLISM IN NONNEURAL AD TISSUES

Interpretation of biochemical or immunohistochemical abnormalities in damaged tissues is complicated by the "chicken-and-egg" question. Do the abnormalities contribute to the tissue damage or do they simply reflect the damage? Or are both effects operating, in a deleterious cycle? This chicken-and-egg problem can be approached experimentally by examining histologically normal tissues. Abnormalities that persist in histopathologically normal tissue, such as the deficiencies in PDHC and KGDHC in histopathologically normal regions of AD brain (e.g., caudate nucleus), are more likely to be part of the disease process rather than consequences of tissue damage. A rigorous test is whether the abnormalities are found in other tissues which are both histopathologically normal and also function normally in the disease. Cultured cells provide a particularly rigorous test system.[62] Abnormalities that persist in cultured cells from patients with a disease can be presumed to be due, directly or indirectly, to biological abnormalities that are characteristic of the disease being studied. Other factors associated with the disease such as medications or alterations in nutrition are diluted out during serial cell culture.[60,62]

Studies of the mitochondrial complexes that are deficient in AD brain have been done in cultured fibroblasts. Most studies of PDHC activity in AD fibroblasts have found no deficiency.[63] Deficiency of KGDHC has been found in many, but not all, fibroblasts from sporadic AD patients.[64] In general, KGDHC deficiency has not been found in fibroblasts from patients with early onset familial AD[64,65] associated with known mutations in *APP* or *PS1* (TABLE 1). A recent report describes a deficiency of COX in AD fibroblasts.[66] In intact AD fibroblasts, oxidation of [^{14}C]glutamate to $^{14}CO_2$ is reduced,[67,68] but the contents of glutamate and related amino acids appear normal.[69] These results are consistent with KGDHC being less "rate limiting" (i.e., having a lower control coefficient) in cultured fibroblasts than in brain.

TABLE 1. α-Ketoglutarate dehydrogenase complex (KGDHC) activity in AD fibroblasts[a]

Group	Number	Activity[a]
Controls	45	11.1 ± 1.0
Familial AD	25	12.3 ± 1.9
Sporadic AD	40	6.4 ± 0.8^{b}

SOURCE: Blass *et al.*[64]
[a] Activity in nmol/min/mg protein ± SEM.
[b] $p < 0.05$ vs. controls, by Student's *t*-test.

In platelets, deficiencies in the activities of COX have been reported in some,[70] but not all,[71] studies. The somewhat lower activity of KGDHC in AD than in control platelets was not statistically significant.[37] Platelets from patients with dementia consistently have higher than normal activity of the mitochondrial enzyme, monoamine oxidase (MAO).[72–74]

FURTHER CONSIDERATIONS CONCERNING THE KGDHC DEFICIENCY IN AD

The deficiency of KGDHC in AD has been a particular focus of study by our group for several reasons. Low KGDHC activity is as characteristic a finding in the AD brain as are amyloid, neurofibrillary tangles, and a deficiency in the cholinergic marker enzyme choline acetyltransferase.[18,29,35,37–39,60,62–65,75] KGDHC activity is low even in the brains of patients with a primary mutation in *APP*.[75] The KGDHC deficiency in the AD brain occurs in histopathologically normal regions of the AD brain such as caudate nucleus as well as in pathologically damaged areas such as parietal and frontal cortex.[37] The KGDHC deficiency occurs in some although not all cultured AD fibroblasts.[64,65] The measured activity of KGDHC in brain is lower than the activities of other enzymes of the Krebs cycle and electron transport, suggesting that even partial impairment of KGDHC activity might impair overall energy/oxidative metabolism.[60] Recent data indicate that in a subgroup of AD patients defined by molecular genetics, reductions in the activity of KGDHC correlate better with the degree of cognitive impairment than does the amount of amyloid plaques or neurofibrillary tangles.[76]

Attempts to elucidate the mechanism(s) that reduces KGDHC in AD are being made. Studies to date have associated AD with polymorphisms in the *DLST* gene that encodes the core component of KGDHC, but as discussed below a plausibly pathogenetic mutation in this gene has not been described. Oxidative damage to KGDHC may be an important nongenetic mechanism of its inactivation.[77–79] Genetic and nongenetic factors may interact—for instance, genetic variations in a KGDHC protein might sensitize it to damage by free radicals.

Genetic studies related to KGDHC in AD have focused on the *DLST* gene,[80,81] which encodes the core protein of the complex, namely, dihdrolipoyl succinyl transferase (E2k). This gene is located on chromosome 14q24.3, in a region associated with familial AD.[80,81] A *DLST* pseudogene is located on chromosome 1 and is tran-

TABLE 2. Association of a *DLST* genotype with reduced risk for AD[a]

DLST Genotype	AD n (%)	Controls n (%)	Odds Ratio (95% CI)	p Value (χ^2)
A,T/A,T	2 (4%)	24 (22%)	0.16 (0.042–0.611)	0.014 (6.04)
A,T/x	19 (40%)	36 (32%)	1.41 (0.698–2.044)	0.434 (0.61)
Non A,T	26 (55%)	51 (46%)	1.46 (0.733–2.893)	0.366 (0.82)

NOTE: Data are for subjects who do not possess an ε4 allele of the *ApoE* gene (i.e., who carry *ApoE$_3$* and/or *ApoE$_2$* alleles). See Sheu *et al.*[84] for details.

ABBREVIATION: A,T = A119,117/T19, 183.

SOURCE: Sheu *et al.*[84]

scribed.[81,82] It can lead to artifacts in the study of *DLST*. Investigations at Burke and the Karolinska Institute[83–85] have demonstrated the association of specific polymorphisms in *DLST* with a higher risk of AD in patients who also carry the −4 allele of the *APOE* gene (TABLE 2). Associations have been found in very elderly Ashkenazi Jews,[83] in the general, white American population,[84] and in a population sample in Sweden.[85] An association of AD with other polymorphisms of *DLST* was reported from a large series in Japan and was reportedly independent of *APOE* status.[81] A shorter series from Japan in which patients and controls were not matched for age and sex did not replicate the larger Japanese study.[86] An association of AD with polymorphisms in *DLST* has also been found in Swedish families who have been found to be free of known mutations in *APP*, *PS1*, or *PS2*.[85] Recent data indicate that a majority of patients with chromosome 14q24.3-linked early onset familial AD do *not* have mutations in the *PS1* gene.[87] Because the *DLST* gene is located in this region of chromosome 14, the observations on the Swedish families reopen the question of whether some 14q24.3-linked familial AD may be due to mutations in *DLST*.

Problems with the current data on the association of *DLST* with AD should be recognized. No plausibly pathogenetic mutation has as yet been found. The specific polymorphisms associated with AD in the U.S., Swedish, and Japanese populations differ from each other. The molecular genetic data by themselves are consistent with an as yet unidentified pathogenetic mutation in *DLST* itself, but do not provide compelling data. The reported associations can, however, also be plausibly interpreted as clinically unimportant variations in the genome.[83–86] The combination of the molecular genetic data and the robust biochemical data on KGDHC deficiency in AD continue to make *DLST* an interesting gene to investigate in relation to AD, but compelling proof of an association has not been published.

Nongenetic damage to KGDHC also appears to occur in AD. The deficiency of KGDHC occurs in the brains of patients carrying the 670/671 ("Swedish") mutation in *APP*.[75] That finding indicates that the deficiency of KGDHC can occur in the AD brain even when the primary, disease-causing mutation is not in a gene encoding one of the components of KGDHC. In the brains of patients with the 670/671 mutation, immunochemical measurements indicated reductions in the amounts of the E1k (−51%) and E2k (−76%) subunits of KGDHC, but not that of the E3 subunit.[75] In sporadic AD brains, the reduction in KGDHC activity was associated with a reduction in the amounts of the E1k and E2k, but not in E3 protein components; the reductions in protein, however, were small compared to the reductions in activity.[38]

A relevant "nongenetic" mechanism that damages KGDHC is oxidation by free radicals.[77–79,89] It is well documented that the AD brain is under oxidative stress.[88] Several kinds of free radicals (reactive oxygen species; ROS) can inativate KGDHC.[77–79,88] The most extensive studies are of nitric oxide (NO). This species leads to the nitrotyrosylation of KGDHC in intact cells.[77] Nitrosylation of the purified enzyme complex *in vitro* inactivates it.[77] Both the E1k and E2k components of KGDHC are nitrotyrosinated, but the E3 component is not.[77] KGDHC can also be inactivated by H_2O_2 [78] and by hydroxynonenal, [79] but studies with these ROS are less extensive. Another Krebs cycle enzyme reported to be sensitive to ROS is aconitase.[89] One may speculate that sensitivity of specific mitochondrial proteins to elevations of ROS may vary with the species of ROS and with relatively small genetic variations in the enzyme, even if those genetic variations are silent in the presence of normal levels of ROS. KGDHC activity was reduced in cultured skin fibroblasts from familial AD patients carrying a pathogenic mutation in *PS1* by a mild stress, which did not reduce the activity of KGDHC in similarly treated control fibroblasts.[89]

INTERACTIONS BETWEEN CEREBROVASCULAR COMPROMISE AND INHERENT BRAIN ABNORMALITIES

The data discussed above lead to the hypothesis[64] that cerebrovascular compromise and inherent abnormalities in the brain's ability to oxidize substrates can interact with each other in the causation of Alzheimer's disease.

The early clinicopathological descriptions of AD emphasized the role of the vascular component in this disorder.[12] For many years "senile psychosis" was attributed to "hardening of the arteries." A large body of data, summarized elsewhere in this volume (see Snowdon *et al.* and other papers in Part II, this volume), indicates that when compromise of the cerebral circulation occurs, it can contribute to the development of AD. However, severe AD can occur in people who have no evidence of vascular disease of the heart or brain, such as younger people with early onset forms of AD.[90]

As discussed elsewhere in this volume, both macrovascular compromise and microvascular disease including "amyloid angiopathy" have been suggested to contribute to AD. Epidemiological studies suggest that cardiac disease can also be a risk factor for AD.[91–94] Oxidative stress occurs in the AD brain[88] and, as previously discussed, may well contribute to the brain damage in this disease. Extensive studies indicate that reperfusion injury is an important mechanism of brain injury in stroke, and oxidative stress appears to be a major factor in reperfusion injury.[95] It is attractive to postulate that a common factor in the contribution of cerebrovascular compromise to the development of AD is oxidative stress related to reperfusion injury. Reperfusion injury may follow strokes or transient ischemic attacks (TIAs) and can probably also accompany alterations in brain perfusion secondary to cardiac arrhythmias. Irregularities of the heart beat, often episodic, are common in the elderly.[96] Cardiac arrhythmias can compromise the supply of blood to the brain because they can cause dizziness and loss of consciousness (Stokes-Adams attacks). It is therefore reasonable to postulate that certain cardiac arrhythmias can cause reperfusion injuries, particularly episodic arrhythmias which decrease cardiac output. The resultant oxidative stress may damage brain tissues, including mitochondria and KGDHC.[77–79,88] Compromise of the cerebral circulation may contribute to the development of AD in people predisposed to develop that syndrome.

The role of microvascular disease, including amyloid angiopathy of small blood vessels, in the causation of AD is a subject of active investigation.[97,98] In many, although not all, AD patients, the extent of small vessel damage more or less parallels the accumulation of plaques and other histopathological abnormalities.[97,98] The flow of substrate into brain cells may be reduced in AD.[99] However, the mutation in the *APP* gene which leads to the most marked cerebrovascular amyloid angiopathy is associated with cerebral hemorrhages and is distinct clinically and pathologically from the common forms of late-onset AD.[100] It is intuitively attractive to propose that amyloid microangiopathy impairs the flow of substrate to the brain and thereby contributes to the development of AD pathology. A quantitatively important role of microvascular damage in causing the common forms of AD has, however, not yet been demonstrated compellingly.

Many postulates can be made about why cerebral circulatory compromise is associated with AD in some but not other elderly people (see Hachinski & Munoz, this volume). One set of possibilities relates to the precise forms of the circulatory compromise, discussed extensively in other articles in this volume. For instance, repetitive reperfusion injury may contribute to the development of AD more than do major strokes. Another promising set of possibilities relates to genetic variations in the patients. Genetic background is well known to influence the phenotypic, "clinical" effects of many insults to organisms including people.[101–103] Clinically, the field of pharmacogenetics provides many examples,[101,102] such as genetically determined sensitivity to phenytoin (dilantin).[101] Experimentally, a particularly clear example is the effect of a mutant superoxide dismutase (SOD) gene in transgenic mice of different genetic backgrounds.[103] The identical SOD transgene induces three different phenotypes ("clinical syndromes") in three different strains of mice.[103]

Genetic variation may also be important in the interaction between AD and cerebral circulatory impairments. Compromise of energy/oxidative metabolism, including impairments in cerebral circulation, can induce dementia even in people who do not develop AD.[1,13,18,104] The difference between dementia with the histopathological hallmarks of AD and that without histopathological evidence of AD may relate in part to the genetic predisposition of the afflicted persons to develop plaques and tangles. The pathoanatomic change in AD that has been reported to correlate most closely with the degree of dementia is loss of synaptic markers in the AD hippocampus.[105] However, prolonged cerebral hypoperfusion secondary to cardiac arrest can induce bilateral hippocampal damage and dementia without plaques and tangles.[104] Hippocampal sclerosis without plaques and tangles can be very hard to distinguish clinically from classical AD.[106] AD is distinguished from other dementias largely by the presence of adequate numbers of neuritic plaques at autopsy.[1,48] We postulate that impairments of energy/oxidative metabolism, including compromises of the cerebral circulation, may favor the development of AD primarily in people who are genetically predisposed to develop neuritic plaques.

ENERGY/OXIDATIVE METABOLISM AND
THE PATHOPHYSIOLOGY OF AD

The relationships between impairments of energy/oxidative metabolism and the manifestations of AD have been the object of extensive study, and have been reviewed elsewhere.[4,5,18,29] Impairment of energy metabolism can be linked to the major manifestations of AD by plausible hypotheses for which there is extensive evidence. This is not surprising because energy metabolism is critical for maintaining brain cell function. The brain accounts for 2% of human body weight but uses 20% of the oxygen, under physiological conditions.[13] The brain has a second-to-second requirement for intact oxidation of substrates to maintain function, including higher functions such as memory and even consciousness.[13, 107–109]

Interference with energy metabolism can lead to clinical and biological abnormalities associated with AD. Impairment of glucose oxidation by the brain leads to impairments in memory, judgment, and other higher functions which resemble the neuropsychological impairments in dementia.[107–109] In fact, impairment of substrate oxidations is a characteristic finding in the "metabolic encephalopathies," that is, in delirium.[101,102] Cholinergic function is exquisitely sensitive to impairments in energy metabolism, [108,109] and cholinergic function is characteristically impaired in AD.[4] Synaptic function is particularly sensitive to impairments of oxidative metabolism, [110] and synaptic damage correlates better with clinical impairment in AD than do other neuroanatomical abnormalities.[105,111] Impairment of energy metabolism can lead to exquisitely selective loss of vulnerable neurons, for instance, in the four-vessel occlusion model of cerebral ischemia[112] or in thiamine deficiency.[113,114] Selective loss of certain populations of neurons is a characteristic of AD. Impairment of energy metabolism leads to disorganization of the cytoskeleton, and cytoskeletal abnormalities are characteristic of AD.[4]

The accumulation of Alzheimer amyloid (A) also interacts with energy/oxidative metabolism. These interactions are of particular interest because of the current interest in the role of amyloid in AD.[115] Impairments of energy/oxidative metabolism, including impairments of the cerebral circulation[116] and thiamine deficiency,[117] typically lead to the accumulation of APP in the brain. This finding is not surprising because the promotor for the *APP* gene contains consensus sequences which are expected to respond to stress, for example, a *cfos*-responsive element.[118] Harmful fragments of APP—A and the 25–35 amino acid fragment of A—appear to damage tissue by free radical mechanisms.[119–124] Free radical scavengers largely abolish A toxicity.[121–124] The toxic 25–35 peptide spontaneously forms a free radical on methionine residue 35, while the nontoxic scramble or reverse peptides do not.[119] Free radicals can also be formed by the longer APP proteins, perhaps through a mechanism requiring copper.[121,125]

CONCLUSION

The considerations developed above suggest the following hypothesis: Cerebrovascular compromise and inherent abnormalities in the brain's ability to oxidize

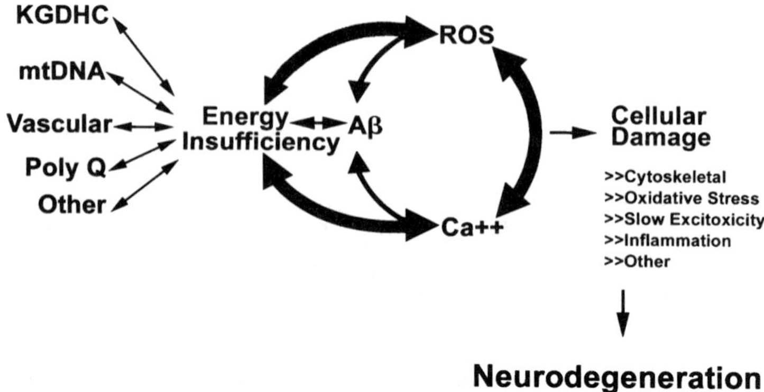

FIGURE 2. Impairments of energy metabolism and brain damage. The cycle shown with the heaviest line occurs in many disorders in which energy metabolism is impaired, including hypoxic/ischemic brain damage. Amyloid (APP and Aβ) can interact with this cycle (*medium heavy lines*). Aβ accumulation is by definition associated with AD. The *narrowest arrows* indicate some of the variety of contributing causes to the cycle, and some of the many consequences which result from compromise of the metabolic pathways by which brain oxidizes substrates to yield energy. (Adapted from Blass *et al.*[126])

substrates can interact to favor the development of AD in individuals who are genetically predisposed to develop neuritic plaques.

A deleterious spiral involving impaired energy metabolism, free radical damage, and impaired cellular calcium homeostasis (FIG. 2) appears to occur in many conditions, including stroke and AD.[119] In AD, neuritic amyloid plaques are also present and may exacerbate this spiral. Neuritic amyloid plaques may therefore contribute to brain damage in individuals who are genetically predisposed to develop them.

Abnormalities in enzymes of energy metabolism can be expected to potentiate the effect of circulatory compromises which reduce the supply of glucose and oxygen to the brain and lead to increased oxidative stress during reperfusion.[4,64,126] Deficiencies of KGDHC, which are characteristically found in the AD brain, may play such a role, whether the deficiencies are due to genetic variations, or to nongenetic factors such as oxidative stress, or to combinations of genetic and nongenetic factors. It will be of interest to explore the effect of compromises of circulation or other impairments of energy/oxidative metabolism in aging transgenic animals who carry specific genes that have been associated with AD, including mutant *APPs* associated with AD.

<h2 style="text-align:center">ACKNOWLEDGMENTS</h2>

This work was supported in part by grants from the Overbrook Foundation, the Winifred Masterson Burke Relief Foundation, and the National Institute on Aging (AG 09014, AG 14930, AG 14600).

REFERENCES

1. TUCKER, G.J., M. POPKIN, E.D. CAINE, M. FOLSTEIN, G.L. GOTTLIEB, I. GRANT & B. LIPTZIN. 1993. Dementia. *In* DSM-IV (Diagnostic and Statistical Manual of Mental Disorders), 4th edit. American Psychiatric Association.: 133–155. Washington, DC.
2. ERKINJUNTTI, T., T. OSTBYE, R. STEENHUIS & V. HACHINSKI. 1997. The effect of different diagnostic criteria on the prevalence of dementia. N. Engl. J. Med. **337:** 1667–1674.
3. NOLAN, K.A., M.M. LINO, A.W. SELIGMANN & J.P. BLASS. 1998. Absence of vascular dementia in an autopsy series from a dementia clinic. J. Am. Geriatr. Soc. **46:** 597–604.
4. BLASS, J.P. 1993. Pathophysiology of the Alzheimer's syndrome. Neurology **43**(Suppl. 4): S25–S38.
5. BLASS, J.P. 1996. Alzheimer's disease: melting pot or mosaic? Alzheimer's Dis. Rev. **1:** 17–20.
6. WALLIN, A. & K. BLENNOW. 1996. Clinical subtypes of the Alzheimer syndrome. Acta Neurol. Scand. Suppl. **165:** 51–57.
7. LOPEZ-ALBEROLA, R.F., W.W. BARKER, D.G. HARWOOD, D.A. LOWEWENSTEIN, P.H. ST. GEORGE-HYSLOP, T. TSUDA, E.A. ROGAEVA & R. DUARA. 1997. Interfamilial and intrafamilial phenotypic heterogeneity in familial Alzheimer's disease. J. Geriatr. Psych. Neurol. **10:** 1–6.
8. DAW, E.W., S.C. HEATH & E.M. WIJSMAN. 1999. Multipoint oligogenic analysis of age-at-onset data with applications to Alzheimer disease pedigrees. Am. J. Hum. Genet. **64:** 839–851.
9. HARWOOD, D.G., W.W. BARKER, D.A. LOEWENSTEIN, R.L. OWNBY, P. ST. GEORGE-HYSLOP, M. MULLAN & R. DUARA. 1999. A cross-ethnic analysis of risk factors for AD in white Hispanics and white non-Hispanics. Neurology **52:** 551–556.
10. EDELBERG, H.K. & J.Y. WEI. 1996. The biology of Alzheimcr's Disease. Mech. Ageing Dev. **91:** 95–114.
11. BLASS, J.P. & F.H. MCDOWELL, Eds. 1999. Mitochondrial/Energy Metabolism in Neurodegenerative Disorders. Ann. N.Y. Acad. Sci., vol. 893.
12. BICK, K., L. AMADUCCI & G. PEPEU. 1987. The Early Story of Alzheimer's Disease. Lavinia Press. Padua, Italy.
13. SOKOLOFF, L. 1989. Circulation and energy metabolism of the brain. *In* Basic Neurochemistry, 4th edit. G. Siegel, B. Agranoff, R.W. Albers & P. Molinoff, Eds.: 565–590. Raven Press. New York.
14. BARCLAY, L., A. ZEMCOV, J.P. BLASS & F. MCDOWELL. 1984. Rates of decrease of cerebral blood flow in progressive dementias. Neurology **34:** 1555–1560.
15. PIETRINI, P., M.L. FUREY, G.E. ALEXANDER, M.J. MENTIS, A. DANI, M. GUAZZELLI, S.I. RAPOPORT & M.B. SCHAPIRO. 1999. Association between brain functional failure and dementia severity in Alzheimer's disease: resting versus stimulation PET study. Am. J. Psychol. **156:** 470–473.
16. SMALL, S.A., G.M. PERERA, R. DELAPAZ, R. MAYEUX & Y. STERN. 1999. Differential regional dysfunction of the hippocampal formation among elderly with memory decline and Alzheimer's disease. Ann. Neurol. **45:** 466–472.
17. MURPHY, D.G.M., P.A. BOTTOMLEY, J.A. SALERNO, C. DECARLI, M.J. MENTIS, C.L. GRADY, D. TEICHBERG, K.R. GIACOMETTI, J.M. ROSENBERG, C.J. HARDY, M.B. SCHAPIRO, S.I. RAPOPORT, J.R. ALGER & B. HORWITZ. 1993. An *in vivo* study of phosphorus and glucose metabolism in Alzheimer's disease using magnetic resonance spectroscopy and PET. Arch. Gen. Psychol. **50:** 341–349.
18. BLASS, J.P. 1997. Cerebral metabolic impairments. *In* Alzheimer's Disease: Cause(s), Diagnosis, Treatment, and Care. Z.S. Khachaturian & T.S. Radebaugh, Eds.: 187–206. CRC Press. Boca Raton, FL.
19. IBÁÑEZ, V., P. PIETRINI, G.E. ALEXANDER, M.L. FUREY, M.S. TEICHBERG, J.C. RAJAPAKSE, S.I. RAPOPORT, M.D. SCHAPIRO & B. HORWITZ. 1998. Regional glucose metabolic abnormalities are not the result of atrophy in Alzheimer's disease. Neurology **50:** 1585–1593.
20. SMALL, G.W., J.C. MAZZIOTTA, M.T. COLLINS, L.R. BAXTER, M.E. PHELPS, M.A. MANDELKERN, A. KAPLAN, A. LARUE, C.F. ADAMSON, L. CHANG, B.H. GUZE, E.H. CORDER, A.M. SAUNDERS, J.L. HAINES, M.A. PERICAK-VANCE & A.D. ROSES. 1995.

Apolipoprotein E type 4 allele and cerebral glucose metabolism in relatives at risk for familial Alzheimer disease. J. Am. Med. Assoc. **273:** 942–947.

21. KENNEDY, A.M., R.S.J. FRACKOWIAK, S.K. NEWMAN, P.M. BLOOMFIELD, J. SEAWARD, P. ROQUES, G. LEWINGTON, V.J. CUNNINGHAM & M.N. ROSSER. 1995. Deficits in cerebral glucose metabolism demonstrated by positron emission tomography in individuals at risk of familial Alzheimer's disease. Neurosci. Lett. **186:** 17–20.

22. REIMAN, E.M., R.J. CASELLI, L.S. YUN, K. CHEN, D. BANDY, S. MINOSHIA, S.N. THIBODEAY & D. OSBORNE. 1996. Preclinical evidence of Alzheimer's disease in persons homozygous for the 4 allele for apolipoprotein E. N. Engl. J. Med. **334:** 752–758.

23. WHITE, H., C. PIEPER, K. SCHMADER & G. FILLENBAUM. 1996. Weight change in Alzheimer's disease. J. Am. Geriatr. Soc. **44:** 265–272.

24. WOLF-KLEIN, G.P. & F.A. SILVERSTONE. 1994. Weight loss in Alzheimer's disease: an international review of the literature. Int. Psychogeriatr. **6:** 135–142.

25. TARIOT, P.N., M.A. OGDEN, C. COX & T. F. WILLIAMS. 1999. Diabetes and dementia in long-term care. J. Am. Geriatr. Soc. **47:** 423–429.

26. ADOLFSSON, R., G. BUCHT, F. LITHNER & B. WINBLAD. 1980. Hypoglycemia in Alzheimer's disease. Acta Med. Scand. **208:** 387–388.

27. MENEILLY, G.S. & A. HILL. 1993. Alterations in glucose metabolism in patients with Alzheimer's disease. J. Am. Geriatr. Soc. **41:** 710–714.

28. DONALDSON, K.E., W.H. CARPENTER, M.J. TOTH, M.I. GORAN, P. NEWHOUSE & E.T. POEHLMAN. 1996. No evidence for a higher resting metabolic rate in noninstitutionalized Alzheimer's disease patients. J. Am. Geriatr. Soc. **44:**1232–1234.

29. GIBSON, G.E., K.-F.R. SHEU & J.P. BLASS. 1998. Abnormalities in mitochondrial enzymes in Alzheimer disease. J. Neural Transm. **105:** 855–870.

30. LIGURI, G., N. TADDEI, P. NASSI, S. LATORRACA, C. NEDIANI & S. SORBI. 1990. Changes in Na^+, K^+-ATPase, Ca^{2+}-ATPase and some soluble enzymes related to energy metabolism in brains of patients with Alzheimer's disease. Neurosci. Lett. **112:** 338–342.

31. BOWEN, D.M., P. WHITE, J.A. SPILLANE, M.J. GOODHARDT, G. CURZON, P. IWANGOFF, W. MEIER-RUGE & A.N. DAVISON. 1979. Accelerated ageing or selective neuronal loss as an important cause of dementia? Lancet **1:**11–14.

32. SIMS, N.R., J.P. BLASS, C. MURPHY, D.M. BOWEN & D. NEARY. 1987. Phosphofructokinase activity in the brain in Alzheimer's disease. Ann. Neurol. **21:** 509–510.

33. PERRY, E.K., R.H. PERRY, B.E. TOMLINSON, G. BLESSED & P.H. GIBSON. 1980. Coenzyme-A acetylating enzymes in Alzheimer's disease: possible cholinergic "compartment" of pyruvate dehydrogenase. Neurosci. Lett. **18:** 105–108.

34. SHEU, K.-F.R.,Y.-Y. KIM, J.P. BLASS & M.E. WEKSLER. 1985. An immunochemical study on the deficit of pyruvate dehydrogenase in Alzheimer's disease. Ann. Neurol. **17:** 444–451.

35. BUTTERWORTH, R. & A.M. BESNARD. 1990. Thiamin-dependent enzyme changes in temporal cortex of patients with Alzheimer's disease. Metab. Brain Dis. **4:** 179–182.

36. YATES, C.M., M. BUTTERWORTH, M.C. TENNANT & A. GORDON. 1991. Enzyme activities in relation to pH and lactate in post-mortem brain in Alzheimer and other dementias. J. Neurochem. **55:** 1624–1631.

37. GIBSON, G.E., K.-F.R. SHEU, J.P. BLASS, A. BAKER, K.C. CARLSON, B. HARDING & P. PERRINO. 1988. Reduced activities of thiamin-dependent enzymes in the brains and peripheral tissues of patients with Alzheimer's disease. Arch. Neurol. **35:** 312–317.

38. MASTROGIACOMO, F., C. BERGERON & S.J. KISH. 1993. Brain–ketoglutarate dehydrogenase complex activity in Alzheimer's disease. J. Neurochem. **61:** 2007–2011.

39. TERWEL, D., J. BOTHMER, E. WOLF, F. MENG & J. JOLLES. 1998. Affected enzyme activities in Alzheimer's disease are sensitive to antemortem hypoxia. J. Neurol. Sci. **161:** 47–56.

40. SCHAPIRA, A.H. 1996. Oxidative stress and mitochondrial dysfunction in neurodegeneration. Curr. Opin. Neurol. **9:** 260–264.

41. MUTSIYAMA, E.M., A.C. BOWLING & M.F. BEAL. 1994. Cortical cytochrome oxidase activity is reduced in Alzheimer's disease. J. Neurochem. **63:** 2179–2184.

42. PARKER,W.D., J. PARKS, C.M. FILLEY & B.K. KLEINSCHMIDT-DEMASTERS. 1994. Electron transport chain defects in Alzheimer's disease brain. Neurology **44:** 1090–1096.

43. WONG-RILEY, M., P. ANTUONO, K.C. HO, R. EGAN, R. HEVNER, W. LIEBL, Z. HUANG, R. RACHEL & J. JONES. 1997. Cytochrome oxidase in Alzheimer's disease: biochemical, histochemical, and immunohistochemical analyses of the visual and other systems. Vision Res. **37:** 3593–3608.

44. KISH, S.J., F. MASTROGIACOMO, M. GUTTMAN, Y. FURUKAWA, J.W. TAANMAN, S. DOZIC, M. PANDOLFO, J. LAMARCHE, L. DISTEFANO & L.J. CHANG. 1999. Decreased brain protein levels of cytochrome oxidase subunits in Alzheimer's disease and in hereditary spinocerebellar disorders: a nonspecific change? J. Neurochem. **72:** 700–707.

45. CAVELIER, L., E.E. JAZIN, I. ERIKSSON, J. PRINCE, U. BAVE, L. ORELAND, & U. GYLLENSTEN. 1995. Decreased cytochrome-c oxidase activity and lack of age-related accumulation of mitochondrial DNA deletions in the brains of schizophrenics. Genomics **29:** 217–224.

46. COOPER, J.M., C. WISCHIK & A.H.V. SCHAPIRA. 1993. Mitochondrial function in Alzheimer's disease. Lancet **341:** 969–970.

47. HEVNER, R.F. & M.T.T. WONG-RILEY. 1993. Mitochondrial and nuclear gene expression for cytochrome oxidase subunits are disproportionately regulated by functional activity in neurons. J. Neurosci. **13:** 1805–1819.

48. SIMONIAN, N.A. & B.T. HYMAN. 1995. Functional alterations in neural circuits in Alzheimer's disease. Neurobiol. Aging **16:** 305–309.

49. HATANPAA, K., D.R. BRADY, J. STOLL, S.I. RAPOPORT & K. CHANDRASEKARAN. 1996. Neuronal activity and early neurofibrillary tangles in Alzheimer's disease. Ann. Neurol. **40:** 411–420.

50. DAVIS, R.E., S. MILLER, C. HERRNSTADT, S.S. GHOSH, E. FAHY, M.F. BEAL, N. HOWELL & W.D. PARKER. 1997. Mutations in mitochondrial cytochrome c oxidase genes segregate with late-onset Alzheimer disease. Proc. Natl. Acad. Sci. USA **94:** 4526–4531.

51. DAVIS, R.E. & W.D. PARKER. 1998. Evidence that two reports of mtDNA cytochrome oxidase "mutations" in Alzheimer's disease are based on nDNA pseudogenes of recent evolutionary origin. Biochem. Biophys. Res. Commun. **244:** 877–883.

52. HIRANO, M., A. SHTILBANS, R. MAYEUX, M.M. DAVIDSON, S. DIMAURO, J.A. KNOWLES & E.A. SCHON. 1997. Apparent mtDNA heteroplasmy in Alzheimer's disease patients and in normals due to PCR amplification of nucleus-embedded mtDNA pseudogenes. Proc. Natl. Acad. Sci. USA **94:** 14894–14899.

53. WALLACE, D.C., C. STUGARD, D. MURDOCK, T. SCHURR & M.D. BROWN. 1997. Ancient mtDNA sequences in the human nuclear genome: a potential source of errors in identifying pathogenic mutations. Proc. Natl. Acad. Sci. USA **94:** 14900–14905.

54. CASSARINO, D.S., R.H. SWERDLOW, J.K. PARKS, W.D. PARKER & J.P. BENNETT. 1998. Cyclosporin A increases resting mitochondrial membrane potential in SYSY cells and reverses the depressed mitochondrial membrane potential of Alzheimer's disease cybrids. Biochem. Biophys. Res. Commun. **248:** 168–173.

55. SHEEHAN, J.P., R.H. SWERDLOW, S.W. MILLER, R.E. DAVIS, J. PARKS, W.D. PARKER & J.B. TUTTLE. 1997. Calcium homeostasis and reactive oxygen species production in cells transformed by mitochondria from individuals with sporadic Alzheimer's disease. J. Neurosci. **17:** 4612–4622.

56. SCHON, E.A., E.A. SHOUBRIDGE & C.T. MORAES. 1998. Cybrids in Alzheimer's disease: a cellular model of the disease? Neurology **51:** 326.

57. ITO, S., S. OHTA, K. NISHIMAKI, Y. KAGAWA, R. SOMA, S.Y. KUNO, Y. KOMATSUZAKI, H. MIZUSAWA & J. HAYASHI. 1999. Functional integrity of mitochondrial genomes in human platelets and autopsied brain tissues from elderly patients with Alzheimer's disease. Proc. Natl. Acad. Sci. USA **96:** 2099–2103.

58. SWERDLOW, R.H., J.K. PARKS, S.W. MILLER, J.B. TUTTLE, P.A. TRIMMER, J.P. SHEEHAN, J.P. BENNET, R.E. DAVIS & W.D. PARKER. 1996. Origin and functional consequences of the complex I defect in Parkinson's disease. Ann. Neurol. **40:** 663–671.

59. GU, M., J.M. COOPER, J.W. TAANMAN & A.H. SCHAPIRA. 1998. Mitochondrial DNA transmission of the mitochondrial defect in Parkinson's disease. Ann. Neurol. **44:** 177–186.

60. BLASS, J.P. 1993. Metabolic alterations common to neural and non-neural cells in Alzheimer's disease. Hippocampus **3:** 45–54.

61. BLASS, J.P., K.-F.R. SHEU & L. KO. 1993. Chemical neuroanatomy and selective vulnerability in relation to disorders of energy metabolism. J. Neurochem. **61:** S249.
62. HUANG, H.-M., R. MARTINS, S. GANDY, R. ETCHEBERRIGARATY, E. ITO, D.L. ALKON, J.P. BLASS & G.E. GIBSON. 1995. Use of cultured fibroblasts in elucidating the pathophysiology and diagnosis of Alzheimer's disease. Ann. N.Y. Acad. Sci. **747:** 225–244.
63. SHEU, K.-F.R., A.J.L. COOPER, J.G. LINDSAY & J.P. BLASS. 1994. Abnormality of the α-ketoglutarate dehydrogenase complex in fibroblasts from familial Alzheimer's disease. Ann. Neurol. **35:** 312–318.
64. BLASS, J.P., K.-F.R. SHEU, S. PIACENTINI & S. SORBI. 1997. Inherent abnormalities in oxidative metabolism in AD: interaction with vascular abnormalities. Ann. N.Y. Acad. Sci. **826:** 382–385.
65. GIBSON, G.E., H. ZHANG, K.F. SHEU, N. BOGDANOVICH, J.G. LINDSAY, L. LANNFELT, M. VESTLING & R.F. COWBURN. 1998. Alpha-ketoglutarate dehydrogenase in Alzheimer brains bearing the APP670/671 mutation. Ann. Neurol. **44:** 676-681.
66. CURTI, D., F. ROGONI, L. GASPARINI, A. CATTANEO, M. PAOLILLO, M. RACCHI, L. ZANI, A. BIANCHETTI, M. TRABUCCHI, S. BERGAMASCHI & S. GOVONI. 1997. Oxidative metabolism in cultured fibroblasts derived from sporadic Alzheimer's disease patients. Neurosci. Lett. **236:** 13–16.
67. SIMS, N.R., J.M. FINEGAN & J.P. BLASS. 1987. Altered metabolic properties of cultured skin fibroblasts in Alzheimer's disease. Ann. Neurol. **21:** 509–510.
68. PETERSON, C. & J.E. GOLDMAN. 1986. Alterations in calcium content and biochemical processes in cultured skin fibroblasts from aged and Alzheimer donors. Proc. Natl. Acad. Sci. USA **83:** 2758–2762.
69. COOPER, A.J.L., K.-F.R. SHEU & J.P. BLASS. 1996. Normal glutamate metabolism in Alzheimer's disease fibroblasts deficient in α-ketoglutarate dehydrogenase activity. Dev. Neurosci. **18:** 499–504.
70. PARKER, W.D., N.J. MAHR, C.M. FILLEY, J.K. PARKS, D. HUGHES, D.A. YOUNG & C.M. CULLUM. 1994. Reduced platelet cytochrome c oxidase activity in Alzheimer's disease. Neurology **44:** 1086–1090.
71. VAN ZUYLEN, A.J., G.J. BOSMAN, W. RUITENBEEK, P.J. VAN KALMTHOUT & W.J. DE GRIP. 1992. No evidence for reduced thrombocyte cytochrome oxidase activity in Alzheimer's disease. Neurology **42:** 1246–1247.
72. ADOLFSSON, R., C.-G GOTTFRIES, L. ORELAND, A. WIBERG & B. WINBLAD. 1980. Increased activity of brain and platelet monoamine oxidase in dementia of Alzheimer type. Life Sci. **27:** 1029–1034.
73. ALEXOPOULOS, G.S., R.C. YOUNG, K.W. LIEBERMAN & C.A. SHAMOIAN. 1987. Platelet MAO activity in geriatric patients with depression and dementia. Am. J. Psychiatr. **144:** 1480–1483.
74. BONGIOVANNI, P., F. GEMIGNANI, B. BOCCARDI, M. BORGNA & B. ROSSI. 1997. Platelet monoamine oxidase molecular activity in demented patients. Ital. J. Neurol. Sci. **18:** 151–156.
75. GIBSON, G.E., H. ZHANG, K.F. SHEU, N. BOGDANOVICH, J.G. LINDSAY, L. LANNFELT, M. VESTLING & R.F. COWBURN. 1998. α-Ketoglutarate dehydrogenase in Alzheimer brains bearing the APP670/671 mutation. Ann. Neurol. **44:** 676–681.
76. GIBSON, G.E., V. HAROUTUNIAN, L.C.H. PARK, H. ZHANG, R. MOHS, R.K.F. SHEU & J.P. BLASS. 1999. Reductions in a key mitochondrial enzyme in brains from Alzheimer's correlate with a clinical dementia rating. J. Neurochem. **73:** S23.
77. PARK, L.C.H., H. ZHANG, R.K.-F. SHEU, N.Y. CALINGSAN, B.S. KRISTAL, J.G. LINDSAY & G.E. GIBSON. 1999. Metabolic impairment induces oxidative stress, compromises inflammatory responses, and inactivates a key mitochondrial enzyme in microglia. J. Neurochem. **72:** 1948–1958.
78. CHINOPOULOS, C., L. TRETTER & V. ADAM-VIZI. 1999. Depolarization of *in situ* mitochondria due to hydrogen peroxide-induced oxidative stress in nerve terminals: inhibition of α-ketoglutarate dehydrogenase. J. Neurochem. **73:** 220–228.
79. HUMPHRIES, K.M. & L.I. SZWEDA. 1998. Selective inactivation of α-ketoglutarate dehydrogenase and pyruvate dehydrogenase: reaction of lipoic acid with 4-hydroxy-2-nonenal. Biochemistry **37:** 15835–15841.

80. ALI, G., W. WASCO, X. CAI, P. SZABO, K.-F. SHEU, A.J. COOPER, S.M. GASTON, J.F. GUSELLA, R. TANZI & J.P. BLASS. 1994. Isolation, cloning, and localization of the gene for the E2k component of the human ketoglutarate dehydrogenase complex. Somatic Cell Mol. Genet. **20:** 190–199.

81. NAKANO, K., C. TAKASE, K. NISHIMAKI, T. MIKI & S. MATUDA. 1997. Alzheimer's disease and *DLST* genotype. Lancet **350:** 1367–1368.

82. CAI, X., P. SZABO, G. ALI, R.F. TANZI & J.P. BLASS. 1994. A pseudogene of dihydrolipyl succinyltransferase (E2k) found by PCR amplification and direct sequencing of rodent-human cell hybrid DNAs. Somatic Cell Mol. Genet. **20:** 339–343.

83. SHEU, K.-F.R., A.M. BROWN, V. HAROUTUNIAN, B.S. KRISTAL, H. THALER, M. LESSER, R. N. KALARIA, N.R. RELKIN, R.C. MOHS, L. LILIUS, L. LANNFELT & J.P. BLASS. 1999. Modulation by *DLST* of the genetic risk of Alzheimer's disease in a very elderly population. Ann. Neurol. **45:** 48–53.

84. SHEU, K.-F.R., A.M. BROWN, B.S. KRISTAL, R.N. KALARIA, L. LILIUS, L. LANNFELT & J.P. BLASS. A *DLST* genotype associated with reduced risk for Alzheimer's Disease. Neurology 1999; **52:** 1505–1507.

85. LILIUS, L, K.-F.R. SHEU, L. LANNFELT & J.P. BLASS. 1998. Association of *DLST* polymorphisms with familial Alzheimer's disease. Neurosci. Abstr. **24:** 255.

86. KUNUGI, H., S. NANKO, A. UEKI, K. ISSE & H. HIRASAWA. 1998. *DLST* gene and Alzheimer's disease. Lancet **351:** 1584–1585.

87. CRUTS, M., C.M. VAN DUIJN, H. BACKHOVENS, M. VAN DEN BROECK, A. WEHNERT, S. SERNEELS, R. SHERRINGTON, M. HUTTON, J. HARDY, P.H. ST. GEORGE-HYSLOP, A. HOFMAN & C. VAN BROECKHOVEN. 1998. Estimation of the genetic contribution of presenilin-1 and -2 mutations in a population-based study of presenile Alzheimer disease. Hum. Mol. Genet. **7:** 43–45.

88. BEAL, M.F. 1998. Mitochondrial dysfunction in neurodegenerative diseases. Biochim. Biophys. Acta **1366:** 211–223.

89. GIBSON, G.E., L.C.H. PARK, H. ZHANG, S. SORBI & N.Y. CALINGASAN. Oxidative stress and a key metabolic enzyme in Alzheimer brains, cultured cells, and an animal model of chronic oxidative deficits. Ann. N.Y. Acad. Sci. In press.

90. GARDNER, P.R., I. RAINERI, L.B. EPSTEIN & C.W. WHITE. 1995. Superoxide radical and iron modulate aconitase activity in mammalian cells. J. Biol. Chem. **270:** 13399–13405.

91. MULLER, H.F., F. ENGELSMANN, N.P. NAIR & Y. ROBITAILLE. 1997. Psychogeriatric clinical,electro-encephalographic and autopsy findings. Neuropsychobiology **35(2):** 95–101.

92. DE PEDIS, G., K. HEDNER, B.W. JOHANSSON & B. STEEN. 1987. Cardiac arrhythmia in geriatric patients with organic dementia. Compr. Gerontol. Sect. A, Clin. Lab. Sci. **1:**115–117.

93. MARIN, D.B., B. BREUER, M.L. MARIN, J. SILVERMAN, J. SCHMEIDLER, D. GREENBERG, S. FLYNN, M. MARE, M. LANTZ, L. LIBOW, R. NEUFELD, L. ALTSTIEL, K.L. DAVIS & R.C. MOHS. 1998. The relationship between apolipoprotein E, dementia, and vascular illness. Atherosclerosis **140:**173–180.

94. SPARKS, D.L. 1997. Coronary artery disease, hypertension, ApoE, and cholesterol: a link to Alzheimer's disease? Ann. N.Y. Acad. Sci. **826:** 128–146.

95. TRAYSTMAN, R.J., J.R. KIRSCH & R.C. KOEHLER. 1991. Oxygen radical mechanisms of brain injury following ischemia and reperfusion. J. Appl. Physiol. **71:**1185–1195.

96. DUNCAN, A.K., J. VITTONE, K.C. FLEMING & H.C. SMITH. 1996. Cardiovascular disease in elderly patients. Mayo Clin. Proc. **71:** 184-196.

97. BUEE, L., P.R. HOF & A. DELACOURTE. 1997. Brain microvascular changes in Alzheimer's disease and other dementias. Ann. N.Y. Acad. Sci. **826:** 7-24.

98. KALARIA, R.N. 1997. Cerebrovascular degeneration is related to amyloid-beta protein deposition in Alzheimer's disease. Ann. N.Y. Acad. Sci. **826:** 263-271.

99. SIMPSON, I.A., K.R. CHUNDU, T. DAVIES-HILL, W.G. HONER & P. DAVIES. 1994. Decreased concentrations of GLUT1 and GLUT3 glucose transporters in the brains of patients with Alzheimer's disease. Ann. Neurol. **35:** 546-551.

100. NATTE, R., H.V. VINTERS, M.L. MAAT-SCHIEMAN, M. BORNEBROEK, J. HAAN, R.A. ROOS & S.G. VAN DUINEN. 1998. Microvasculopathy is associated with the number of

cerebrovascular lesions in hereditary cerebral hemorrhage with amyloidosis, Dutch type. Stroke **29:** 1588–1594.

101. MAMIYA, K., I. IEIRI, J. SHIMAMOTO, E. YUKAWA, J. IMAI, H. NINOMIYA, H. YAMADA, K. OTSUBO, S. HIGUCHI & M. TASHIRO. 1998. The effects of genetic polymorphisms of CYP2C9 and CYP2C19 on phenytoin metabolism in Japanese adult patients with epilepsy: studies in stereoselective hydroxylation and population pharmacokinetics. Epilepsia **39:** 1317–1323.

102. LINDER, M.W., R.A. PROUGH & R. VALDES, JR. 1997. Pharmacogenetics: a laboratory tool for optimizing therapeutic efficiency. Clin. Chem. **43:** 254–266.

103. EPSTEIN, C.J. Phenotypes of Cu,Mn-SOD transgenic mice. Ann. N.Y. Acad. Sci. In press.

104. VOLPE, B.T. & C.K. PETITO. 1985. Dementia with bilateral medial temporal lobe ischemia. Neurology **35:** 1793–1797.

105. SZE, C.-I., J.C. TRONCOSO, C. KAWAS, P. MOUTON, D.L. PRICE & L.J. MARTIN. 1997. Loss of the presynaptic vesicle protein synaptophysin correlates with cognitive decline in Alzheimer's disease. J. Neuropathol. Exp. Neurol. **8:** 933–934.

106. COREY-BLOOM, J., M.N. SABBAGH, M.W. BONDI, L. HANSEN, M.F. ALFORD, E. MASLIAH & L.J. THAL. 1997. Hippocampal sclerosis contributes to dementia in the elderly. Neurology **48:**154–160.

107. BLASS, J.P., K.A. NOLAN, R.S. BLACK & A. KURITA. 1992. Delirium: phenomenology and diagnosis—A neurobiological view. Int. Psychogeriatr. **3:** 121–134.

108. BLASS, J.P. & G.E. GIBSON. Cerebrometabolic aspects of delirium in relationship to dementia. Dementia Other Cogn. Disord. In press.

109. BLASS, J.P., H.-M. HUANG & G.B. FREEMAN. 1992. The cellular basis of delirium and its relevance to age related disorders including Alzheimer's disease. Int. Psychogeriatr. **3:** 373–396.

110. FREEMAN, G.B. & G.E. GIBSON. 1988. Dopamine, acetylcholine and glutamate interactions in aging: behavioral and biochemical correlates. Ann. N.Y. Acad. Sci. **515:** 191–202.

111. TERRY, R.D., E. MASLIAH, D.P. SALMON, N. BUTTERS, R. DETERESA, R. HILL, L.A. HANSEN & R. KATZMAN. 1991. Physical basis of cognitive alterations in Alzheimer's disease: synapse loss is the major correlate of cognitive impairment. Ann. Neurol. **30:** 572–580.

112. MCBEAN, D.E. & P.A. KELLY. 1998. Rodent models of global cerebral ischemia: a comparison of two-vessel occlusion and four-vessel occlusion. Gen. Pharmacol. **30:** 431–434.

113. CALINGASAN, N.Y. & G.E. GIBSON. 1999. Vascular endothelium is a site of free radical production and inflammation in areas of neuronal loss in thiamine-deficient brain. Ann. N.Y. Acad. Sci. In press.

114. CALINGASAN, N.Y., W.J. CHUN, L.C.H. PARK, K. UCHIDA & G.E. GIBSON. Oxidative stress is associated with region-specific neuronal death during thiamine deficiency. J. Neuropathol. Exp. Neurol. In press.

115. HARDY, J., K. DUFF, K.G. HARDY, J. PEREZ-TUR & M. HUTTON. 1998. Genetic dissection of Alzheimer'sdisease and related dementias: amyloid and its relationship to tau. Nature Neurosci. **1:** 355–358.

116. JENDROSKA, K., O.M. HOFFMANN & S. PATT. 1997. Amyloid beta peptide and precursor protein (APP) in mild and severe brain ischemia. Ann. N.Y. Acad. Sci. **826:** 401–405.

117. CALIGNASAN, N.Y., S.E. GANDY, H. BAKER, K.-F. SHEU, J.D. SMITH, B.T. LAMB, J.D. GEARHART, J.D. BUXBAUM, C. HARPER, D.J. SELKOE, D.L. PRICE, S.S. SISODIA & G.E. GIBSON. 1996. Novel neuritic clusters with accumulations of amyloid precursor protein and amyloid precursor-like protein 2 immunoreactivity in brain regions damaged by thiamine deficiency. Am. J. Pathol. **149:** 1063–1071.

118. BEYREUTHER, K., P. POLLWEIN, G. MULTHAUP, U. MONNING, G. KONIG, T. DYRKS, W. SCHUBERT & C.L. MASTERS. 1993. Regulation and expression of the Alzheimer's beta/A4 amyloid /A4 amyloid precursor protein in health, disease, and Down's syndrome. Ann. N.Y. Acad. Sci. **695:** 91–102.

119. YATIN, S.M., M. YATIN, T. AULICK, K.B. AIN & D.A. BUTTERFIELD. 1999. Alzheimer's amyloid beta-peptide associated free radicals increase rat embryonic neuronal

polyamine uptake and ornithine decarboxylase activity: protective effect of vitamin E. Neurosci. Lett. **263:**17–20.

120. GUO, Q., L. SEBASTIAN, B.L. SOPHER, M.W. MILLER, C.B. WARE, G.M. MARTIN & M.P. MATTSON. 1999. Increased vulnerability of hippocampal neurons from presenilin-1 mutant knock-in mice to amyloid beta-peptide toxicity: central roles of superoxide production and caspase activation. J. Neurochem. **72:** 1019–1029.

121. DIKALOV, S.I., M.P. VITEK, K.R. MAPLES & R.P. MASON. 1999. Amyloid beta peptides do not form peptide-derived free radicals spontaneously, but can enhance metal-catalyzed oxidation of hydroxylamines to nitroxides. J. Biol. Chem. **274:** 9392–9399.

122. BRUCE-KELLER, A.J., J.G. BEGLEY, W. FU, D.A. BUTTERFIELD, D.E. BREDESEN, J.B. HUTCHINS, K. HENSLEY & M.P. MATTSON. 1998. Bcl-2 protects isolated plasma and mitochondrial membranes against lipid peroxidation induced by hydrogen peroxide and amyloid beta-peptide. J. Neurochem. **70:** 31–39.

123. IADECOLA, C., F. ZHANG, K. NIWA, C. ECKMAN, S.K. TURNER, E. FISCHER, S. YOUNKIN, D.R. BORCHELT, K.K. HSIAO & G.A. CARLSON. 1999. SOD1 rescues cerebral endothelial dysfunction in mice overexpressing amyloid precursor protein. Nature Neurosci. **2:** 157–161.

124. SUBRAMANIAM, R., T. KOPPAL, M. GREEN, S. YATIN, B. JORDAN, J. DRAKE & D.A. BUTTERFIELD. 1998. The free radical antioxidant vitamin E protects cortical synaptosomal membranes from amyloid beta-peptide(25–35) toxicity but not from hydroxynonenal toxicity: relevance to the free radical hypothesis of Alzheimer's disease. Neurochem. Res. **23:**1403–1410.

125. MULTHAUP, G. & C.L. MASTERS. 1999. Metal binding and radical generation of proteins in human neurological diseases and aging. Metal Ions Biol. Systems **36:** 365–387.

126. BLASS, J.P., G.E. GIBSON & S. HOYER. 1997. Metabolism of the aging brain. *In* The Aging Brain. M.P. Mattson, J.W. Geddes, P. Tamiras, E.E. Bittar, Eds.: 109–128. JAI Press. London.

Insulin Effects on Glucose Metabolism, Memory, and Plasma Amyloid Precursor Protein in Alzheimer's Disease Differ According to Apolipoprotein-E Genotype

SUZANNE CRAFT,[a,c,h] SANJAY ASTHANA,[a,d] GERARD SCHELLENBERG,[a,d,e,f] LAURA BAKER,[a,c] MONIQUE CHERRIER,[c] ADAM A. BOYT,[g] RALPH N. MARTINS,[g] MURRAY RASKIND,[b,c] ELAINE PESKIND,[b,c] AND STEPHEN PLYMATE[a,d]

[a]*Geriatric Research, Education, and Clinical Center and* [b]*Mental Health Services, VA Puget Sound Health Care System, Seattle, Washington 98108, USA*

Departments of [c]*Psychiatry and Behavioral Sciences,* [d]*Medicine,* [e]*Neurology, and* [f]*Pharmacology, University of Washington School of Medicine, Seattle, Washington 98108, USA*

[g]*Sir James McCusker Alzheimer's Disease Research Unit, Department of Surgery, The University of Western Australia, Perth, Australia*

ABSTRACT: Higher fasting plasma insulin levels and reduced CSF-to-plasma insulin ratios, suggestive of insulin resistance, have been observed in patients with Alzheimer's disease (AD) who do not possess an apolipoprotein E (ApoE)-ε4 allele. Insulin has also been implicated in processing of β-amyloid and amyloid precursor protein (APP). We examined the effects of intravenous insulin administration while maintaining euglycemia on insulin-mediated glucose disposal, memory, and plasma APP in patients with AD and normal adults of varying ApoE genotypes. AD subjects without an ε4 allele had significantly lower insulin-mediated glucose disposal rates than did AD patients with an ε4 allele ($p < 0.03$) or than did normal adults without an ε4 allele ($p < 0.02$). AD subjects without an ε4 allele also showed significant memory facilitation with insulin administration ($p < 0.04$), whereas the AD-ε4 group did not. Insulin reduced APP levels for AD patients without an ApoE ε4 allele, but raised APP for AD patients with an ApoE εH4 allele These results document ApoE-related differences in insulin metabolism in AD that may relate to disease pathogenesis.

INTRODUCTION

Patients with AD who are not homozygous for the ApoE ε4 allele have higher fasting plasma insulin levels and reduced brain insulin uptake, as reflected by a lower CSF-to-plasma insulin ratio, than do other patients with AD.[1] These results sug-

[h]Address for correspondence: Suzanne Craft, GRECC 182B, VA Puget Sound Health Care System, 1660 South Columbian Way, Seattle, Washington 98108. Tel.: 206-764-2308; fax: 206-764-2569.
e-mail: scraft@u.washington.edu

"

gest that defective insulin action may be of particular pathophysiologic significance for patients with sporadic AD who do not possess an ApoE ε4 allele. Such a defect may be of considerable import, given accruing evidence that insulin affects function in brain regions such as the hippocampus that are known to be compromised at the earliest stages of AD.[2] Furthermore, a recent neuropathological study documented increased insulin receptor numbers and reduced tyrosine kinase activity in AD brains relative to age-matched controls, which the authors interpreted as indicative of defective insulin signal transduction.[3]

Although our previous finding of higher fasting plasma insulin levels in non-ε4 homozygotes is suggestive of insulin resistance, no metabolic studies were conducted to definitively determine the presence of resistance or to quantify insulin sensitivity in these patients. In recent studies, we examined peripheral insulin action in a new sample of patients with AD of differing ApoE genotypes using a hyperinsulinemic–euglycemic infusion protocol that is a sensitive measure of insulin-mediated glucose disposal. We also determined the degree of memory facilitation shown by patients at a hyperinsulinemic–euglycemic steady-state level that has been shown previously to enhance memory in patients with insulin resistance.[4] The degree of memory facilitation reflects direct or indirect insulin effects on the hippocampus and medial temporal memory system.[4] In addition, given that insulin has also been implicated in processing of β–amyloid and amyloid precursor protein (APP),[5,6] we measured the effects of infusing insulin *in vivo* on plasma APP levels in normal adults and in AD patients with and without the ApoE ε4 allele.

METHODS

Subjects

This study was approved by the Human Subjects Committee of the University of Washington. Participants were 31 patients with AD (10 women, 21 men) and 26 healthy age-matched adults (11 women, 15 men). Patients with mild to moderate AD met NINCDS-ADRDA criteria. All subjects were free from any significant medical, neurological, or psychiatric illness other than AD, as determined by a detailed history, medical, neurological, and neuropsychological examination. Subjects were not receiving any cognition-enhancing or other CNS medication. Demographic data are presented in TABLE 1.

Procedure

Each fasting subject participated in two metabolic conditions on separate mornings in counterbalanced order: (1) *Hyperinsulinemia with plasma glucose maintained at baseline levels.* Subjects were maintained at plasma insulin levels of about 80 μU/ml using an insulin infusion dose of $1.0 \text{ mU} \cdot \text{kg}^{-1} \cdot \text{min}^{-1}$. A 20% dextrose solution (D20) was infused as needed to keep plasma glucose at baseline levels of 100 mg/dl. (2) *Baseline insulin and glucose.* Both plasma glucose and insulin remained at fasting baseline levels (insulin levels of ~10 μU/ml and glucose levels of ~100 mg/dl) with accompanying saline infusion.

TABLE 1. Clinical and demographic characteristics (means and standard deviation)

	Normal		AD	
	With ε4	Without ε4	With ε4	Without ε4
n	9	17	19	12
Age (in years)	69.4 (7.7)	71.2 (6.7)	71.6 (9.5)	73.1 (8.0)
Body mass index (kg/m^2)	25.2 (5.7)	24.4 (2.5)	25.2 (2.9)	22.8 (1.8)
Dementia rating scale	141.2 (2.6)	137.1 (12.0)	109.7 (16.1)	113.3 (19.2)
Plasma glucose (mg/dl)				
With saline infusion	102.8 (8.8)	96.5 (8.6)	99.4 (12.2)	98.7 (10.9)
With insulin infusion	104.9 (7.2)	105.6 (6.0)	103.5 (7.6)	98.4 (5.4)
Plasma insulin (μU/ml)				
With saline infusion	8.5 (2.6)	7.6 (2.7)	9.4 (3.4)	10.6 (4.3)
With insulin infusion	80.3 (15.5)	83.4 (15.6)	83.8 (16.9)	72.6 (20.9)

Subjects rested with i.v. lines in place for a 30-min habituation period. Insulin and D20 infusions were then begun. Plasma glucose was measured at 5- to 10-min intervals using a glucose analyzer (Beckman Instruments, Fullerton, CA), and the D20 infusion rate was adjusted periodically to maintain euglycemia. After 90 min, a 30-min stabilization period occurred. Following this stabilization period, a 30-min cognitive protocol was administered, and blood samples were obtained through an in-dwelling catheter at 0, 15, and 30 min during the protocol to measure insulin, glucose, and APP. Insulin-mediated glucose disposal was calculated as the amount of D20 infused to maintain euglycemia during the 30-min cognitive protocol in the hyperinsulinemic condition (cc per 30 min), as described by Bergman *et al.*[7] Larger insulin-mediated glucose disposal values reflected greater insulin sensitivity (e.g., more D20 was required to maintain euglycemia during the insulin infusion), whereas smaller values reflected less insulin sensitivity.

Two comparable versions of a cognitive protocol were used, consisting of a story recall measure and a measure of selective attention. Subjects heard a narrative story containing 44 informational bits and were asked to recall as much as possible both immediately and after a 10-min delay period. Subjects received credit for each informational bit recalled verbatim or for accurate paraphrases. The selective attention task (Stroop Color-Word Interference test) had three conditions.[8] In the first two conditions, subjects were asked to read color words and to name colors. In the third condition, subjects were required to name the ink color of color names printed in discordant colors (e.g., the word "red" printed in the green ink). Thus, to respond correctly subjects were required to selectively attend to the color of the word and inhibit the prepotent reading response. Time to complete each condition and number of errors was recorded and summed across conditions.

APP Measurement and Quantification

As described by Martins and colleagues,[6,9] aprotinin (30 U/ml of plasma) was added to plasma samples, and APP was partially purified using a Heparin-Sepharose (HS) gel (50% slurry in 50 mM Tris-HCl, pH 7.4; 150 mM NaCl). Plasma (100 ml) was incubated with an equal volume of HS overnight at 4°C, buffered with 1.5 ml of isotonic Tris buffer. Plasma APP, a serine protease inhibitor, is stable overnight under these conditions.[6,9] The IIS gel was then washed three times in the same buffer and boiled in tricine sample buffer (containing 5% β-mercaptoethanol) to elute all bound protein. The samples were run on 8% Tris-tricine polyacrylamide gels, then electroblotted for 6 Amp hours onto nitrocellulose membrane. APP standard was included on each gel, to ensure between-gel reliability and for standard curve generation.[6,9] The membranes were blocked for 1 hour at room temperature, with 5% milk in Tris-buffered saline (TBS; 50 mM Tris-HCl, pH 8; 150 mM NaCl) then incubated for 2 hours at room temperature with 22C11 antibody, diluted 1000-fold in TBST (TBS with 0.05Tween 20). The membranes were then washed for three 10-min periods with TBST, then incubated for 2 min in chemiluminescent substrate before being exposed to ECL film. APP was quantitated by transmission-scanning the developed film (gray-scale 600 dpi) using a UMAX scanner and measuring the total density of APP with NIH Image v1.60 software. Linearity of densitometric data was ensured by comparison with 5 APP standards on each gel, ranging over one and a half orders of magnitude.[6,9] APP densitometry values were calculated twice for each subject in each condition. Intermeasurement reliability as estimated with Pearson product moment correlations were high for both the saline ($r = 0.74$, $p < 0.0001$) and insulin ($r = 0.83$, $p < 0.0001$) conditions.

Statistical Analysis

AD and normal subjects were divided into two ApoE groups: subjects with an ε4 allele and subjects without an ε4 allele. Insulin-mediated glucose disposal rates, cognitive scores, and plasma APP values were subjected to repeated measures—analysis of variance, with condition (insulin or saline) as a within-subjects factor and diagnosis and ApoE genotype as between-subjects factors.

RESULTS

Plasma insulin levels during insulin infusion were similar for AD and normal groups (AD mean ± standard error = 80.5 μU/ml ± 3.1; normal = 82.2 μU/ml ± 3.6). AD subjects without an ε4 allele had significantly lower insulin-mediated glucose disposal rates than AD patients with an ε4 allele [FIG. 1, $F(1,25) = 5.11$, $p < 0.03$], or than normal adults without an ε4 allele ($p < 0.02$). No effects for ApoE genotype were observed for normal adults. AD subjects without an ε4 allele also showed sig-

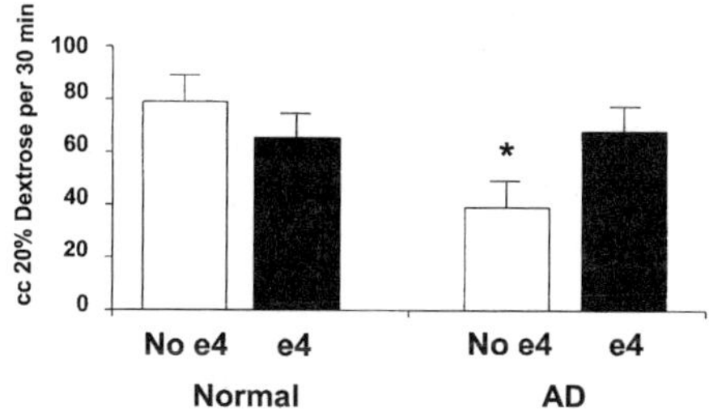

FIGURE 1. Mean insulin-mediated glucose disposal rates with standard errors for AD and normal subjects with and without an ApoE ε4 allele. AD patients without an ε4 allele had lower insulin-mediated glucose disposal rates than AD patients with an ε4 allele or than normal subjects without an ε4 allele ($p < 0.03$ and $p < 0.02$, respectively).

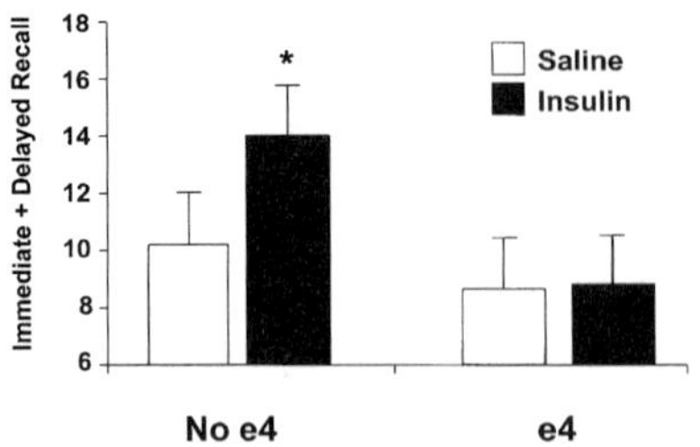
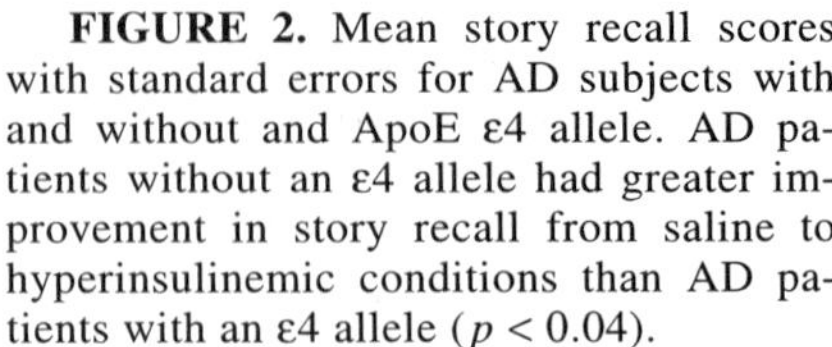

FIGURE 2. Mean story recall scores with standard errors for AD subjects with and without and ApoE ε4 allele. AD patients without an ε4 allele had greater improvement in story recall from saline to hyperinsulinemic conditions than AD patients with an ε4 allele ($p < 0.04$).

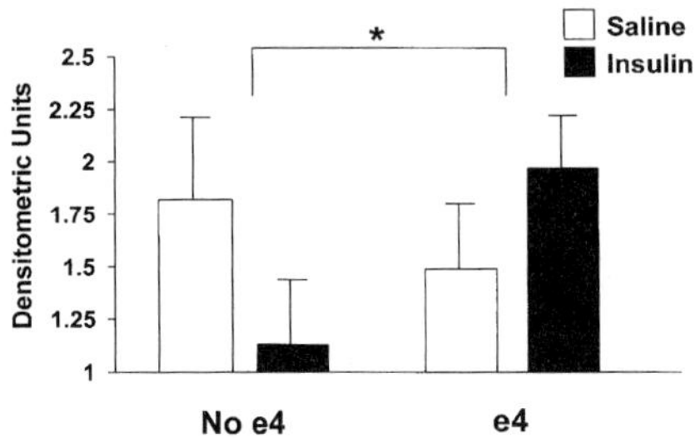

FIGURE 3. Mean plasma APP concentrations (optical densitometric units) with standard errors for AD patients with and without the ApoE ε4 allele during saline and insulin infusions. AD patients without an ε4 allele had reduced plasma APP concentrations, whereas AD patients with an ε4 allele had increased plasma APP concentrations during insulin infusions relative to saline infusions ($p < 0.05$).

nificant memory facilitation in the hyperinsulinemic condition [FIG. 2, $F(1,29) = 4.78, p < 0.04$], whereas the AD group with the ε4 allele did not. Normal adults' performance did not differ between the two conditions.

AD patients without an ε4 allele showed different effects of insulin on APP than did AD patients with an ε4 allele or than did normal adults, as reflected in a significant condition by diagnosis by ApoE interaction [$F (1,53) = 6.42, p < 0.02$]. As can be seen in FIGURE 3, insulin infusion reduced plasma APP levels for AD patients without an ε4 allele, but raised APP for patients with an ε4 allele [$F(1,29) = 4.40, p < 0.05$]. Two-thirds (8 of 12) AD subjects without an ε4 allele had lower APP in the insulin condition than in the saline condition. For AD subjects with an ε4 allele, 10 of 19 subjects had higher APP in the insulin condition; interestingly however, four of five ApoE-ε4 homozygotes had higher APP levels during insulin infusion than during saline infusion. Normal adults showed no significant change in plasma APP in response to insulin infusion (mean APP densitometric units ± standard error during saline and insulin infusions 1.27 ± 0.24 and 1.02 ± 0.23, respectively).

DISCUSSION

These results confirm that patients who are not apoE-ε4 homozygotes have insulin resistance as measured by a sensitive index of insulin-mediated glucose disposal. In addition, the finding that patients without an ε4 allele demonstrated significantly greater hyperinsulinemic memory facilitation and lowered APP levels than did other patients provides further *in vivo* evidence of differences in insulin metabolism between ε4 and non-ε4 disease. Links between insulin and ApoE have been established in studies of lipid metabolism. Insulin reduces ApoE mRNA translation and plays a role in the degradation of ApoE in hepatic cell lines.[10] Interestingly, one mechanism through which insulin affects degradation of ApoE is by increasing low-density lipoprotein receptor-related protein (LRP) promoted uptake of ApoE-enriched lipoprotein.[11] LRP has been strongly implicated in CNS ApoE metabolism and has been identified in dentate granule and pyramidal hippocampal neurons, as well as in senile plaques.[12] LRP also degrades the APP isoform that is present in both plasma and brain.[13] This action may have implications for the present findings that adults with AD without the ApoE-ε4 allele had reduced levels of plasma APP in response to intravenous insulin infusion, whereas APP levels were increased for other AD patients. These results suggest a role for insulin in systemic APP processing. Patients with AD without an ε4 allele have demonstrated insulin resistance in this and previous studies[4]; administering exogenous insulin may have overcome this resistance and effectively mobilized LRP-mediated APP degradation. A pattern of lowered APP in response to increased plasma glucose and insulin has been observed in normal adults at lower insulin levels than were achieved in this study.[6] The failure to observe this pattern for normal adults in this study is likely a dose effect, given that normal adults who are not insulin resistant show insulin effects on memory and metabolism at lower doses of insulin than do adults with AD.[4]

Insulin resistance may interfere with APP processing in adults without the ε4 allele, leading to chronic elevations in plasma APP such as have been identified in some forms of familial AD. The present results may also account for inconsistent reports of plasma APP elevations in adults with sporadic AD. Such findings may be expected to differ according to ApoE status of the AD and control groups. In the present sample, AD patients without an ε4 allele had greater APP levels than did normal adults without an ε4 allele, although this effect only approached statistical significance ($p < 0.10$).

For patients with AD with an ε4 allele, insulin did not lower plasma APP, and in fact raised APP levels. In particular, four of the five AD subjects who were ApoE-ε4 homozygotes had higher APP levels in the insulin condition than in the saline condition. Although the cause and significance of this finding is unclear at this time, it provides further support for ApoE-related differences in insulin metabolism in AD.

ACKNOWLEDGMENTS

This study was supported by the Department of Veterans Affairs, NIA AG-10880 (S.C.), AG-05136 (G.S.), and Alzheimer's Association IIRG-95-1151 (S.C). In Australia, support was provided by Sir James McCusker and the Department of Veterans Affairs (A.A.B., R.N.M). The authors would like to thank Cassin Lofgreen, R.N., Shawn Latendresse, Andreana Petrova, Karla Grimwood, M.S., Colby Wait, Lindel Cubberly, R.N., and Maria Gonzales for their excellent technical assistance.

REFERENCES

1. CRAFT, S., E. PESKIND, M.W. SCHWARTZ *et al.* 1998. Cerebrospinal fluid and plasma insulin levels in Alzheimer's disease: relationship to severity of dementia and apolipoprotein E genotype. Neurology **50:** 164–168.

2. MARFAING, P., L. PENICAUD, Y. BROER *et al.* 1990. Effects of hyperinsulinemia on local cerebral insulin binding and glucose utilization in normoglycemic awake rats. Neurosci. Lett. **115:** 279–285.
3. FROLICH, L., D. BLUM-DEGEN, H.G. BERNSTEIN *et al.* 1998. Brain insulin and insulin receptors in aging and sporadic Alzheimer's disease. J. Neural Trans. **105:** 423–438.
4. CRAFT, S., J. NEWCOMER, S. KANNE *et al.* 1996. Memory improvement following induced hyperinsulinemia in Alzheimer's disease. Neurobiol. Aging **17:** 123–130.
5. QIU, W.Q., D.M. WALSH, Z. YE *et al.* 1998. Insulin-degrading enzyme regulates extracellular levels of amyloid β-protein by degradation. J. Biol. Chem. **273:** 32730–32738.
6. BOYT, A.A., K. TADDEI, J. HALLMEYER *et al.* The effect of insulin and glucose on the plasma concentration of Alzheimer's amyloid precursor protein. Submitted manuscript.
7. BERGMAN, R.N., Y.Z. IDER, C.R. BOWDEN & C. COBELLI. 1979. Quantitative estimation of insulin sensitivity. Am. J. Physiol. **236:** E667–677.
8. PERRET, E. 1974. The left frontal lobe of man and the suppression of habitual responses in verbal categorical behavior. Neuropsychologia **12:** 323–330.
9. MARTINS, R.N., J. MUIR, W.S. BROOKS *et al.* 1993. Plasma amyloid precursor protein is decreased in Alzheimer's disease. Clin. Neurol. Neuropathol. **4:** 757–759.
10. OGBONNA, G., A. THERIAULT & K. ADELI. 1993. Hormonal regulation of human apolipoprotein E gene expression in HepG2 cells. Int. J. Biochem. **25:** 635–640.
11. DESCAMPS, O., D. BILHEIMER & J. HERZ. 1993. Insulin stimulates receptor-mediated uptake of ApoE-enriched lipoproteins and activated α_2-macroglobulin in adipocytes. J. Biol. Chem. **268:** 974–981.
12. REBECK, W.G., S.D. HARR, D.K. STRICKLAND & B.T. HYMAN. 1995. Multiple, diverse senile plaque-associated proteins are ligands of an apolipoprotein E receptor, the α_2-macroglobulin receptor/low-density-lipoprotein receptor-related protein. Ann. Neurol. **37:** 211–217.
13. KOUNNAS, M.Z., R.D. MOIR, G.W. REBECK *et al.* 1995. LDL receptor-related protein, a multifunctional ApoE receptor, binds secreted β-amyloid precursor protein and mediates its degradation. Cell **82:** 331–340.

Interface between Vascular Dementia and Alzheimer Syndrome

Nosologic Redefinition

V. OLGA EMERY,[a,b,d] EDWARD X. GILLIE,[b,c] AND JOSEPH A. SMITH[c]

[a]Department of Psychiatry, Dartmouth Medical School,
Lebanon, New Hampshire 03756, USA

[b]Department of Medicine, Beth Israel-Deaconess Hospitals, Harvard Medical School,
Boston, Massachusetts 02114, USA

[c]Veterans Affairs Medical Center, Manchester, New Hampshire 03104, USA

ABSTRACT: Vascular dementia is redefined so as to include noninfarct vascular dementia: vascular dementia caused by underlying vascular factors other than cerebral infarction. Data are presented that bring into focus the interface between vascular dementia and Alzheimer syndrome, and the ambiguous transition between multifocality and diffuse or generalized disease. By cross-cutting both stroke and nonstroke vascular groups, arteriosclerosis, abnormal blood pressure, abnormal electrocardiogram, and other vascular factors are implicated in the distal causality of both infarct and noninfarct vascular dementia.

INTRODUCTION

In this paper the construct of vascular dementia is reconceptualized and broadened to include what we term "noninfarct vascular dementia."[1-3] How vascular dementia is defined is critical for understanding clinicopathophysiological features of the syndrome. Definition, nomology, and nosology are crucial methodological components for understanding mechanisms underlying vascular dementia.[4] Further, valid clinical diagnosis and rationally based treatment are in large measure a function of the validity and reliability of medical constructs and their operationalization and classification.[5-8] An analysis of the nosologic history of vascular dementia during the 1900s uncovers a constant error of the misidentification of the overarching category of vascular dementia, first with one and then with some other of its subtypes. Overall, the classificatory history of vascular dementia indicates a failure to place the construct of vascular dementia in a superordinate hierarchical position, with a number of subtypes comprising the broader category. The results of our investigations of a broad spectrum of vascular disorders suggest that the term vascular dementia should not be regarded as coextensive nor be used interchangeably with any of its subtypes.

To be more specific, in analyzing the evolution of the construct of vascular dementia during the 20th century, one sees that during the mid-1900s the term vascular

[d]Address for correspondence: V.O. Emery, Ph.D., Dept. of Psychiatry, HB7750, Dartmouth Medical School, Lebanon, NH 03756. Tel.: (603) 774-4933; (603) 668-4079; fax: (603) 625-8199.

dementia was equated with arteriosclerotic psychosis or cerebral arteriosclerosis.[9,10] Following this, there has been an equation between vascular dementia and multiinfarct dementia for the past 25 years.[1,2,11–14] These two terms became virtually synonymous, and this equation between vascular dementia and multiinfarct dementia has been reflected in formal classification.[15–19] The DSM-III and DSM-III-R specifically and DSM-IV more generally and with less closure, have equated vascular dementia with multiinfarct dementia.[15–17] In contrast, ICD-10[18] placed vascular dementia in what we regard the correct superordinate position with a number of subtypes comprising the broader category. Conflictually, however, in its actual research criteria, the ICD-10 requires cerebral infarction for diagnosis of vascular dementia,[19] thus contradicting what potentially could and should have been a broader, hierarchical categorization of the vascular dementias.

We will suggest that the construct validity[2,4,20,21] of vascular dementia would have been better served had multiinfarct dementia been conceptualized as an additional subtype of vascular dementia rather than as a replacement for all previous subtypes. Our data point to the idea that multiinfarct dementia is only one subtype of vascular dementia, although possibly the most prevalent one, and that vascular dementia is broader than multiinfarct dementia.[1–3] Further, our data will suggest that the nosologic entity of vascular dementia must be extended beyond the infarct concept, because there appear to exist noninfarct vascular dementing conditions.[1–3] Vascular dementia is redefined to include a new category of vascular dementia, which we have termed noninfarct vascular dementia.[1–3,22] The nosologic construct of noninfarct vascular dementia would be useful for clinicians as well as researchers, because a diagnosis of vascular dementia would not, and in fact should not, be discounted in the absence of actual cerebral infarction. Our data, as well as the data from several other investigators,[23–26] point to some noninfarct factors that appear to be critical in the genesis of vascular dementia. There are pathophysiologic mechanisms underlying vascular dementia that are as yet unidentified.

Finally, this discussion will focus on the ambiguous transitions between the spectra of the vascular dementias and Alzheimer syndrome. We will suggest that a subtype of the overarching category of vascular dementia is "Alzheimerized vascular dementia," in which two pathogenic disease sequences intersect, overlap, and in some ways trigger one another. This interface between vascular dementia and generalized degenerative dementia represents a critical research area that must be studied to understand unknown characteristics of both syndromes.

Our ongoing investigation of the vascular dementias arose from frustration in attempting to diagnosis patients with long-standing histories of vascular disorders who were cognitively impaired but who met neither criteria for vascular dementia, i.e., patients without cerebral infarction, nor that for probable Alzheimer's disease (AD), e.g., patients with higher ischemia scores than criteria permit and/or gait or seizure disorder early in illness.[27–30] The investigation to be reported tests the following null hypotheses/hypotheses: (1) The cognitive impairment of infarct and noninfarct vascular patients is not/is significantly greater than and outside the range of normal aging, as indicated by performance on mental status and other cognitive measures; and (2) there are/are not significant differences between patients with cerebral infarction and noninfarct vascular patients on measures of mental status and other cognitive measures. When these hypotheses are plugged into a deductive paradigm, the data will provide information on the relation between the broader construct of vascular dementia and its subtypes. If the infarct and noninfarct vascular groups do not differ significantly from one another, then vascular dementia cannot validly be equated with just one of these groups while excluding the other subgroup from the possibility of being classified as vascular dementia.

METHOD

This report involves a total of 117 elderly participants: 81 vascular patients and 36 normal controls. The 81 vascular patients formed two vascular samples: cerebral infarction sample ($n = 43$) and noninfarct sample ($n = 38$). The cerebral infarct, noninfarct, and normal elderly samples had mean ages of 71.9, 77.1, and 70.2 years, respectively. Mean education of infarct, noninfarct, and normal elderly samples was 11.3, 11.8, and 11.9 years, respectively. Variables of race, native birth, native language, and occupation were also comparable across the three samples.

Vascular patients were recruited through the geriatric service of a Veterans Affairs Medical Center (VAMC). The vascular samples were comprised of 81 consecutive vascular patients meeting sample criteria. Excluded from vascular samples were patients with other dementing disorders and patients with major head trauma. The 81 vascular patients were being evaluated through the VAMC geriatric evaluation unit for medical problems of a noncognitive nature related to vascular disorders (e.g., hypertension, hypotension, high cholesterol, bradycardia, abnormal electrocardiogram (ECG), peripheral vascular disease, coronary disease). Screening procedures included medical examination, medical history, and physical, neurologic, psychiatric, and psychosocial assessments. All vascular patients had laboratory tests, chest radiography, ECG, and computed tomographic (CT) scanning of brain; some patients also underwent magnetic resonance imaging (MRI). CT scans were performed without contrast enhancement with 10-mm continuous slices using Phillips Tomo Scan 60. All scans were reexamined for this research by the same neuroradiologist without knowledge of clinical diagnosis. Morphologic changes analyzed included (a) focal/localized changes suggesting cerebral infarction, (b) white-matter changes/white matter low attenuation,[14,23–26] and absence or presence of cerebral atrophy. Gray-matter and white-matter changes were noted.

Vascular patients were selected for infarct and noninfarct samples on the basis of brain scan/imaging evidence for cerebral infarction (gray-matter or white-matter) and on the basis of clinical history. Patients in the infarct sample had to have both clinical and CT evidence of infarction. The following disorders were included in the category of cerebral infarction: (a) transient ischemic attacks (TIA), (b) reversible ischemic neurological deficit (RIND), and (c) prolonged neurologic deficit or completed stroke.[31,32]

Inclusion in the cerebral noninfarct sample required that vascular patients had a long-standing history (minimum of 5 years) of vascular disorders and that there existed neither clinical nor CT or MRI evidence of cerebral infarction of either gray-matter or white-matter. Of these patients without cerebral infarction, 97% had abnormal blood pressure, 84% had an abnormal ECG, 84% had arteriosclerosis, 79% had ischemic heart disease, 55% had myocardial infarction, 53% had peripheral vascular disease, 47% had chronic obstructive pulmonary disease, and 42% had diabetes mellitus (TABLE 1). Other conditions of these cerebral noninfarct patients included

TABLE 1. Vascular factors in vascular patients with cerebral infarction and without cerebral infarction

	Vascular Group	
Vascular Factor	With Cerebral Infarction ($n = 43$)	Without Cerebral Infarction ($n = 38$)
Cerebral infarction	100%	0%
Myocardial infarction	33%	55%
Heart block	28%	24%
Cardiomegaly	21%	24%
Ischemic heart disease	58%	79%
Arteriosclerosis	77%	84%
Abnormal electrocardiogram	72%	84%
Abnormal blood pressure	86%	97%
Hypertension[a]	86%	79%
Hypotension	0%	18%
Diabetes mellitus	37%	42%
Peripheral vascular disease	40%	53%
Chronic obstructive pulmonary disease	47%	47%

[a]Hypertension ($160\ \text{mmHg}^+/90\text{mmHg}^+$).

vascular collagen disease, aortic aneurysm, uncontrolled hypertension, atrial fibrillation, left ventricular hypertrophy, bradycardia, cardiomegaly, carotid stenosis, pacemaker complications, hypercholesterolemia, and calcified iliac heart vessels. All cerebral noninfarct subjects had Hachinski Ischemia Scale scores of 7 or higher, thereby not meeting exclusionary criteria for probable Alzheimer's disease.[27–30]

Mental status and cognitive function were screened and assessed with the Mini-Mental State Examination (MMSE)[33] and Dementia Rating Scale (DRS).[34] The suggested cut-off point between normal aging and organic brain syndromes on the MMSE is 23 out of a 30-point total.[33] The DRS, which was designed to provide a measure of cognitive status in persons with known dementing disorders, has a 144-point total, with a cut-off score of 123 for the boundary between normal aging and dementia.[34] The DRS assesses the five cognitive factors of attention, initiation, memory, conceptualization, and construction.[34]

Language processing was assessed by subtests from the Western Aphasia Battery[35] and Boston Naming Test.[36] Formal language variable assessed were repetition, naming, auditory verbal comprehension, grammatical-syntactic processing, and reading comprehension; more detailed descriptions of these language parameters are reported elsewhere.[21,35–37]

RESULTS

Results are organized to address the research null hypotheses/hypotheses: (1) the cognitive impairment of cerebral infarct and noninfarct vascular patients is not/is significantly greater than and outside the range of normal aging; and (2) there are/

TABLE 2. Comparisons of means by sample on measures of mental status and language processing

Measure (Maximal Score)	Infarct (1) $n = 43$		Noninfarct (2) $n = 38$		Normal (3) $n = 36$		Group Comparisons[a]
	M	SD	M	SD	M	SD	
Mini-Mental State Exam (30)	22.38	4.14	21.95	5.33	29.37	1.39	1,2<3
Dementia Rating Scale (144)	112.39	25.54	115.36	22.12	141.75	3.92	1,2<3
Boston Naming Test (15)	12.46	2.39	12.41	2.08	14.97	0.12	1,2<3
WAB Repetition (100)	87.67	11.86	89.12	11.44	95.92	7.56	1,2<3
WAB Sentence Completion (10)	9.68	1.12	9.79	0.63	9.90	0.47	
WAB Responsive Speech (10)	9.84	0.62	9.89	0.44	10.00	0.00	
WAB Word Fluency (20)	9.69	5.50	10.01	5.71	17.71	3.68	1,2<3
WAB Yes/No Questions (60)	59.70	0.86	59.35	1.89	60.00	0.00	
WAB Sequential Commands (80)	66.24	19.87	65.46	22.62	79.55	1.88	1,2<3
WAB Reading Comprehension (40)	30.39	11.14	34.08	7.48	38.17	3.72	1,2<3

[a]Results of *t*-test comparisons. Degrees of freedom for the respective comparisons are: 79 (1 vs. 2), 77 (1 vs. 3), and 72 (2 vs. 3). Differences are significant at $p \leq .005$.

are not significant differences between patients with cerebral infarction and non-infarct vascular patients on measures of mental status and other cognitive measures.

Analyzing first research results relating to mental status, comparisons between the 43 patients with cerebral infarcts and 36 normal elderly on both the Mini-Mental State Exam and Dementia Rating Scale are all significant at the 0.0001 level (TABLES 2 and 3). Similarly, comparisons between the 38 noninfarct patients and 36 normal elderly also are all significant at the 0.0001 level (TABLES 2 and 3). Comparisons between both vascular samples and normals on Dementia Rating Scale factors of attention, memory, initiation, conceptualization, construction were all significant at the 0.0001 level. Thus, the data indicate that a broad spectrum of vascular disorders result in significantly impaired mental status when contrasted with deficits of normal aging.

Looking next at language measures, both the infarct and noninfarct samples were significantly impaired at the 0.0001 level when contrasted to normal elderly on the Boston Naming Test (TABLES 2 and 3). Turning now to the seven subtests of the Western Aphasia Battery,[35] both vascular samples had deficits at the 0.0001 level when compared to normal elderly on the word fluency task, which is a meta-naming[38] task assessing capability for generative naming (e.g., "name as many foods as you can"). The infarct sample was also impaired at the 0.0001 level when compared to normal elderly on reading comprehension and sequential commands tasks, whereas the noninfarct sample was impaired in relation to normals on these tasks at the 0.004 and 0.0004 levels (TABLE 3). Comparisons between the two vascular samples and normals on repetition and auditory comprehension were also statistically significant (TABLE 3). Of the eight language assessments made, only two were not statistically significant (TABLE 3). There were no significant differences on responsive speech and sentence completion tasks, which are the simplest of language tasks

TABLE 3. Difference of means on measures of mental status and language processing

Measure	Infarct vs. Noninfarct		Infarct vs. Normal		Noninfarct vs. Normal	
	t-Value	P	t-Value	P	t-Value	P
Mini-Mental State Exam	0.41	0.68	−9.68	0.0001	−8.09	0.0001
Dementia Rating Scale	−0.56	0.58	−6.82	0.0001	−7.05	0.0001
Boston Naming Test	0.10	0.92	−6.29	0.0001	−7.37	0.0001
WAB Repetition	−0.56	0.58	−3.60	0.0006	−3.00	0.004
WAB Sentence Completion	−0.54	0.59	−1.10	0.28	−0.85	0.40
WAB Responsive Speech	−0.41	0.68	−1.55	0.13	−1.50	0.14
WAB Word Fluency	−0.26	0.80	−7.50	0.0001	−6.85	0.0001
WAB Yes/No Questions	1.09	0.28	−2.09	0.04	−2.06	0.04
WAB Sequential Commands	0.17	0.87	−4.00	0.0001	−3.72	0.0004
WAB Reading Comprehension	−1.73	0.09	−4.00	0.0001	−2.95	0.004

NOTE: Degrees of freedom for the respective comparisons are: infarct vs. noninfarct (79); infarct vs. normal (77); noninfarct vs. normal (72).

involving overlearned language sequences (e.g., "roses are red, violets are what?").[8,37–39]

In sum, the data suggest that patients with a broad spectrum of vascular disorders have significant disadvantage in relation to demographically comparable normal elderly on assessments of mental status, language processing and other cognitive parameters.

Finally, looking at comparisons between infarct and noninfarct groups, there are no significant differences between these two groups of vascular patients on any of the mental status measures nor on any of the language assessments (TABLES 2 and 3).

This report has described the meta-analytic or combined results from smaller, independent studies[1–3,40] of our ongoing investigation of cognitive deficits in vascular dementia.

CONCLUSIONS

In comparing two groups of vascular patients (infarct and noninfarct) with demographically comparable normal elderly, the vascular patients performed significantly worse on all measures of mental status as well as on all measures of language assessment except two. Thus, in addressing the first research question of how patients with a spectrum of vascular disorders compare with normal controls, we conclude that vascular disorders involve decrements in higher cortical processing that are reliably greater and outside the range of normal aging. This is not to say, however, that all patients with vascular disorders have vascular dementia. Elsewhere the relevance of the continuum concept for medical diagnostics has been pointed out.[1,21,41] The cognitive impairments of vascular disorders can be conceptualized as a continuum, with minimal cognitive impairment on one end and vascular dementia on the other end.

If one adds a diachronic dimension, then the possibility of progression from the mild to the severe end of this cognitive-impairment continuum comes into focus.

Turning now to the second research question relating to comparisons between the cerebral infarct and noninfarct patients, the data show there are no significant differences between these two groups of vascular patients on any of the mental status, language, and other cognitive assessments. How then can one explain the overall similarity in cognitive deficits between stroke patients and vascular patients with no stroke? This question requires further work and also a new perspective on vascular dementia. We have introduced the concept of noninfarct vascular dementia: vascular dementia caused by underlying vascular factors other than cerebral infarction. The introduction of noninfarct vascular dementia as a nosologic entity presents a changed paradigm from which to work. However, some tentative directions follow from the data presented. The data suggest that the distinction of focal versus diffuse or generalized cerebral dysfunction has less explanatory significance for understanding cognitive impairment in vascular disorders than do some shared factors of vascular abnormality. Vascular abnormalities cross-cutting both the cerebral infarct and noninfarct groups include abnormal blood pressure, abnormal ECG, arteriosclerosis, ischemic heart disease, peripheral vascular disease, chronic obstructive pulmonary disease, and other pathogenic vascular factors (TABLE 1). The pathogenetic mechanisms underlying these disorders that cross-cut both vascular groups have yet to be defined. Although vascular dementia has by convention been associated with focality, focal lesions are in reality not purely localized. Focal lesions, such as stroke, may precipitate a diffuse encephalopathy or dementia in the aging brain.[42] The distinction between focal and generalized or diffuse disease is in reality not clear-cut. Focal lesions may disrupt functions of other areas of the brain through a number of mechanisms, including edema, disruption of cortical connections, and diaschisis (i.e., reduced metabolic activity of distant but synaptically connected areas of the brain).[23–26,42,43] Further, multiinfarct dementia, the definitional and nosologic prototype of focal vascular disorder is, in reality, a multifocal (i.e., multiple infarction equals multiple focality) disorder. Where is the line drawn between multifocality and diffuse or generalized disease? These issues are at the core of questions pertaining to the lack of cognitive processing differences between stroke and nonstroke vascular patients. These issues are also at the core of questions pertaining to the interface between vascular dementia and Alzheimer syndrome.

During the 1950s and 1960s it was believed that the cognitive decrements of vascular disorders were caused by arteriosclerosis.[9,10] This line of explanation was abandoned when vascular dementia became equated with multiinfarct dementia.[12–19] We submit it was an error to completely throw out the arteriosclerotic explanation in favor of the concept of multiinfarct dementia. We propose that multiple infarction be considered only one proximal cause of vascular dementia, while the arteriosclerotic process be considered a major vascular variable in the distal causality of what appears to be a substantial percentage of cases of vascular dementia. By cross-cutting both stroke and nonstroke groups, arteriosclerosis is implicated in the causal chain of vascular events related to cognitive decline in both vascular populations. This same reasoning should be applied to abnormalities of blood pressure. Our data, as well as the data of others,[24,25] indicate that hypertension and/or hypotension are distal factors in the vascular chain of events leading to many cases of cognitive impairment in vascular patients.

Vascular dementia has the characteristics of a syndrome and appears to be caused by a number of vascular disorders with a number of underlying mechanisms. Thus, to equate vascular dementia with any single subtype would appear to be invalid. Accordingly, the classification of vascular dementia should not be delimited by the infarct concept. There should be a formal provision for the classification of noninfarct vascular dementias. Vascular dementia is a broad overarching category comprised of a number of subtypes.

Finally, looking again at the interface between vascular dementia and Alzheimer syndrome, the ambiguous transition between these two syndromes parallels the ambiguous transitions between multifocality and diffuse or generalized disease. Further, the discussion related to arteriosclerosis in the distal causality of vascular dementia is of interest here. Atherosclerosis, a subtype of the broader category of arteriosclerosis,[32] is basically an inflammatory disease, which can lead to ischemia of the brain, heart, or extremities.[25] The underlying mechanisms of atherosclerosis are fundamentally no different than those in other inflammatory syndromes.[25,44–48] The role of inflammation in Alzheimer syndrome has recently been brought into focus.[49–51] Thus, the common function of inflammation is relevant for future research at the interface between vascular dementia and Alzheimer syndrome. Similarly, future research should investigate the amyloid interface between vascular dementia and Alzheimer syndrome. Specifically, the role of cystatin C amyloid appears to play a prominent role at the interface between these two syndromes[24,41,52] and needs to be investigated further.

To conclude, we have examined the ambiguous relationships between vascular disorders and normal aging, infarct and noninfarct vascular patients, and patients at the interface of vascular dementia and Alzheimer syndrome, i.e., "Alzheimerized vascular dementia" and have made some nosologic suggestions, developed some heuristic paradigms, and have pointed toward some future research directions.

REFERENCES

1. EMERY, V.O.B., E.X. GILLIE & P. RAMDEV. 1994. Vascular dementia redefined. *In* Dementia: Presentation, Differential Diagnosis, and Nosology. V.O.B. Emery & T.E. Oxman, Eds.: 162–194. Johns Hopkins University Press. Baltimore, MD.
2. EMERY, V.O.B., E.X. GILLIE & J.A. SMITH. 1996. Reclassification of the vascular dementias: comparisons of infarct and noninfarct vascular dementias. Int. Psychogeriatr. **8:** 33–61.
3. EMERY, V.O.B., E.X. GILLIE & J.A. SMITH. 1999. Vascular dementia of the noninfarct subtype. Psychosomatics **40:** 141–142.
4. NIEDEREHE, G. & T.E. OXMAN. 1994. The dementias: construct and nosologic validity. *In* Dementia: Presentations, Differential Diagnosis, and Nosology. V.O.B. Emery & T.E. Oxman, Eds.: 19–45. Johns Hopkins University Press. Baltimore, MD.
5. DRACHMAN, D.A. & K.L. NEWELL. 1999. A 67-year-old man with three years of dementia. N. Engl. J. Med. **340:** 1269–1277.
6. SACHDEV, P.S., H. BRODATY & J.C. LOOI. 1999. Vascular dementia: diagnosis, management and possible prevention. Med. J. Aust. **170:** 81–85.
7. WRIGHT, R.A. & E. KOKMEN. 1999. Gradually progressive dementia without discrete cerebrovascular events in a patient with Sneddon's syndrome. Mayo Clin. Proc. **74:** 57–61.
8. EMERY, V.O.B. 1988. Pseudodementia: a theoretical and empirical discussion. Western Reserve Geriatric Education Center Monograph Series, Case Western Reserve University School of Medicine. Cleveland, OH.

9. MAYER-GROSS, W., E. SLATER & M. ROTH. 1960. Clinical Psychiatry. Bailliere, Tindall & Cassell. London.
10. SLATER, E. & M. ROTH. 1969. Clinical Psychiatry. Bailliere, Tindall & Cassell. London.
11. HACHINSKI, V.C., N.A. LASSEN & J. MARSHALL. 1974. Multi-infarct dementia: a cause of mental deterioration in the elderly. Lancet **2:** 207–210.
12. HACHINSKI, V.C., L. ILIFF, M. PHIL, E. ZILHKA, G.H. DUBOULAY *et al.* 1975. Cerebral blood flow in dementia. Arch. Neurol. **32:** 632–637.
13. ROMAN, G.C., T.K. TATEMICHI, T. ERKINJUNTTI, J.L. CUMMINGS, J. MASDEU *et al.* 1993. Vascular dementia: diagnostic criteria for research studies. Report of the NINDS-AIREN International Workshop. Neurology **43:** 250–260.
14. ERKINJUNTTI, T. 1997. Vascular dementia: challenge of clinical diagnosis. Int. Psychogeriatr. **9:** 51–58.
15. American Psychiatric Association. 1980. Diagnostic and Statistical Manual of Mental Disorders. 3rd edit. Author. Washington, DC.
16. American Psychiatric Association. 1987. Diagnostic and Statistical Manual of Mental Disorders. 3rd edit. rev. Author. Washington, DC.
17. American Psychiatric Association. 1994. Diagnostic and Statistical Manual of Mental Disorders. 4th edit. Author. Washington, DC.
18. World Health Organization. 1992. The ICD-10 Classification of Mental and Behavioral Disorders: Clinical Descriptions and Diagnostic Guidelines. Author. Geneva, Switzerland.
19. World Health Organization. 1993. The ICD-10 Classification of Mental and Behavioral Disorders: Diagnostic Criteria for Research. Author. Geneva, Switzerland.
20. CAMPBELL, S. & J.C. STANLEY. 1969. Experimental and Quasi-Experimental Designs for Research. Rand McNally. Chicago, IL.
21. EMERY, V.O.B. 2000. Language impairment in dementia of the Alzheimer type: a hierarchical declinc? Int. J. Psychiatr. Med. **29.** In press.
22. EMERY, V.O.B., E.X. GILLIE & P.T. RAMDEV. 1996. Noninfarct vascular dementia: a new subtype. J. Clin. Geropsychol. **2:** 197–213.
23. ERKINJUNTTI, T., V.C. HACHINSKI & R. SULKAVA. 1994. Alzheimer disease and vascular dementia. *In* Dementia: Presentations, Differential Diagnosis, and Nosology. V.O.B. Emery & T.E. Oxman, Eds.: 208–231. Johns Hopkins University Press. Baltimore, MD.
24. KOBAYASHI, S. 1994. The relation of hypertension to vascular dementia. *In* Dementia: Presentations, Differential Diagnosis, and Nosology. V.O.B. Emery & T.E. Oxman, Eds.: 195–207. Johns Hopkins University Press. Baltimore, MD.
25. ROSS, R. 1999. Mechanisms of disease: atherosclerosis—an inflammatory disease. N. Engl. J. Med. **340:** 115–126.
26. WALLIN, A., K. BLENNOW, P. FREDMAN, C.G. GOTTFRIES, I. KARLSSON & L. SVENNERHOLM. 1990. Blood brain barrier function in vascular dementia. Acta Neurol. Scand. **81:** 318–322.
27. MCKHANN, G., D. DRACHMAN, M. FOLSTEIN, R. KATZMAN, D. PRICE *et al.* 1984. Clinical diagnosis of Alzheimer's disease. Report of the NINCDS-ADRDA Work Group under auspices of Department of Health and Human Services Task Force on Alzheimer's disease. Neurology **34:** 939–944.
28. REISBERG, B., A. BURNS, H. BRODATY, R. EASTWOOD, M. ROSSOR, N. SARTORIUS & B. WINBLAD. 1997. Diagnosis of Alzheimer's disease: report of an International Psychogeriatric Association Special Meeting Work Group under cosponsorship of Alzheimer's Disease International, European Federation of Neurological Societies, World Health Organization, and World Psychiatric Association. Int. Psychogeriatr. **9:** 11–38.
29. HACHINSKI, V.C. 1983. Differential diagnosis of Alzheimer's dementia: multi-infarct dementia. *In* Alzheimer's Disease. B. Reisberg, Ed.: 188–192. The Free Press. New York.
30. WADE, J.P.H. & V.C. HACHINSKI. 1987. Multi-infarct dementia. *In* Dementia. B. Pitt, Ed. Churchill Livingstone. London.
31. National Institute of Neurological and Communicative Disorders and Stroke. 1975. A classification and outline of cerebrovascular disease II. Stroke **6:** 564–616.

32. STEDMAN, T.L. 1990. Stedman's Medical Dictionary. Williams & Wilkins. Baltimore, MD.
33. FOLSTEIN, M.F., S.E. FOLSTEIN & P.R. MCHUGH. 1975. "Mini-Mental State": a practical method for grading the mental state of patients for the clinician. J. Psychiatr. Res. **12:** 189–198.
34. MATTIS, S. 1988. Dementia Rating Scale Professional Manual. Psychological Assessment Resources. Odessa, FL.
35. KERTESZ, A. 1982. Western Aphasia Battery. Grune & Stratton. New York.
36. KAPLAN, E., H. GOODGLASS & S. WEINTRAUB. 1983. Boston Naming Test. Lea & Febinger. Philadelphia, PA.
37. EMERY, V.0.B. 1985. Language and Aging. Exp. Aging Res. Monogr. 11(1).
38. EMERY, V.0.B. & L.D. BRESLAU. 1988. The problem of naming in SDAT: a relative deficit. Exp. Aging Res. **14:** 181–193.
39. EMERY, V.O.B. 1999. On the relationship between memory and language in the dementia spectrum of depression, Alzheimer syndrome, and normal aging. *In* Language and Communication in Old Age: Multidisciplinary Perspectives. H. Hamilton, Ed. Vol. 9: 25–62. Garland Publishing. New York.
40. EMERY, V.O.B., E.X. GILLIE & P.T. RAMDEV. 1995. Noninfarct vascular dementia. *In* Treating Alzheimer's and Other Dementias. M. Bergener & S. Finkel, Eds.: 184–203. Springer Publishing Co. New York.
41. EMERY, V.O.B. & T.E. OXMAN. 1994. The spectra of dementia. *In* Dementia: Presentations, Differential Diagnosis, and Nosology. V.O.B. Emery & T.E. Oxman, Eds.: 384–407. Johns Hopkins University Press. Baltimore, MD.
42. KIRSHNER, H.S. 1994. Progressive aphasia and other focal presentations of Alzheimer disease, Pick disease, and other degenerative disorders. *In* Dementia: Presentations, Differential Diagnosis, and Nosology. V.O.B. Emery & T.E. Oxman, Eds.: 108–122. Johns Hopkins University Press. Baltimore, MD.
43. LURIA, A. 1980. Higher Cortical Functions in Man. Basic Books. New York.
44. ROSS, R. 1993. The pathogenesis of atherosclerosis: a perspective for the 1990s. Nature **362:** 801–809.
45. ROSS. R. 1993. Atherosclerosis: a defense mechanism gone awry. Am. J. Pathol. **143:** 987–1002.
46. TORMEY, V.J., J. FAUL, C. LEONARD, C.M. BURKE, A. DILMEC & L.W. POULTER. 1997. T-cell cytokines may control the balance of functionally distinct macrophage populations. Immunology **90:** 463–469.
47. LUKACS, N.W. & P.A. WARD. 1996. Inflammatory mediators, cytokines, and adhesion molecules in pulmonary inflammation and injury. Adv. Immunol. **62:** 257–304.
48. JOHNSON, R.J. 1997. What mediates progressive glomerulosclerosis? The glomerular endothelium comes of age. Am. J. Pathol. **151:** 1179–1181.
49. ROGERS, J. 1997. Anti-inflammatory approaches to the treatment of Alzheimer's disease. *In* Postgraduate Dementia Course: Heterogeneity of Alzheimer's Disease. Excerpta Medica Medical Communications B.V., Ed.: 32–33. Excerpta Medica. Amsterdam.
50. ROGERS, J., J. LUBER-NAROD, S.D. STYREN & W.H. CIVIN. 1988. Expression of immune-system-associated antigens by cells of the human central nervous system: relationship to the pathology of Alzheimer's disease. Neurobiol. Aging **9:** 339–349.
51. RICH, J.B., D.X. RASMUSSON, M.F. FOLSTEIN *et al.* 1995. Nonsteroidal anti-inflammatory drugs in Alzheimer's disease. Neurology **45:** 51–55.
52. FUJIHARA, S., K. SHIMODE, M. NAKAMURA, S. KOBAYASHI & T. TSUNEMATSU. 1989. Cerebral amyloid angiopathy with the deposition of cystatine C (gammatrace) and B-protein. *In* Alzheimer's Disease and Related Disorders. K. Iqbal, H.M. Wisniewski & B. Winblad, Eds. Vol. 317: 189–205. Alan R. Liss. New York.

Which Vascular Lesions Are of Importance in Vascular Dementia?

MARGARET M. ESIRI[a]

Departments of Clinical Neurology, University of Oxford, and Neuropathology, Radcliffe Infirmary NHS Trust, Oxford, United Kingdom

ABSTRACT: Most necropsy surveys of dementia have found that vascular disease is second only to Alzheimer's disease as a cause of dementia. Alzheimer's disease and cerebrovascular disease also often coexist. The purpose of the present study was to determine the nature of the cerebrovascular lesions that are most significant in producing dementia. These were analyzed in a group of cases of dementia in which only vascular pathology was present and, in particular, no more than trivial amounts of Alzheimer-type pathology were present. The cerebrovascular lesions in this group of cases were compared with those in a group of stroke cases who were nondemented and a group of elderly cases without stroke or dementia. Severe cribriform change and deep white/grey matter microinfarcts were significantly more common in the test group than in either of the control groups, whereas single macroscopic infarcts were more common in the stroke control group than either of the other two groups. Thus, microvascular deep white and grey matter lesions, but not macroscopic infarction, were significant in vascular dementia. The results of this study will be discussed in relation to the view that microvascular lesions may also contribute to dementia in subjects with more extensive Alzheimer-type pathology and thus lower the threshold at which Alzheimer-type pathology becomes clinically manifest.

Large epidemiological surveys show an exponential rise in the prevalence of dementia with age.[1] This rise, coupled with the increased numbers of people surviving into old age and the even larger numbers projected to survive in the next century, accounts for the enormous rise in the number of people suffering from dementia, amounting to a true epidemic, and the urgent concern to find ways to prevent it.

Over the last 30 years or so we have come to recognize Alzheimer's disease (AD) as the leading cause of dementia.[2,3] Vascular causes come second, however, accounting for perhaps one-fifth as many cases as AD.[4] However, the situation is not quite as simple as this breakdown sounds because often these two types of pathology occur together to varying extents, and it can then be difficult to say which type of pathology has played the major part in causing dementia in a particular case. Quite often it is thought to be both.

[a]Address for correspondence: Dr. Margaret M. Esiri, Neuropathology Department, Radcliffe Infirmary, Oxford OX2 6HE, UK. Tel.: 01865 224403; fax: 01865 224508.
e-mail: margaret.esiri@clinical-neurology.ox.ac.uk

We now have a fair idea of how AD-type pathology develops, probably over decades, from occasional diffuse amyloid plaques scattered in neocortex and a few neurofibrillary tangles localized to transentorhinal cortex[5] to widespread amyloid and neurofibrillary pathology; however, we still lack large prospective, community-based surveys of the extent of such pathology at different ages. There is general agreement that clinical dementia appears when these changes attain a threshold level and the severity of the cognitive deficit is largely determined by the extent of neurofibrillary pathology.[6]

In comparison to this reasonable understanding of AD-type pathology in relation to dementia, we know much less about how cerebrovascular pathology relates to dementia. The lesions involved are hypoxic/ischemic and are of two main types: lobar infarcts and subcortical lesions consisting of small infarcts or lacunae[4] in white and deep grey matter and other subcortical damage, falling short of frank infarction but producing loss of myelin and some rarefaction of axons—a type of pathology referred to in severe form as Binswanger's disease.[7]

To try to determine which of these two types of cerebrovascular disease is the more important one in causing dementia, we recently studied some of our archival material.[9] To avoid having to consider the contribution that AD-type pathology might be making, we excluded from the study cases with any more than trivial amounts of AD pathology and compared three groups of cases:

1. Demented subjects with only vascular disease to account for the dementia.

2. Subjects with vascular disease but no dementia. Clinically these were mostly subjects with strokes, but a few had not been recognized as having any neurological disease in life.

3. Subjects with neither dementia nor cerebrovascular disease nor any other neurological disease at autopsy.

There were 18 subjects in the nondemented control group, 19 in the nondemented group with cerebrovascular disease, and 24 in the vascular dementia group. Because full autopsies were performed, we had information on myocardial pathology which revealed myocardial infarction more frequently in the stroke group than in the controls (58% versus 18%, $p = 0.019$). The vascular dementia group showed myocardial infarction in 40% of subjects, but this was not significantly different from controls. No significant differences were found in the proportion of cases with left ventricular hypertrophy, which was found in 41% of nondemented controls, 32% in stroke cases, and 40% of vascular dementia cases.

We had only one cerebral hemisphere fixed from some of these cases so estimation of the extent of macroscopic infarction in the brain was incomplete; in every case, however, we estimated the proportion of at least one cerebral hemisphere that was infarcted by using a point counting technique on 1-cm coronal slices. We also semi-quantitatively estimated the extent of atheroma in the circle of Willis vessels and the extent of small vessel subcortical disease and microinfarction.

The age of the vascular dementia group was slightly lower than the two control groups and significantly lower than the stroke group. Brain weights did not differ between the groups, although weights were lower in the vascular dementia group. Circle of Willis atheroma was modestly but significantly greater ($p = 0.029$) in the stroke group compared with the nondemented controls, with a nonsignificant trend in the same direction for the vascular dementia group.

The control nondemented group had, by definition, no cerebrovascular disease. Comparing the ratios of infarcted/uninfarcted brain tissue in the nondemented and demented vascular disease groups, we found a nonsignificantly higher ratio in the demented than in the nondemented group (2.48 versus 1.93). Single infarcts were significantly more common in the stroke group than in the group with vascular dementia ($p = 0.014$), and absence of any macroscopic infarction was significantly more common in the vascular dementia group than the stroke group ($p = 0.034$).

The most significant differences between the nondemented and demented vascular disease groups were seen when microvascular disease scores were compared. Any cribriform change differed only slightly between the two groups, being present in 63% of the nondemented and 92% of the demented groups, but *severe* cribriform change was much more common in the demented group (71% versus 3%) ($p = 0.0006$). Microinfarction was also significantly more common in the demented vascular group (63% versus 26%) ($p = 0.031$). Congophilic angiopathy was more common in the demented than in the stroke/vascular disease group (33% versus 21%, a nonsignificant difference), but significantly more common for the vascular dementia compared with the nondemented/no vascular disease group ($p = 0.0067$).

Thus, although this study probably cannot rule out a role for major infarction in dementia because study of this aspect was incomplete, one can say that, in this group of cases at least, microvascular brain damage clearly distinguished cases of vascular dementia from cases of cerebrovascular disease that were not demented, suggesting that we need to improve our understanding of how subcortical white and deep grey matter vascular disease contributes to dementia if we want to prevent vascular dementia. Although the most prominent damage in white matter is to myelin, there is some associated axon damage as has been demonstrated in studies that have used immunocytochemistry for APP as a marker of such damage.[10] Although the axon damage and loss are not easy to quantify, it may well be important—recent experience in another demyelinating disorder, multiple sclerosis, indicates that although the most prominent pathological feature is loss of myelin, it is the secondary axonal degeneration associated with this that determines functional deficit.[11] Whether or not this turns out to be the case in vascular dementia, the main mechanism by which this type of vascular disease contributes to dementia seems to be by interrupting functional connections between one part of the cortex and another, between cortex and subcortical nuclei and subcortical nuclei and cortex. Consistent with this suggestion, the cognitive deficits associated with vascular dementia tend to be those related to impaired attention and concentration and delayed motor responses with memory relatively little affected early on. This is in contrast to AD in which memory is affected severely and early, and motor reactions and attention are better preserved.[12]

As well as contributing in a major way to vascular dementia in the absence of AD, subcortical small vessel disease also contributes to dementia by making clinically manifest mild degrees of AD pathology which would not, on their own, be symptomatic. This was made known in a study published in the United States in 1997—the Nun Study.[13] In this study, 61 of 102 elderly nuns were found to have sufficient plaques at autopsy to satisfy Khachaturian criteria for diagnosing AD. Clinical testing of their cognitive status during life showed that the prevalence of dementia in these cases was crucially dependent on how much subcortical small vessel associated vascular disease they had. In the presence of lacunar infarcts, 93% exhibited dementia, whereas in the absence of the infarcts only 57% were demented. Lobar infarcts did not significantly relate to dementia although there was a trend for dementia to be expressed more frequently in their presence. In the presence of lacunae, fewer AD lesions resulted in dementia than in those without lacunae.

In a study of OPTIMA subjects—subjects enrolled in a longitudinal prospective study of dementia in Oxford, published at about the same time as the Nun Study—Nagy[14] showed somewhat similar findings. When the severity of neocortical pathology in frontal, temporal and parietal lobes was compared between subjects with AD alone and those with AD plus vascular disease, it was found that for an equivalent cognitive deficit those with vascular disease had significantly fewer neurofibrillary tangles than those with AD alone. In addition, whereas in AD alone the main determinant of cognitive deficit was the density of neurofibrillary tangles, in the presence of vascular disease it was the amount of amyloid laid down as plaques. These studies suggest that subcortical vascular disease can lower the threshold of AD pathology at which dementia is manifest and can unmask a cognition-impairing effect of amyloid deposits that is scarcely detectable in AD alone. The mechanism by which AD and vascular disease interact seems to be one of simple summation. No evidence exists that the underlying course of AD progression is altered in the presence of vascular disease. On the other hand, there is a potential mechanism by which AD pathology may contribute to cerebrovascular disease and that is the deposition of β-amyloid in the walls of small leptomeningeal arteries and cortical arterioles. However, the contribution of such vascular deposits of β-amyloid to the overall cognitive deficit has not yet been clearly determined.

Finally, a remarkable number of risk factors are apparently shared between AD and vascular dementia of which increasing age is perhaps the most prominent; ApoE4 genotype,[15–18] hypertension,[18] and atherosclerosis[19,20] are others. Although we must take into consideration the capacity of cerebrovascular disease to lower the threshold at which AD-type pathology is clinically manifest as dementia, this effect seems unlikely to account entirely for this commonality of risk factors. To my mind it raises the possibility that AD and cerebrovascular disease have common etiological factors which, if they could be counteracted, might open the way to the prevention of both.

REFERENCES

1. JORM, A.F. & D. JOLLEY. 1998. The incidence of dementia: a meta-analysis. Neurology **51:** 728–33.
2. TOMLINSON, B.E. *et al.* 1970. Observations on the brains of demented old people. J. Neurol. Sci. **11:** 205–42.
3. MORRIS, J.H. 1997. Alzheimer's disease. *In* The Neuropathology of Dementia. M.M. Esiri & J.H. Morris, Eds.: 70–121. Cambridge University Press. Cambridge, UK.
4. MORRIS, J.H. 1997. Vascular dementia. *In* The Neuropathology of Dementia. M.M. Esiri & J.H. Morris, Eds.: 137–171. Cambridge University Press. Cambridge, UK.
5. BRAAK, H. & E. BRAAK. 1991. Neuropathological staging of Alzheimer-related changes. Acta Neuropathol. **82:** 239–259.
6. NAGY, ZS. *et al.* 1995. Relative roles of plaques and tangles in the dementia of Alzheimer's disease. Dementia **6:** 21–31.
7. FISHER, C.M. 1989. Binswanger's encephalopathy: a review. J. Neurol. **236:** 65–79.
8. VAN GIJN, J. 1998. Leukoaraiosis and vascular dementia. Neurology **51**(Suppl. 3): 3–58.

9. Esiri, M.M. *et al.* 1997. Neuropathological assessment of the lesions of significance in vascular dementia. J. Neurol. Neurosurg. Psychiatry **63:** 749–753.
10. Suenaga, T. *et al.* 1994. Bundles of amyloid precursor protein-immunoreactive axons in human cerebrovascular white matter lesions. Acta Neuropathol. **87:** 450–455.
11. Davie, C.A. *et al.* 1995. Persistent functional deficit in multiple sclerosis and autosomal dominant cerebellar ataxia is associated with axon loss. Brain **118:** 1583–1592.
12. Libon, D.J. *et al.* 1998. Declarative and procedural learning, quantitative measures of the hippocampus and subcortical white alterations in Alzheimer's disease and ischaemic vascular dementia. J. Clin. Exp. Neuropsychol. **20:** 30–41.
13. Snowdon, D.A. *et al.* 1997. Brain infarction and the clinical expression of Alzheimer's disease. JAMA **277:** 813–817.
14. Nagy, Zs. *et al.* 1997. The effects of additional pathology on the cognitive deficit in Alzheimer's disease. J. Neuropathol. Exp. Neurol. **56:** 165–170.
15. Marin, D.B. *et al.* 1998. The relationship between apolipoprotein E, dementia and vascular illness. Atherosclerosis **140:** 173–180.
16. Ji, Y. *et al.* 1998. Apolipoprotein E polymorphism in patients with Alzheimer's disease, vascular dementia and ischaemic cerebrovascular disease. Dement. Geriatr. Cogn. Disord. **9:** 243–245.
17. Chapman, J. *et al.* 1998. ACE, MTHFR, factor V Leiden and ApoE polymorphisms in patients with vascular and Alzheimer's dementia. Stroke **29:** 1401–1404.
18. Skoog, I. *et al.* 1996. 15-year longitudinal study of blood pressure and dementia. Lancet **347:** 1141–1145.
19. Hofman, A. *et al.* 1997. Atherosclerosis, apolipoprotein E, and prevalence of dementia and Alzheimer's disease in the Rotterdam study. Lancet **349:** 151–154.
20. Stewart, R. 1998. Cardiovascular factors in Alzheimer's disease. J. Neurol. Neurosurg. Psychiatry **65:** 143–14.

Severity of Cardiovascular Disease, Apolipoprotein E Genotype, and Brain Pathology in Aging and Dementia

IRINA ALAFUZOFF,[a,b,e] SEPPO HELISALMI,[c] ARTO MANNERMAA,[c] AND HILKKA SOININEN[a,d]

[a]*Department of Neuroscience and Neurology, Kuopio University, and*
[b]*Department of Pathology, Kuopio University Hospital, Kuopio, Finland*

[c]*Division of Diagnostic Services, Chromosome and DNA Laboratory, Kuopio University Hospital, Kuopio, Finland*

[d]*Department of Neurology, Kuopio University Hospital, Kuopio, Finland*

ABSTRACT: Neuropathological lesions, essential for the diagnosis of Alzheimer's disease (AD), such as senile-neuritic plaques (SP/NPs), neurofibrillary tangles (NFTs), the beta-amyloid load (Aβ4) and the load of PHF-τ did not increase with increased severity of cardiovascular disease in 126 clinically demented and 303 nondemented aged individuals. In contrast, the extent of AD lesions was greater in nondemented and demented individuals with the ApoE ε4 allele compared to those without this allele. On the other hand, the extent of vascular lesions currently used for the diagnosis of vascular dementia (VaD) showed correlation with the cardiovascular index, whereas ApoE ε4 allele did not seem to influence the extent of vascular lesions. The calculated CVI showed significant correlation with premortem estimated Hachinski score, and both the CVI and Hachinski score were higher in demented patients with extensive vascular lesions. Our results demonstrate that ApoE ε4 allele, a known risk factor for dementia, indeed influences the extent of Alzheimer's lesions seen in the brain tissue of demented patients and asymptomatic controls. The cardiovascular disease again seems to influence the extent of vascular lesions.

INTRODUCTION

In recent years Alzheimer's disease (AD) and vascular dementia (VaD) have been reported to be associated with vascular risk factors including hypertension, coronary heart disease, and atrial fibrillation. An epidemiological study[1] showed that dementia and its two major subtypes, AD and VaD, are associated with atherosclerosis. Furthermore, an interaction between atherosclerosis and the ApoE genotype has been suggested to be of importance in the etiology of AD.[1]

The above findings caused us to study whether the severity of cardiovascular disease shows an association with histopathological changes seen in AD and VaD—

[e]Address for correspondence: Irina Alafuzoff, M.D., Ph.D., Department of Neuroscience and Neurology and Pathology, Kuopio University, P.O.B. 1627, 70 211 Kuopio, Finland. Tel.: 358 17 162877; fax: 358 17 162048.
e-mail: irina.alafuzoff@uku.fi

TABLE 1. Clinical information

Clinical Diagnosis	Σ	Gender F/M	Age at Death m ± SD	Duration Years m ± SD	Hachinski Score (n) m ± SD	MMSE (n) m ± SD	ApoE Genotype		
							εx/x	εx/4	ε4/4
Not demented	303	136/167	70.7 ± 12.9*		4.2 ± 3.4 (40)*	25.3 ± 4.2 (20)*	65%	31%	4%
Demented	126	98/28	82.0 ± 8.5*	9.1 ± 4.8	2.4 ± 3.3 (85)*	3.5 ± 5.8 (92)*	35%	51%	14%
poAD	7	7/0	83.8 ± 5.2	6.7 ± 3.8	1.7 ± 1.9 (7)	1.3 ± 3.3 (6)	71%	29%	
AD	68	61/7	82.9 ± 8.9	10.5 ± 4.1	0.6 ± 1.5 (52)	2.9 ± 5.2 (60)	30%	54%	16%
AD/VaD	29	16/13	80.2 ± 7.9	7.3 ± 5.3	5.7 ± 2.7 (6)	9.8 ± 8.9 (8)	17%	61%	22%
AD/PD	2	1/1	76.6 ± 7.2	11.0 ± 8.5	3.5 ± 4.9 (2)	0.0 ± 0.0 (2)		100%	
VaD	17	12/5	83.3 ± 7.1	7.9 ± 4.2	7.3 ± 2.7 (16)	3.9 ± 5.7 (16)	59%	35%	6%
Others	3	1/2	71.0 ± 10.2	7.3 ± 10.9	2.0 ± 2.8 (2)	0.0 ± 0.0 (3)	100%		

ABBREVIATIONS: AD, Alzheimer's disease; VaD, vascular dementia; PD, Parkinson's disease; F, female; M, male; MMSE, Mini Mental State Examination; ApoE, apolipoprotein E; εx/x, no ApoE ε4 alleles; εx/4, one ApoE ε4 allele; and ε4/4, two ApoE ε4 alleles. m ± SD, mean ± standard deviation.
*p at least <0.05.

TABLE 2. Postmortem findings and clinicopathological correlation

Clinical Diagnosis	n	CVI m ± SD	CERAD Classification (% with vascular lesions: only microscopic[1], microscopic and macroscopic[2])					
			Norm, a	Norm, b	possADb	possADa	proAD	defAD
Not demented	303	8.5 ± 3.2*	210 (6[1], 31[2])	46 (17[1], 22[2])	56 (5[1], 41[2])			
Demented	126	7.6 ± 3.1*				17 (18[1], 47[2])	31 (13[1], 52[2])	78 (2[1], 23[2])
poAD	7	6.0 ± 2.2				1	4 (25[2])	2 (50[2])
AD	68	7.3 ± 3.1				2 (50[2])	10 (20[1] 40[2])	56 (2[1] 16[2])
AD/VaD	29	8.3 ± 3.1				9 (22[1] 44[2])	10 (20[1] 40[2])	10 (20[2])
AD/PD	2	5.5 ± 2.1				1 (100[1])		1
VaD	17	8.5 ± 2.3				2 (100[2])	7 (100[2])	8 (13[1] 75[2])
Others	3	8.3 ± 6.4				2 (50[1])		1

ABBREVIATIONS: AD, Alzheimer's disease; VaD, vascular dementia; PD, Parkinson's disease; n, number of cases; CVI, cardiovascular index; CERAD classes: norm, a, clinically unimpaired without histopathological AD lesions; norm, b and possADb, clinically unimpaired with some, moderate or many AD lesions; possADa, demented with some AD lesions; proAD, demented with moderate number of AD lesions; and defAD, demented with numerous AD lesions. m ± SD, mean ± standard deviation.

*p at least <0.05.

that is, whether there is an association between cardiovascular disease and the final diagnosis of AD and VaD.

MATERIAL AND METHODS

Postmortem brain tissue samples obtained at Kuopio University Hospital were evaluated. All nondemented cases were sampled during the period from 1991 to 1998, and those sampled demented cases that fulfilled histopathological CERAD criteria for possible, probable or definite AD[2] were included. The clinical diagnosis of AD was based on the NINCDS-ADRDA[3] and the DSM-III-R criteria (1987). The ApoE genotype was analyzed using polymerase chain reaction (PCR) as described earlier[4] with the genomic DNA being extracted from blood or brain tissue samples (TABLE 1). At necropsy, a cardiovascular index (CVI) was calculated.[5] The CVI was a score ranging from 0 to 15, based on a semiquantitative estimation of grossly notable cardiovascular pathology at autopsy. All cases were classified into neuropathological diagnostic groups as recommended by CERAD[2] (TABLE 2). Vascular lesions were graded on a three-step scale (0, no lesions; 1, only microscopic lesions; and 2, microscopically and macroscopically notable lesions). Neurofibrillary tangles (NFTs) and senile-neuritic plaques (SP/NPs) were also quantified, as described previously by Mölsä *et al.*[6] The scoring of lesions (counts of NFTs and SP/NPs) from 0 to 10 was performed under light microscopy with a 100× magnification (area 0.92 mm^2) on five fields selected by chance in each cortical region. The score was the sum of scores in frontal, temporal, and parietal cortices. The Aβ4 aggregates (DAKO, M872) and PHF-τ (Innogenetics BR-03) expression in the gray matter was visualized using immunohistochemical methodology.[5] The quantification of Aβ4 expression was performed under light microscopy at a 40× magnification, using the NIH Image system for PC. The Aβ4 load was estimated as stained area fraction in temporal and parietal cortices. The PHF-τ expression was graded on a four-step scale (0, none; 1, some; 2, moderate extent; and 3, numerous) in frontal, parietal, temporal cortices, and hippocampus. The SPSS program for Windows was used for statistical analysis. The differences were analyzed by Student's *t* test. The correlation between individual variables was estimated using Pearson's correlation tests.

RESULTS

Alzheimer's lesions were noted in 34% of the nondemented elderly controls. In 55% of these, or 18% of all nondemented, the extent of Alzheimer's lesions was sufficient for the histopathological diagnosis of AD (TABLE 2).

Both the Hachinski score and CVI were significantly lower in demented compared to nondemented individuals (TABLE 2), and the CVI showed significant correlation ($r = 0.3$, $p < 0.05$) with a premortem estimated Hachinski score (FIG. 1). In demented and nondemented individuals, the SP/NPs and NFTs scores, the load of Aβ4, and the extent of PHF-τ were influenced by the ApoE genotype (FIGS. 2–5). The extent of these lesions was greater in a patient with ApoE ε4 allele compared to a patient without this allele. In contrast, the CVI did not reveal any major influence

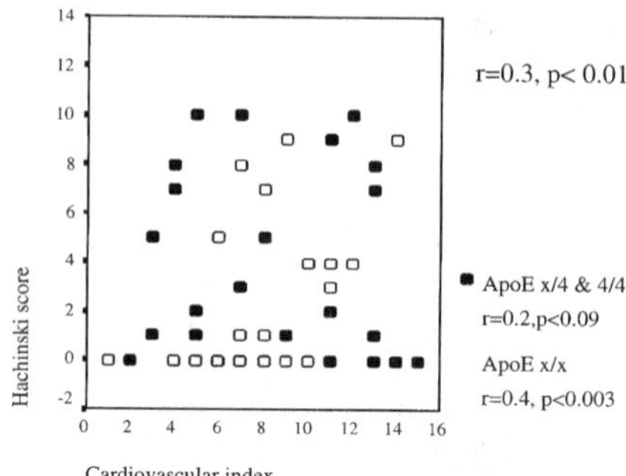

FIGURE 1. Cardiovascular index/Hachinski score.

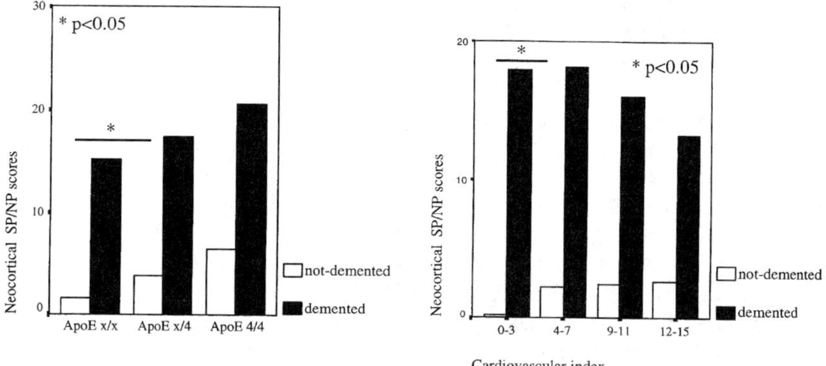

FIGURE 2. Neocortical SP/NP scores in relation to ApoE genotype (*left*) and cardiovascular index (*right*).

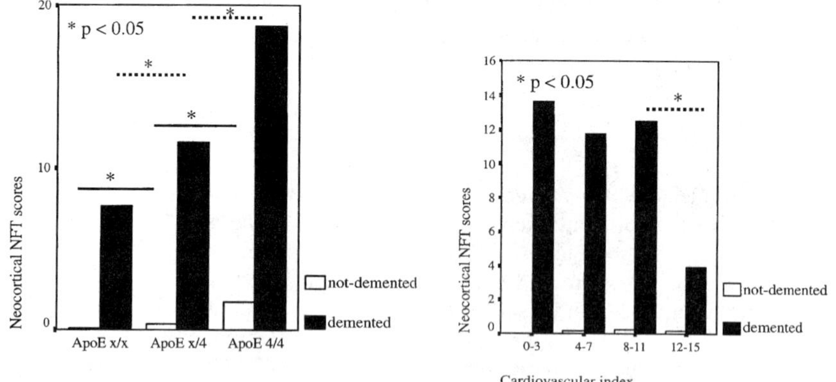

FIGURE 3. Neocortical NFT scores in relation to ApoE genotype (*left*) and cardiovascular index (*right*).

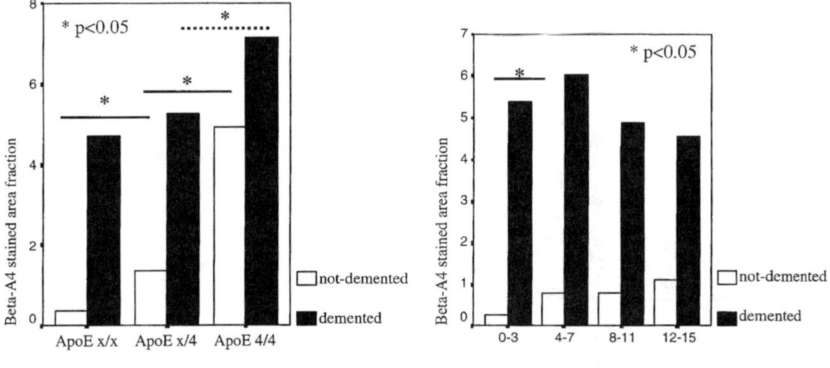

FIGURE 4. Beta-amyloid load in temporal and parietal cortices in relation to ApoE genotype (*left*) and cardiovascular index (*right*).

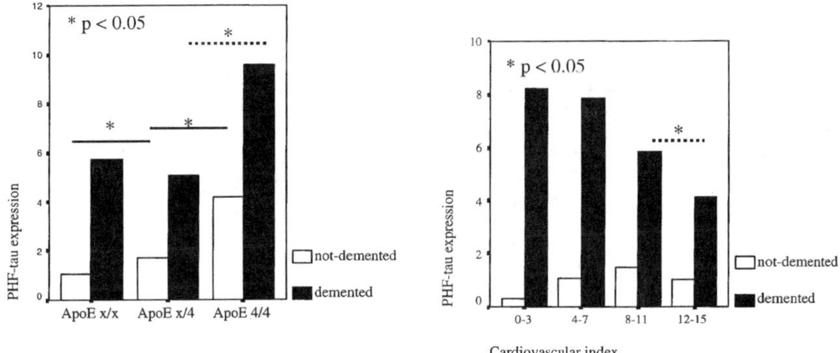

FIGURE 5. PHF-tau expression in relation to ApoE genotype (*left*) and cardiovascular index (*right*).

on the extent of AD lesions. The extent of vascular lesions increased both with the addition of the ApoE ε4 allele and significantly so with an increase in the value of the CVI (FIGS. 6 and 7).

DISCUSSION

Recent reports have proposed that AD may be associated with vascular risk factors including hypertension, coronary heart disease, and atrial fibrillation. In the present study, the calculated CVI was based on autopsy findings where both the presence of atherosclerosis and the state of the myocardium were estimated. According

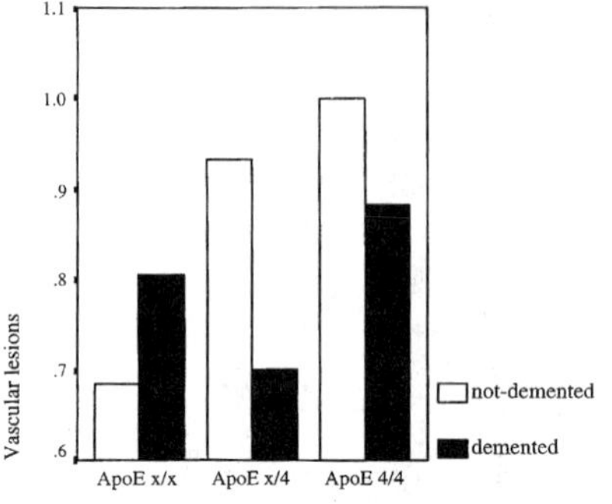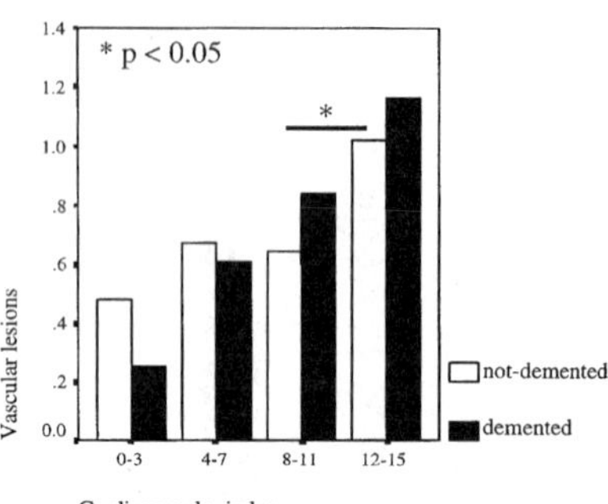

FIGURE 6. Vascular lesions in relation to ApoE genotype (*left*) and cardiovascular index (*right*).

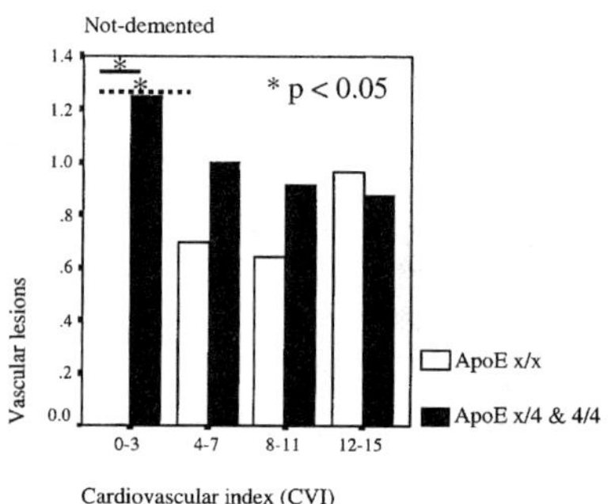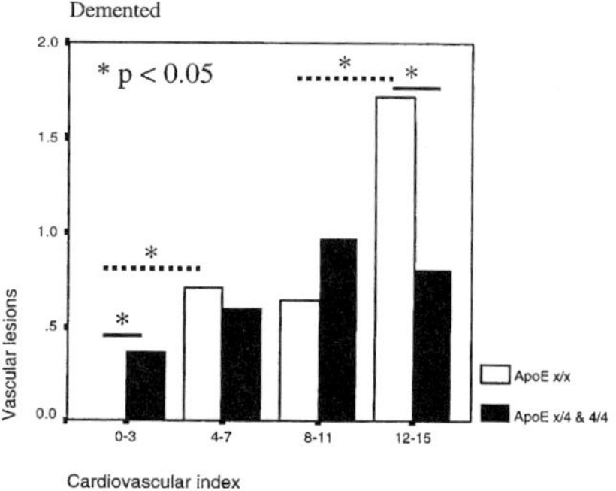

FIGURE 7. Vascular lesions in relation to cardiovascular index/ApoE genotype.

to our results, the essential neuropathological lesions, that is, those fundamental for a definite diagnosis of AD such as SP/NP, NFT, Aβ4 and PHF-τ load, did not increase significantly with elevation of the CVI. In contrast, when the AD lesions were related to the ApoE ε4 allele, both nondemented and demented individuals with the ApoE ε4 allele had significantly more lesions compared to those without this detrimental allele. The influence of the ApoE ε4 allele was most significant on neuronal degeneration estimated by NFT counts or PHF-τ load. Contrary to the influence of the ApoE 4 genotype on the extent of AD lesions, the increase in CVI was associated with some decrease in the extent of AD lesions. We conclude that aggregation of Aβ4 in the brain tissue, development of PHF-τ, and the formation of SP/NPs and NFTs are not directly dependent on the patient's cardiovascular status, whereas the ApoE ε4 allele is linked with the development of Alzheimer's lesions. These findings emphasize the need for identifying specific and reproducible histopathological lesions to be detected in the brain tissue of demented individuals resulting from cardiovascular dysfunction.

ACKNOWLEDGMENTS

This study was supported by the Health Research Council of the Academy of Finland and EVO grant Nos. 5018 and 5105. We thank Hannu Tiainen, Heikki Luukkonen, Tarja Kauppinen, and Tarja Tuunanen for their skillful technical help.

REFERENCES

1. HOFMAN, A., A. OTT, M.M. BRETELER, A.J. SLOOTER, F. VAN HARSKAMP, C.N. VAN DUIJN, C. VAN BROECKHOVEN & D.E. GROBBEE. 1991. Atherosclerosis, apolipoprotein E, and prevalence of dementia and Alzheimer's disease in the Rotterdam Study. Lancet **349:** 151–154.
2. MIRRA, S.S., A. HEYMAN, D. MCKEEL, S.M. SUMI, B.J. CRAIN, L.M. BROWNLEE, F.S. VOGEL, J.P. HIGHES, G. VAN BELLE & L. BERG. 1991. The consortium to establish a registry for Alzheimer's disease (CERAD). Part II. Standardization of the neuropathologic assessment of Alzheimer's disease. Neurology **4:** 479–486.
3. MCKHANN, G., D. DRACHMAN, M. FOLSTEIN, R. KATZMAN, D. PRICE & E.M. STADLAN. 1984. Clinical diagnosis of Alzheimer's disease: Report of the NINCDS-ADRDA Work Group under the auspices of the Department of Health and Human Task Force of Alzheimer's Disease. Neurology **34:** 939–944.
4. TSUKAMOTO, K., T. WATANABE, T. MATSUSHIMA, M. KINOSHITA, H. KATO, Y. HASHIMOTO, K. KUROKAWA & T. TERAMOTO. 1993. Determination by PCR-RFLP of apoE genotype in a Japanese population. J. Lab. Clin. Med. **121:** 598–602.
5. ALAFUZOFF, I., S. HELISALMI, A. MANNERMAA, P. RIEKKINEN, SR. & H. SOININEN. 1999. β-amyloid load is not influenced by the severity of cardiovascular disease in aged and demented patients. Stroke **30:** 613–618.
6. MÖLSÄ, P.K., E. SÄKÖ, L. PALJÄRVI, J.O. RINNE & U.K. RINNE. 1987. Alzheimer's disease: neuropathological correlation of cognitive and motor disorders. Acta Neurol. Scand. **75:** 376–384.

Can PET Data Differentiate Alzheimer's Disease from Vascular Dementia?

KEN NAGATA,[a,f] HIROSHI MARUYA,[a] HIROMICHI YUYA,[b] HIROO TERASHI,[c] YASUNORI MITO,[a] HARUHISA KATO,[a] MIKA SATO,[a] YUICHI SATOH,[a] YASUHITO WATAHIKI,[a] YUTAKA HIRATA,[a] ERIKO YOKOYAMA,[d] AND JUN HATAZAWA[e]

[a]*Department of Neurology, Research Institute for Brain and Blood Vessels, Akita, Japan*

[b]*Shiranuka Medical Office, Shiranuka, Japan*

[c]*The Third Department of Medicine, Tokyo Medical University, Tokyo, Japan*

[d]*Akita Prefectural Medical Center of Rehabilitation and Mental Health, Akita, Japan*

[e]*Department of Radiology and Nuclear Medicine, Research Institute for Brain and Blood Vessels, Akita, Japan*

ABSTRACT: The present study endeavored to differentiate Alzheimer's disease (AD) from vascular dementia (VaD) by comparing the metabolic and hemodynamic parameters. Positron emission tomographic (PET) studies were carried out in 13 patients with probable AD and 20 patients with VaD. PET findings were not included in the diagnostic criteria of AD or VaD. Using oxygen-15 labeled compounds, cerebral blood flow (CBF), cerebral metabolic rate of oxygen ($CMRO_2$), oxygen extraction fraction (OEF), cerebral blood volume, and vascular transit time (VTT) were measured quantitatively during the resting state. To evaluate vascular reactivity (VR), CBF was also measured during 7% CO_2 inhalation. Regional CBF from the parietal cortex positively correlated with the neuropsychological scores in both AD and VaD groups. The typical parietotemporal pattern of hypoperfusion and hypometabolism was observed in the AD group, whereas the frontal lobe including the cingulate and superior frontal gyri were predominantly affected in the VaD group. The occipital cortex was preserved in both groups. A significant increase of the OEF was found in the parietotemporal areas in the AD group. No significant prolongation was seen with VTT. There was a marked difference in VR between the two groups: VR was depleted in the VaD group, whereas VR was normal in the AD group. The increased OEF with preserved vascular reserve seen in AD may implicate participation of a vascular factor in the pathogenesis of AD, possibly at the capillary level. Thus, PET provides important functional information in discriminating AD from VaD by comparing the patterns of hypoperfusion and/or hypometabolism, and in the understanding of the underlying hemodynamic pathophysiology.

[f]Address for correspondence: Ken Nagata, M.D., Department of Neurology, Research Institute for Brain and Blood Vessels, 6-10 Senshu-Kubota-Machi, Akita 010-0874, Japan. Tel.: +81-18-833-0115; fax: +81-18-833-2104.

e-mail: nagata@akita-noken.go.jp

INTRODUCTION

Vascular dementia (VaD) due to multiple small infarction constitutes a small, but significant, part of mental deterioration in the elderly population, as compared to Alzheimer's disease (AD), which is the most common cause. In many cases, AD and VaD share behavioral and neuropsychological manifestations, and furthermore the ischemic vascular lesions in VaD patients often coexists with pathological characteristic features of AD in postmortem studies.[1] Accordingly, difficulties may exist in the differential diagnosis of AD from VaD clinically. Structural neuroimaging techniques, such as X-ray computerized tomography (CT) and magnetic resonance (MR) imaging, have been used in the detection of organic changes including large or small lacunar infarcts and leukoaraiosis. However, mild ischemia may cause partial neuronal loss and consequently result in undetectable structural changes on such neuroimagings.

Functional neuroimaging techniques, including single photon emission computerized tomography (SPECT) and positron emission tomography (PET), provide quantitative measures of brain function; the pattern of hypoperfusion and hypometabolism in AD is assumed to be different from that of VaD.

The previous studies with PET and SPECT demonstrated characteristic hypoperfusion and hypometabolism patterns in AD patients. The reduction of cerebral blood flow (CBF) and energy metabolism was more pronounced in the parietotemporal-associated neocortical areas and correlated with the distribution of neuropathological features such as senile plaques, neurofibrillary tangles, vascular amyloid deposits, and neuronal cell loss, whereas the primary sensorimotor and visual neocortical areas, basal ganglia, thalamus, and cerebellum are relatively preserved in AD.[2–9]

In VaD patients, functional imagings revealed even more heterogeneous patterns of hypoperfusion or hypometabolism. The reduction was observed in the frontal, temporal, and parietal lobes, which are within the territory of the middle cerebral artery and/or basal ganglionic areas, irrespective of localization of small infarcts or white matter lesions, and correlated with the degree of neuropsychological deficit.[9–11] The occipital cortex was relatively spared in the majority of VaD patients. Thus, the typical cases of dementia due to either pathology can be readily distinguished by the patterns of hypoperfusion and/or hypometabolism visualized on PET or SPECT images.

Besides the patterns of hypoperfusion and hypometabolism, PET studies with oxygen-15 compounds also provide important information concerning vascular and metabolic reserve, including the balance between blood flow and energy metabolism of the brain. In patients with VaD, reduction of blood flow may theoretically first occur because of occlusive vascular lesions or hypotension, and the depression of energy metabolism follows subsequently.[2,3] In contrast, in dementia due to the degenerative process such as in AD, fallout of neuronal cells can primarily be caused by the energy failure. In that case, PET is expected to reveal such pathogenetic differences between AD and VaD.

Our previous report on AD patients showed that the reduction of CBF was significantly greater than that of oxygen metabolism as compared with the age-matched normal controls.[12] This seems to make the relationship between AD and VaD somewhat complicated, but may indicate a possible participation of vascular factors in

AD. The present study was conducted to compare the hemodynamic parameters, including oxygen extraction fraction (OEF), vascular transit time (VTT), and vascular reactivity (VR) to carbon dioxide inhalation between those with probable AD and those with VaD.

SUBJECTS

The study included 13 patients with probable AD and 20 patients with VaD. All patients underwent neuropsychological assessment, X-ray CT, MRI, and PET studies. The diagnosis of probable AD was made based on performance on the neurological and neuropsychological test, including the Japanese version of the Mini-Mental State Exam (MMSE)[13] and the Alzheimer's Disease Assessment Scale (ADAS)[14] with reference to the criteria proposed by NINCDS-ADRDA[15] and the Clinical Dementia Rating.[16] The diagnosis of VaD was based on the MR T2-weighted images, the risk factors of stroke including hypertension, diabetes, hyperlipidemia and history of previous stroke, and the modified Hachinski ischemic score.[17,18] The severity of dementia was also evaluated in VaD patients by using the MMSE. The mean age for AD and VaD group was 60 ± 8 years and 64 ± 9 years, respectively. The PET or SPECT findings were not included in the diagnostic criteria for AD or VaD in this study.

METHODS

PET

According to the $H_2^{15}O$ intravenous bolus injection method, CBF was measured quantitatively. Cerebral metabolic rate of oxygen ($CMRO_2$), and OEF were measured by the $^{15}O_2$ single-breath method. In addition, CBV was measured by inhalation of $C^{15}O$ for the correction for contamination from ^{15}O in the vascular compartment.[19] VTT was calculated by dividing CBV with CBF. We used HEAD-TOME IV,[20] a seven-slice tomograph, with a translation in the Z-direction providing fourteen slices parallel to the anterior commissure/posterior commissure (AC-PC) plane. For the evaluation of vascular reactivity to hyper- or hypocapnia, CBF was also measured during 7% CO_2 inhalation or hyperventilation, respectively. Then CBF was compared between resting state and CO_2 inhalation, and between resting state and hyperventilation. The vascular reactivity was evaluated as $\Delta\%CBF/PaCO_2$ mmHg.[12,21] Quantitative image analysis was performed on a Titan 750 workstation (Kubota Company, Tokyo, Japan), using the Dr.View image processing package (Asahi-Kasei Information, Tokyo, Japan). By referring to each subject's MR images, which were obtained in the same imaging plane, regions of interest were determined on the CBF images in 20 regions including the cerebellar hemispheres, hippocampi, thalami, and superior temporal, inferior and superior frontal, cingulate, angular (parietal), occipital and paracentral (rolandic) cortices on both sides. In addition to the raw values, regional CBF and $CMRO_2$ values were normalized as relative to the whole-brain mean values. The normal values were collected from 20 age-matched normal volunteers. The mean regional values of CBF, $CMRO_2$, OEF, VTT, and VR were compared between AD and VaD patient groups by ANOVA with Bonferoni-Dunn correction. By use of linear regression analysis, the regional values of CBF from the parietal lobes were compared with the scores on the MMSE in both patient groups.

RESULTS

The reduction of CBF was generally greater in the VaD group than in the AD group. Hypoperfusion was pronounced in the parietal cortex and the inferior frontal gyri in AD group, whereas it was marked in the frontal cortices including cingulate, superior frontal, and inferior frontal gyrus in the VaD group (FIG. 1). In both patient groups, the occipital cortex was well preserved.

In the comparison of $CMRO_2$, a severe reduction was seen in the hippocampus and parietal cortex in the AD group, whereas hypometabolism was pronounced in the cingulate gyrus and hippocampus; the angular and superior temporal gyrus were less affected in the VaD group (FIG. 2). The occipital cortex was again preserved in both groups.

Because the mean values for OEF range between 0.38 and 0.50, a significant increase in OEF was found in the angular and superior temporal gyri, and it was relatively decreased in the hippocampus and thalamus in the AD group (FIG. 3). In the VaD group, by contrast, OEF did not significantly increase, and there was a relative decrease in the thalamus, hippocampus, and cingulate gyrus (FIG. 3).

A mild prolongation of VTT in the hippocampus was found in the AD group, whereas VTT was mildly prolonged in the hippocampus and cingulate gyrus in the VaD group (FIG. 4).

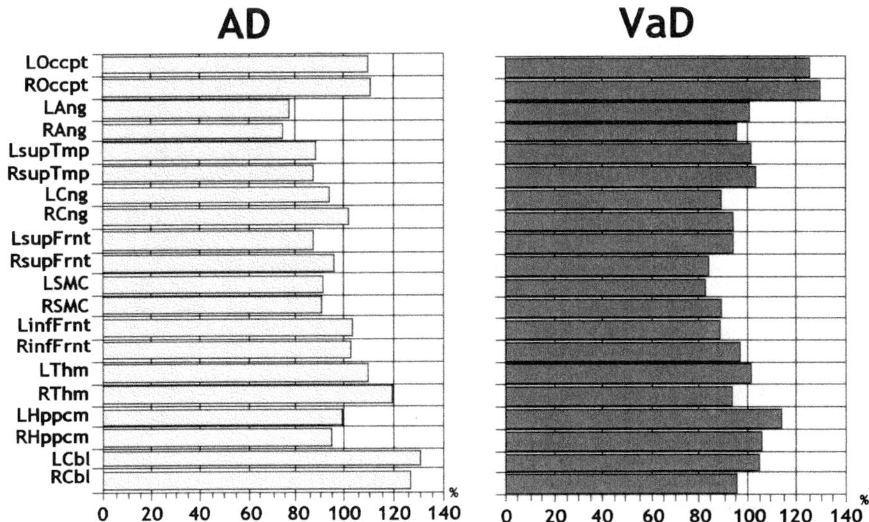

FIGURE 1. Comparison of normalized regional CBF between the AD and VaD groups.

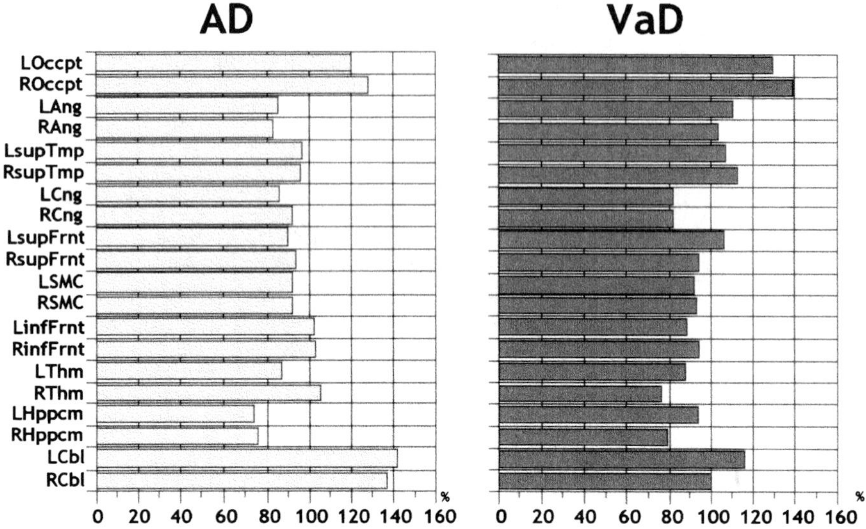

FIGURE 2. Comparison of normalized regional $CMRO_2$ between the AD and VaD groups.

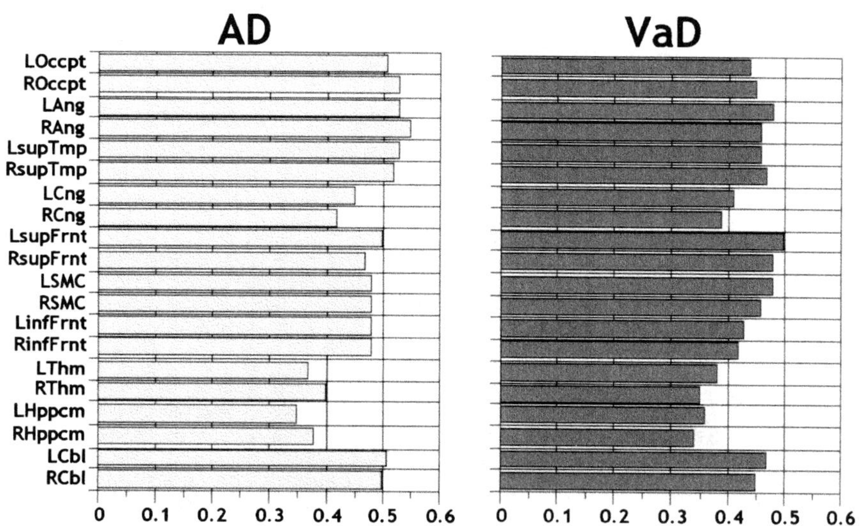

FIGURE 3. Comparison of regional OEF between the AD and VaD groups.

In the analysis of VR versus CO_2 inhalation, a marked difference existed between the two patient groups. In the VaD group, VR was markedly exhausted in the hippocampus and frontal lobe, including cingulate, superior frontal and inferior frontal gyri, whereas VR was not significantly depressed in the AD group (FIG. 5).

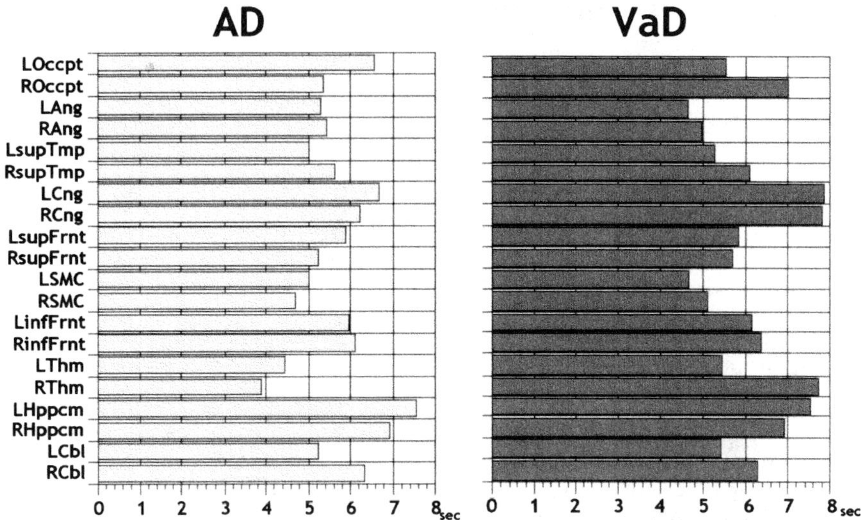

FIGURE 4. Comparison of regional VTT between the AD and VaD groups.

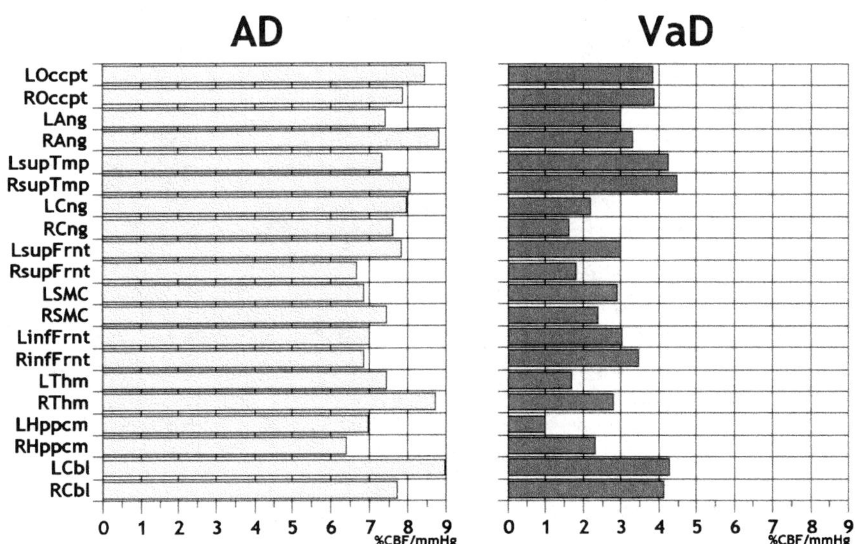

FIGURE 5. Comparison of VR to CO_2 inhalation between the AD and VaD groups.

The scores on the MMSE correlated positively with the regional CBF from the parietal cortex in both the AD and VaD groups ($p < 0.05$).

DISCUSSION

As suggested in previous PET studies,[7–10,22,23] the typical parietotemporal pattern of hypoperfusion and hypometabolism was observed in the AD group, whereas an even more heterogeneous pattern was seen in the VaD group with the present results. In the recent report in which PET with fluorodeoxyglucose (FDG) was used, patients with probable AD showed a typical parietotemporal pattern of hypometabolism with relative sparing of primary cortical areas, whereas VaD patients exhibited scattered areas with a reduction of CMRGlu extending over the cortical and subcortical structures.[24] In terms of the pattern of hypoperfusion and hypometabolism, functional neuroimaging such as PET is expected to be helpful in the differential diagnosis between VaD and AD, at least on the level of patient groups.[24]

The early PET studies on the ischemic pathogenesis of VaD focused on the relationship between CBF and $CMRO_2$ and the subsequent changes in the OEF.[3] It was concluded that no evidence existed for the alteration of the normal balance between CBF and $CMRO_2$ in either the AD or VaD patient group.[3] Since then, the changes in the OEF have been almost ignored in the PET studies in AD patients.

In the present results, the OEF was mildly increased also around the parietotemporal regions in AD patients. Similar results were obtained from the recent PET studies based on patients with senile dementia of the Alzheimer's type (SDAT) and those with diffuse white-matter lesions on MR images.[25] The authors speculated that the increase of the OEF seen in patients with SDAT might be associated with the reduction in CBV resulting from the impaired cholinergic vasodilatory function, whereas the increased OEF observed in the demented patients with diffuse white matter lesions was caused by the relative preservation of oxidative metabolism as compared to decreased perfusion; they have not tested vascular reactivity in their patient groups.[25] In our results, however, the increase of the OEF was not accompanied by prolongation of VTT, and the VR was not disturbed in AD patients. In contrast, the pathophysiological significance of the increase of the OEF seen in AD patients seems to differ from that usually observed in stroke patients.

The increase of the OEF due to the disproportionate fall of blood flow to oxygen metabolism is known as a misery perfusion syndrome,[26] and is usually regarded as a compensatory phase of recent cerebral ischemia. From observation in ischemic stroke patients, the misery perfusion syndrome mostly appears immediately after the insult and can be sometimes observed in the chronic stage.[27,27] In cases with chronic ischemia due to occlusive vascular lesions, VR was significantly depressed and the increase of the OEF correlates with the prolongation of VTT.[28] A change inVR to vasodilating agents such as CO_2 is assumed to be mediated at the level of the arteriole, which is known as a vascular resistance vessel (FIG. 6). Depletion of VR is assumed to be caused by either the maximal dilatation by exposure to ischemia or the impaired arteriolar vasculature due to advanced arteriosclerosis, as seen in VaD patients.[29,30] Because VR was well preserved in AD patients, the angioarchitectural integrity of the arteriole is considered to remain normal in the AD brain. These

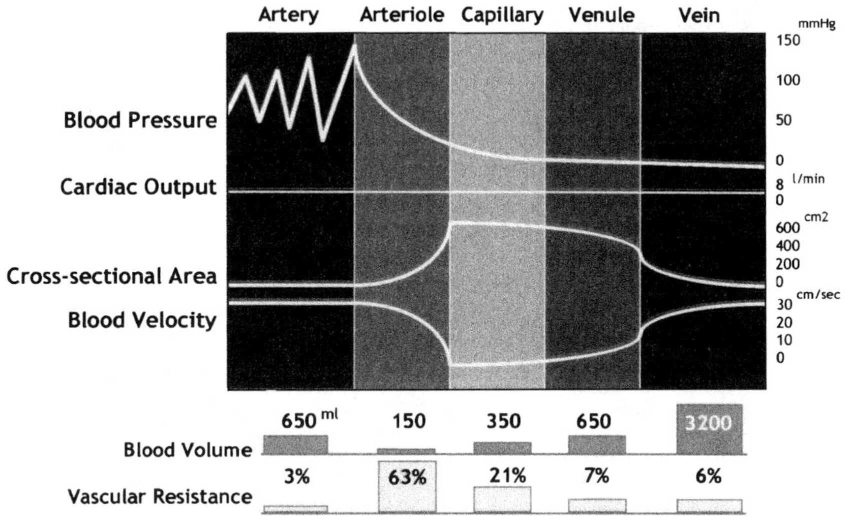

FIGURE 6. Outline of vasculature in systemic circulation with reference to blood pressure, cross-sectional area, blood velocity, blood volume, and vascular resistance.

evidences may suggest a cerebrovascular involvement underlying AD, possibly at the level of capillary and blood-brain barrier, not at the level of arteriole.

Besides the larger cerebral vessels comprising penetrating arteries and arterioles with degenerative smooth muscle,[31–33] recent ultrastructural studies demonstrate characteristic angioarchitecural abnormalities in the capillaries and sites of the blood-brain barrier.[34–37] It was also speculated that the structural alterations of microvasculature can initiate interference with the fluid dynamics, hemorrhagic compromise resulting in the increased resistance, the increased blood viscosity, and changes in shear stress.[38–40] Extensive abnormalities in the capillaries and blood-brain barrier may cause hemorrhagic and hemodynamic changes that will alter the delivery of energy nutrients to the brain.

In conclusion, PET provides important functional information in discriminating AD patients from VaD patients, by comparing the patterns of hypoperfusion and/or hypometabolism, and by understanding the hemodynamic pathophysiology underlying AD and VaD.

REFERENCES

1. TOMLINSON, B.E. *et al.* 1970. Observation on the brains of demented old people. J. Neurol. Sci. **11:** 205.
2. GRUBB, R. *et al.* 1977. Cerebral blood flow, oxygen utilization and blood volume in dementia. Neurology **27:** 905–910.
3. FRACKOWIAK, R.S.J. *et al.* 1981. Regional cerebral oxygen supply and utilization in dementia. A clinical and physiological study with oxygen-15 and positron tomography. Brain **104:** 753–778.

4. FRIEDLAND, R.P. *et al.* 1985. Alzheimer's disease: anterior-posterior and lateral hemispheric alterations in cortical glucose utilization. Neurosci. Lett. **53:** 235–240.
5. NEARY, D. *et al.* 1987. Single photon emission tomography using ^{99m}Tc-HM-PAO in the investigation of dementia. J. Neurol. Neurosurg. Psychiatry **50:** 1101–1109.
6. RAPOPORT, S.T. 1990. Positron emission tomography in Alzheimer's disease in relation to disease pathogenesis: a critical view. Cerebrovasc. Brain Metab. Rev. **3:** 297–335.
7. SALMON, E. *et al.* 1994. Differential diagnosis of Alzheimer's disease with PET. J. Nucl. Med. **35:** 391–398.
8. FUKUYAMA, H. *et al.* 1994. Altered cerebral energy metabolism in Alzheimer's disease. a PET study. J. Nucl. Med. **35:** 1–6.
9. MIELKE, R. *et al.* 1994. HMPAO SPECT and FDG PET in Alzheimer's disease and vascular dementia: comparison of perfusion and metabolic pattern. Eur. J. Nucl. Med. **21:** 1052–1060.
10. TERAYAMA, Y. *et al.* 1992. Patterns of cerebral hypoperfusion compared among demented and nondemented patients with stroke. Stroke **23**(5): 686–692.
11. SABRI, O. *et al.* 1999. Neuropsychological impairment correlates with hypoperfusion and hypometabolism but not with severity of white matter lesions on MRI in patients with cerebral microangipathy. Stroke **30**(3): 556–566.
12. NAGATA, K. *et al.* 1997. Misery perfusion with preserved vascular reactivity in Alzheimer's disease. Ann. N.Y. Acad. Sci. **826:** 272–281.
13. MORI, E. *et al.* 1985. Usefulness of Japanese version of the Mini-Mental State test in neurological patients. Jpn. J. Neuropsychiatry **1:** 82–90.
14. HONMA, A. *et al.* 1992. Development of a Japanese version of Alzheimer's disease assessment scale. Jpn. J. Geriatr. Psychiatry **5:** 647–655.
15. MCKHANN, G. *et al.* 1984. Clinical diagnosis of Alzheimer's disease: report of the NINCDS-ADRDA working group under the auspices of department of health and human services task force on Alzheimer's disease. Neurology **5:** 2801–2808.
16. MORRIS, J.C. 1993. The clinical dementia rating: current version and screening rules. Neurology **43:** 2412–2414.
17. HACHINSKI, V.C. 1974. Multi-infarct dementia: a cause of mental deterioration in the elderly. Lancet **2:** 207–210.
18. LOEB, C. *et al.* 1983. Diagnostic evaluation of degenerative and vascular dementia. Stroke **14:** 399–401.
19. LAMMERTSMA, A.A. & T. JONES. 1983. Correction for the presence of intravascular oxygen-15 in the steady-state technique for measuring regional oxygen extraction ratio in the brain: 1. Description of the method. J. Cereb. Blood Flow Metab. **3:** 416–424.
20. IIDA, H. *et al.* 1989. Design of evaluation of HEADTOME IV: a whole body PET. IEEE Trans. Nucl. Sci. **36:** 1006–1010.
21. NAGATA, K. *et al.* 1993. Effects of fasudil hydrochloride on cerebral blood flow in patients with chronic cerebral infarction. Clin. Neuropharmacol. **16**(6): 501–510.
22. SALMON, E. *et al.* 1994. Differential diagnosis of Alzheimer's disease with PET. J. Nucl. Med. **35**(3): 391–398.
23. HERHIOLZ, K. 1995. FDG PET and differential diagnosis of dementia. Alzheimer Dis. Assoc. Disord. **9**(1): 6–16.
24. HEISS, M.R. 1988. Positron emission tomography for diagnosis of Alzheimer's disease and vascular dementia. J. Neural Transm. Suppl. **53:** 237–250.
25. TOHGI, H. *et al.* 1998. Cerebral blood flow and oxygen metabolism in senile dementia of Alzheimer's type and vascular dementia with deep white matter changes. Neuroradiology **40**(39): 131–137.
26. BARON, J.C. *et al.* 1980. Human hemispheric infarction studied with positron emission tomography and the ^{15}O continuous inhalation technique: *In* Computerized Tomography. J.M. Cailler & G. Salamon, Eds.: 231–237. Springer. Berlin.
27. Baron, J.C. *et al.* 1981. Reversal of focal "misery-perfusion syndrome" by extra-intracranial arterial bypass in hemodynamic cerebral ischemia. Stroke **12:** 454–459.
28. TSUTSUMI, K. & K. NAGATA. 1998. Misery perfusion syndrome in the chronic stage of cerebral infarction. Jpn. J. Stroke **20:** 489–499.
29. DE REUCK, J. *et al.* 1998. Positron emission tomography in vascular dementia. J. Neurol. Sci. **154**(1): 55–61.

30. DE REUCK, J. *et al.* 1999. Acetazolamide vascular reactivity in vascular dementia: a positron emission tomographic study. Eur. Neurol. **41**(1): 31–36.
31. SHOJI, M. *et al.* 1990. The amyloid-protein precursor is localized in smooth muscle cells of leptomeningeal vessels. Brain Res. **530:** 113–116.
32. KAWAI, M. *et al.* 1993. Degeneration of amyloid precursor protein-containing smooth muscle cells in cerebral amyloid angiopathy. Brain Res. **623:** 142–146.
33. TAGLIAVINI, F. *et al.* 1991. Coexistence of Alzheimer's amyloid precursor protein and amyloid protein in cerebral vessel walls. Lab. Invest. **62:** 761–767.
34. YAMAGUCHI, H. *et al.* 1992. Beta amyloid is fally deposited within the outer basement membrane in the amyloid angiopathy of Alzheimer's disease. Am. J. Pathol. **141:** 249–259.
35. WISNIEWSKI, H. *et al.* 1991. Ultrastructural studies of the cell forming amyloid in the cortical vessel wall in Alzheimer's disease. Acta Neuropathology **84:** 117–127.
36. JAGUAST, W.J. *et al.* 1991. Diminished glucose transport in Alzheimer's disease: dynamic PET studies. J. Cereb. Blood Flow. Metab. **11:** 323–330.
37. KONDOH, Y. *et al.* 1997. Dynamic FDG-PET study in probable Alzheimer's disease. Ann. N.Y. Acad. Sci. **826:** 406–409.
38. DE LA TORRE, J.C. & T. MUSSIVAND. 1993. Can disturbed brain microcirculation use Alzheimer's disease. Neurol. Res. **15:** 146–153.
39. KALARIA, R.N. *et al.* 1992. The blood-brain barrier and cerebral microcirculation in Alzheimer's disease. Cerebovasc. Brain Metab. Rev. **4:** 226–260.
40. DE LA TORRE, J.C. 1994. Impaired brain microcirculation may trigger Alzheimer's disease. Neuro. Biobehav. Rev. **18**(3): 397–401.

Limitations of Clincal Criteria for the Diagnosis of Vascular Dementia in Clinical Trials

Is a Focus on Subcortical Vascular Dementia a Solution?

TIMO ERKINJUNTTI,[a,g] DOMENICO INZITARI,[b] LEONARDO PANTONI,[b] ANDERS WALLIN,[c] PHILIP SCHELTENS,[d] KENNETH ROCKWOOD,[e] AND DAVID W. DESMOND[f]

[a]*Department of Clinical Neurosciences, Helsinki University Central Hospital, Helsinki, Finland*

[b]*Department of Neurological and Psychiatric Sciences, University of Florence, Florence, Italy*

[c]*Institute of Clinical Neuroscience, Gothenburg University, Mölndal, Sweden*

[d]*Department of Neurology, Academisch Ziukenhuis VU, Amsterdam, the Netherlands*

[e]*Divisions of Geriatric Medicine and Neurology, Department of Medicine, Dalhousie University, Halifax, Nova Scotia, Canada*

[f]*Department of Neurology, Columbia University, College of Physicians and Surgeons, New York, New York, USA*

ABSTRACT: Vascular dementia (VaD) includes several different vascular mechanisms and changes in the brain, and has different causes and clinical manifestations. Critical to its conceptualization and diagnosis are definitions of the cognitive syndrome, vascular etiologies, and changes in the brain. Variation in these has resulted in different definitions of VaD, estimates of prevalence, and types and distribution of brain lesions. This defintional heterogeneity may have been a factor for negative results in prior clinical trials on VaD. We propose that the division of VaD into subtypes can identify a more homogenous group of patients for drug trials. A so-called "subcortical" VaD could incorporate two old clinical entities "Binswanger's disease" and "the lacunar state." Small vessel disease is the primary vascular etiology, lacunar infarcts and ischemic white matter lesions are the primary type of brain lesions, the subcortical areas and frontal connections are the primary location of lesions, and a subcortical syndrome as the primary clinical manifestation. The clinical syndromes are likely more variable, and urgently need to be categorized. Selection of these patients for clinical trials could mainly be based on brain imaging features, where the essential changes and the main aspects of the lesions include extensive ischemic white matter lesions and lacunar infarcts in the deep gray and white matter structures. Subcortical VaD is expected to show a more predictable clinical picture, natural history, outcomes, and treatment responses.

[g]Address for correspondence: Timo Erkinjuntti, M.D., Ph.D., Chief, Memory Research Unit, Department of Clinical Neurosciences, Helsinki University Central Hospital, P.O. Box 300, 00290 HYKS, Finland. Tel.: +358-9-471 72353; fax: +358-9-471 72352.
e-mail: timo.erkinjuntti@huch.fi

INTRODUCTION

VaD cannot be wholly identified by the traditional multiinfarct dementia.[1–3] VaD includes several different vascular mechanisms and changes in the brain, and has different causes and clinical manifestations. Current criteria for VaD, however, select an etiologically and clinically heterogeneous group.[4] As vascular causes of cognitive impairment are common, and may be preventable, and as patients could benefit from therapy, early detection and diagnosis of VaD is a challenge.[5] VaD research, until recently overshadowed by that into Alzheimer's disease (AD), is now developing rapidly, as it is an area that holds great promise for intervention. Here, we review the concepts and criteria of VaD, and propose subcortical VaD as a more homogenous group of patients for clinical trials.

CONCEPTUAL ISSUES

The critical elements in analyzing the concept and diagnosis of VaD include *the cognitive syndrome* and *the vascular etiologies and changes in the brain.* Variation in defining these two critical elements has namely caused that different definitions in use give different point prevalence estimates, identify different groups of subjects, and consequently also identify different types and distribution of brain lesions.[6–10] Further, this heterogeneity may have been a factor for negative results in prior clinical trials on VaD.[11]

Cognitive Syndrome

The traditional concept of dementia has been based on the clinical features of AD, such as early episodic memory impairment, global cognitive syndrome, progressive course, and major impairment in the activities of daily living (ADL). These features rather select an end-stage of VaD.[12] Moreover, the conventionally used criteria of dementia identify different proportions and clusters of patients.[6,7,9] This syndrome, however, is present in only a minority of patients affected with vascular cognitive impairment (VCI).[5] While international consensus in defining the syndrome and stages of VCI has yet to be achieved, clinical studies and trials of defined subsets of patients could be undertaken. Such an approach must clarify the selection, defining, and measuring of domains related to the VCI construct including cognitive functions (e.g., memory, executive functions, aphasia, apraxia, agnosia), behavioral and psychological symptoms (e.g., depression, anxiety, psychotic symptoms, apathy, emotional control, personality), and social functions (e.g., work, executive ADL, instrumental ADL and basic ADL).[13,14]

Vascular Cause

Primary vascular mechanisms related to VaD include large artery disease (artery-to-artery embolism, occlusion of an extra- or intracranial artery), cardiac embolic events, small vessel disease (ischemic white matter lesions, lacunar infarcts), and hemodynamic mechanisms.[15–19] Still, the individual roles that these factors play in causation have not been identified in detail.[1,2,19–22] The secondary vascular factors

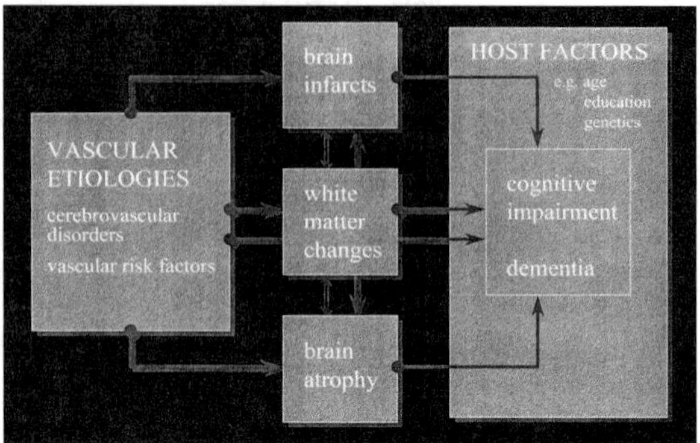

FIGURE 1. Pathophysiology of vascular dementia incorporates interactions between vascular etiologies, changes in the brain, host factors, and cognition.

include risk factors for CVD, stroke, and white matter lesions, but, at the same time, also those of any cognitive decline and AD.[23] *Changes in the brain* related to VaD include arterial territorial infarcts, distal field (watershed) infarcts, lacunar infarcts, ischemic white matter lesions (WMLs), and incomplete ischemic injury.[15,16,20,21] Incomplete ischemic injury incorporates laminar necrosis, focal gliosis, granular atrophy, and incomplete white matter infarction.[24,25] In addition, both focal (around the ischemic lesion) and remote (disconnection, diaschisis) functional ischemic changes relate to VaD.[26] An obstacle has been our limited technologies to detect and verify lesions of incomplete ischemic injury and functional ischemic changes in routine clinical work-up.[27]

The relationship between vascular factors and cognition is vital. The clinical issues to be solved include whether the identified vascular factors cause, compound, or only coexist with the VaD syndrome,[28,29] whether they contribute to the risk and clinical picture of AD,[22,30] and which type, extent, side, site, and tempo of vascular lesions in the brain relates to different types of VaD.[15,20,21,31]

In summary, the pathophysiology of VaD incorporates interactions between vascular etiologies (cerebrovascular disorders and vascular risk factors), changes in the brain (infarcts, WMLs, atrophy), host factors (age, education), and cognition[20–23,31] (FIG. 1).

INTERACTIONS OF BRAIN LESIONS IN VaD

VaD has been related to the volume of brain infarcts (size reaching a critical threshold), the number of infarcts (additive, synergistic), the site of infarcts (bilateral, strategic cortical or subcortical sites), the ischemic WMLs (extent, site, type, density), the other ischemic factors (incomplete ischemic injury, delayed neuronal death, functional changes), the atrophic changes (origin, location, extent), and finally the additive effects of other pathologies (e.g., AD, Lewy body dementia, frontal lobe dementias).[15,20,21,31]

A current review on the subject indicates that incident VaD might relate to complex interactions between infarct features, extent of WMLs, medial temporal lobe atrophy, and host features.[10] This review concluded that: (1) Not a single feature, but a combination of infarct features, extent and type of WMLs, degree and site of atrophy, and host factors are correlates of VCI/VaD; (2) Infarct features favoring VaD include bilaterality, multiplicity (>1), and location in the dominant hemisphere and in the limbic structures (fronto-limbic or prefrontal-subcortical and medial-limbic or medial-hippocampal circuits); (3) WML features favoring VaD are extensive WMLs (extending periventricular WMLs and confluent to extending WMLs in the deep WM) on computerized tomography (CT) and magnetic resonance imaging (MRI); (4) While it is arguable whether only a single small lesion on imaging could support an imaging evidence for a diagnosis of VaD, such lesions may well identify patients at risk for further progression of cognitive impairment of vascular origin. By contrast, the heterogeneity of the patients with so-called "strategic infarct dementia" may obviate their value as objects of clinical trials; and (5) The absence of cerebrovascular disease (CVD) lesions on CT or MRI is evidence against a vascular etiology.

CURRENT CLINICAL CONCEPTS AND CRITERIA

As reviewed, growing evidence indicates that VaD relates to different vascular mechanisms and changes in the brain, has different causes and clinical manifestations, and, accordingly, includes an etiologically and clinically heterogeneous group of patients. The currently used clinical criteria are consensus criteria, which are neither derived from prospective community-based studies on vascular factors affecting the cognition, nor based on detailed natural histories.[32–36] They are mainly based on the ischemic infarct concept and designed to have high specificity, although they have been poorly implemented and validated.[32,33]

As outlined, variations in defining the dementia syndrome,[7,9] and the vascular cause,[6,8] have caused that the criteria identify different numbers and cluster of patients labeled as VaD and are not interchangeable. The DSM-IV criteria are less restrictive compared to the ICD-10, the ADDTC and the NINDS-AIREN criteria.[6,37] The NINDS-AIREN criteria are currently most widely used in clinical drug trials on VaD. In a neuropathological series their sensitivity was 58%, their specificity was 80%, they successfully excluded AD in 91% of cases, and the proportion of combined cases misclassified as probable VaD was 29%.[38] Compared to the ADDTC criteria, the NINDS-AIREN criteria were more specific, and they better excluded combined cases (54% vs. 29%).[38]

THE NEED FOR AN UPDATED SYSTEMATIZATION OF VaD

The heterogeneity of patient populations derived by using the current criteria has created a need for an updated systematization. One suggestion has been that, by dividing VaD into subtypes, a more homogenous group of patients could be identified.

Classification of VaD may be based on (1) the primary vascular etiology, (2) the primary type of ischemic brain lesions, (3) the primary location of brain lesions, and (4) the primary clinical syndrome.[15] The currently proposed subtypes of VaD incorporate a variable combination of the given categories. The proposed types of VaD

TABLE 1. Vascular mechanisms and changes in the brain in main subtypes of vascular dementia

Vascular Mechanisms	Changes in the Brain
Cortical Vascular Dementia or Multiinfarct Dementia	
Large vessel disease	Arterial territorial infarct
Cardiac embolic events	Distal field (watershed) infarct
Hypoperfusion	
Subcortical Vascular Dementia or *Small Vessel Dementia*	
Small vessel disease	Lacunar infarct
Hypoperfusion	Focal and diffuse white matterlesions
	Incomplete ischemic injury
Strategic Infarct Dementia	
Large vessel disease	Arterial territorial infarct
Cardiac embolic events	Distal field (watershed) infarct
Small vessel disease	Lacunar infarct
Hypoperfusion	Focal and diffuse white matterlesions

include the cortical VaD or multiinfarct dementia, the subcortical VaD or the small vessel dementia, and the strategic infarct dementia,[16,18,35,39–42] and many include also the hypoperfusion dementia.[16,35,41,43] Further subtypes suggested include hemorrhagic dementia, hereditary vascular dementia, and combined or mixed dementia (AD with CVD).

A question being debated is whether these suggested subtypes are distinct disorders, having pathological and clinical features, as well as response to therapy of their own.[18] However, the goal is to identify homogenous subtypes, which would improve comparability of independent studies and benefit multicenter collaboration.[36]

MAIN SUBTYPES OF VASCULAR DEMENTIA

The multiinfarct dementia or cortical VaD, the strategic infarct dementia, and the small vessel dementia or the subcortical VaD are the three common types, but the frequency of these varies in different series.[16,40,41]

Cortical VaD

Cortical VaD relates to large vessel disease, cardiac embolic events, and also hypoperfusion (TABLE 1). It shows predominantly cortical and cortico-subcortical arterial territorial and distal field (watershed) infarcts. Typical clinical features are lateralized sensorimotor changes and abrupt onset of cognitive impairment and aphasia.[40] In addition, some combination of different cortical neuropsychological syndromes has been suggested to be present in cortical VaD.[44] This group shows heterogeneity with regard to the etiologies, vascular mechanisms, changes in the brain, as well as clinical manifestations.

Strategic Infarct Dementia

Focal, often small, ischemic lesions involving specific sites critical for higher cortical functions have been classified separately. Of the cortical sites, the hippocampal formation and angluar gyrus are examples. The subcortical sites include thalamus, cyrus cinguli, fornix, basal forebrain, caudate, globus pallidus and the genu or anterior limb of the internal capsule.[1,15,20] This group shows most heterogeneity (TABLE 1).

Subcortical VaD

Subcortical VaD incorporates the old entities "the lacunar state" and "Binswanger's disease," relates to small vessel disease and hypoperfusion, and from the pathological point of view is predominately characterized by lacunar infarcts, focal and diffuse ischemic WMLs, and incomplete ischemic injury.[40,44,45] Clinically, small vessel dementia is characterized classically by pure motor hemiparesis, bulbar signs and dysarthria, gait disorder, depression and emotional lability, and, especially, deficits in executive functioning.[44–48] Such clinical findings, however, frequently do not occur together, and these patients often have AD type clinical features also (see Rockwood *et al.*, this volume).

CHALLENGING NEW CLINICAL CRITERIA FOR VaD

A need for international agreement within clinical criteria for VaD in clinical trials exists. The constructs should be based on *homogeneity* in the (1) etiologies (primary vascular mechanism/etiology), (2) changes in the brain (type and location of brain lesions), and (3) the clinical syndrome. They should show a *predictable* (1) phenomenology and clinical picture, (2) clinical course and natural history, as well as (3) outcomes and treatment responses. They should further be *reproducible* (intra- and inter-rater reliability), and *practical* in various clinical settings. In this way, they should be able to identify homogenous and representative patient samples.

SUBCORTICAL VaD: A SOLUTION?

A proposal for a more homogenous subtype with a more predictable outcome is the subcortical VaD. The subcortical VaD incorporate small vessel disease as primary vascular etiology, lacunar infarcts and ischemic WMLs as primary types of brain lesions, and subcortical location as the primary location of lesions. A clinical subcortical syndrome, when present, offers a specific primary clinical manifestation (TABLE 2). The ischemic lesions in VaD affect especially the prefrontal subcortical circuit,[49] which explains the main cognitive, behavioral, and clinical neurological features (TABLE 2).

Selection of patients with subcortical VaD for clinical studies and trials could be mainly based on brain imaging features, as these seem to be the most consistent findings and can be easily fit to multicenter use. The brain imaging requirements of the criteria should reflect the essential changes (construct validity) and all the main aspects

TABLE 2. Etiology, brain changes, and clinical syndrome of the subcortical vascular dementia

Etiology

Primary vascular mechanisms

- *Small vessel disease*: obliteration and occlusion, increased resistance, decreased auto-regulation, cerebral blood flow fluctuation, endothelial changes, -blood-brain-barrier and -carrier changes, perivascular changes

Primary risk factors

- Arterial hypertension, age

Secondary vascular mechanisms

- Hemodynamic changes of systemic vascular, cardiac and carotid origin

Secondary risk factors

- Arterial hypotension, hypoxic-ischemic events, blood pressure fluctuations, diabetes, hyperlipidemia, low education

Brain changes

Primary type

- *Ischemic white matter lesions (WMLs)*: araiosis, état crible, demyelination, axonal loss, changes in oligodendrocytes and glial cells, incomplete infarcs
- Lacunar infarcts
- *Incomplete ischemic injury*: laminar necrosis, focal gliosis, granular atrophy, incomplete white matter infarcts

Primary location

- *WMLs*: extending periventricular and deep WML's affecting especially the genu or anterior lim of the internal capsule, anterior corona radiata and anterior centrum semiovale
- *Lacunes*: lacunes in the caudate, globus pallidus, thalamus, internal capsule, corona radiata, frontal white matter

Clinical syndrome

Cognitive syndrome

- *Dysexecutive syndrome*: impairment in goal formulation, initiation, planning, organizing, sequencing, executing, set-sifting and -maintenance, abstracting
- *Memory deficit* (may be mild): impaired recall, relative intact recognition, less severe forgetting, benefit from cues
- Interfering with complex (executive) social activities not due to physical effects of cerebrovascular disease alone

Behavioral and psychological symptoms

- *Depression, personality change, emotional incontinence,* psychomotor retardation

NOTE: Clinical neurological findings early in the course: episodes of mild upper motor neuron signs (drift, reflex assymetry, incoordination), gait disorder, imbalance and falls, urinary frequency and incontinence, dysarthria, dysphagia, extrapyramidal signs (hypokinesia, rigidity).

Features making the diagnosis uncertain: early onset and progressive worsening of memory deficit or some other cognitive cortical deficit in the absence of corresponding focal lesions on brain imaging. Absence of focal neurological signs, other than cognitive disturbance.

of the changes (content validity). In subcortical VaD the essential changes, as well as the main aspects of the lesions, include (1) extensive ischemic WMLs and (2) lacunar infarcts in the deep grey and white matter structures. A proposal for brain imaging requirements for subcortical VaD is given in TABLE 3.[50–53] The brain imaging criteria

TABLE 3. Proposed bran maging criteria for subcortical vascular dementia

A. Computed tomography
  • Extending periventricular and deep white matter lesions: patchy or diffuse symmetrical areas of low attenuation (intermediate density between that of normal white matter and that of intraventricular cerebrospinal fluid) with ill-defined marigins extending to the centrum semiovale, *and* at least one lacunar infarct; and
  • Absence of cortical and/or cortico-subcortical nonlacunar territorial infarcts and watershed infarcts, hemorrhages, signs of normal pressure hydrocephalus, and specific causes of white matter lesions (e.g., multiple sclerosis, sarcoidosis, brain irradiation).

B. Magnetic resonance imaging
  • To include predominantly "white matter cases": extending periventricular and deep white matter lesions: extending caps (>10 mm as measured parallel to ventricle) or irregular halo (>10 mm broad, irregular margins and extending into deep white matter) *and* diffusely confluent hyperintensities (>25 mm, irregular shape) or extensive white matter change (diffuse hyperintensity without focal lesions), *and* lacune(s) in the deep grey matter; or
  • To include predominantly "lacunar cases": multiple lacunes (e.g., >5) in the deep gray matter *and* at least moderate white matter lesions: extending caps or irregular halo or diffusely confluent hyperintensities or extensive white matter change; and
  • Absence of cortical and/or cortico-subcortical nonlacunar territorial infarcts and watershed infarcts, hemorrhages, signs of normal pressure hydrocephalus, and specific causes of white matter lesions (e.g., multiple sclerosis, sarcoidosis, brain irradiation).

should cover both cases having predominantly WMLs ("the Binswanger type"), as well as those with predominantly lacunar infarcts ("the lacunar state type").

GOALS FOR FURTHER STUDIES

Subcortical VaD offers a solution to identify more homogenous and representative groups of patients, which would improve comparability of independent studies and benefit multicenter collaboration.

Further empirical research and international debate is especially needed (1) to define the cognitive syndrome and stages of VCI , including that of VaD, (2) to refine selection, definitions and measures of domains related to the construct including cognitive functions (e.g., memory, executive functions, aphasia, apraxia, agnosia), behavioral and psychological symptoms (e.g., depression, anxiety, psychotic symptoms, apathy, emotional control, personality), and social functions (e.g., work, executive ADL, instrumental ADL and basic ADL), (3) to validate further the proposed brain imaging criteria for subcortical VaD, (4) to characterize in large community samples the natural history and outcomes of the syndrome, (5) to identify the outcome measures for clinical trials (cognition, behavioral and psychological symptoms, functional and social activities) and length of follow-up, and (6) to investigate biochemical correlates of WMLs in blood and cerebrospinal fluid.

REFERENCES

1. ERKINJUNTTI, T. & V.C. HACHINSKI. 1993. Hachinski. Rethinking vascular dementia. Cerebrovasc. Dis. **3:** 3–23.

2. CHUI, H.C. 1998. Rethinking vascular dementia: moving from myth to mechanism. *In* The Dementias. J.H. Growdon & M.N. Rossor, Eds.: 377–401. Butterworth-Heinemann. Boston.

3. WALLIN, A. & K. BLENNOW. 1993. Heterogeneity of vascular dementia: mechanisms and subgroups [review; 184 refs.]. J. Geriatr. Psychiatry Neurol. **6:** 177–188.

4. ERKINJUNTTI, T. 1999. Cerebrovascular dementia. Pathophysiology, diagnosis and treatment. CNS Drugs **12:** 35–48.

5. BOWLER, J.V. & V. HACHINSKI. 1995. Vascular cognitive impairment: a new approach to vascular dementia [review; 75 refs.]. Baillieres Clin. Neurol. **4:** 357–376.

6. WETTERLING, T., R.D. KANITZ & K.J. BORGIS. 1996. Comparison of different diagnostic criteria for vascular dementia (ADDTC, DSM-IV, ICD-10, NINDS-AIREN). Stroke **27:** 30–36.

7. ERKINJUNTTI, T., T. OSTBYE, R. STEENHUIS & V. HACHINSKI. 1997. The effect of different diagnostic criteria on the prevalence of dementia. N. Engl. J. Med. **337:** 1667–1674.

8. SKOOG, I., L. NILSSON, B. PALMERTZ, L.A. ANDREASSON & A. SVANBORG. 1993. A population-based study of dementia in 85-year-olds [see comments]. N. Engl. J. Med. **328:** 153–158.

9. POHJASVAARA, T., T. ERKINJUNTTI, R. VATAJA & M. KASTE. 1997. Dementia three months after stroke. Baseline frequency and effect of different definitions of dementia in the Helsinki Stroke Aging Memory Study (SAM) cohort. Stroke **28:** 785–792.

10. ERKINJUNTTI, T., J.V. BOWLER, C. DECARLI *et al.* 1999. Imaging of static brain lesions in vascular dementia: implications for clinical trials. Alzheimer Dis. Assoc. Disord. **13**(Suppl. 3): S81–S90.

11. INZITARI, D., T. ERKINJUNTTI, A. WALLIN, T. DEL SER, M. ROMANELLI & L. PANTONI. 1999. Subcortical vascular dementia as a specific target for clinical trials. This volume.

12. BOWLER, J.V., M. ELIASZIW, R. STEENHUIS *et al.* 1997. Comparative evolution of Alzheimer's disease, vascular dementia, and mixed dementia. Arch. Neurol. **54:** 697–703.

13. DESMOND, D.W., T. ERKINJUNTTI, M. SANO *et al.* 1999. The cognitive syndrome of vascular dementia: implications for clinical trials. Alzheimer Dis. Assoc. Disord. **13**(Suppl. 3): S21–S29.

14. GAUTHIER, S., K. ROCKWOOD, I. GÉLINAS *et al.* 1999. Outcome measures for the study of activities of daily living in vascular dementia. Alzheimer Dis. Assoc. Disord. **13**(Suppl. 3): S143–S147.

15. ERKINJUNTTI, T. 1996. Clinicopathological study of vascular dementia. *In* Vascular Dementia. Current Concepts. I. Prohovnik, J. Wade, S. Knezevic, T.K. Tatemichi & T. Erkinjuntii, Eds.: 73–112. John Wiley & Sons. Chichester.

16. BRUN, A. 1994. Pathology and pathophysiology of cerebrovascular dementia: pure subgroups of obstructive and hypoperfusive etiology. Dementia **5:** 145–147.

17. AMAR, K. & G. WILCOCK. 1996. Vascular dementia [review; 65 refs.]. BMJ **312:** 227–231.

18. WALLIN, A. & K. BLENNOW. 1994. The clinical diagnosis of vascular dementia [review; 11 refs.]. Dementia **5:** 181–184.

19. PANTONI, L. & J.H. GARCIA. 1995. The significance of cerebral white matter abnormalities 100 years after Binswanger's report. A review [164 refs.]. Stroke **26:** 1293–1301.

20. TATEMICHI, T.K. 1990. How acute brain failure becomes chronic. A view of the mechanisms and syndromes of dementia related to stroke. Neurology **40:** 1652–1659.

21. CHUI, H.C. 1989. Dementia: a review emphasizing clinicopathologic correlation and brain-behavior relationships. Arch. Neurol. **46:** 806–814.

22. PASQUIER, F. & D. LEYS. 1997. Why are stroke patients prone to develop dementia? [review; 94 refs.]. J. Neurol. **244:** 135–142.

23. SKOOG, I. 1998. Status of risk factors for vascular dementia [review; 89 refs.]. Neuroepidemiology **17:** 2–9.

24. PANTONI, L. & J.H. GARCIA. 1997. Pathogenesis of leukoaraiosis: a review [114 refs.]. Stroke **28:** 652–659.

25. ENGLUND, E., A. BRUN & C. ALLING. 1988. White matter changes in dementia of Alzheimer's type. Biochemical and neuropathological correlates. Brain **111:** 1425–1439.

26. MIELKE, R., K. HERHOLZ, M. GROND, J. KESSLER & W.D. HEISS. 1992. Severity of vascular dementia is related to volume of metabolically impaired tissue. Arch. Neurol. **49:** 909–913.
27. GARCIA, J.H., N.A. LASSEN, C. WEILLER, B. SPERLING & J. NAKAGAWARA. 1996. Ischemic stroke and incomplete infarction. Stroke **27:** 761–765.
28. TATEMICHI, T.K., M. PAIK, E. BAGIELLA *et al.* 1994. Risk of dementia after stroke in a hospitalized cohort: results of a longitudinal study. Neurology **44:** 1885–1891.
29. ERKINJUNTTI, T., M. HALTIA, J. PALO, R. SULKAVA & A. PAETAU. 1988. Accuracy of the clinical diagnosis of vascular dementia: a prospective clinical and post-mortem neuropathological study. J. Neurol. Neurosurg. Psychiatry **51:** 1037–1044.
30. SNOWDON, D.A., L.H. GREINER, J.A. MORTIMER, K.P. RILEY, P.A. GREINER & W.R. MARKESBERY. 1997. Brain infarction and the clinical expression of Alzheimer disease. The Nun Study [see comments]. JAMA **277:** 813–817.
31. DESMOND, D.W. 1996. Vascular dementia: a construct in evolution [review; 215 refs.]. Cerebrovasc. Brain Metab. Rev. **8:** 296–325.
32. ERKINJUNTTI, T. 1997. Vascular dementia: challenge of clinical diagnosis. Int. Psychogeriatr. **9:** 51–58.
33. ROCKWOOD, K., I. PARHAD, V. HACHINSKI *et al.* 1994. Diagnosis of vascular dementia: Consortium of Canadian Centres for Clinical Cognitive Research concensus statement [review; 60 refs.]. Can. J. Neurol. Sci. **21:** 358–364.
34. ERKINJUNTTI, T. 1994. Clinical criteria for vascular dementia: The NINDS-AIREN criteria. Dementia **5:** 189–192.
35. ROMAN, G.C., T.K. TATEMICHI, T. ERKINJUNTTI *et al.* 1993. Vascular dementia: diagnostic criteria for reserach studies. report of the NINDS-AIREN International Work Group. Neurology **43:** 250–260.
36. CHUI, H.C., J.I. VICTOROFF, D. MARGOLIN, W. JAGUST, R. SHANKLE & R. KATZMAN. 1992. Criteria for the diagnosis of ischemic vascular dementia proposed by the State of California Alzheimer's Disease Diagnostic and Treatment Centers [see comments]. Neurology **42:** 473–480.
37. VERHEY, F.R., J. LODDER, N. ROZENDAAL & J. JOLLES. 1996. Comparison of seven sets of criteria used for the diagnosis of vascular dementia. Neuroepidemiology **15:** 166–172.
38. GOLD, G., P. GIANNAKOPOULOS, J.C. MONTES-PAIXAO *et al.* 1997. Sensitivity and specificity of newly proposed clinical criteria for possible vascular dementia. Neurology **49:** 690–694.
39. KONNO, S., J.S. MEYER, Y. TERAYAMA, G.M. MARGISHVILI & K.F. MORTEL. 1997. Classification, diagnosis and treatment of vascular dementia [review; 83 refs.]. Drugs Aging **11:** 361–373.
40. ERKINJUNTTI, T. 1987. Types of multi-infarct dementia. Acta Neurol. Scand. **75:** 391–399.
41. CUMMINGS, J.L. 1994. Vascular subcortical dementias: clinical aspects [review; 25 refs.]. Dementia **5:** 177–180.
42. LOEB, C. & J.S. MEYER. 1996. Vascular dementia: still a debatable entity? [review; 50 refs.]. J. Neurol. Sci. **143:** 31–40.
43. SULKAVA, R. & T. ERKINJUNTTI. 1987. Vascular dementia due to cardiac arrhythmias and systemic hypotension. Acta Neurol. Scand. **76:** 123–128.
44. MAHLER, M.E. & J.L. CUMMINGS. 1991. The behavioural neurology of multi-infarct dementia. Alzheimer Dis. Assoc. Disord. **5:** 122–130.
45. ROMAN, G.C. 1987. Senile dementia of the Binswanger type. A vascular form of dementia in the elderly. JAMA **258:** 1782–1788.
46. BABIKIAN, V. & A.H. ROPPER. 1987. Binswanger's disease: a review. Stroke **18:** 2–12.
47. ISHII, N., Y. NISHIHARA & T. IMAMURA. 1986. Why do frontal lobe symptoms predominate in vascular dementia with lacunes? Neurology **36:** 340–345.
48. WALLIN, A., K. BLENNOW & C.G. GOTTFRIES. 1991. Subcortical symptoms predominate in vascular dementia. Int. J. Geriatr. Psychiatry **6:** 137–146.
49. CUMMINGS, J.L. 1993. Fronto-subcortical circuits and human behavior. Arch. Neurol. **50:** 873–880.
50. ERKINJUNTTI, T., F. GAO, D.H. LEE, M. ELIASZIW, H. MERSKEY & V.C. HACHINSKI. 1994. Lack of difference in brain hyperintensities between patients with early Alzheimer's disease and control subjects. Arch. Neurol. **51:** 260–268.

51. MANTYLA, R., T. ERKINJUNTTI, O. SALONEN *et al.* 1997. Variable agreement between visual rating scales for white matter hyperintensities on MRI. Comparison of 13 rating scales in a poststroke cohort [review; 61 refs.]. Stroke **28:** 1614–1623.
52. PANTONI, L., M. CAROSI, S. AMIGONI, M. MASCALCHI & D. INZITARI. 1996. A preliminary open trial with nimodipine in patients with cognitive impairment and leukoaraiosis. Clin. Neuropharmacol. **19:** 497–506.
53. SCHELTENS, P., F. BARKHOF, J. VALK *et al.* 1992. White matter lesions on magnetic resonance imaging in clinically diagnosed Alzheimer's disease: evidence for heterogeneity. Brain **115:** 735–748.

CADASIL: Hereditary Arteriopathy Leading to Multiple Brain Infarcts and Dementia

MATTI VIITANEN[a] AND HANNU KALIMO[b,c]

[a]*Division of Geriatric Medicine, Karolinska Institutet, Huddinge Hospital, SE-141 86 Huddinge, Sweden*

[b]*Department of Pathology, Turku University Hospital and University of Turku, FIN-20520 Turku, Finland*

ABSTRACT: Cerebral autosomal dominant arteriopathy with subcortical infarcts and leukoencephalopathy (CADASIL) often begins with migraine with aura. Recurrent strokes usually appear between 30 and 50 years of age. The arteriopathy develops slowly, resulting in destruction of smooth muscle cells and thickening and fibrosis of the walls of small and medium-sized penetrating arteries with consequent narrowing of the lumen. This impairs cerebral blood flow, visible in PET, and produces characteristic white-matter hyperintensities in T2-weighted MRI on the basis of which CADASIL may be diagnosed well before the first stroke. Multiple lacunar infarcts, mainly in the frontal white matter and basal ganglia, lead to progressive permanent brain damage manifested as cognitive decline and finally as dementia. At present, no specific therapy is available.

Infarcts result from thickening and fibrosis of the walls of small and medium-sized penetrating arteries with consequent obliteration and/or thrombosis. Although the symptoms are almost exclusively neurological, the arteriopathy is generalized and diagnosis can be made on the basis of accumulation of pathognomonic basophilic, PAS-positive and in electron microscopy osmiophilic material between degenerating smooth muscle cells in dermal arteries. CADASIL is caused by missense point mutations in the Notch3 gene, which encodes a transmembrane receptor protein with an important signaling function during development. The gene defects lead to either a gain or loss of a cysteine residue in the extracellular N-terminal part of the molecule, most probably causing a conformational and functional alteration. The function of Notch3 in adults and the definite pathogenesis of CADASIL are still unknown, but interestingly its intramembranous proteolytic cleavage may be regulated or implemented by presenilin similarly as cleavage of amyloid precursor protein in Alzheimer's disease.

INTRODUCTION

In 1977 Sourander and Wålinder described a new entity, an autosomally dominantly inherited multi-infarct dementia.[1] Thereafter, families with similar clinical pictures and pathological findings were described in the European literature under

[c]Address for correspondence: Hannu Kalimo, M.D., Department of Pathology, Turku University Hospital, FIN-20520 Turku, Finland. Tel.: +358-2-2611685; fax: +358-2-3337459.

e-mail: hannu.kalimo@utu.fi

several names, including chronic familial cerebral atherosclerosis or vascular encephalopathy, familial disorder with subcortical ischemic strokes, dementia, leukoencephalopathy, and familial Binswanger's syndrome.[2] In 1993 the disease was given a new, accurate yet extensive name, cerebral autosomal dominant arteriopathy with subcortical infarcts and leukoencephalopathy, but fortunately its acronym—CADASIL—is easy to remember.[3]

In 1993 CADASIL was first linked to chromosome 19, in 1996 the defective gene was reported to be *Notch3*,[4] and the next year the mutations were described in detail.[5] Now that the gene analysis allows definite diagnosis, it is apparent that CADASIL is surprisingly common.[6] CADASIL should always be taken into consideration in the differential diagnosis of patients examined for strokes at a young age or for suspected vascular dementia or for strokes associated with migraine.

CLINICAL PICTURE

Epidemiology

CADASIL occurs worldwide and in many different ethnic populations, although the greatest number of families identified thus far have been among European Caucasians. To date, two large reports on the clinical aspects of CADASIL have been published, comprising 45 members from seven French families[6] and 102 patients from 28 families of German ancestry and one of Austrian.[7] In Finland, with a population of about 5 million, we have so far diagnosed (gene defect identified in the patient or a near relative) about 80 individuals derived from one very large and ten smaller families.

Clinical Symptoms

The four principal symptoms of CADASIL are (1) migraine with aura, (2) ischemic strokes, (3) psychiatric symptoms, and (4) cognitive decline and dementia. CADASIL is slowly progressive with exacerbations associated with recurrent strokes. Death most often ensues after 10 to 30 years of illness, with early onset often predicting longer duration.

Migraine

Recurrent headache, most frequently in the form of migraine with aura, is frequent in patients with CADASIL, and it may begin even before the age of 10 years. Approximately one-third of the patients (22 to 38%) have suffered from it, the mean age of onset being 26 to 38 years.[6,7] The aura may be common visual or sensory disturbances, but often it is atypical, long-lasting or exceptionally severe even including symptoms of hemiplegia.[6] This association may be explained by the fact that the gene for hemiplegic migraine (encoding for the α1A-subunit of P/Q-type calcium channel) is located close to *Notch3*.[8] Interestingly, in the majority of German/Austrian patients with migraine and stroke, migraine attacks either ceased or became markedly less frequent after the first stroke.[7]

Strokes

The most common manifesting symptom is a transient ischemic attack (TIA) or stroke; in 71% of the German/Austrian patients the disease began by TIA or stroke.[7] Patients with CADASIL may already have had their first ischemic symptoms before the age of 30 (in a patient of the original Swedish family and in the Finnish homozygote at the age of 28 years). The peak is around 40–50 years of age. The strokes are most often focal (lacunar), such as pure motor or pure sensory strokes, dysarthria or diplopia. Lacunar infarcts are almost invariably subcortical, located in the white matter or basal ganglia, sometimes in the brain stem, and rarely in the spinal cord. Recurrent infarcts may lead to pseudobulbar paresis, difficulties in locomotion, and finally the patients are completely unable to move.

Psychiatric Symptoms

Mood disturbances are present in 20% of CADASIL patients. Most common is depression, especially in those patients who are at risk of this disease. Manic episodes are rare.

Cognitive Decline and Dementia

Cognitive decline becomes clinically manifest between 40 and 70 years of age. Frontal-lobe cognitive functions are predominantly and progressively affected. Patients develop impaired executive and organizing functions, general mental slowing, poor concentration, and slowing of motor functions. Memory is impaired later on, when the cumulative tissue destruction has progressed. The dementia is of subcortical type,[9,10] and four out of five CADASIL patients aged over 65 years are demented. In 10–15% of the patients dementia develops without a history of clinical strokes[7,11] (K. Vahedi, personal communication).

Additional Clinical and Laboratory Findings

Partial or generalized epileptic seizures occur in 6–7% of the patients. Absence of vascular risk factors has been emphasized, but recently certain vascular risk factors, such as smoking, high serum cholesterol or use of contraceptive pills or even high blood pressure, have been reported to occur at a low frequency among CADASIL patients.[12,13] Routine laboratory examinations are usually normal.

IMAGING

Even in asymptomatic carriers of the gene defect, T2-weighted MRI reveals changes that are highly suggestive of, though not entirely specific for, CADASIL. These are small periventricular or white-matter hyperintense areas, which may be described as leukoaraiosis and/or are reminiscent of multiple sclerosis (FIG. 1A and 1B). Involvement of capsula interna appears to be very typical of CADASIL (P. Scheltens, personal communication). Chabriat *et al.*[12] suggested that the periventricular hyperintesities (called frontal and occipital caps) are so common—present in 96% of CADASIL patients—that their absence virtually excludes the diagnosis of

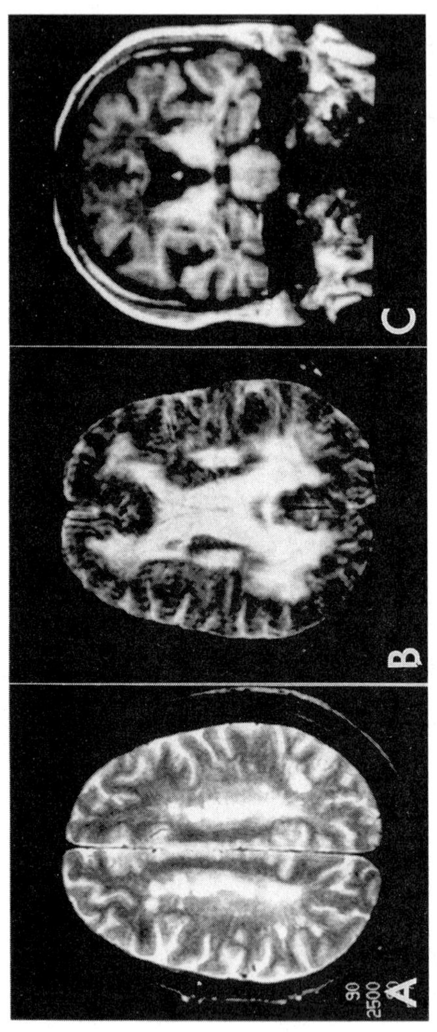

FIGURE 1. (**A**) A T2-weighted MR image of a 39-year-old, subjectively healthy male CADASIL patient, whose neuropsychological examination, however, revealed mild cognitive decline, mainly impaired executive functions. The image shows typical nodular hyperintensities in the white matter, predominantly around the ventricles. (**B**) A T2-weighted MR image of a 53-year-old, male CADASIL patient, who is moderately demented (MMSE 19/30) and homozygous for the C475T/R133C mutation, and has had several stroke episodes. Severe confluent white-matter hyperintensities are present. (**C**) A T1-weighted MR image of the same 53-year-old male as in **B** reveals marked hypointensities of the white matter including several infarcts.

CADASIL. In symptomatic patients who have sustained strokes (in 10–15% of cases clinically silent episodes), one or multiple small infarcts can be identified in T1-weighted MRI (FIG. 1C) and CT. The infarcts are most commonly located in the basal ganglia, cerebral white matter or brain stem, whereas the cortex is spared.

Reduction of cerebral blood flow (CBF) has been reported with SPECT in six patients and with PET in two CADASIL patients.[11,14] In the PET study the oxygen extraction fraction was also increased in the asymptomatic patient, whereas oxygen consumption was decreased only in the demented person, indicating that the decrease in CBF precedes tissue destruction. Concordantly, in five Finnish clinically asymptomatic CADASIL patients, an approximately 20% generalized decrease of the CBF was recorded by PET (J.O. Rinne, Turku, Finland, unpublished observations), indicating that brain tissue can still compensate for such a decrease in CBF by increasing the oxygen extraction fraction.[14] At the later stage, when the infarcts have appeared, the oxygen and glucose consumptions decrease in parallel to tissue loss and development of dementia.[14]

Conventional cerebral angiography is generally considered a noncontributing examination; instead it is actually contraindicated, because it has been reported to carry a considerably increased risk of complication[15] (S. Tuisku, Kokkola, Finland, unpublished observation).

PATHOLOGY

Even though the symptoms of CADASIL are almost solely neurological, vascular changes were found to be generalized, present in medium-sized and small arteries of almost all organs, including tissues available for *intra vitam* diagnostic biopsies. In electron microscopic analyses of nerve, muscle, and skin biopsies, it was noticed that granular osmiophilic material (GOM), not found in any other disease entity than CADASIL, is present in the arterial walls in these tissues, usually without causing any obvious clinical symptoms. Identification of GOM in these biopsies, skin being the easiest source of tissue, offers a histopathological possibility for specific diagnosis.[2,16,17] GOM is located free either between degenerating smooth muscle cells or in indentations of these cells, often within the thickened basal lamina (FIG. 2). The composition of GOM has not yet been reported, even though the Notch3 protein is suspected to be one component.

In postmortem neuropathological examinations, in accordance with the imaging findings, small multiple infarcts are detected in the white matter or deep grey matter (FIG. 3), and the brain stem is also frequently affected. On the other hand, the cerebral cortex is usually remarkably well preserved. Unlike in congophilic angiopathies, the arterial walls in CADASIL are not prone to rupture and hence intracerebral hemorrhages are uncommon, mainly as complications of anticoagulant or antiaggregant therapy.

Histologically, the walls of small- and medium-sized leptomeningeal and penetrating arteries are markedly thickened. Hematoxylin-and-eosin and Herovici stainings reveal the accumulation of characteristic basophilic granular material in the thickened, fibrotic tunica media (FIG. 4A). The presence of granular material, which is usually positive in PAS staining (FIG. 4B), distinguishes CADASIL from the fi-

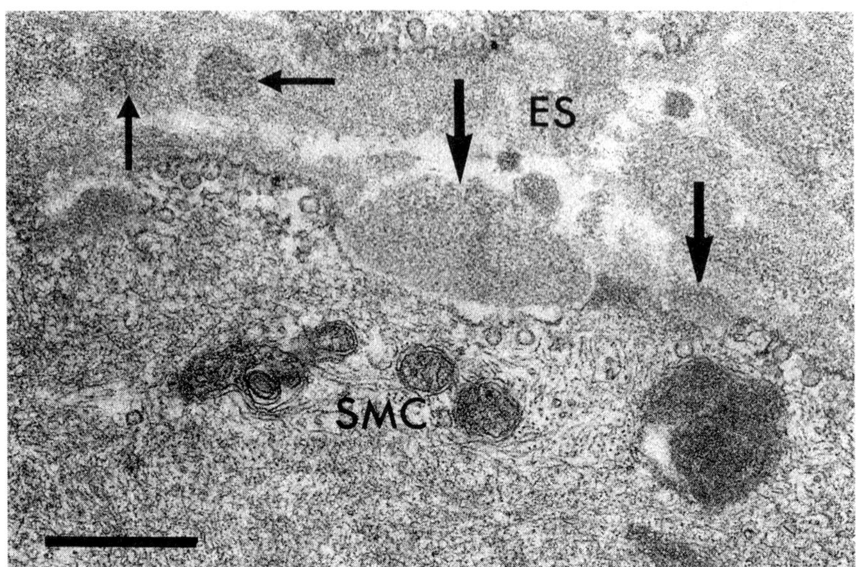

FIGURE 2. Electron microscopic findings in a skin biopsy from the CADASIL patient in FIGURE 1B and C. There are deposits of characteristic granular osmiophilic material in the indentations of the degenerative smooth muscle cell (*large arrows*) and free in the extracellular space (*small arrows*). ES, extracellular space; SMC, smooth muscle cell. Bar: 500 nm.

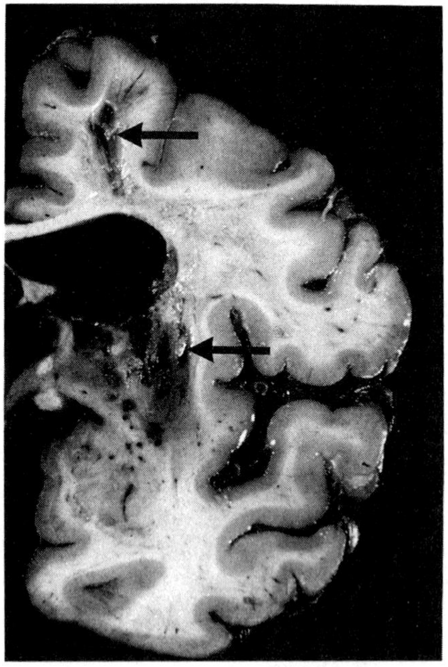

FIGURE 3. Numerous, mainly lacunar, infarcts are seen in the basal ganglia and white matter (*arrows*) in the brain of a CADASIL patient, who died at the age of 63 years.

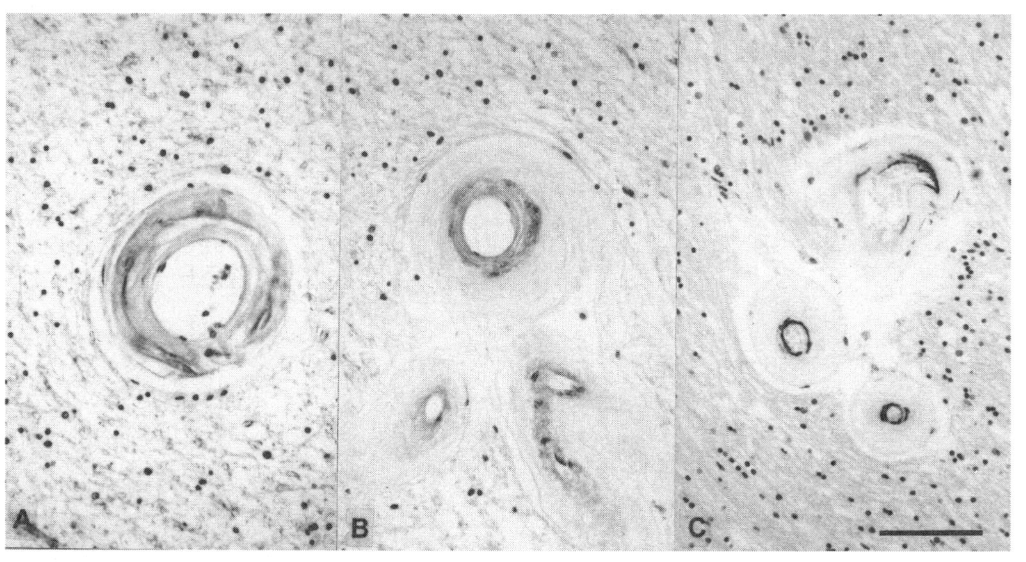

FIGURE 4. Histopathological changes in the medium-sized cerebral penetrating arteries deep in the white matter from the patient in FIGURE 3. (**A**) The wall of the artery is markedly thickened, fibrotic with accumulation of basophilic granular material. (**B**) The material accumulated is PAS-positive. (**C**) Immunohistochemical staining demonstrates that only remnants of smooth muscle cells (*arrows*) are left in the fibrotic arterial walls. A: Herovici; B: PAS; C. Anti-smooth muscle actin and hematoxylin counterstain. Bar: 40 μm.

brotic vasculopathy occurring in arterial hypertension. The thickened arteries of CADASIL are negative in stainings for amyloid. Destruction of the smooth muscle cells can be verified immunohistochemically with antibody to smooth muscle actin (FIG. 4C) and in greater detail by electron microscopy. The basophilic and PAS-positive granular material in the arterial walls corresponds to the above-described GOM (cf. FIG. 2).

GENETICS

The CADASIL gene is located at 19p13.1-13.2 and the defective gene is *Notch3*, which encodes a transmembrane receptor protein[3,4,18] (FIG. 5). *Notch* genes are highly conserved during evolution and corresponding genes with a high degree of homology have been identified from nematodes to man.[18,19] During development, genes of the *Notch* family regulate differentiation of cells via the so-called lin-12/sel-12 signaling pathway,[18,19] but the function of *Notch* genes in adult animals is still unknown.

The human *Notch3* gene has 33 exons encoding the Notch3 protein of 2,321 amino acids with a single transmembrane domain. The extracellular N-terminal part of the molecule contains 34 epidermal growth factor (EGF)-type repeats followed by three notch/lin-12 repeats. On the cytoplasmic side, there are six cdc10/ankyrin repeats[5] (FIG. 5). Over 90% of CADASIL cases are due to missense point mutations in the extracellular domain of the EGF repeats, with marked clustering at the 5′ end of the *Notch3* gene.[5] At least 26 different point mutations have been identified, but

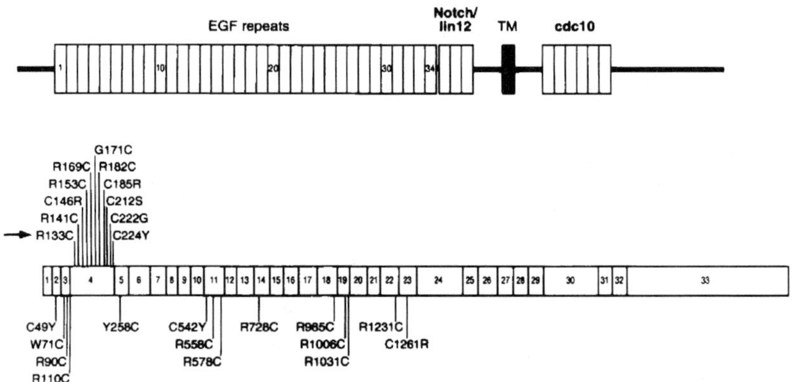

FIGURE 5. The *Notch3* gene (*bottom*) and its protein product (*top*), a type 1 integral-membrane molecule with presumptive receptor function. The *Notch3* gene has 33 exons. The extracellular part of the molecule is composed of 34 epidermal growth factor-like (EGF) repeats, followed by three Notch3/lin-12 repeats. The cytoplasmic domain is composed of six cdc10 repeats. Most mutations are located at the 5′ end of the gene (the amino acid substitution of each mutation has been marked in the picture). The mutation R133C, which has occurred as a homozygous mutation in one Finnish patient, is marked with an arrow. TM, transmembrane domain. (Modified from Joutel *et al.*[5])

in about 70% of patients the mutation is located within exons 3 and 4, which encode for the first five EGF repeats (FIG. 5). The multitude of mutations makes the detection of the mutation in new families somewhat cumbersome, but, to a considerable extent, the clustering helps in the search. All these mutations result either in replacement of a wild-type cysteine with another amino acid or vice versa. Thus, instead of the normal number of six cysteines in the normal EGF repeat, the mutated repeat contains either five or seven cysteines. Joutel *et al.* confirmed the pathogenicity of these mutations by their absence in 100 control persons and by linkage of the mutation to the disease in all affected families.[5] In a few families (including the original family of Sourander and Wålinder[1]), the gene defects have not been identified; hence other disease entities with a similar clinical picture may exist. Definite sporadic cases of CADASIL have not been diagnosed. Interestingly, in one family with genetically verified CADASIL, two family members had similar clinical and MRI findings as the diseased members, but because they had no gene defect or GOM in the skin biopsy, they were classified as CADASIL phenocopies.[20] Recently, we found a Finnish patient who is homozygous for the R133C mutation.[21]

PATHOGENESIS

It is very likely that the alteration in the number of cysteine residues affects the formation of sulfur bridges and thereby the three-dimensional structure of the extracellular part of the Notch3 receptor. Consequently, dimerization of Notch3 molecules, binding of ligands, induction of the cleavage of Notch intracellular domain or other molecular interactions may be affected.[5] Mutations may thereby lead to altered signaling in vascular smooth cells which express Notch3 receptors. The exact pathogenetic mechanism is not known, but in an autosomally dominantly inherited disease the two main alternatives are gain of function (i.e., hyperactivity of Notch3 receptors) or loss of function (i.e., so-called haploinsufficiency).

Because GOM is closely associated with smooth muscle cells, the primary damage is assumed to be directed against these cells. Alternatively, damage to endothelial cells has also been suggested to cause the breakdown of the blood-brain barrier and secondary destruction of smooth muscle cells.[16] The destruction of smooth muscle cells induces secondary fibrosis with consequent thickening of the walls and narrowing of the lumen of cerebral arteries. These vascular changes must finally lead to either thrombosis or severe obliteration, which reduces blood flow to a sufficient degree to cause focal ischemic infarcts with cognitive impairment and, finally, dementia as the clinical consequence. The preponderant localization of infarcts to the white matter and deep gray matter depends on these areas being supplied by relatively long, penetrating arteries of the end-artery type.

The discovery of the *Notch3* gene has also raised an interesting association with Alzheimer's disease (AD). Notch gene products are engaged in the same signaling pathway as presenilin 1 (PS1). After ligand binding, γ-secretase appears to cleave the Notch intracellular domain (NICD), similarly as it cleaves β-amyloid precursor protein (APP) to produce Aβ peptide (FIG. 6). This cleavage of both APP and Notch is presumed to be regulated or possibly even implemented by presenilin-1.[22] NICD is liberated to the cytoplasm and is translocated to the nucleus to bind DNA as a transcription factor.

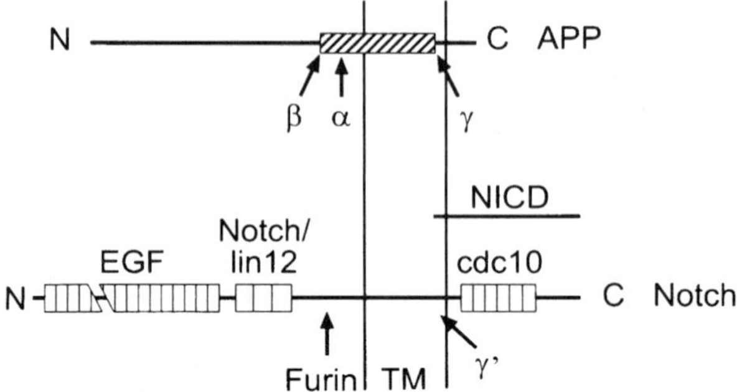

FIGURE 6. The presumptive proteolytic cleavage of the Notch molecule— similar to γ-secretase as β-amyloid precursor protein (APP) in Alzheimer's disease—within the plasma membrane. This cleavage has been suggested to be regulated or possibly even implemented by presenilin 1.[22] The cleavage product, Notch intracellular domain (NICD), is translocated to the nucleus to modify transcription of its target genes. EGF, epidermal growth factor-like repeats; TM, transmembrane domain. α, β, cleavage sites of respective secretases. (Modified from De Strooper *et al.*[22])

DIAGNOSIS AND DIFFERENTIAL DIAGNOSIS IN CADASIL

Diagnosis

CADASIL should be always considered in cases of minor cerebrovascular accidents at an exceptionally young age—all the more so if similar events have occurred in the family, because all CADASIL cases diagnosed thus far have been familial. MRI examination should be performed to search for the white-matter changes, though alternative diagnoses must also be considered. History of migraine with aura provides strong further support for CADASIL.

In patients with white-matter MRI findings, an electron microscopic examination of skin biopsy should be performed. Detection of GOM in the arterial walls makes the diagnosis of CADASIL virtually certain, because GOM has not been reported in any other disease. Failure to find GOM, however, does not definitely exclude CADASIL,[2] because GOM deposits may be too focal or the biopsy too superficial. Molecular genetic identification of a pathogenic *Notch3* mutation gives the definite diagnosis. However, the great number of different mutations (at least 26 at present) may make the search relatively cumbersome in new families and, furthermore, gene defects were detected in only 90% of the cases.[5]

Differential Diagnosis

Migraine is associated with stroke-like symptoms also in rare autosomal dominant familial hemiplegic migraine.[23] Stroke may also be associated with "independent" migraine, and migraine is included among risk factors for stroke in young women.[24] White-matter infarcts are also caused by the somewhat equivocal entity of Binswanger's disease, which is commonly associated with hypertension, whereas

CADASIL patients are most often normotensive.[12] Finally, strokes in young persons may also be caused by a mitochondrial encephalopathy, especially MELAS, though these infarcts are usually cortical and located in occipital lobes.[25,26]

THERAPEUTIC POSSIBILITIES

At present, only symptomatic therapy is available. Anticoagulant therapy and antiaggregant therapy have been tried without definite positive effects. Rather, in two cases these treatments may have caused intracerebral hemorrhage. The slow and unpredictable progression of CADASIL makes evaluation of therapeutic effects very difficult.

REFERENCES

1. SOURANDER, P. & J. WÅLINDER. 1977. Hereditary multi-infarct dementia. Morphological and clinical studies of a new disease. Acta Neuropathol. **39:** 247–254.
2. RUCHOUX, M.-M.& C.A. MAURAGE. 1997. CADASIL: Cerebral autosomal dominant arteriopathy with subcortical infarcts and leukoencephalopathy. J. Neuropathol. Exp. Neurol. **56:** 947–964.
3. TOURNIER-LASSERVE, E., A. JOUTEL, J. MELKI, *et al.* 1993. Cerebral autosomal dominant arteriopathy with subcortical infarcts and leukoencephalopathy maps to chromosome 19q12. Nature Genet. **3:** 256–259.
4. JOUTEL, A., C. CORPECHOT, A. DUCROS, *et al.* 1996. *Notch3* mutations in CADASIL, a hereditary late-onset condition causing stroke and dementia. Nature **383:** 707–710.
5. JOUTEL, A., K. VAHEDI, C. CORPECHOT, *et al.* 1997. Strong clustering and stereotyped nature of Notch3 mutations in CADASIL patients. Lancet **350:** 1511–1515.
6. CHABRIAT, H., K. VAHEDI, M. IBA-ZIZEN, *et al.* 1995. Clinical spectrum of CADASIL: a study of 7 families. Lancet **346:** 934–939.
7. DICHGANS, M., M. MAYER, D.P. UTTNER, *et al.* 1998. The phenotypic spectrum of CADASIL: clinical findings in 102 cases. Ann. Neurol. **44:** 731–739.
8. OPPHOFF, R.A., G.M. TERWINDT, M.N. VERGOUWE, *et al.* 1997. Wolff Award 1997. Involvement of a Ca^{2+} channel gene in familial hemiplegic migraine and migraine with and without aura. Headache **37:** 479–485.
9. AMBERLA, K., H. MONONEN, M. REPO & M. VIITANEN. 1998. Cognitive decline in members of a Finnish CADASIL family. Neurobiol. Aging **19:** S86.
10. TAILLIA, H., H. CHABRIAT, A. KUETZ, *et al.* 1998. Cognitive alterations in non-demented CADASIL patients. Cerebrovasc. Dis. **8:** 97–101.
11. MELLIES, J.K., T. BÄUMER, J.A. MÜLLER, *et al.* 1998. SPECT study of a German CADASIL family. A phenotype with migraine and progressive dementia only. Neurology **50:** 1715–1721.
12. CHABRIAT, H., C. LEVY, H. TAILLIA, *et al.* 1998. Patterns of MRI lesions in CADASIL. Neurology **51:** 452–457.
13. DAVOUS, P. 1998. CADASIL: a review with proposed diagnostic criteria. Eur. J. Neurol. **5:** 219–233.
14. CHABRIAT, H., M.-G. BOUSSER & S. PAPPATA. 1995. Cerebral autosomal dominant arteriopathy with subcortical infarcts and leukoencephalopathy: a positron emission tomography study in two affected family members. Stroke **26:** 1729–1730.
15. DICHGANS, M. & D. PETERSEN. 1997. Angiographic complications in CADASIL. Lancet **349:** 776–777.
16. RUCHOUX, M.-M. & C.A. MAURAGE. 1998. Endothelial changes in muscle and skin biopsies in patients with CADASIL. Neuropathol. Appl. Neurobiol. **24:** 60–65.
17. SCHRÖDER, J.M., B. SELLHAUS & J. JORG. 1995. Identification of the characteristic vascular changes in a sural biopsy of a case with cerebral autosomal dominant arteriop-

athy with subcortical infarcts and leukoencephalopathy (CADASIL). Acta Neuropathol. **89:** 116–121.

18. ARTAVANIS-TSAKONAS, S., M.D. RAND & R.J. LAKE. 1999. Notch signaling: cell fate control and signal integration in development. Science **284:** 770–776.

19. JOUTEL, A. & E. TOURNIER-LASSERVE. 1998. Notch signalling pathway and human diseases. Semin. Cell Dev. Biol. **9:** 619–625.

20. FURBY, A., K. VAHEDI, M. FORCE, S. LARROUY, M.-M. RUCHOUX, A. JOUTEL & E. TOURNIER-LASSERVE. 1998. Differential diagnosis of a vascular leukoencephalopathy within a CADASIL family: use of skin biopsy electron microscopy study and direct genotypic screening. J. Neurol. **245:** 734–740.

21. JUVONEN, V., S. TUOMINEN, T. JOLMA, *et al.* 1999. A CADASIL patient with homozygous R133C Notch3 mutation. Alzheimer's Rep. **2**(S1)**:** 35.

22. DE STROOPER, B., W. ANNAERT, P. CUPERS, *et al.* 1999. A presenilin-1-dependent γ-secretase-like protease mediates release of Notch intracellular domain. Nature **398:** 518–522.

23. CHABRIAT, H., E. TOURNIER-LASSERVE, K. VAHEDI, D. LEYS, A. JOUTEL, A. NIBBIO, J.P. ESCAILLAS, M.T. IBA-ZIZEN, S. BRACARD, A. TEHINDRAZANARIVELO, *et al.* 1995. Autosomal dominant migraine with MRI white-matter abnormalities mapping to the CADASIL locus. Neurology **45:** 1086–1091.

24. TZOURIO, C., A. TEHINDRAZANARIVELO, S. IGLÉSIAS, *et al.* 1995. Case-control study of migraine and risk of ischaemic stroke in young women. Br. Med. J. **310:** 830–833.

25. ALLARD, J.C., S. TILAK & A.P. CARTER. 1988. CT and MR of MELAS syndrome. Am. J. Neuroradiol. **9:** 1234–1238.

26. MAJAMAA, K., J. TURKKA, M. KÄRPPÄ, S. WINQVIST & I.E. HASSINEN. 1997. The common MELAS mutation A3243G in mitochondrial DNA among young patients with an occipital brain infarct. Neurology **49:** 1331–1334.

Skin Biopsy Value and Leukoaraiosis

M.M. RUCHOUX,[a] P. BRULIN, E. LETEURTRE, AND C.A. MAURAGE

Laboratoire de Neuropathologie, Hôpital Roger Salengro, EA 2691 MENRT, University of Lille, F-59037 France

ABSTRACT: In the field of leukoaraiosis, the identification of CADASIL and its link to Notch 3 mutation has shed light on the pathogenesis of white matter (WM) abnormalities related to small-vessel disease. Since 1993, its systemic vascular involvement allows skin biopsy diagnosis and research on tissues before postmortem examination. We received 160 skin biopsies from patients presenting subcortical dementia, recurrent strokes, behavioral disturbances or migraines, and suspected CADASIL. Almost all the patients lacked the well-known vascular risk factors. The ultrastructural study was systematically carried out looking at the vessel walls and the other components found in skin. In a third, we found endothelial changes, destruction of vascular smooth muscle cells (VSMCs), and characteristic granular osmiophilic material (GOM). In these cases, the genetic analysis confirmed the Notch 3 mutation. Curiously, the skin biopsies from the other two thirds presented marked alterations within the vessel walls. Such changes included destruction of VSMCs, lack of GOM, and replacement of these cells by an extracellular matrix. Frequently, we noticed endothelial pathological changes as well as other tissue impairments. By now, we are able to describe eight different groups of lesions according to either the prevalence of a lesion or the asssociation of different lesions.

The skin biopsy ultrastructural study seems to be highly informative given that we can observe vessel lesions and association of impairments in various tissues that might, in part, explain the brain vessel involvement and then the leukoaraiosis and probably some clinical symptoms. Moreover, these vessel lesions often belonged to young people (30–50 years old), and many of them seemed to run in families. These new data associated with early onset of clinical symptoms and leukoaraiosis would be extremely valuable in clarifying the wide field of leucoencephalopathy and might provide genetic research with new issues.

INTRODUCTION

From the very beginning, the significance of cerebral white matter (WM) changes have been dealt with in research. Moreover, cerebral hemispheric WM changes are detected with increasing frequency by CT and MRI even among people older than 60. So we are confronted with MRI changes that are probably either physiologic in the very elderly or pathologic with clinical and histopathological relevance. Therefore, the lack of knowledge of the pathogenesis associated with the various etiologies hinders classification.[1] Actually, it seems illusory to value original changes with lesions observed 20–30 years after onset. In 1993, a new disease named CADASIL

[a]Address for correspondence: Prof. M.M. Ruchoux, Laboratoire de Neuropathologie, Hôpital Roger Salengro, EA 2691 MENRT, University of Lille, F-59037 France. Tel. and fax: +33 3 20 44 64 21.
e-mail: mmruchoux@chru-lille.fr

(cerebral autosomal dominant arteriopathy with subcortical infarcts and leukoencephalopathy) was defined by Tournier-Lasserve.[2] CADASIL is considered to be a disease predominantly affecting the small vessels of the brain WM with an autosomal transmission linked to chromosome 19p13.[2] The linkage was later confirmed in a large number of families. CADASIL patients carry mutation within the Notch 3 gene.[3] Moreover Estes,[4] Baudrimont,[5] and Guttierrez-Molina[6] described an osmiophilic material surrounding the VSMCs of the arteries located in the WM and in the meninges in patients belonging to CADASIL families. Then, we also found this osmiophilic material in the muscle biopsy and in the skin biopsy of a Lille patient and also in six other patients from the first family.[7] We called this deposit granular osmiophilic material (GOM), and we observed it surrounding the VSMCs of the whole arterial tree in an autopsic case.[8] So CADASIL became a systemic disease. Later Ebke[9] confirmed the value of studying the skin biopsy of symptomatic patients and their relatives in a new German family. With the discovery of CADASIL as a systemic vascular disease, a new approach was opened owing to skin biopsy diagnosis confirmed by genetic analysis. As a matter of fact, we have to remind ourselves that skin is a true tissue with many components, which allows a wide range of analyses. There were an epithelial coating and divers glands with different metabolisms, several neurotransmitters in myelinic or amyelinic nerves and specialized cells, capillaries, arterioles, veins and lymphatics at different levels, different sorts of extracellular matrix according to their location, and inflammatory cells. Consequently, skin biopsy allows a wide analysis, which has proved useful in the field of subcortical dementia with leukoaraiosis.

MATERIALS AND RESULTS

In the field of CADASIL, we received 160 skin biopsies from patients presenting a leukoaraiosis without risk factors (e.g., hypertension, dyslipidemia, smoking, heavy drinking, myocardial infarction, chronic arteriopathy, or homocysteinuria), before the normal age, which is around 30–60. These skin biopsies were sent for an ultrastructural study with only one question: Is it CADASIL or not CADASIL? In one third we found GOMs surrounding the VSMCs, and in the other two thirds we were surprised to observe various changes, which are summarized in TABLE 1.

The first group corresponds to the CADASIL cases, which were diagnosed thanks to the presence of GOM in 53 patients. The average age was 50. The statistical morphometric analysis (data not published) showed that there was a destruction of the VSMCs leading to a slight decrease in vessel wall thickness and not an increase. There was no more than the extra cellular matrix, just a sort of replacement of the VSMCs. Actually, the same observation was made in the brain, where the vessel walls were either devoid of VSMCs or could show disappearing VSMCs. As a matter of fact, the vessel walls in the brain seemed to have thickened, because there is a possibility of expansion owing to the formation of a lacune following the ischemic destruction surrounding the vessel.

The second group ($n = 34$) includes patients without obvious vascular risk factors, in which the vessel walls presented a dramatic extracellular matrix and a lumen stenosis either with or without a fragmentation of the VSMCs. This group has to be

TABLE 2. Different types of vascular changes observed in skin biopsies from patients presenting with leuckoaraiosis in the field of CADASIL-like diseases

Morphology	n	Family Cases		Age
		n	%	
CADASIL(GOM)	53	45	84%	25<**50**<72
Increase in extra cellular matrix	34	18	52%	36>**59**<75
VSMC fragmentation	23	17	73%	25>**44**<70
Increase in elastica lamina area	9	5	55%	37>**57**<79
AHT + miscellaneous cases	22	15	64%	34>**50**<77
Controls	10	—	—	18>**40**<72
ND + age >75 years	12	—	—	24>**68**<89

divided into two, given that some patients showed an increase in extracellular matrix both in their vessel walls and in their smooth muscle fascicle. In these cases, the pathology concerned both types of smooth muscle: the vessel type and the fascicle type. This group probably belongs to a pathology of the extracellular matrix. On the other hand, the other patients presented normal erectile smooth muscle fascicles. Consequently, the modifications only involved the vessel wall, so the pathology seems linked to vessel wall components.

The third group ($n = 23$) includes patients presenting vessel walls with a fragmentation of the VSMCs owing to the formation of voluminous holes within their cytoplasms. There was no increase in extracellular matrix, and the vessel wall seems thin and weak. In this group, the patients were particularly young, the average age being 44. Other members of his family are affected in 73% of the cases.

The next group includes patients in whom the vessel walls showed an increase in the elastica lamina areas. Many of them presented migrains without leukoaraiosis and belonged to families of familial hemiplegic migraine mapping to chromosome 19. The following groups include some hypertensive patients and elderly people whose vessel walls were interpretable, and then a control group.

DISCUSSION

Medical opinion shares the idea of an ischemic origin to the leukoaraiosis (LA) in subcortical vascular dementia. Long and different types of reviews have been written concerning this fascinating subject.[10,11] Various and well-known pathogeneses are proposed as being most likely responsable for these WM changes. The unique pattern of blood supply to the WM which could be both a predisposing and a localizing factor is noticed firstly.[12] In addition, arteriolosclerosis in the hypertension, tortuosity, and elongation of these vessels in aging impair WM irrigation. In contrast, the U-fibers benefit from the distinctive arterial supply from the cortex and are spared in cases of ischemic leukoencephalopathies. In addition to an elevated blood pressure that does not exist in all symptomatic patients with LA,[13,14] a blood pressure dysregulation might also contribute to the pathogenesis of LA. Abnormal circadian rhythm and high blood pressure values are often observed in persons with LA compared to matched control subjects.[15,16] Another group of symptomatic patients with LA presents frequent hypotensive crises.[17,18] The general effect of blood pressure dysregulation is determined by the inability of sclerotic vessels either to dilate or to contract. There are no autoregulatory responses in the vessels. Evidently due to the WM blood pattern evocated in the first part, the decrease in blood flow is more prononced in the WM than in the gray matter. Interestingly, cerebral blood flow (CBF) studies showed whole brain or gray matter alterations in the CBF of patients with LA.[19,20] This point seems of great interest, since the vessel walls in these vascular pathologies are impaired as well in the gray matter as in the WM. A systematic ultrastructural study carried out with gray matter vessels and WM matter proved this (data not published). Similarly in CADASIL, we have intentionally shown vessel walls located within the gray matter and in the cerebellum as well as in the WM to demonstrate the gray and WM vessel involvement. The whole arterial tree (including arteries, arterioles, and capillaries) harbors VSMCs or pericytes; consequently, they unfortunately suffer from the same VSMC destruction. In the other vascular pathologies presenting with modifcation of the blood pressure, it is inconceivable that the complex alterations due to blood pressure dysregulation do not involve the first part of the WM blood supply, which is located in the gray matter. The histological descriptions were numerous, and the ultrastructural study was convincing. The unique difference is the formation of lacunes surrounding the vessel in the WM, which is so easy and obvious to observe, but with ultrastructural study the vessel walls are involved in the cortical gray matter as well as in the WM (data not published).

Another hypothesis about ischemia, which seems to be interrelated with the ischemic origine of LA, is the disturbances of cerebrospinal fluid (CSF).[21] Increased ventricular pressure may cause ischemic changes in the WM. This is supported by observations showing that among patients with normal pressure hydrocephalus, blood flow in the WM returns to normal after a shunting procedure that lowers the intraventricular pressure. This is accompanied with parallel clinical improvement and reduction in the severity of LA.[22] Finally, in hypertension the blood-brain barrier (BBB) may be leaky, and the capillary permeability to proteins may be increased in patients with systemic hypertension.[23] In addition to the effects of sustained hypertension, hypertensive bouts of short duration could cause fluid transudation and protein leakage.

The pathological research on the mechanismes for human leukoaraiosis up to now has been carried out on brain lesions observed after death. Previously, it was impossible to have an idea of the first vascular lesion leading to leukoaraiosis and to follow the evolution of the process. After death, the brain presents several intricate lesions, and we are unable to differentiate between the first vascular lesion, the lesions corresponding to a normal evolution or the lesions raised by the side effects of so many symptomatic drugs received by the patients.

In contrast, examination of the skin vessel walls in CADASIL and in other conditions leading to leukoaraiosis demonstrated that it is possible to observe various changes in peripheral vessel walls besides CADASIL. These changes, particularly observed in young patients, are so marked that it seems relevant to think that the brain vessels could also be involved in the same mechanisms.

Considering the different skin vessel wall lesions, we propose classifying them into two main types according to the presence or the destruction of the VSMCs. The

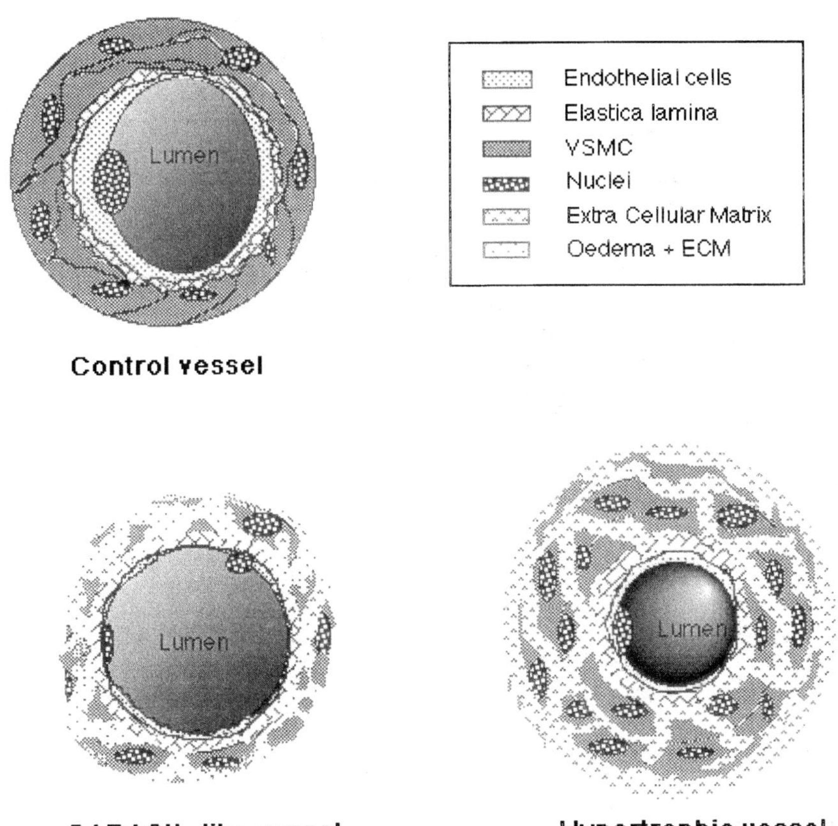

FIGURE 1. Schematic representation of the two main types of vessels observed in vascular subcortical dementia.

first type corresponds to a thickening of the vessel wall and narrowing of vascular lumen that we observe in Binswanger dementia or in the type with an increase in extracellular matrix without hypertension (FIG. 1). Hemodynamic troubles might be the first and major reason that the blood supply to the WM is altered (FIG. 2). The second type corresponds to a pseudothickening of the vessel wall, which becomes empty of VSMCs without a real increase in extracellular matrix as we saw in CADASIL and in the group of patient with VSMC fragmentation (FIG. 1). In this second type, we hypothesize that another mechanism might be involved (FIG. 2). The endothelial permeability primarily depends on vascular endothelial growth factor (VEGF) and histamine. In the brain, there are rare mast cells, and the histaminergic neurons are localized in the thalamomamillary tracts with a diffused distribution that may be involved during the evolution of the disease. VEGF is five hundred thousand

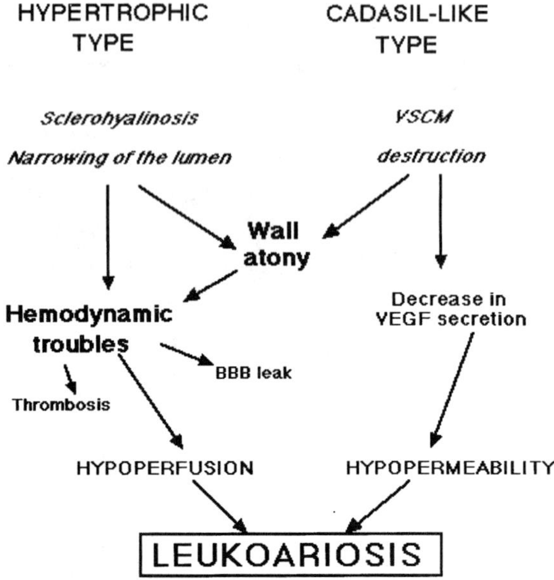

FIGURE 2. Proposed mechanisms for cerebral lesions according to their type of vascular changes.

times more potent than histamine. VEGF is first secreted by vascular VSMCs, and its receptors are localized on the endothelial cells.[24] During deep hypoxia, VEGF is also secreted by astrocytes. When we observed CADASIL vessel walls, we noticed that endothelial cells look modified and show changes that are likely to lead to a decrease in permeability.[25,26] In addition, the fragmentation and the general aspect of the VSMCs do not seem to be favorable to a normal secretion. Consequently, we suppose that the VSMC destruction leads first to an atony which might be the major cause of hemodynamic troubles and thrombosis in the capillary ends and secondly to a decrease in VEGF secretion leading to a decrease in endothelial permeability, which worsen the VSMC pathology.

CONCLUSION

In the field of CADASIL-like diseases associated with leukoaraiosis, the study of skin biopsies allows the diagnosis of CADASIL patients and individualization of several different types of vascular lesions during life and even early in life if we want it. As in CADASIL, the vessel lesions observed in the skin are probably nothing compared to the lesions of the brain vessels because of the blood-brain barrier endothelial cells. Up to now, the examination of vascular walls in vascular dementia has only been done with postmortem samples, and consequently old and new lesions were concerned. With this new approach, we are able to define which type of vessel lesion might be responsible for leukoaraiosis and then probably brain disease. Moreover, the identification of the different changes of skin vessel walls correlated with clinical symptoms and MRI features will provide further insight into the classification of subcortical vascular dementia that was proposed by Roman *et al.* in 1993.[1] According to either the presence or the absence of VSMCs within the vessel walls, continued research into the biochemical and physiological processes that cause subcortical vascular dementia will help us to understand the pathogenesis of this group of disorders, and this together with genetic research and the use of animal models may allow potential therapies to be designed.

ACKNOWLEDGMENTS

The authors thank the clinicians and neuropathologists who have kindly sent us excellent documents from numerous countries. They also thank Mmes. Limol, Henneron, Goetinck, and Delpierre for their technical and typing assistance. Financial support was received in part from a Lille University Hospital grant.

REFERENCES

1. ROMAN, G.C., T.K. TATEMICHI, T. ERKINJUNTTI, J.L. CUMMINGS, J.C. MASDEU, J.H. GARDIA, L. AMADUCCI, J.M. ORGOGOZO, A. BRUN, A. HOFMAN, D.M. MOODY, M.D. O'BRIEN, T. YAMAGUCHI, J. GRAFMAN, B.P. DRAYER, D.A. BENNETT, M. FISHER, J. OGATA, E. KOKMEN, F. BERMEJO, P.A. WOLF, P.B. GORELICK, K.L. BICK, A.K. PAJEAU, M.A. BELL, C. DE CARLI, A. CULEBRAS, A.D. KORCZYN, J. BOGOUSSLAVSKY, A. HARTMANN & P. SCHEINBERG. 1993. Vascular dementia: diagnostic criteria for research studies. Report on the NINDS-AIREN international workshop. Neurology **43:** 250–260.
2. TOURNIER-LASSERVE, E., A. JOUTEL, J. MEKLI, J. WEISSENBACH, G.M. LATHROP, H. CHABRIAT, J.L. MAS, E.A. CABANIS, M. BAUDRIMONT, J. MACIAZEK, M.A. BACH & M.G. BOUSSER. 1993. Cerebral autosomal dominant arteriopathy with subcortical infarcts and leukoencephalopathy maps, to chromosome 19q12. Nat. Genet. **3:** 256–259.
3. JOUTEL, A., C. CORPECHOT, A. DUCROS, K. VAHEDI, H. CHABRIAT, P. MOUTON, S. ALAMOWITCH, V. DOMENGA, M. CECILLION, E. MARECHAL, J. MACIAZEK, C. VAYSSIERE, D.C. CRUAU, E.A. CABANIS, M.M. RUCHOUX, J. WEUSSENBACH, J.F. BACH, M.G. BOUSSER & E. TOURNIER-LASSERVE. 1996. Notch 3 mutations in CADASIL, a hereditary adult-onset condition causing stroke and dementia. Nature **383:** 707–710.
4. ESTES, M.L., M.I. CHIMOWITZ, I.A. AWAD, J.T. MCMAHON, A.J. FURLAN & N.B. RATLIFF. 1991. Sclerosing vasculopathy of the central nervous system in nonelderly demented patients. Arch. Neurol. **48:** 631–636.
5. BAUDRIMONT, M., F. DUBAS, A. JOUTEL, E. TOURNIER-LASSERVE & M.G. BOUSSER. 1993. Autosomal dominant leucoencephalopathy and subcortical ischemic infarcts: a clinicopathological study. Stroke **24:** 122–125.
6. GUTIERREZ-MOLINA, M., A. CAMINERO-RODRIGUEZ, C. MARTINEZ-GARCIA, J. ARPA-GUTIERREZ, C. MORALES-BASTOS & G. AMER. 1994. Small arterial granular degeneration in familial Binswanger's syndrome. Acta Neuropathol. **87:** 98–105.
7. RUCHOUX, M.M., H. CHABRIAT, M.G. BOUSSER, M. BAUDRIMONT & E. TOURNIER-LASSERVE. 1994. Presence of ultrastructural arterial lesions in muscle and skin vessels of patient with CADASIL. Stroke **25:** 2291–2292.
8. RUCHOUX, M.M., D. GUEROUAOU, B. VANDENHAUTE, J.P. PRUVO, P. VERMERSCH & D. LEYS. 1995. Systemic vascular VSMC impairment in cerebral autosomal dominant arteriopathy with subcortical infarct and leucoencephalopathy. Acta Neuropathol. **89:** 500–512.

9. EBKE, M., M. DICHGANS, M. BERGMANN, H.U. VOELTER, P. RIEGER, T. GASSER & G. SCHWENDEMANN. 1997. CADASIL: skin biopsy allows diagnosis in early stages. Acta Neurol. Scand. **95:** 351–357.

10. PANTONI, L. & J.H. GARCIA. 1997. Pathogenesis of leukoaraiosis: a review. Stroke **28**(3): 652–659.

11. VAN GIJN, J. 1998. Leukoaraiosis and vascular dementia. Neurology **51**(Suppl. 3): S3–S8.

12. DE REUCK, J. 1971. The human periventricular arterial blood supply and the anatomy of cerebral infarctions. Eur. Neurol. **5:** 321–334.

13. IIJIMA, M., H. ISHINO, T. INGAKI & S. HARUKI. 1993. An autopsic case of Binswanger disease without hypertension and associated with cerebral infarction in the terminal stage. Jpn. J. Psychiatry Neurol. **47:** 901–907.

14. RÄIHÄ, I., S. TARVOREN, T. KURKI, T. RAJALA & L. SOURANDER. 1993. Relationship between vascular factors and white matter low attenuation of the brain. Acta Neurol. Scand. **87:** 286–289.

15. SHIMADA, K., A. KAWAMOTO, K. MATZUBAYASHI, M. NISHINAGA, S. KIMURA & T. OZAWA. 1992. Diurnal blood pressure variations and silent cerebrovascular damage in elderly patients with hypertension. J. Hypertens. **10:** 875–878.

16. TOHGI, H., K. CHIBA & M. KIMURA. 1991. Twenty-four-hour variation of blood pressure in vascular dementia of the Binswanger type. Stroke **22:** 603–608.

17. MCQUINN, B.A. & D.H. O'LEARY. 1987. White matter lucencies on computed tomography, subacute arteriosclerotic encephalopathy (Binswanger's disease), and blood pressure. Stroke **18:** 900–905.

18. HARRISON, M.J.G. & J. MARSHALL. 1984. Hypoperfusion in the etiology of subcortical arteriosclerotic encephalopathy (Binswanger type). J. Neurol. Neurosurg. Psychiatry **47:** 754.

19. FAZEKAS, F., K. NIEDERKORN, R. SCHMIDT, H. OFFENBACHER, S. HORNER, G. BERTHA & H. LECHNER. 1988. White matter signal abnormalities in normal individuals: correlation with carotid ultrasonography, cerebral blood flow measurements and cerebrovascular risk factors. Stroke **19:** 1285–1288.

20. SULZER, D.L., M.E. MAHLER, J.L. CUMMINGS, W.G. VAN GORP, C.H. HINKIN & C. BROWN. 1995. Cortical abnormalities associated with subcortical lesions in vascular dementia: clinical and positron emission tomographic findings. Arch. Neurol. **52:** 773–780.

21. ROMAN, G.C. 1991. White matter lesions and normal-pressure hydrocephalus: Binswanger's disease or Hakim syndrome? Am. J. Neuroradiol. **12:** 40–41.

22. KIMURA, M., A. TANAKA & S. YOSHINAGA. 1992. Significance of periventricular hemodynamics in normal pressure hydrocephalus. Neurosurgery **30:** 701–705.

23. NAG, S. 1984. Cerebral changes in chronic hypertension: combined permeability and immunohistochemical studies. Acta Neuropathol. (Berl.) **62:** 178–184.

24. FERRARA, N., J. WINER & T. BURTON. 1991. Aortic VSMCs express and secrete vascular endothelial growth factor. Growth Factors **5:** 141–148.

25. RUCHOUX, M.M. & C.A. MAURAGE. 1997. Endothelial changes in muscle and skin biopsies in patients with CADASIL. Neuropathol. Appl. Neurobiol. **23:** 60–65.

26. RUCHOUX, M.M. & C.A. MAURAGE. 1998. CADASIL: cerebral autosomal dominant arteriopathy with subcortical infarcts and leukoencephalopathy. J. Neuropathol. Exp. Neurol. **56**(9): 947–964.

Hereditary Vascular Dementia Linked to Notch 3 Mutations

CADASIL in British Families

N.J. THOMAS,[a] C.M. MORRIS,[a] F. SCARAVILLI,[b] J. JOHANSSON,[b]
M. ROSSOR,[b] R. DE LANGE,[c] D. ST CLAIR,[c] J. NICOLL,[d] C. BLANK,[a]
A. COULTHARD,[a] K. BUSHBY,[a] P.G. INCE,[a] D. BURN,[a] AND R.N. KALARIA[a,e]

[a]*Institute for the Health of the Elderly, University of Newcastle,
Newcastle upon Tyne, United Kingdom*

[b]*Institute of Neurology, Queen Square, London, United Kingdom*

[c]*University of Aberdeen, Aberdeen, United Kingdom*

[d]*University of Glasgow, Glasgow, United Kingdom*

ABSTRACT: The most common form of familial vascular dementia is considered
to be CADASIL or cerebral autosomal dominant arteriopathy with subcortical
infarcts and leukoencephalopathy, which is now also increasingly manifest in
the United Kingdom. CADASIL has been previously dubbed as a familial form
of Binswanger disease. However, unlike in Binswanger disease CADASIL does
not involve hypertension or other risk factors associated with cardiovascular
disease. CADASIL appears to be essentially a disorder of the arteries that is
linked to single missense mutations in the *NOTCH* 3 gene locus on chromosome 19. The pathogenesis of the disorder or the genetic mechanism leading to
brain infarcts and dementia is not known. The elucidation of the microvascular
pathology evident in CADASIL may be an interesting way to delineate effects
of defective genes on brain cells from systemic vascular influences.

INTRODUCTION

The second most common cause of dementing illness in the elderly is designated
to cerebrovascular disease. How does cerebrovascular disease cause cognitive disability or dementia? Current studies show that several chromosome loci or genes are
linked to disorders involving cerebrovascular disease or stroke. The hereditary cerebral amyloid angiopathies which invariably result in strokes and hemorrhagic
infarcts have increased our knowledge on the biology of the genes and their products
such as the gamma trace and amyloid precursor proteins.[1,2] Similarly, it is recognized that genetic mutations or polymorphisms involved in other brain vascular disorders such as cavernous angiomas and hypertensive encephalopathies will no doubt
be applicable in evaluating genetic factors and the pathogenesis of cerebrovascular
disease. In light of this, the elucidation of the pathogenesis of cerebral autosomal

[e]Address for correspondence: Prof. R.N. Kalaria, CBV Group, Wolfson Research Centre,
Institute for the Health of the Elderly, Newcastle General Hospital, Westgate Road, Newcastle
upon Tyne NE4 6BE, UK. Tel.: (0191) 273 8811; fax: (0191) 272-5291.
e-mail: r.n.kalaria@ncl.ac.uk

dominant arteriopathy with subcortical infarcts and leukoencephalopathy (CADASIL) will be important to understand the primary vascular mechanisms that lead to ischemic blood flow and its consequences on neuronal vulnerability.

CADASIL is an autosomal dominantly inherited disorder that has been linked to single missense mutations in the *NOTCH* 3 gene.[3,4] CADASIL and its close variants consistently presenting with recurrent strokes and progressive dementia likely exist in over 250 families worldwide including Western Europe, the Americas, Japan, Australia, the Caribbean, and North Africa.[5–16] Prevalence rates of CADASIL yet remain to be determined. The earlier studies did not confirm CADASIL by screening the then unknown *NOTCH* 3 gene, but recent reports have established these suspected cases were indeed *bona fide* CADASIL.[6–8] In the United Kingdom, we are aware of several families and individuals with CADASIL. While many of these are currently under genetic scrutiny we have clinical and pathological assessments on cases from Aberdeen, Bristol, Glasgow, London, Oxford, and Newcastle. Here, we review progress and consider some of our interests in the genetics and microvascular pathology of a disorder apparently not influenced by risks factors for cardiovascular disease or stroke.

LEUKOENCEPHALOPATHIES, FEATURES OF CADASIL, AND BRAIN IMAGING

Hereditary forms of leukoencephalopathies similar to Binswanger disease[17] as well as other familial variants have previously been described.[18–20] These disorders exhibit autosomal dominant dementia, profound white matter lesions, and small arterial granular degeneration. However, they do not appear to be linked to the *NOTCH* 3 type of CADASIL strongly implying that a non-*NOTCH* type of CADASIL or its variant may exist. The first cases of hereditary multiinfarct dementia (MID) were described in a family living in Sweden by Sourander and Walinder.[21] The cerebrovascular pathology described by Olsson and colleagues[22] is essentially similar to CADASIL, but this Swedish disorder has not yet been genetically confirmed as the *NOTCH* 3 type (Kalaria *et al.*, unpublished observations). However, it is expected that the recognition of CADASIL will increase steadily.

Current trends reveal that CADASIL appears to be far more common than previously perceived. It may be overlooked and possibly misdiagnosed, because the phenotype of CADASIL can bear considerable variability.[5,6,23,24] It is characterized by the remarkable absence of identifiable risk factors for cerebrovascular disease such as hypertension or hypercholesterolemia. Even in British patients the average age of onset for CADASIL is 45 years.[5] The disorder is invariably preceded by a history of severe headaches leading to migraine, followed by recurrent subcortical lacunar infarcts, signs of mood disorder in the form of depression, and cognitive disabilities. Neocortical strokes are rare and if they occur they usually do not cover a wide territory. The described features collectively lead to a rapidly progressing dementia, which appears severely manifest in the older patients. It is likely that other modifying factors either epigenetic or genetic contribute to the phenotypic variations in age at onset, number of cerebrovascular incidents, degree of dementia, and general morbidity. While these variable features seem unlikely to be due to an incomplete penetrance of the defective gene, the presence of migraine with visual aura in CADASIL along with a history of recurrent strokes are critical for the differential diagnosis of the disorder and distinguish CADASIL from multiple sclerosis, atypical Alzheimer's disease, and Binswanger disease, which also exhibit white matter abnormalities upon magnetic resonance imaging.

Magnetic resonance images reveal profound hyperintensities as white matter lesions and periventricular abnormalities in the basal ganglia, thalamus, and external capsules.[25–28] Our recent investigation of a large family from northeast England with confirmed exon 4 mutation (R153C) has revealed profound hyperintensities in the deep white matter in affected patients compared to the unaffecteds.[28] These lesions also observed in the corpus callosum appear secondary to small vessel disease.[28] The hypersignals interpreted as ischemic infarcts, lacunes, and a diffuse leukoencephalopathy increase exponentially after the age of 40.[29] Ventricular dilatation similar to that seen in Alzheimer's and Binswanger diseases is not usually evident in CADASIL.

MICROVASCULAR PATHOLOGY

Although abnormalities appear in blood vessels of peripheral tissues[30,31] CADASIL bears distinct brain microvascular pathology. At autopsy the brain almost always shows multiple infarcts, lacunes and regions of edema and myelin damage.[12] While we have noted cerebral atrophy upon brain imaging[28] cerebral atrophy at autopsy has been described in some cases but not widely confirmed.[30] The arteriopathy is in many ways different from the vascular lesions in other cerebral degenerative diseases currently under intense study. Our observations based on brain tissue from a few cases and those of others show the absence of cerebral amyloid angiopathy or evident accumulation of amyloid fibrils in CADASIL. However, unlike amyloid angiopathy where the extracellular matrix is profoundly disrupted, in CADASIL the lumen of the microvessels is consistently narrowed with considerable eosinophilic deposits in the medial sheath and accompaniment of profound intimal thickening.[6] Despite the notable degeneration of arterial smooth muscle cells, hemorrhages seem rare in CADASIL. This was also testified in the brains we have examined. The perivascular fibrosis and intimal thickening presumably fortify and reseal the vessel wall preventing breakdown or indiscriminate leakage of the lumen contents.

Analyses of serial sections from brains of our CADASIL patients obtained at autopsy and by biopsy indicate marked degeneration and paucity of vascular smooth muscle cells in both the adventitial and medial layers. This was preceded by prominent discontinuity and disruption of the layering of smooth muscle cells as revealed by disarray and depletion of α-actin immunoreactivity in vascular smooth cells within the medial layers. We have also observed endothelial abnormalities and blebbing that was evident by immunostaining with antibodies to the glucose transporter. In a large proportion of the vessels (40%) destruction of the walls was marked by the deposition of diffuse ubiquitin reactivity, which was seldom seen over cells. The muscular and endothelial abnormalities in cerebral vessels in both the subcortical grey and white matter would predictably result in breach of the barrier properties, and severe repercussions on cerebral blood flow particularly in the arteries and arterioles supplying the white matter. Such profound ischemic blood flow would undoubtedly contribute to the characteristic neurological sequelae of CADASIL. The extracellular deposits found in cerebral as well as vessels of peripheral tissues constitute granular osmiophilic material. However, we have observed more amorphous material in brain biopsies.[6] Evidence from electron microscopy suggests that these 1–2 nm densities largely restricted to arterial vessels are secreted by smooth muscle cells. The nature of granular or amorphous material is not known. Whether these contain components of the basement membrane and secretions or products of disordered or prematurely dying smooth muscle cells bearing the mutant Notch 3 protein fragments is yet to be known.[30] The cerebrospinal fluid (CSF) from CADASIL patients reveals oligoclonal bands, but these seem undistinguishable from those in other disorders. However, there may be important CSF proteins[32] that may underlie key features of the pathogenesis.

NOTCH 3 MUTATIONS IN BRITISH FAMILIES

Our French colleagues suggest that the inheritance patterns of CADASIL in an autosomal dominant manner may not be obvious. More than 80% of the identified familial cases with atypical headache or stroke in young adults were thought to be sporadic. Current observations reveal that CADASIL may occur in multiple generations involving large pedigrees with a male to female ratio of 1 among the probands.[4] Affected members of several French families have shown to bear single missense mutations in the *NOTCH* 3 gene pathogenically linked to the disease condition.[33] A large number of the mutations is clustered in exon 4 of the gene that encodes one of the 34 epidermal growth factor (EGF) repeat domains in the extracellular arm of the protein. Like others[5,7,9,13] we also confirm such clustering in six British families to date. While the majority of the mutations in the British families[15,16] are in exons 4 and 5 of *NOTCH* 3 we have recently identified a new mutation in exon 8 of the gene that involves an arginine to cysteine change (R449C) at codon 449. This patient presented with severe neurological symptoms, and memory lapses had marked small vessel disease and white matter ischemia.[6] As in the French families polymorphisms[33] were also evident in the British families, but it is unclear how these substitutions relate to phenotype.[34]

The strong coexpression of Notch 3 and the presenilins in the adult CNS and vascular smooth muscle cells (T. Mizuno and R. Kalaria, unpublished observations) secondary to development suggests an essential role for Notch 3 in a different capacity such as programmed cell death. The repeat EGF domains in the extracellular arm and other conserved motifs including the cysteine-rich regions located immediately downstream may be negatively or positively regulated by various ligands at the cell surface. That the 34 EGF repeats in Notch 3 each bear about 40 residues implies that the spatial arrangement of the repeats is vital to its function of ligand binding and protein-protein interactions. Similar to our experience most *NOTCH* 3 mutations result in a change to or from a cysteine residue suggesting occurrence of highly specified genetic events[34] and implicating changes in activation of the receptor protein by disruption of the nuclear translocation of the intracellular carboxyl-terminal fragment and its interaction with a delta, serrate, or line ligand. Given that the *NOTCH* signaling pathway may strongly interact with the presenilins associated with familial Alzheimer's disease it is likely that interest in this order will grow considerably.[35] The elucidation of these issues and the vascular pathology will not only provide further understanding of this devastating vascular disease afflicting the young and old but also knowledge of the Notch receptor and its interaction with related cell signaling systems in brain vascular cells. CADASIL has important relevance not only to cerebrovascular disorders leading to stroke or dementing disorders in the elderly but also to Alzheimer's disease where impaired cerebral blood flow encroaches upon cognitive function.

ACKNOWLEDGMENTS

The work was supported by a Zenith Award from the National Alzheimer's Association, Chicago, USA, and grants from the NINDS (NIH) and UK MRC.

REFERENCES

1. PREMKUMAR, D.L., D. COHEN, R.P. FRIEDLAND *et al.* 1996. Apolipoprotein E ε4 alleles in cerebral amyloid angiopathy and cerebrovascular pathology in Alzheimer's disease. Am. J. Pathol. **148:** 2083–2095.
2. KALARIA, R.N. 1996. Cerebral vessels in ageing and Alzheimer's disease. Pharmacol. Ther. **72:** 193–214.
3. TOURNIER-LASSERVE, E., A. JOUTEL, J. MELKI *et al.* 1993. Cerebral autosomal dominant arteriopathy with subcortical infarcts and leukoencephalopathy maps to chromosome 19q12. Nat. Genet. **3:** 256–259.
4. JOUTEL, A., C. CORPECHOT, A. DUCROS *et al.* 1996. Notch 3 mutations in CADASIL, a hereditary adult-onset condition causing stroke and dementia. Nature **383:** 707–710.
5. CHABRIAT, H., K. VAHEDI, M.T. IBA-ZIZEN *et al.* 1995. Clinical spectrum of CADASIL: a study of 7 families. Lancet **346:** 934–939.
6. LAMMIE, G.A., J. RAKSHI, M.N. ROSSOR *et al.* 1995. Cerebral autosomal dominant arteriopathy with subcortical infarcts and leukoencephalopathy (CADASIL)—confirmation by cerebral biopsy in 2 cases. Clin. Neuropathol. **14:** 201–206.
7. BERGMANN, M., M. EBKE, Y. YUAN *et al.* 1996. Cerebral autosomal dominant arteriopathy with subcortical infarcts and leukoencephalopathy (CADASIL): a morphological study of a German family. Acta Neuropathol. **92:** 341–350.
8. HEDERA. P. & R.P. FREIDLAND. 1997. CADASIL: study of two American families with predominant dementia. J. Neurol. Sci. **146:** 27–33.
9. DESMOND, D.W., J.T. MORONEY, T. LYNCH *et al.* 1998. CADASIL in a North American family: clinical, pathologic, and radiologic findings. Neurology **51:** 844–899.
10. CARONTI, B., L. CALANDRIELLO, A. FRANCIA *et al.* 1998. Cerebral autosomal dominant arteriopathy with subcortical infarcts and leucoencephalopathy (CADASIL). Neuropathological and *in vitro* studies of abnormal elastogenesis. Acta Neurol. Scand. **98:** 259–267.
11. DICHGANS, M., M. MAYER, I. UTTNER *et al.* 1998. The phenotypic spectrum of CADASIL: clinical findings in 102 cases. Ann. Neurol. **44:** 731–739.
12. KALIMO, H., M. VIITANEN, K. AMBERLA *et al.* 1999. CADASIL: hereditary disease of the arteries causing brain infarcts and dementia. Neuropathol. Appl. Neurobiol. **25:** 257–265.
13. OBERSTEIN, S.A., M.D. FERRARI, E. BAKKER *et al.* 1999. Diagnostic Notch 3 sequence analysis in CADASIL: three new mutations in Dutch patients. Neurology **52:** 1913–1915.
14. KAMIMURA, K., K. TAKAHASHI, E. UYAMA *et al.* 1999. Identification of a Notch 3 mutation in a Japanese CADASIL family. Cerebral autosomal dominant arteriopathy with subcortical infarcts and leukoencephalopathy. Alzheimer Dis. Assoc. Disord. **13:** 222–225.

15. BLANK, C., R. LYALL, K.M.D. BUSHBY *et al.* 2000. CADASIL in a British family: a multidisciplinary approach with NOTCH 3 mutation analysis. Brain. Submitted.

16. DE LANGE, R.P.J., J. BOLT, C. SCHANEN *et al.* 1999. Screening British CADASIL families for mutations in NOTCH 3 gene. J. Med. Genet. In press.

17. ROMAN, G.C. 1999. New insight into Binswanger disease. Arch. Neurol. **56:** 1061–1062.

18. FUKUTAKE, T. 1999. Young-adult-onset hereditary subcortical vascular dementia: cerebral autosomal recessive arteriosclerosis with subcortical infarcts and leukoencephalopathy. Rinsho Shinkeigaku **39:** 50–52.

19. UTATSU, Y., H. TAKASHIMA, K. MICHIZONO *et al.* 1997. Autosomal dominant early onset dementia and leukoencephalopathy in a Japanese family: clinical neuroimaging and genetic studies. J. Neurol. Sci. **147:** 55–62.

20. JEN, J., A.H. COHEN, Q. YUE *et al.* 1997. Hereditary endotheliopathy with retinopathy, nephropathy, and stroke (HERNS). Neurology **49:** 1322–1330.

21. SOURANDER, P. & J. WALINDER. 1977. Hereditary multi-infarct dementia. Acta Neuropathol. **39:** 247–254.

22. ZHANG, H., P. SOURANDER & Y. OLSSON. 1994. The microvascular changes in cases of hereditary multi-infarct disease of the brain. Acta Neuropathol. **87:** 317–324.

23. DESMOND, D.W., J.T. MORONEY, T. LYNCH *et al.* 1999. The natural history of CADASIL. A pooled analysis of previously published cases. Stroke **30:** 1230–1233.

24. MALANDRINI, A., P. CARRERA, G. CIACCI *et al.* 1997. Unusual clinical features and early brain MRI lesions in a family with cerebral autosomal dominant arteriopathy. Neurology **48:** 1200–1203.

25. CHABRIAT, H., C. LEVY, H. TAILLIA *et al.* 1998. Patterns of MRI lesions in CADASIL. Neurology **51:** 452–457.

26. YOUSRY, T.A., K. SEELOS, M. MAYER *et al.* 1999. Characteristic MR lesion pattern and correlation of T1 and T2 lesion volume with neurologic and neuropsychological findings in cerebral autosomal dominant arteriopathy with subcortical infarcts and leukoencephalopathy (CADASIL). Am. J. Neuroradiol. **20:** 91–100.

27. DICHGANS, M., M. FILIPPI, R. BRUNING *et al.* 1999. Quantitative MRI in CADASIL: correlation with disability and cognitive performance. Neurology **52:** 1361–1367.

28. COULTHARD, A., S.C. BLANK, K.M.D. BUSHBY *et al.* 1999. Distribution of cranial MRI abnormalities in patients with symptomatic and subclinical CADASIL. Br. J. Radiol. In press.

29. FILLEY, C.M., L.L. THOMPSON, C.I. SZE *et al.* 1999. White matter dementia in CADASIL. J. Neurol. Sci. **163:** 163–167.

30. RUCHOUX, M.M. & E. MAURAGE. 1997. Review on CADASIL. J. Neuropathol. Exp. Neurol. **56:** 947–964.

31. RUCHOUX, M.M., H. CHABRIAT, M.G. BOUSSER *et al.* 1994. Presence of ultrastructural arterial lesions in muscle and skin vessels of patients with CADASIL. Stroke **25:** 2291–2292.

32. DICHGANS, M., M. WICK & T. GASSER. 1999. Cerebrospinal fluid findings in CADASIL. Neurology **39:** 110–112.

33. JOUTEL, A., K. VAHEDI, C. CORPECHOT *et al.* 1997. Strong clustering and stereotyped nature of Notch 3 mutations in CADASIL patients. Lancet **350:** 1511–1515.

34. JOUTEL, A. & E. TOURNIER-LASSERVE. 1998. Notch signalling pathway and human diseases. Semin. Cell Dev. Biol. **9:** 619–625.

35. RAY, W.J., M. YAO, P. NOWOTNY *et al.* 1999. Evidence for a physical interaction between presenilin and Notch. Proc. Natl. Acad. Sci. USA **96:** 3263–3268.

Linear Relation between Cerebral Phosphocreatine Concentration and Memory Capacities during Permanent Brain Vessel Occlusions in Rats

KONSTANZE PLASCHKE,[a] SEONG-WOOK YUN,[b] EIKE MARTIN,[a] SIEGFRIED HOYER,[b] AND HUBERT J. BARDENHEUER[a,c]

[a]Anesthesiology Clinic, and [b]Department of Pathochemistry and General Neurochemistry, University of Heidelberg, Germany

ABSTRACT: The present study investigates the interrelation between cerebral energy state and memory capacities in a rat model of stepwise cerebral vessel occlusions. After acute and subchronic permanent vessel occlusions, cortical energy metabolites (ATP, phosphocreatine, ADP, AMP) were detected by high-pressure liquid chromatography (HPLC) analysis, and the effects on learning, memory, and cognitive behavior were evaluated using a holeboard test. The results of the study demonstrated a drastic decrease in energy-rich phosphates by 33% for phosphocreatine and by 44% for ATP after acute vessel occlusions. In addition, rat working and reference memories were strikingly decreased to about 5% of controls. In contrast, two weeks after four-vessel occlusion, the energy state was almost completely restored to control levels. However, a significant decrease in memory capacities was observed in subchronic state. In summary, this study has demonstrated a close linear relationship ($p < 0.001$) between an impaired cerebral energy state and brain memory dysfunction after acute and permanent cerebral four-vessel occlusion. Thus, this animal model of stepwise reduction of the cerebral blood supply may reflect some clinically relevant processes occurring during cerebrovascular and neurodegenerative diseases.

Chronic, progressive, age-related dementias are characterized by decreased brain glucose and oxygen metabolism.[1] Energy-rich compounds are essential to maintain cellular structure and cellular functions. The reduced availability of energy-rich phosphates, and in particular of phosphocreatine (PCr), reduces cellular function and subsequently cellular integrity.[2] Thus, when the energy state of the brain is compromised, long-lasting disturbances in brain function may develop.

In the past, animal models of either acute incomplete or acute complete cerebral ischemia have been used to investigate the interrelation between disturbances in

[c]Address for correspondence: Prof. Dr. med. H.J. Bardenheuer, Anesthesiology Clinic, University of Heidelberg, Im Neuenheimer Feld 110, D-69120 Heidelberg, Germany. Tel.: 49-6221-568263; fax: 49-6221-565531.

e-mail: hubert_bardenheuer@med.uni-heidelberg.de

brain circulation and morphologic and metabolic abnormalities.[3,4] In a few chronic studies only, a permanent hypoperfusion was induced to produce a state approximating vascular-type dementia with resulting cholinergic dysfunction and discrimination learning deficits.[4,10,12] Thus far, no detailed studies are available on the effect of graded cerebral ischemia on cerebral energy metabolism and its relationship to learning and memory abilities in permanent ischemia. It was, therefore, our intention to study the effects of reduction in brain energy metabolism on rat behavior, with the aim of establishing a long-term alteration in the cerebrovascular system, which might adequately reflect disturbances related to cerebrovascular and neurodegenerative diseases.

METHODS

Animal Procedure

Sixty one-year-old male Wistar rats (breeder: Centre d'Elevage R. Janvier, France) weighing 450–660 g were housed in a temperature-controlled animal room with a reversed 12 h : 12 h light/dark cycle. All animals underwent psychometric testing with handling three times within 5 days. During the habituation and training periods and 2 days before retest, food restriction (5 g/day) was imposed to enhance the motivation of rats to perform the holeboard tests. Three rats died in the course of the operation for vessel occlusion. After a handling and training period, rats were divided into two subgroups with 30 rats each for biochemical and psychometric testing. Each subgroup was divided into three smaller groups ($n = 10$ each): controls (**A**), rats subjected to acute (**B**), and to long-term (**C**) brain-vessel occlusion.

Experimental scheme for stepwise brain vessel occlusion (vo):

```
       ∇        ∇∇
  B: |------------|⇓

       ∇        ∇∇
  C: |------------||------------||------------ |⇓
     1st week   2nd week   3rd week
```

∇: occlusion of *A.vertebralis dextra* and *A. carotis comm. sinistra;*
∇∇: occlusion of *A. vertebralis sinistra* and *A. carotis comm. dextra;*
⇓: steady state experiment.

Vessel Occlusions

Forty adult male Wistar rats underwent stepwise and crosswise occlusion of the common carotid arteries by ligation, and the vertebral arteries by electrocoagulation, as previously described[8] for acute ($n = 20$) and chronic ($n = 20$) ischemic studies. Corresponding control groups of adult rats for acute ($n = 10$) and long-term ($n = 10$) experiments underwent surgical intervention without vessel occlusions.

Holeboard Test

Habituation, training, and retests for memory measurements were performed in a holeboard box as described in detail by Lannert and Hoyer.[9] Working and reference memories were calculated according to van der Staay *et al.*[13]

Steady-State Experiment

Animals were kept under general anesthesia induced by 0.5 vol% halothane and nitrous oxide/oxygen (70:30) to obtain cerebral tissue samples for biochemical analysis of high-energy phosphates. After tracheotomy, rats were artificially ventilated during muscle relaxation with pancuronium bromide (2 mg/kg body weight), and a 20-min steady state of arterial normotension, normocapnia, normoxemia, and normothermia was established. Thereafter, the brains were frozen *in situ* by means of liquid nitrogen poured into a skin funnel formed from the sagittally incised galea. The animals were decapitated, the brains were chiseled out of the skulls under liquid nitrogen and stored at −80°C. The cerebral parietotemporal cortex was prepared at −20°C.

Energy-rich Phosphates

Tissue samples for biochemical analyses were obtained after 20 min of hemodynamic steady state immediately after acute and permanent four-vessel occlusion.

Adenosine 5′-triphosphate, adenosine 5′-diphosphate, adenosine 5′-monophosphate, PCr, and adenosine were determined by high-pressure liquid chromatography (HPLC) analysis after disruption of brain cell membranes with an ultraturrax in a chloroform–acetic acid mixture (1:2) at −20°C, as previously described.[8]

Statistical Analysis

Statistical analysis was performed by ANOVA following the post hoc Tukey test for biochemical analysis. To compare the effects of permanent vessel occlusions on psychometric parameters with those of the related acute experiments, the Mann-Whitney U test was used. Data in the tables and figures are expressed as means ± SD and means ± SEM, respectively. Significant differences were assumed at $p < 0.05$. Linear correlation was analyzed according to the Pearson correlation coefficient using the SPSS statistic program; the coefficient was considered significant at $p < 0.001$.

RESULTS

Energy State

As shown in TABLE 1, the concentration of energy-rich phosphates is striklingly decreased after acute cerebral vessel occlusion by 33% for PCr and by 44% for ATP, respectively. In contrast, cortical AMP was increased fivefold, and adenosine was enhanced from 4.75 ± 0.9 to 35.37 ± 5.67 nmol/g.

After two weeks of permanent four-vessel occlusion, the concentration of energy metabolites in rat cerebral cortex was almost completely restored to control levels.

TABLE 1. Effect of brain vessel occlusion on cortical energy state in adult rat brain

μmol/g	Sham	Vessel Occlusion	
		Acute	Permanent
PCr	6.52 ± 1.24	1.99 ± 1.45	5.01 ± 0.65[a,b]
ATP	2.38 ± 0.39	1.70 ± 0.55	2.16 ± 0.15[a]
ADP	0.48 ± 0.09	0.31 ± 0.17	0.33 ± 0.08[a]
AMP	0.01 ± 0.01	0.05 ± 0.03	0.02 ± 0.01[a]

NOTE: The data are shown as mean ± SD, $n = 10$ per group. Significant differences ($p < 0.05$) between the following groups are determined by ANOVA following the Tukey test: (a) sham vs. acute; (b) sham vs. permanent.

Memory Capacities

All animals improved their abilities in learning, memory, and cognition after a 7-day training period. Acute vessel occlusion severely decreased working and reference memories (FIG. 1A and B). The partial improvement in brain energy metabolism was accompanied by a relative improvement in memory capacities, although both functional parameters remained lower than in the control experiments.

Correlation

The data of the present study demonstrate a linear relationship ($p < 0.001$) between cortical PCr concentration and working memory (FIG. 2A) as well as reference memory (FIG. 2B); the correlation coefficients of both were calculated as $r = 0.849$ and $r = 0.765$, respectively, after acute and permanent brain vessel occlusions in rats.

DISCUSSION

During acute ischemia, ATP metabolism is upset because the energy stores in the tissue are rapidly depleted at a rate determined by (i) the metabolic activity of the tissue, (ii) its capacity for anaerobic energy production, and (iii) by the availability of substrates that can by metabolized anaerobically. Consequently, there was a significant fall in the concentrations of ATP and PCr in the parietotemporal cerebral cortex, resulting in a reduction of the energy load by more than 50%. Acute impairment of tissue oxygenation following four-vessel occlusion was associated with a tremendous increase in the cortical concentration of adenosine. In this way, adenosine fulfils an important regulatory role as an ischemic marker during acute cerebral ischemia.

In rats with permanent four-vessel occlusion, the concentrations of energy-rich phosphates exhibited a tendency toward near-complete restoration. Several compensatory mechanisms might be responsible for the improvement in the brain energy metabolism during permanent vessel occlusion. On the one hand, pronounced vasodilation of cerebral arteries can occur to improve cerebral blood flow, thereby preserving energy metabolites.[11] On the other hand, recruitment of preexisting

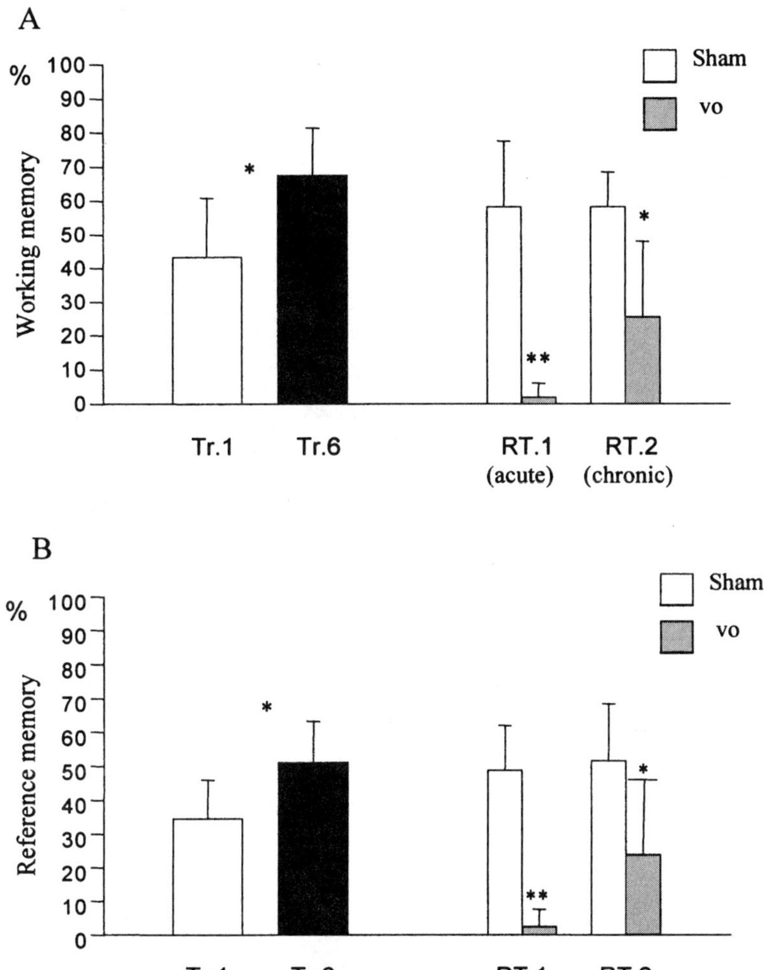

FIGURE 1. Effect of permanent vessel occlusion on working (**A**) and reference (**B**) memories. The rats were trained (Tr.) six times before operation (*gray bars*). After sham operation and four-vessel occlusion, the memory capacities were measured in the acute (RT.1) and chronic (RT.2) state. $^*p < 0.05$; $^{**}p < 0.001$ (retest 1 vs. retest 2); vo, vessel occlusion.

collaterals can improve cerebral perfusion. Coyle and Panzerbeck[12] reported enhanced collateral circulation in the ipsilateral hemisphere within six weeks after unilateral carotid artery ligation. In addition, using an arteriovenous fistula model Sekhon *et al.*[4] described enhanced capillary density as a result of neovascularization in response to chronic cerebral ischemia. Moreover, because the rat anatomy pro-

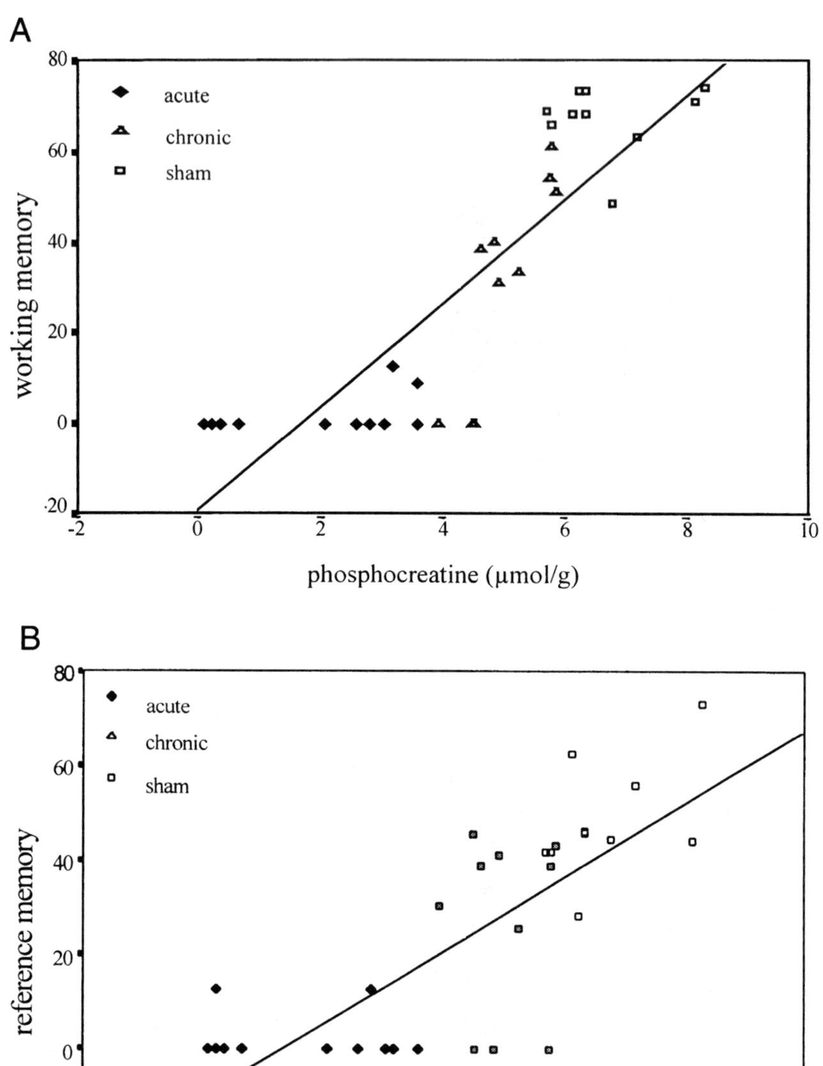

FIGURE 2. Interrelation between rat memory capacities and cortical phosphocreatine concentration. Linear correlation coefficient was according to Pearson ($n = 30$ animals) and was calculated as $r = 0.849$ for working memory (**A**) and $r = 0.765$ for reference memory (**B**) in cerebral cortex ($p < 0.001$).

vides a well-developed spinal circulation,[13] it is likely that the significant improvement in cerebral energy metabolism is caused by adaptive processes of collateral circulation after permanent four-vessel occlusion.

In parallel with the severe reduction in brain-energy metabolism, complex cerebral functions had significantly deteriorated after acute vessel occlusion (−95%). Although memory capacities did not reach the preoperative conditions seen in trained rats, the increase in energy load during permanent vessel occlusion was associated with significant increases in both memory capacities. These data indicate that such cerebral functions, which are characterized by a high degree of complexity, improved over time despite permanent cerebral hypoperfusion.

In the present study, under conditions of permanent brain ischemia, a close relationship was obtained between the cortical PCr concentration on the one side, and working and reference memories on the other. Interestingly, the rank order of statistical significance of the relation between memory capacities and energy compounds was generally higher in the case of PCr and follows the sequence: working memory > reference memory ≫ locomotor activity (data not shown). These data can be interpreted to mean that brain activities with higher functional complexity necessarily require an intact cerebral energy metabolism.

In summary, this study has demonstrated a close correlation between an impaired cerebral energy state and brain memory dysfunction after acute and permanent cerebral four-vessel occlusion. Thus, this occlusion model of stepwise reduction of the cerebral blood supply may reflect some clinically relevant processes occurring during cerebrovascular and neurodegenerative diseases. Furthermore, this rat model might be suited to characterize new strategies in neuroprotective targeting to enhance cerebral energy metabolism after global cerebral hypoperfusion.

REFERENCES

1. SWERDLOW, R., D.L. MARCUS, J. LANDMAN, D. KOOBY, W. FREY & M.L. FREEDMAN. 1994. Brain glucose metabolism in Alzheimer's disease. Am. J. Med. Sci. **308:** 141–144.
2. BUTTGEREIT, F. & M.D. BRAND. 1995. A hierarchy of ATP-consuming process in mammalian cells. Biochem. J. **312:** 163–167.
3. NI, J.W., K. MATSUMOTO, H.B. LI, Y. MARAKAMI & H. WATANABE. 1995. Neuronal damage and decrease of central acetylcholine level following permanent occlusion of bilateral common carotid arteries in rat. Brain Res. **673:** 290–296.
4. SEKHON, L.H.S., M.K. MORGAN, I. SPENCE & N.C. WEBER. 1994. Chronic cerebral hypoperfusion and impaired neuronal function in rats. Stroke **25:** 1022–1027.
5. DE LA TORRE, J.C., A. CADA, N. NELSON, G. DAVIS, R.J. SUTHERLAND & F. GONZALEZ-LIMA. 1997. Reduced cytochromoxidase and memory dysfunction after chronic brain ischemia in aged rats. Neurosci. Lett. **223:** 165–168.
6. SEKHON, L.H., M.K. MORGAN & I. SPENCE. 1997. Normal perfusion pressure breakthrough: the role of capillaries. J. Neurochem. **86:** 519–524.
7. TANAKA, K., N. OGAWA, M. ASANUMA, Y. KONDO & M. NOMURA. 1996. Relationship between cholinergic dysfunction and discrimination learning disabilities in Wistar rats following chronic cerebral hypoperfusion. Brain Res. **729:** 55–65.
8. PLASCHKE, K., H.J. BARDENHEUER, M.A. WEIGAND, E. MARTIN & S. HOYER. 1998. Increased ATP production during long-term brain ischemia in rats in the presence of propentofylline. Eur. J. Pharmacol. **349:** 33–40.
9. LANNERT, H. & S. HOYER. 1998. Intracerebroventricular administration of streptozotocin causes long-term diminutions in learning and memory abilities and in cerebral energy metabolism in adult rats. Behav. Neurosci. **112:** 1199–1208.

10. VAN DER STAAY, F.J., J. VAN NIESAND & W. RAAIJMAKERS. 1990. The effects of aging in rats on working and reference memory performance in a spatial holeboard discrimination task. Behav. Neural Biol. **53:** 356–370.

11. BRONNER, G., K. MITCHELL & F.A. WELSH. 1998. Cerebrovascular adaption after unilateral carotid artery ligation in th rat: preservation of blood flow and ATP during forebrain ischemia. J. Cereb. Blood Flow Metab. **18:** 118–121.

12. COYLE, P. & M.J. PANZENBECK. 1990. Collateral development after artery occlusion in Fisher 344 rats. Stroke **21:** 316–321.

13. EKLÖF, B. & B.K. SIESJÖ. 1972. The effect of bilateral carotid ligation upon the blood flow and energy state of the rat brain. Acta Physiol. Scand. **86:** 155–165.

Mechanisms of Cerebrovascular Amyloid Deposition

Lessons from Mouse Models

PATRICK BURGERMEISTER, MICHAEL E. CALHOUN, DAVID T. WINKLER, AND MATHIAS JUCKER[a]

Department of Neuropathology, Institute of Pathology, University of Basel, CH-4003 Basel, Switzerland

ABSTRACT: Cerebrovascular deposition of amyloid is a frequent observation in Alzheimer's disease patients. It can also be detected sporadically in normal aged individuals and is further found in familial diseases linked to specific gene mutations. The source and mechanism of this pathology are still unknown. It has been suggested that amyloidogenic proteins are derived from blood, the vessel wall itself, or from the central nervous system. In this article evidence is reviewed for and against each of these hypotheses, including new data obtained from transgenic mouse models. In APP23 transgenic mice that develop cerebral amyloid angiopathy (CAA) in addition to amyloid plaques, the transport and drainage of neuronally produced amyloid-β (Aβ) seem to be responsible for CAA rather than vascular Aβ production or blood uptake. Although a number of mechanisms may contribute to CAA in humans, these results suggest that a neuronal source of Aβ is sufficient to induce vascular amyloid deposition. The possibility to cross genetically defined mouse models of CAA with other mutant mice now has the potential to identify molecular mechanisms of CAA.

INTRODUCTION

Cerebral amyloid angiopathy of the amyloid-β type (Aβ-CAA) occurs sporadically in the elderly and can be detected in up to 90% of patients with Alzheimer's disease (AD).[1,2] Aβ-CAA affects primarily leptomeningeal and cortical vessels and is associated with degeneration of smooth muscle cells, pericytes, endothelial cells, and blood-brain barrier (BBB) damage.[1,3] Severe Aβ-CAA can cause fatal cerebral hemorrhage and increases the risk of cerebral microinfarcts.[1,4,5] In normal aging and AD, Aβ-CAA occurs in conjunction with parenchymal Aβ plaques. However, Aβ-CAA can also occur in the absence of amyloid plaques. For example, patients with hereditary cerebral hemorrhage with amyloidosis-Dutch type (HCHWA-D), an autosomal dominant severe form of Aβ-CAA caused by a point mutation at codon 693 of the β-amyloid precursor protein (APP), exhibit very few amyloid plaques.[6]

Although the most common form of cerebrovascular amyloid is Aβ-CAA, there are other proteins that have been linked to familial forms of CAA. Hereditary cere-

[a]Address for correspondence: Mathias Jucker, Ph.D., Neuropathology, Institute of Pathology, University of Basel, Schönbeinstrasse 40, CH-4003 Basel, Switzerland. Tel.: 41-61-265 2894; fax: 41-61-265 3194

e-mail: mjucker@uhbs.ch

bral hemorrhage with amyloidosis-Iceland type (HCHWA-I) is caused by a mutation in the cystatin C gene (ACys-CAA), and leads to dementia and severe, early-onset hemorrhage.[7,8] A familial British dementia with CAA (ABri-CAA) is caused by a mutation in the *BRI* gene, and notably is also characterized by parenchymal ABri deposits.[9] In addition, familial CAA has been linked to specific mutations in prion protein, gelsolin, and transthyretin.[10–14]

The origin and mechanism of cerebral amyloid deposition remains puzzling. APP, cystatin C, BRI, prion protein, gelsolin, and transthyretin are biochemically different proteins with expression in many tissues, including brain.[7–9,11,12,15,16] Most of these proteins and/or their amyloidogenic fragments can also be detected in cerebrospinal fluid (CSF) and blood. Thus, a common denominator responsible for their predominant brain-specific deposition is likely.

A long-held hypothesis suggests that amyloidogenic proteins circulate in blood, pass through the vascular endothelium and get deposited in the vessel wall. Alternatively, a local production of amyloid by vascular smooth muscle cells, pericytes and/ or perivascular microglia has been suggested. A more recent hypothesis follows the idea that amyloid has its origin in the central nervous system (CNS) and that drainage and transport mechanisms may play a role in cerebrovascular amyloid. By far, the most research in terms of mechanisms has been done for Aβ-CAA. Thus, in the following report, we focus on Aβ-CAA and summarize some arguments in favor and against these three mechanistic hypotheses.

The Blood Hypothesis

APP is expressed in megakaryocytes and is present in platelets.[17] In blood, Aβ is found in concentrations of 0.3–0.9 ng/ml.[18–20] Evidence exists that circulating Aβ can damage the endothelium and compromise BBB function.[21] Leakage of BBB may then allow increased amounts of Aβ to pass from the blood into the vessel wall. This BBB leakage is consistent with the frequent finding of serum proteins, such as amyloid P-component, associated with cerebrovascular amyloid.[1,22]

The hematogenous origin of amyloid has gained some attention from studies of peripheral injections of Aβ in blood. After intra-arterial infusion with [^{125}I]Aβ in squirrel monkeys, essentially every existing amyloid deposit was also labeled by [^{125}I]Aβ.[23] Further study in a similar infusion model indicated increased BBB permeability and accumulation of Aβ in the vessel wall in the presence of significant amounts of CAA.[24] The uptake of Aβ from the blood has also been shown to be very efficient, suggestive of a receptor-mediated process.[25,26] These observations have sustained the hypothesis that blood-borne amyloid is the cause of Aβ-CAA (TABLE 1).

The blood hypothesis, however, fails to explain why deposition of Aβ occurs exclusively in brain. Patients with systemic amyloidosis of the AA- and AL-type show some vascular amyloid in choroid plexus, infundibulum, area postrema, pineal body, and subfornical organ.[27] This distribution corresponds to areas with incomplete BBB, consistent with a hematogenic origin of AA and AL.[27] This pattern, however, is different from that in Aβ-CAA where mainly cortical and leptomeningeal vessels are affected.

An argument often used against the hematogenous hypothesis is the observation that the Aβ concentration in brain and CSF are significantly higher than in blood (see below). However, a recent study using chromatographic separation of plasma pro-

TABLE 1. Hematogenous origin

In Favor of Hematogenous Origin	Against Hematogenous Origin
Aβ is found in blood	Circulating Aß does not easily explain exclusive cerebral deposition
Aβ injected in blood is transported through the BBB	Blood Aß is relatively low compared to CNS Aβ
Other amyloidoses are caused by a blood-borne precursor protein	First occurrence of Aß in abluminal part of vessel wall

teins followed by Aβ quantification suggests a previously unrecognized pool of Aβ bound to plasma proteins in blood which is 100 times more than previously suggested.[28] Moreover, the same study suggests that $A\beta_{1-42}$ in blood of AD patients is significantly higher than in controls. However, the large pool of bound Aβ in blood may have a much lower BBB transport rate than free or injected Aβ.[29]

A further argument against the blood hypothesis is the finding that the first detectable amyloid deposits in the vessel wall are confined to the abluminal basement membrane.[30,31] This observation is not easily explained with a blood origin of Aβ unless one assumes significant differences among endothelial, smooth muscle, and parenchymal basement membranes, which would cause the transported Aβ to accumulate in the outer basement membrane. Although there are molecular differences among vessel basement membranes (e.g., in laminin subunit composition[32]), it is not clear whether these differences are significant in terms of Aβ sequestration.

The Vessel Wall Hypothesis

Smooth muscle cells, endothelial cells, pericytes, and perivascular microglia are all intimately associated with the deposition of cerebrovascular amyloid, raising the possibility that Aβ is locally produced and deposited (TABLE 2). Aβ production has been demonstrated in isolated brain microvessels and meningeal vessels, and APP is expressed in smooth muscle cells, pericytes, and endothelial cells.[33–36] Moreover, degenerating smooth muscle cells and pericytes overproduce Aβ and have been implicated in the deposition and progression of cerebrovascular amyloid.[34,35,37–39]

A local production of Aβ by smooth muscle cells would explain the predilection of arteries compared to veins[31,38] and the observation that CAA occurs most often in vessels outside the CNS parenchyma proper, i.e., pia, fissures. A local production of amyloid in the vessel wall is also consistent with the infiltration of fine radiating amyloid fibrils into the neuropil in more advanced stages of CAA (dyshoric amyloid). Finally, it has elegantly been shown that amyloid fibrils assemble on the surface of vascular smooth muscle cells supporting a role of smooth muscle cells in cerebrovascular amyloidosis.[40]

However, if Aβ is produced locally by the vascular smooth muscle cells, it is not clear why amyloid deposition is restricted to cortical and leptomeningeal vessels and not to all vessels with smooth muscle cells.[41] An explanation for this might be differences in APP processing between leptomeningeal/cortical smooth muscle cells and other arterial smooth muscle cells.[42] However, the observation that larger arteries that have several layers of smooth muscle cells are in fact less affected than smaller arteries does not support a primary role of smooth muscle cells.[31]

TABLE 2. Vessel wall origin

In Favor of Vessel Wall Origin	Against Vessel Wall Origin
Production of Aβ by vascular cells	Extracranial arteries are not affected
Smooth muscle origin explains predilection for arterioles/arteries compared to veins	Smooth muscle cell origin does not explain amyloid in capillary and predilection for smaller arteries compared to large arteries
Amyloid fibrils assemble on smooth muscle cell surface	

The initial observation that cerebrovascular amyloid consists of $A\beta_{1-39}$[43] and thus is different from the plaque amyloid has sustained the hypothesis that CAA is an independent and local process within the vasculature. However, later studies have not confirmed these findings and report chemical similarities between vascular and plaque amyloid with $A\beta_{1-40}$ being the major component of CAA.[44,45]

The Drainage Hypothesis

This hypothesis suggests that Aβ is produced in the CNS and drains with the brain interstitial fluid (ISF) along perivascular spaces surrounding intracortical and leptomeningeal arteries, finally reaching the cervical lymph nodes and the venous circulation.[31] It is suggested that amyloid fibrils begin to accumulate and that deposition of Aβ along this drainage pathway is the major contributor to CAA.[31] Age-related pathological changes such as thickening of the vascular basement membrane, atherosclerosis, and hypertension could comprise the normal flow of ISF and thus lead to Aβ accumulation. The hypothesis explains CAA localization to the adventitia and outermost smooth muscle basement membrane, the site of the putative periarterial ISF drainage pathway. It also provides an explanation why arteries are affected and not veins, and why Aβ deposition is specific to the brain (TABLE 3). To date, however, the drainage of Aβ along this pathway has been a subject of debate. The experimental evidence thus far has been limited to an anatomical description of the pathway using the injection of nonphysiological tracers (e.g., India ink).

TABLE 3. ISF drainage hypothesis

In Favor of ISF Drainage Hypothesis	Against ISF Drainage Hypothesis
Selectivity for arteries versus veins	Experimental support still lacking
First deposits in abluminal vessel wall	
High levels of Aβ in CSF	
Regional distribution of CAA	

LESSONS FROM TRANSGENIC MOUSE MODELS

Aβ-CAA occurs naturally in some dogs and monkeys, but has not been observed in rodents.[46] In addition, co-deposition of Aβ and cystatin C has been reported in aged monkeys with significant cerebrovascular amyloid.[47] Because mouse models of amyloidogenesis offer distinct advantages to study CAA pathogenesis, transgenic mice overexpressing a variety of wild-type and mutant APP constructs have been produced. Although early studies did not reproduce amyloid pathology because transgene expression levels were not high enough, more recent efforts have succeeded in producing mice that develop cerebral β-amyloidosis, including Aβ-CAA, as they age (see below). No transgenic mouse models of CAA other than of the Aβ-type have yet been reported.

Mouse Models of Aβ-CAA

Games and collaborators[48] generated transgenic mice with a platelet-derived growth factor-β chain (PDGF) promoter to drive the expression of a human APP minigene encoding the V717F mutation linked to familial AD. These PDAPP mice express human APP on a mixed genetic background at levels four to six times the endogenous APP levels found in mice or humans.[49] At 6–8 months of age, the mice develop amyloid plaques, which are composed mainly of Aβ_{1-42}.[50] No significant amount of vascular amyloid has been reported in these mice. The same construct was later used to produce transgenic mice on a B6D2 background.[51] Consistently, these mice also developed parenchymal amyloid plaques with little cerebrovascular amyloid deposition. Interestingly, however, when these mice were crossed with transgenic mice overexpressing TGFβ1, vascular amyloid was present even in young mice with no concomitant acceleration of parenchymal plaque formation.[52] TGFβ1 increases production of basement membrane proteins, which can act as seeds for amyloid deposition.[30,53,54] Thus, increased CAA in TGFβ1 $\times$ APP transgenic mice may be the result of increased Aβ seeding. Alternatively, a thickened basement membrane has been described in TGFβ1 transgenic mice[55] and may compromise periarterial ISF drainage and thus accelerate Aβ accumulation around the vessels.[31]

Hsiao and collaborators[56] and Stürchler-Pierrat and colleagues[57] overexpressed human APP with the Swedish double mutation (K670N, M671L). Hsiao and collaborators used a prion protein promoter and expressed the APP$_{695}$-isoform in B6SJL mice (Tg2576 mice), while Stürchler-Pierrat and colleagues used a Thy-1 promoter element and expressed the APP$_{751}$-isoform in B6D2 mice (APP23 mice). Both transgenic lines develop cerebral amyloidosis with onset at 11 and 6 months for Tg2576 and APP23, respectively. This difference in onset may at least partly be a reflection of the level of human APP expression which, in Tg2576 mice, is five to six times, and in APP23 mice, at least seven times APP levels of wild-type mice.[56,57]

An interesting difference between Tg2576 and APP23 mice appears to be the development of CAA. Although cerebrovascular amyloid deposition in vessels has been noted in Tg2576 mice,[58] it is not a prominent feature of this transgenic mouse model. In contrast, a significant amount of cerebrovascular amyloid has been reported in APP23 mice.[59] CAA in APP23 mice is very similar to that found in human aging and in AD. Many vessels were affected with arterioles and capillaries showing the earliest and most severe deposits. Initial deposition was noted in the outer vessel wall. CAA in APP23 mice was associated with local neuron loss, synaptic alterations, microglia activation, and microhemorrhage.[59] The reason for the significant occurrence of CAA in APP23 mice and the relatively rare occurrence in Tg2576

TABLE 4. Aβ in body fluids of humans and APP transgenic mice

	Plasma Aβ (ng/ml)	CSF Aβ (ng/ml)	CAA
Humans[18–20,62,63]	0.3–0.9[a]	2.5–16	frequently
Tg mouse[61]	9.6	N/A	no
Tg mouse[60]	30	N/A	no
APP23 tg mice[59]	<5	40	yes

[a]A recent study[28] suggests a previously unrecognized pool of Aβ bound to plasma proteins in blood which is 100 times more than reported here.

mice is not clear. Expression levels and genetic background of the transgenic lines may be important.

The presence of CAA in APP23 mice is particularly interesting because of the brain and neuron-specific Thy-1 promoter element used to express human APP.[59] This suggests that a neuronal source of APP is sufficient to induce cerebrovascular amyloid deposition in these mice. This conclusion is further substantiated by the finding that APP23 mice on an *App*-null background develop a similar degree of CAA, demonstrating that endogenous mouse Aβ and smooth muscle cell APP production are not necessary for cerebrovascular amyloid deposition in these mice.[59]

Further clues regarding the mechanism of deposition come from the analysis of human Aβ levels CSF and blood plasma of APP23 mice. Results revealed about 10 times higher human Aβ levels in mouse CSF compared to Aβ levels in CSF of normal human subjects and patients with AD. In contrast, only trace amounts of human Aβ were found in the blood of APP23 mice.[59] This finding is interesting in light of two previously established transgenic mouse lines that show exceptionally high levels of Aβ in the plasma (TABLE 4), but do not develop CAA.[60,61] Both of these mouse lines overexpress the C-terminal 99-amino-acid of human APP under the control of a cytomegalovirus enhancer/chick β-actin promoter. These results argue against a hematogenous origin of cerebrovascular amyloid in the APP23 mice.

The ISF drainage hypothesis of Weller and colleagues[31,64] could provide an explanation for CAA in APP23 mice. Aβ released from neurons into the ISF may drain along periarterial spaces into the cervical lymph nodes or may diffuse first into the CSF and then drain along the same pathway. Along this drainage pathway, Aβ then begins to accumulate and forms cerebrovascular amyloid. The preferential localization of CAA in APP23 mice is similar to the vessels implicated in ISF drainage pathway—the arterioles supplying regions with the highest levels of APP production (neocortex and adjacent regions) are affected. Although the blood supply to the thalamus (which also shows significant CAA in APP23 mice) is not derived from regions of high APP expression, corticothalamic axonal transport and release of Aβ is a possible mechanism by which Aβ reaches the thalamus before draining along the thalamic arteries.[59]

CONCLUSION AND OUTLOOK

A number of mechanisms may contribute to CAA in humans, and the mechanisms may be different from those seen in APP overexpressing transgenic mice. Nevertheless, APP transgenic mouse models provide strong evidence for a predominant neuronal origin of cerebrovascular Aβ. Moreover, from the study of such mouse models, Aβ transport and drainage along the perivascular space have been suggested as mechanisms of CAA. Smooth muscle cells and other vascular components may play an important role in Aβ sequestration and fibril formation.[3,40,65]

It is tempting to speculate that mechanisms of ACys-CAA and ABri-CAA, as well as the other rarer forms of CAA (see above), are similar to mechanisms of Aβ-CAA. For most of these amyloid proteins or precursors, a neuronal expression and/ or high CSF levels have been demonstrated. Unfortunately, no transgenic mouse models of CAA other than the Aβ-type have yet been reported; several groups, however, have recently succeeded in producing cystatin C and BRI transgenic mice, which now await analysis as they age. To further understand the mechanisms and significance of Aβ-CAA, it will also be important to study mouse models with Aβ-CAA in the absence of amyloid plaques. To this end we have recently produced new APP transgenic mice harboring the HCHWA-D mutation.

Last, but not least, to study the mechanism of CAA at the molecular level, it will be crucial to crossbreed mouse models of CAA with transgenic or null mice of putative risk factors for CAA. Breeding of TGFβ1 transgenic mice with APP transgenic mice has already identified TGFβ1 as a putative risk factor for Aβ-CAA. Overall, we believe that the further analysis and development of transgenic mouse models of CAA will provide the tools to advance the study of the pathopsyphysiology and significance of CAA.

ACKNOWLEDGMENTS

We are grateful to D. Abramowski, A. Phinney, A. Probst, B. Sommer, M. Stalder, M. Staufenbiel, C. Stürchler-Pierrat, M. Tolnay, and K.-H. Wiederhold for experimental help and comments on this manuscript. This work was supported by grants from the Swiss National Foundation, Roche Foundation, A&D-Foundation of the Swiss Academy of Medical Sciences, and the Fritz Thyssen Foundation.

REFERENCES

1. VINTERS, H.V. 1987. Cerebral amyloid angiopathy. A critical review. Stroke **18:** 311–324.
2. YAMADA, M. *et al.* 1987. Cerebral amyloid angiopathy in the aged. J. Neurol. **234:** 371–376.
3. KALARIA, R.N. 1996. Cerebral vessels in ageing and Alzheimer's disease. Pharmacol. Ther. **72:** 193–214.
4. VONSATTEL, J.P. *et al.* 1991. Cerebral amyloid angiopathy without and with cerebral hemorrhages: a comparative histological study. Ann. Neurol. **30:** 637–649.
5. ITOH, Y. *et al.* 1993. Cerebral amyloid angiopathy: a significant cause of cerebellar as well as lobar cerebral hemorrhage in the elderly. J. Neurol. Sci. **116:** 135–141.
6. LEVY, E. *et al.* 1990. Mutation of the Alzheimer's disease amyloid gene in hereditary cerebral hemorrhage, Dutch type. Science **248:** 1124–1126.
7. GHISO, J. *et al.* 1986. Amyloid fibrils in hereditary cerebral hemorrhage with amyloidosis of Icelandic type is a variant of γ-trace basic protein (cystatin C). Proc. Natl. Acad. Sci. USA **83:** 2974–2978.
8. ABRAHAMSON, M. *et al.* 1990. Structure and expression of the human cystatin C gene. Biochem. J. **268:** 287–294.
9. VIDAL, R. *et al.* 1999. A stop-codon mutation in the *BRI* gene associated with familial British dementia. Nature **399:** 776–781.

10. HALTIA, M. *et al.* 1990. Amyloid in familial amyloidosis, Finnish type, is antigenically and structurally related to gelsolin. Am. J. Pathol. **136:** 1223–1228.

11. KIURU, S. *et al.* 1999. Gelsolin-related spinal and cerebral amyloid angiopathy. Ann. Neurol. **45:** 305–311.

12. PETERSEN, R.B. *et al.* 1997. Transthyretin amyloidosis: a new mutation associated with dementia. Ann. Neurol. **41:** 307–313.

13. VIDAL, R. *et al.* 1996. Meningocerebrovascular amyloidosis associated with a novel transthyretin mis-sense mutation at codon 18 (TTRD186). Am. J. Pathol. **148:** 361–366.

14. GHETTI, B. *et al.* 1996. Vascular variant of prion protein cerebral amyloidosis with tau-positive neurofibrillary tangles: the phenotype of the stop codon 145 mutation in PRNP. Proc. Natl. Acad. Sci. USA **93:** 744–748.

15. SELKOE, D.J. 1994. Normal and abnormal biology of the β-amyloid precursor protein. Annu. Rev. Neurosci. **17:** 489–517.

16. RAEBER, A.J. *et al.* 1998. Transgenic and knockout mice in research on prion diseases. Brain Pathol. **8:** 715–733.

17. GARDELLA, J.E. *et al.* 1992. Characterization of Alzheimer amyloid precursor protein transcripts in platelets and megakarocytes. Neurosci. Lett. **138:** 229–232.

18. SEUBERT, P. *et al.* 1992. Isolation and quantification of soluble Alzheimer's β-peptide from biological fluids. Nature **359:** 325–327.

19. IDA, N. *et al.* 1996. Analysis of heterogeneous βA4 peptides in human cerebrospinal fluid and blood by a newly developed sensitive Western blot assay. J. Biol. Chem. **271:** 22908–22914.

20. SCHEUNER, D. *et al.* 1996. Secreted amyloid β-protein similar to that in the senile plaques of Alzheimer's disease is increased in *vivo* by the presenilin 1 and 2 and APP mutations linked to familial Alzheimer's disease. Nature Med. **2:** 864–870.

21. THOMAS, T. *et al.* 1997. *In vivo* vascular damage, leukocyte activation and inflammatory response induced by β-amyloid. J. Submicrosc. Cytol. Pathol. **29:** 293–304.

22. VERBEEK, M.M. *et al.* 1998. Distribution of A beta-associated proteins in cerebrovascular amyloid of Alzheimer's disease. Acta Neuropathol. (Berl.) **96:** 628–636.

23. GHILARDI, J.R. *et al.* 1996. Intra-arterial infusion of $[^{125}I]A\beta_{1-40}$ labels amyloid deposits in the aged primate brain *in vivo*. Neuroreport **7:** 2607–2611.

24. MACKIC, J.B. *et al.* 1998. Cerebrovascular accumulation and increased blood-brain barrier permeability to circulating Alzheimer's amyloid beta peptide in aged squirrel monkey with cerebral amyloid angiopathy. J. Neurochem. **70:** 210–215.

25. PODUSLO, J.F. *et al.* 1997. Permeability and residual plasma volume of human, Dutch variant, and rat amyloid β-protein 1–40 at the blood-brain barrier. Neurobiol. Dis. **4:** 27–34.

26. MACKIC, J.B. *et al.* 1998. Human blood-brain barrier receptors for Alzheimer's amyloid-β_{1-40}. J. Clin. Invest. **102:** 734–743.

27. SCHRÖDER, R. & R.P. LINKE. 1999. Cerebrovascular involvement in systemic AA and AL amyloidosis: a clear haematogenic pattern. Virchows Arch. **434:** 551–560.

28. KUO, Y.M. *et al.* 1999. High levels of circulating Aβ42 are sequestered by plasma proteins in Alzheimer's disease. Biochem. Biophys. Res. Commun. **257:** 787–791.

29. SHAYO, M. *et al.* 1997. The putative blood-brain barrier transporter for the beta-amyloid binding protein apolipoprotein J is saturated at physiological concentrations. Life Sci. **60:** 115–118.

30. YAMAGUCHI, H. *et al.* 1992. Beta amyloid is focally deposited within the outer basement membrane in the amyloid angiopathy of Alzheimer's disease. An immunoelectron microscopic study. Am. J. Pathol. **141:** 249–259.

31. WELLER, R.O. *et al.* 1998. Cerebral amyloid angiopathy: Amyloid β accumulates in putative interstitial fluid drainage pathways in Alzheimer's disease. Am. J. Pathol. **153:** 725–733.

32. TIAN, M. *et al.* 1996. Dystroglycan in the cerebellum is a laminin α2-chain binding protein at the glial-vascular interface and is expressed in Purkinje cells. Eur. J. Neurosci. **8:** 2739–2747.

33. KALARIA, R.N. *et al.* 1996. Production and increased detection of amyloid β protein and amyloidogenic fragments in brain microvessels, meningeal vessels and choroid plexus in Alzheimer's disease. Brain Res. Mol. Brain Res. **35:** 58–68.

34. VERBEEK, M.M. *et al.* 1997. Rapid degeneration of cultured human brain pericytes by amyloid β protein. J. Neurochem. **68:** 1135–1141.
35. WISNIEWSKI, H.M. & J. WEGIEL. 1994. β-amyloid formation by myocytes of leptomeningeal vessels. Acta Neuropathol. **87:** 233–241.
36. NATTE, R. *et al.* 1999. Amyloid β precursor protein-mRNA is expressed throughout cerebral vessel walls. Brain Res. **828:** 179–183.
37. KAWAI, M. *et al.* 1993. Degeneration of vascular muscle cells in cerebral amyloid angiopathy of Alzheimer disease. Brain Res. **623:** 142–146.
38. WISNIEWSKI, H.M. *et al.* 1994. Vascular β-amyloid in Alzheimer's disease angiopathy is produced by proliferating and degenerating smooth muscle cells. Amyloid: Int. J. Exp. Clin. Invest. **1:** 8–16.
39. DAVIS-SALINAS, J. *et al.* 1995. Amyloid β-protein induces its own production in cultured degenerating cerebrovascular smooth muscle cells. J. Neurochem. **65:** 931–934.
40. VAN NOSTRAND, W.E. *et al.* 1998. Pathologic amyloid β-protein cell surface fibril assembly on cultured human cerebrovascular smooth muscle cells. J. Neurochem. **70:** 216–223.
41. SHINKAI, Y. *et al.* 1995. Amyloid β-proteins 1–40 and 1–42(43) in the soluble fraction of extra- and intracranial blood vessels. Ann. Neurol. **38:** 421–428.
42. VAN NOSTRAND, W.E. *et al.* 1994. Amyloid β-protein precursor in cultured leptomeningeal smooth muscle cells. Amyloid: Int. J. Exp. Clin. Invest. **1:** 1–7.
43. PRELLI, F. *et al.* 1988. Differences between vascular and plaque core amyloid in Alzheimer's disease. Neurochemistry **51:** 648–651.
44. ROHER, A.E. *et al.* 1993. β-Amyloid-(1–42) is a major component of cerebrovascular amyloid deposits: implications for the pathology of Alzheimer disease. Proc. Natl. Acad. Sci. USA **90:** 10836–10840.
45. VERBEEK, M.M. *et al.* 1997. Differences between the pathogenesis of senile plaques and congophilic angiopathy in Alzheimer disease. J. Neuropathol. Exp. Neurol. **56:** 751–761.
46. WALKER, L.C. 1997. Animal models of cerebral β-amyloid angiopathy. Brain Res. Brain Res. Rev. **25:** 70–84.
47. WEI, L.H. *et al.* 1996. Cystatin C: Iceland-like mutation in an animal model of cerebrovascular β-amyloidosis. Stroke **27:** 2080–2085.
48. GAMES, D. *et al.* 1995. Alzheimer-type neuropathology in transgenic mice overexpressing V717F β-amyloid precursor protein. Nature **373:** 523–527.
49. ROCKENSTEIN, E.M. *et al.* 1995. Levels and alternative splicing of amyloid β protein precursor (APP) transcripts in brains of APP transgenic mice and humans with Alzheimer's disease. J. Biol. Chem. **47:** 28257–28267.
50. JOHNSON-WOOD, K. *et al.* 1997. Amyloid precursor protein processing and Aβ$_{42}$ deposition in a transgenic mouse model of Alzheimer disease. Proc. Natl. Acad. Sci. USA **94:** 1550–1555.
51. HSIA, A.Y. *et al.* 1999. Plaque-independent disruption of neural circuits in Alzheimer's disease mouse models. Proc. Natl. Acad. Sci. USA **96:** 3228–3233.
52. WYSS-CORAY, T. *et al.* 1997. Amyloidogenic role of cytokine TGF-β1 in transgenic mice and in Alzheimer's disease. Nature **389:** 603–606.
53. SNOW, A.D. *et al.* 1994. An important role of heparan sulfate proteoglycan (perlecan) in a model system for the deposition and persistence of fibrillar Aβ-amyloid in rat brain. Neuron **12:** 219–234.
54. NARINDRASORASAK, S. *et al.* 1995. An interaction between the basement membrane and Alzheimer precursor proteins suggests a role in the pathogenesis of Alzheimer's disease. Lab. Invest. **72:** 272–282.
55. WYSS-CORAY, T. *et al.* 1995. Increased central nervous system production of extracellular matrix components and development of hydrocephalus in transgenic mice overexpressing transforming growth factor β1. Am. J. Pathol. **147:** 53–67.
56. HSIAO, K. *et al.* 1996. Correlative memory deficits, Aβ elevation, and amyloid plaques in transgenic mice. Science **274:** 99–102.
57. STÜRCHLER-PIERRAT, C. *et al.* 1997. Two amyloid precursor protein transgenic mouse models with Alzheimer disease-like pathology. Proc. Natl. Acad. Sci. USA **94:** 13287–13292.

58. WALKER, L.C. *et al.* 1999. Cerebrovascular amyloidosis: experimental analysis *in vitro* and *in vivo*. Histol. Histopathol. **14:** 827–837.
59. CALHOUN, M.E. *et al.* 1999. Neuronal overexpression of mutant amyloid precursor protein results in prominent deposition of cerebrovascular amyloid. Proc. Natl. Acad. Sci. USA **96:** 14088–14093.
60. KAWARABAYASHI, T. *et al.* 1996. Accumulation of beta-amyloid fibrils in pancreas of transgenic mice. Neurobiol. Aging **17:** 215–222.
61. FUKUCHI, K. *et al.* 1996. High levels of circulating β-amyloid peptide do not cause cerebral β-amyloidosis in transgenic mice. Am. J. Pathol. **149:** 219–227.
62. NAKAMURA, T. *et al.* 1994. Amyloid β protein levels in cerebrospinal fluid are elevated in early-onset Alzheimer's disease. Ann. Neurol. **36:** 903–911.
63. NITSCH, R.M. *et al.* 1995. Cerebrospinal fluid levels of amyloid β-protein in Alzheimer's disease: inverse correlation with severity of dementia and effect of apolipoprotein E genotype. Ann. Neurol. **37:** 512–518.
64. WELLER, R.O. 1998. Pathology of cerebrospinal fluid and interstitial fluid of the CNS: significance for Alzheimer disease, prion disorders and multiple sclerosis. J. Neuropathol. Exp. Neurol. **57:** 885–894.
65. URMONEIT, B. *et al.* 1997. Cerebrovascular smooth muscle cells internalize Alzheimer amyloid beta protein via a lipoprotein pathway: implications for cerebral amyloid angiopathy. Lab. Invest. **77:** 157–166.

Alzheimer's Disease–like Cerebrovascular Pathology in Transforming Growth Factor-β1 Transgenic Mice and Functional Metabolic Correlates

T. WYSS-CORAY,[a,b,e] C. LIN,[a] D. VON EUW,[c] E. MASLIAH,[d] L. MUCKE,[a,b] AND P. LACOMBE[c]

[a]*Gladstone Institute of Neurological Disease and* [b]*Department of Neurology, University of California, San Francisco, California 94141, USA*

[c]*Laboratoires de Recherches Cérébrovasculaires, Centre Nationale de la Recherche Scientifique, UPR 646, Paris, France*

[d]*Departments of Neurosciences and Pathology, University of California at San Diego, La Jolla, California 92093, USA*

ABSTRACT: Alzheimer's disease (AD) is frequently associated with cerebrovascular changes, including perivascular astrocytosis, amyloid deposition, and microvascular degeneration, but it is not known whether these pathological changes contribute to functional deficits in AD. To characterize the temporal relationship between amyloid deposition, cerebrovascular abnormalities, and potential functional changes, we studied transgenic mice that express transforming growth factor-β1 (TGF-β1) at low levels in astrocytes. TGF-β1 induced a prominent perivascular astrocytosis, followed by the accumulation of basement membrane proteins in microvessels, thickening of capillary basement membranes, and later, around 6 months of age, deposition of amyloid in cerebral blood vessels. At 9 months of age, various AD-like degenerative alterations were observed in endothelial cells and pericytes. Associated with these morphological changes were changes in regional cerebral glucose utilization. Preliminary results showed that TGF-β1 mice had significantly decreased glucose utilization in the mammillary bodies, structures involved in mnemonic and learning processes. Glucose utilization tended to be decreased in several other brain regions as well; however, in the inferior colliculus, it was markedly higher in TGF-β1 mice than in controls. We conclude that chronic overproduction of TGF-β1 triggers a pathogenic cascade leading to AD-like cerebrovascular amyloidosis, microvascular degeneration, and local alterations in brain metabolic activity. Similar mechanisms may be involved in AD pathogenesis.

INTRODUCTION

The central nervous system (CNS) requires an efficient vasculature to supply metabolic substrates to brain cells. A decrease in cerebrovascular function could reduce brain perfusion, limit the metabolic rate, and impair cognitive abilities. In Alzheimer's

[e]Address for correspondence: Dr. Tony Wyss-Coray, Gladstone Institute of Neurological Disease, P.O. Box 419100, San Francisco, CA 94141-9100. Tel.: (415) 826-7500; fax: (415) 826-6541.
e-mail: twysscoray@gladstone.ucsf.edu

disease (AD), progressive dementia is accompanied both by neurodegenerative changes and distinct cerebrovascular abnormalities (for review, see Refs. 1–4) and by functional impairments of cerebral blood flow and glucose utilization.[5–7]

The most apparent cerebrovascular change in AD is cerebral amyloid angiopathy (CAA), the deposition of amyloid-β peptide (Aβ) in cerebral blood vessel walls. Found in most AD cases, CAA is in its severest forms also a major cause of normotensive intracerebral hemorrhage in the elderly.[8–11] AD and CAA are associated with other changes in the cerebrovasculature, including alterations in smooth muscle cells and pericytes, endothelial cell thinning, and loss of endothelial mitochondria (for review, see Refs. 1, 12, and 13). Most consistently noted was a thickening of the vascular basement membrane, probably resulting from the accumulation of basement membrane proteins.[1,14,15] The cause and the functional consequences of these microvascular abnormalities are unclear. Likewise, the temporal relationships between basement membrane accumulation, amyloid deposition, and other microvascular changes are also unknown.

Recently, we reported that overexpression of transforming growth factor-β1 (TGF-β1) in transgenic mice results in age-related cerebrovascular amyloid deposits.[16] These mice develop amyloid deposits in cerebral blood vessels in the absence of amyloid plaques, and thus, cerebrovascular amyloid deposition can be studied independent of plaque formation. In addition, TGF-β1 overexpression results in cerebral amyloid deposition without the need to overexpress the amyloid precursor protein. Here we used TGF-β1 transgenic mice to study the temporal development of cerebrovascular pathology and to assess the possible functional consequences of these pathological changes by measuring cerebral glucose utilization.

METHODS

Specimens of frontal cortex (midfrontal gyrus) from AD and CAA cases and nondemented controls were obtained from the Alzheimer's Disease Research Center at the University of California San Diego. Tissue blocks were fixed in freshly prepared 4% paraformaldehyde in 0.1 M phosphate buffer (pH 7.4) at 4°C for 48 h. Transgenic mice overexpressing TGF-β1 in astrocytes under the control of regulatory elements of the glial fibrillary acidic protein (GFAP) gene have been described.[17] Brains from 3- or 15-month-old TGF-β1 heterozygous mice (low-expresser line) or nontransgenic controls were obtained after transcardiac perfusion of anesthetized animals.

Brain sections from human or mouse tissues were generated (40 μm thickness) and stained with antibodies against GFAP (DAKO), TGF-β1 (G4 antiserum[17]) or latent TGF-β1 (R&D Systems). Species-matched secondary antibodies and avidin-biotin complex/immunoperoxidase techniques or fluorescein isothiocyanate–labeled secondary antibodies were used to reveal immunoreactive proteins.[16] Some sections were stained with thioflavin-S as described.[16]

Glucose utilization was measured by the quantitative autoradiographic method of Sokoloff,[18] with [14C]-deoxyglucose as a tracer, in 13–15-month-old TGF-β1 heterozygous mice ($n = 6$) and age-matched nontransgenic controls ($n = 5$). Mice were anesthetized with halothane, catheterized in the femoral vein and artery, and placed in a hammock; lidocaine was used for local anesthesia at the femoral level. The mice were allowed to recover from anesthesia for 90 min. Then, [14C]-deoxy-

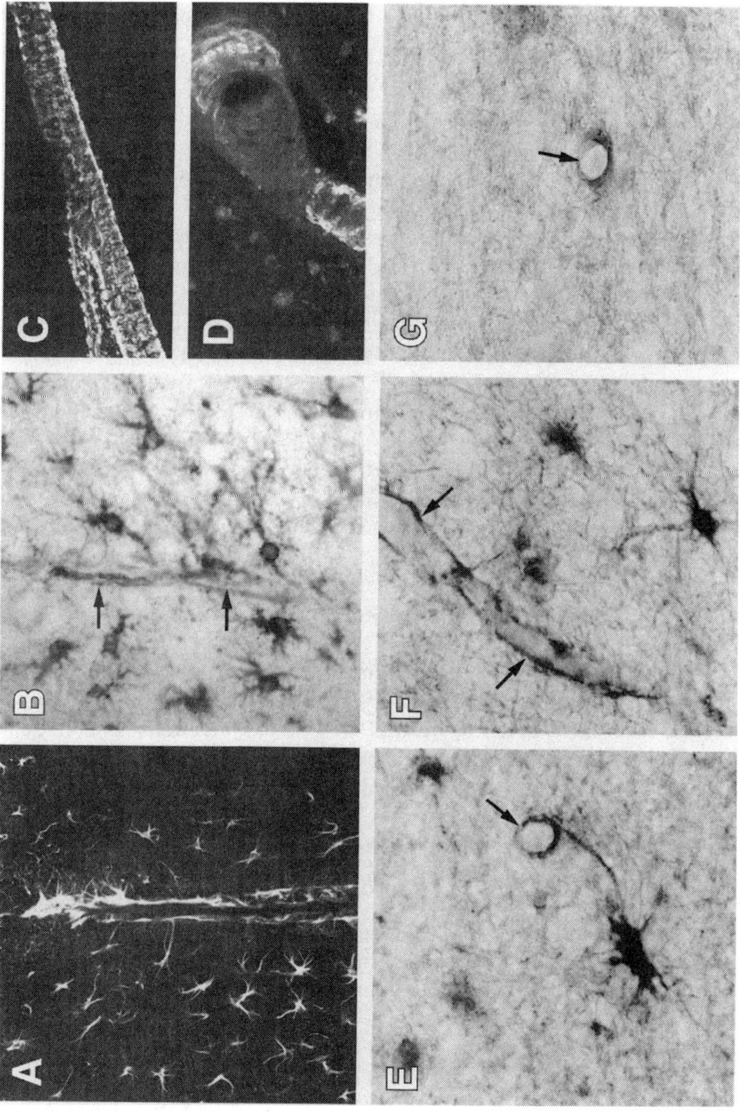

FIGURE 1. Amyloid deposition and TGF-β1 immunostaining of perivascular astrocytes in TGF-β1 mice and AD cases. Cortical brain sections from TGF-β1 mice (**A–C**) and humans with AD (**D–F**) or no dementia (**G**) were stained with antibodies against astrocytes (GFAP, A), TGF-β1 (B, E–G), or with thioflavin-*S* (C,D). Note the similarity in staining for TGF-β1 and amyloid in TGF-β1 mice and AD cases, and the absence of TGF-β1 immunopositive astrocytes in a control case without dementia.

glucose (150 µCi/kg in 0.1 ml) was administered by intravenous infusion, and cerebral glucose utilization measurements were recorded for 45 min. Small amounts of arterial blood were obtained serially to determine tracer and glucose concentrations in plasma during the experiment. At the end of the experiments, mice were anesthetized again, brains were removed and cut sagitally into 20-µm sections. Tracer concentrations in various brain regions were quantitated by autoradiography as previously described.[19]

RESULTS

The first pathological change detected in brains of TGF-β1 mice was a strong activation of perivascular astrocytes. These astrocytes were intensely immunopositive for TGF-β1 (FIGS. 1A and B) and were seen as early as 7 days postnatally. At 3–4 months of age, basement membrane proteins, including perlecan and fibronectin, were considerably increased in isolated microvessels from the cortex and hippocampus of TGF-β1 mice.[27] This increase was accompanied by a thickening of cortical basement membranes, as measured by ultrastructural morphometry. Amyloid deposition was first detected in 6–9-month-old TGF-β1 mice, predominantly in small to medium-sized cerebral vessels and in the meninges (FIG. 1C). Nontransgenic mice showed none of these cerebrovascular changes (data not shown). In 9–18-month-old TGF-β1 mice, evidence of vascular injury and degeneration was observed in microvascular cells. Capillary endothelial cells in TGF-β1 mice were thin and displayed microvilli-like protrusions and blebs not seen in nontransgenic controls. Occasionally, chromatin condensation was noted in transgenic endothelial cell nuclei, but not in controls. In capillary profiles, the area occupied by pericytes was significantly smaller in TGF-β1 transgenic mice than in controls.[27]

These pathological changes in TGF-β1 mice are similar to cerebrovascular abnormalities in AD brains (FIGS. 1D–F). Perivascular astrocytosis is observed frequently in AD brain,[20,21] and here we show that perivascular astrocytes in AD express TGF-β1. The close interaction of astrocyte endfeet with vascular cells is depicted in FIGURES 1E and F. Brain sections from non-demented control cases immunostained for TGF-β1 showed only faint labeling of blood vessels but not of astrocytes (FIG. 1G).

To relate the cerebrovascular pathological alterations in TGF-β1 mice to functional changes we measured cerebral glucose utilization, a marker of brain metabolic activity. Preliminary results showed that TGF-β1 mice had significantly decreased glucose utilization in mammillary bodies, structures involved in mnemonic and learning processes. Glucose utilization tended to be decreased in several other brain regions as well; however, in the inferior colliculus, it was markedly higher in TGF-β1 mice than in controls.

DISCUSSION

Our study describes the temporal development of cerebrovascular amyloidosis and degeneration *in vivo* and establishes an association with functional changes reflected in the rate of glucose utilization. Cerebrovascular amyloidosis and degener-

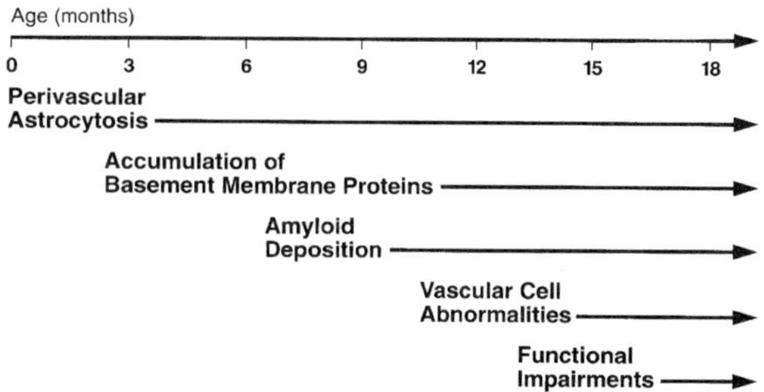

FIGURE 2. Temporal development of cerebrovascular pathology and functional deficits in TGF-β1 mice.

ation are frequently reported in AD, but their possible contribution to AD pathogenesis is unknown.[1,3,4,22] In addition, glucose metabolism is decreased in specific cortical brain regions in AD.[5–7] Our findings show that chronic elevation of TGF-β1 production in the CNS of transgenic mice leads to a prominent astrocytosis and accumulation of basement membrane proteins,[27] which is followed by amyloid deposition. With increasing age, degenerative changes in cerebrovascular cells were noted (FIG. 2). In many aspects, these pathological changes in TGF-β1 mice resemble those found in AD and CAA (for review, see Ref. 1).

Although more experiments are required to correlate the pathological alterations with regional metabolic changes, our current findings suggest a cause-effect relationship between TGF-β1-induced cerebrovascular pathology and brain metabolic activity and function. Energy is delivered to the brain in the form of glucose mainly through perivascular astrocytes and their endfeet on the microvasculature (for review, see Ref. 23). These astrocytes are thought to be actively involved in regulating brain energy metabolism[24,25] and have also been suspected to play a pathogenic role in neurodegenerative disorders.[20,21] The combination of perivascular astrocytosis, abnormal levels of basement membrane proteins, and amyloid deposits in the vascular wall idenified in TGF-β1 mice could lead to a disruption of normal glucose transport into the brain. The cerebrovascular abnormalities observed in TGF-β1 mice could also lead to impaired neurogenic control of cerebral blood flow at the capillary level,[19,26] which may cause changes in glucose utilization and deficits in brain function. Experiments to further assess these possibilities are in progress.

In conclusion, overexpression of TGF-β1 in mouse astrocytes resulted in AD-like cerebrovascular pathology and functional metabolic changes. TGF-β1 mice represent a good *in vivo* model to dissect the pathogenetic interactions between cerebrovascular amyloidosis, degeneration, and functional CNS impairments.

ACKNOWLEDGMENTS

This work was supported by the NIH (AG11385) and by the Alzheimer's Disease Program of the State of California (98-15724).

REFERENCES

1. KALARIA, R.N. 1996. Cerebral vessels in ageing and Alzheimer's disease. Pharmacol. Ther. **72:** 193–214.
2. VINTERS, H.V. 1992. Cerebral amyloid angiopathy and Alzheimer's disease: two entities or one? J. Neurol. Sci. **112:** 1–3.
3. PLASSMAN, B.L. & J.C.S. BREITNER. 1996. Recent advances in the genetics of Alzheimer's disease and vascular dementia with an emphasis on gene-environment interactions. J. Am. Geriatr. Soc. **44:** 1242–1250.
4. VERBEEK, M.M., P. EIKELENBOOM & R.M.W. DE WAAL. 1997. Differences between the pathogenesis of senile plaques and congophilic angiopathy in Alzheimer disease. J. Neuropathol. Exp. Neurol. **56:** 751–761.
5. FRACKOWIAK, R.S.J., G. POZZILLI, N.J. LEGG, G.H. DUBOULAY, J. MARSHALL, G.L. LENZI & T. JONES. 1981. Regional cerebral oxygen supply and utilization in dementia. Brain **104:** 753–778.
6. FOSTER, N.L., T.N. CHASE, L. MANSI, R. BROOKS, P. FEDIO, N.J. PATRONAS & G. DICHIRO. 1984. Cortical abnormalities in Alzheimer's disease. Ann. Neurol. **16:** 649–654.
7. RAPOPORT, S.I., K. HATANPÄÄ, D.R. BRADY & K. CHANDRASEKARAN. 1996. Brain energy metabolism, cognitive function and down-regulated oxidative phosphorylation in Alzheimer disease. Neurodegeneration **5:** 473–476.
8. VINTERS, H.V. 1987. Cerebral amyloid angiopathy: a critical review. Stroke **18:** 311–324.
9. ITOH, Y., M. YAMADA, M. HAYAKAWA, E. OTOMO & T. MIYATAKE. 1993. Cerebral amyloid angiopathy: a significant cause of cerebellar as well as lobar cerebral hemorrhage in the elderly. J. Neurol. Sci. **116:** 135–141.
10. HAAN, J., M.L.C. MAAT-SCHIEMAN & R.A.C. ROOS. 1994. Clinical aspects of cerebral amyloid angiopathy. Dementia **5:** 210–213.
11. GREENBERG, S.M., J.P. VONSATTEL, J.W. STAKES, M. GRUBER & S.P. FINKLESTEIN. 1993. The clinical spectrum of cerebral amyloid angiopathy: presentations without lobar hemorrhage. Neurology **43:** 2073–2079.
12. VINTERS, H.V., D.L. SECOR, S.L. READ, J.G. FRAZEE, U. TOMIYASU, T.M. STANLEY, J.A. FERREIRO & M.-A. AKERS. 1994. Microvasculature in brain biopsy specimens from patients with Alzheimer's disease: an immunohistochemical and ultrastructural study. Ultrastruct. Pathol. **18:** 333–348.
13. WISNIEWSKI, H.M., J. WEGIEL, K.C. WANG & B. LACH. 1992. Ultrastructural studies of the cells forming amyloid in the cortical vessel wall in Alzheimer's disease. Acta Neuropathol. **84:** 117–127.
14. MANCARDI, G.L., F. PERDELLI, C. RIVANO, A. LEONARDI & O. BUGIANI. 1980. Thickening of the basement membrane of cortical capillaries in Alzheimer's disease. Acta Neuropathol. **49:** 79–83.
15. PERLMUTTER, L.S., H.C. CHUI, D. SAPERIA & J. ATHANIKAR. 1990. Microangiopathy and the colocalization of heparan sulfate proteoglycan with amyloid in senile plaques of Alzheimer's disease. Brain Res. **508:** 13–19.
16. WYSS-CORAY, T., E. MASLIAH, M. MALLORY, L. MCCONLOGUE, K. JOHNSON-WOOD, C. LIN & L. MUCKE. 1997. Amyloidogenic role of cytokine TGF-β1 in transgenic mice and Alzheimer's disease. Nature **389:** 603–606.
17. WYSS-CORAY, T., L. FENG, E. MASLIAH, M.D. RUPPE, H.S. LEE, S.M. TOGGAS, E.M. ROCKENSTEIN & L. MUCKE. 1995. Increased central nervous system production of extracellular matrix components and development of hydrocephalus in transgenic mice overexpressing transforming growth factor-β1. Am. J. Pathol. **147:** 53–67.
18. SOKOLOFF, L., M. REIVICH, C. KENNEDY, M.H. DES ROSIERS, C.S. PATLAK, K.D. PETTIGREW, O. SAKURADA & M. SHINOHARA. 1977. The [^{14}C]deoxyglucose method for the measurement of local cerebral glucose utilization: theory, procedure, and normal values in the conscious and anesthetized albino rat. J. Neurochem. **28:** 897–916.
19. VAUCHER, E., J. BORREDON, G. BONVENTO, J. SEYLAZ & P. LACOMBE. 1997. Autoradiographic evidence for flow-metabolism uncoupling during stimulation of the nucleus basalis of Meynert in the conscious rat. J. Cereb. Blood Flow Metab. **17:** 686–694.
20. MANDYBUR, T.I. & B.A. CHUIRAZZI. 1990. Astrocytes and the plaques of Alzheimer's disease. Neurology **40:** 635–639.

21. CULLEN, K.M. 1997. Perivascular astrocytes within Alzheimer's disease plaques. Neuroreport **8:** 1961–1966.
22. SNOWDON, D.A., L.H. GREINER, J.A. MORTIMER, K.P. RILEY, P.A. GREINER & W.R. MARKESBERY. 1997. Brain infarction and the clinical expression of Alzheimer disease: the nun study. J. Am. Med. Assoc. **277:** 813–817.
23. MAGISTRETTI, P.J., L. PELLERIN, D.L. ROTHMAN & R.G. SHULMAN. 1999. Energy on demand. Science **283:** 496–497.
24. MAGISTRETTI, P.J. & L. PELLERIN. 1996. Cellular basis of brain energy metabolism and their relevance to functional brain imaging: evidence for a prominent role of astrocytes. Cereb. Cortex **6:** 50–61.
25. KACEM, K., P. LACOMBE, J. SEYLAZ & G. BONVENTO. 1998. Structural organization of the perivascular astrocyte endfeet and their relationship with the endothelial glucose transporter: a confocal microscopy study. Glia **23:** 1–10.
26. VAUCHER, E. & E. HAMEL. 1995. Cholinergic basal forebrain neurons project to cortical microvessels in the rat: electron microscopic study with anterogradely transported *Phaseolus vulgaris* leucoagglutinin and choline acetyltransferase immunocytochemistry. J. Neurosci. **15:** 7427–7441.
27. WYSS-CORAY, T., C. LIN, D. SANAN, L. MUCKE & E. MASLIAH. 2000. Chronic overproduction of TGF-β1 in astrocytes promotes Alzheimer's disease-like microvascular degeneration in transgenic mice. Am. J. Pathol. **156:** 139–150.

The Role of Apolipoprotein E in the Deposition of β-Amyloid Peptide during Ischemia-Reperfusion Brain Injury

A Model of Early Alzheimer's Disease

RYSZARD PLUTA[a]

Department of Neuropathology, Medical Research Center, Polish Academy of Sciences, Warsaw, Poland

ABSTRACT: Transient brain ischemia in the rat produces a stereotyped pattern of selective neuronal degeneration which simulates early Alzheimer's disease (AD) pathology. The aim of the present study was to determine if apolipoprotein E (ApoE) variables are related to alterations in other proteins which play a central role in the pathogenesis of AD; amyloid precursor protein (APP) and β-amyloid peptide (Aβ). The postischemic time course of ApoE and APP and Aβ immunoreactivity in brain was examined at survival time from 2 days to 1 year in rats subjected to 10 min cardiac arrest. These data indicate that there are long lasting alterations of ApoE and Aβ after brain ischemia. The most likely stimulus for promoting increase of both ApoE and Aβ expression are ischemic-reperfusion processes. Our data suggest that ApoE modulates the outcome following cerebral ischemia via molecular events in common with AD pathogenesis. We propose that ischemic-reperfusion processes in brain are the fountainhead of a cycle of molecular and cellular events that have neurodegenerative consequences which finally lead to AD.

INTRODUCTION

Involvement in Alzheimer's disease (AD) research includes clinical and epidemiological studies, neuroimaging, neuropathology, molecular genetics, neurochemistry, disease models and neuronal degeneration, and currently also a transgenic program related to understanding risk genes and disease progression and lately new environmental risk factors.[1–3] In the past twenty years, we have developed approximately 8 different models in areas of neuroscience related to brain ischemia. Our last data provide further characterization of a new and unique chronic model of brain ischemia that can be applied to relevant clinical studies.[4] We are interested in the pathophysiology, pathology, and consequences of mild ischemic brain injury, since

[a]Address for correspondence: Ryszard Pluta, M.D., Ph.D., Department of Neuropathology, Medical Research Center, Polish Academy of Sciences, Pawiñskiego 5 Str., 02-106 Warsaw, Poland. Fax: (48-22) 668-5532.
e-mail: rp@ibbrain.ibb.waw.pl

such lesions are frequently encountered in the clinic and carry considerable morbidity including long lasting cognitive and emotional disturbances. By using simple techniques without extensive surgical preparation and pharmacological manipulations, we produce an impact trauma induced by cardiac arrest (CA)[4] to the rat brain characterized by loss of some cortical and hippocampal neurons and a mild delayed brain atrophy.[5]

The vascular abnormalities observed in AD are usually neglected or considered incidental to neuronal degeneration. But recent findings of our group propose an early and significant role for vascular factors (e.g., ischemia) contributing to the neurodegenerative processes.[1,2] A few years ago we demonstrated activation of platelets, adhesion to the vessel wall, and migration to the extravascular space as a striking feature of the *in vivo* vascular response to brain injury during ischemia-reperfusion.[6] We propose that the release of free β-amyloid peptide (Aβ) from platelets and/or other alternative sources[2] will initiate a cascade of events triggered by the production of apolipoprotein E (ApoE) following brain ischemia.[7] Inheritance of the ApoE-4 allele increases the risk of development of AD and reduces the age of onset.[8] Thus investigation of ApoE alterations in rat ischemic brain may provide insight into human neurodegeneration such as AD. This question can be addressed in experimental rat model because all nonhuman creatures have the ApoE-4 allele. After ischemia-reperfusion brain injury, variables in ApoE and its receptor occur[9] very rapidly, and this is accompanied by increased expression of amyloid precursor protein (APP). These both proteins play a key role in the pathogenesis of AD. Recent data indicate that ApoE receptors also interact with APP by binding to secreted APP and mediating its degradation.[10] We suggest that ApoE expression modulates the response to and the neurological outcome following brain ischemia via molecular events in common with AD etiology. So far, however, there are few data available for understanding the biological significance of the association of ApoE with Aβ and neuronal death.[7,11–14] This is because we strongly feel that it is time to develop and present our own unique program in AD research which we have started over the last 10 years. Now we especially hope that during this complex investigation we can conceptually bring together the role of ApoE and APP induced by ischemia and brain injury during ischemia-reperfusion in AD, and discuss whether they offer new leads that could help in understanding the relationships of the various aspects of the AD pathology.

MATERIALS AND METHODS

Female Wistar rats ($n = 25$; 160–180 g; 3 months old) under ether anesthesia, were subjected to 10 min CA.[4] At 2, 7, and 14 days and 6 and 12 months after CA they were perfused with buffered saline followed by 2% paraformaldehyde.[1,4] As controls ($n = 15$) sham operated rats in due time were sacrificed. For immunocytochemistry, we used antibodies raised against synthetic peptides corresponding to the aa residues of APP; monoclonal antibody (mAb) 22C11 against the N-terminal of APP (NAPP), mAb 6E10 recognizing 1–17 aa residues of Aβ, polyclonal antibodies (pAb) SP 28 recognizing 1–28 aa residues of Aβ, and pAb RAS 57 against the C-terminal of APP (CAPP).[1,5,7] Staining with pAb was used for labeling ApoE.[11]

RESULTS

Neuropathological Examination

At 2 days neuronal loss was superimposed with degenerating neurons, which at that time became even more intense and diffuse. In later stages (7–14 days) the number of neurons with pathological changes were reduced being replaced by neuronal loss. The latter was localized in hippocampus, third neocortical layer and striatum. Borderline zones of the brain cortex were also the site of severe changes. Six months after ischemia in addition to localized neuronal loss different types of degenerative changes of neurons were present. The first one took the form of chronic neurons degeneration, and their calcification seemed to represent the residual stage of abnormalities noted in the early postischemic period. Curiously other changes were of a nature typical for the early postischemic stage, but they appeared in those structures and areas of the brain that were not involved early, e.g., the CA2, CA3, and CA4 sectors of hippocampus. In both early and late stages after ischemia disappearing neurons were replaced by naked astrocytic nuclei and glial nodules. Later hypertrophic and proliferating astrocytes were localized in areas of mild and severe neuronal loss. In some rats mixed astrocytic microglial nodules were present. Neuropathological examination performed one year after ischemia revealed hydrocephalic features of brain (FIG. 1). They were expressed by almost complete atrophy of dorsal hippocampus and striatum leading to enlargement of the ventricular system. Brain cortex in most areas was narrow showing increased neuronal density. Frequently small groups of neurons with features of chronic neuronal changes were seen. White matter re-

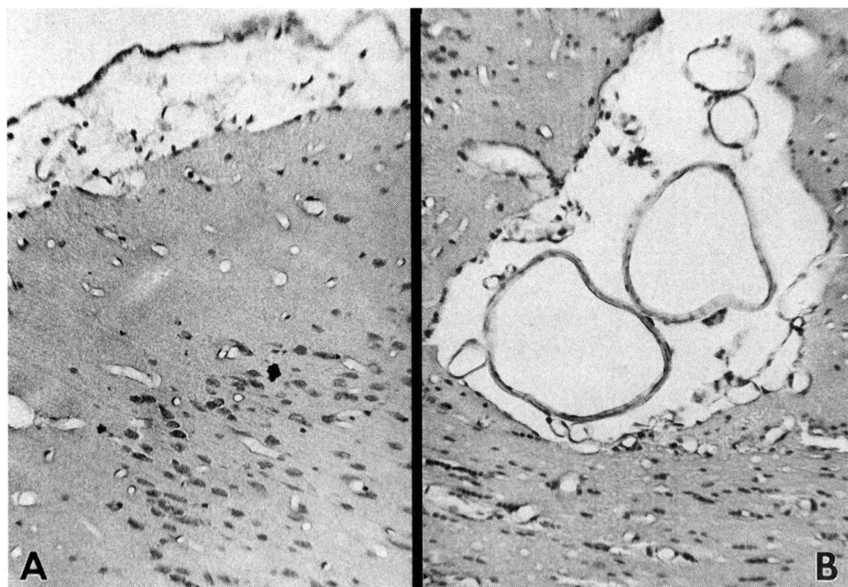

FIGURE 1. Dilatation of subarachnoid space around (**A**) and between brain hemispheres (**B**) after ischemia. One year survival. H&E. ×60.

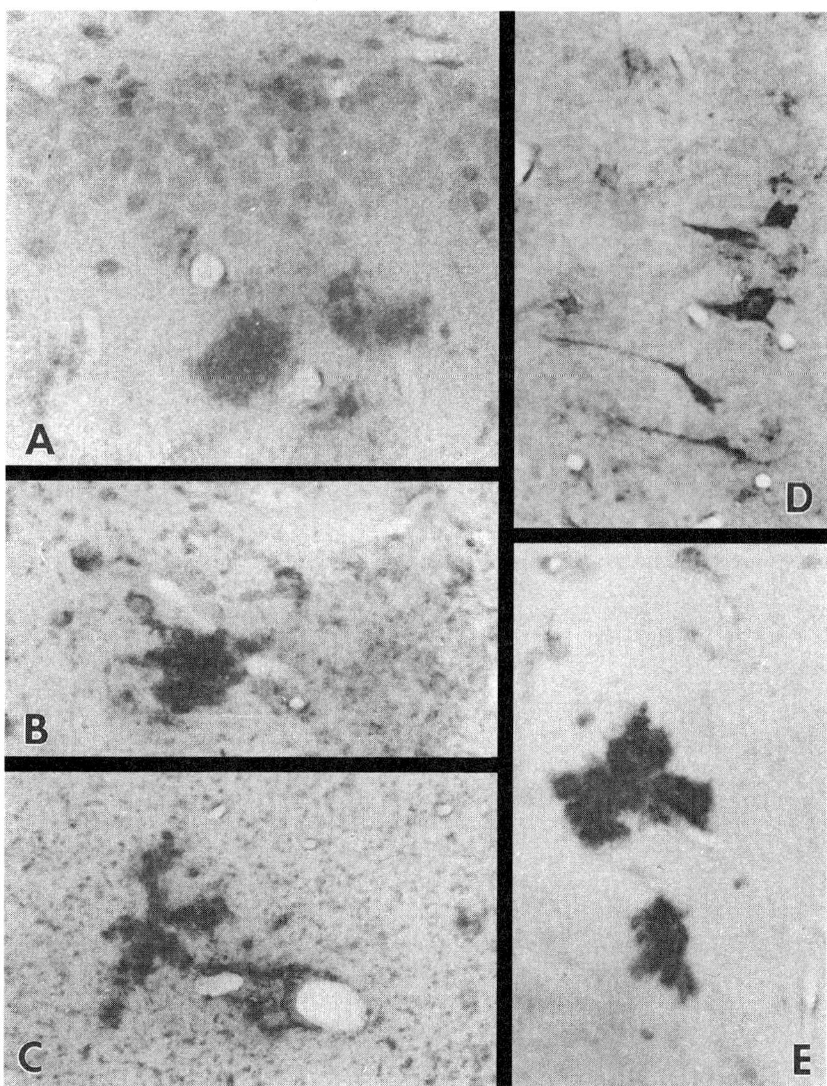

FIGURE 2. Extracellular deposits of NAPP (**A**, hippocampus, 7 days survival; ×400), Aβ (**B**, hippocampus, 7 days survival; ×400), and CAPP (**C**, hippocampus, 2 days survival; ×400) and intra- (**D**, hippocampus, 7 days survival; ×400) and extracellular (**E**, hippocampus, 2 days survival; ×400) expression of ApoE after ischemia.

TABLE 1. Immunohistochemical profile of intra- and extracellular ApoE and different epitopes of APP deposits in brain following ischemia

Group	ApoE	APP		
		N-terminal	βA	C-terminal
Control				
Short-term survival	–/+	–	–	–/+
Long-term survival	–/+	–	–	–/+
Ischemia				
Short-term survival	+++	++	+++	+++
Long-term survival	+++	–	+++	+++

NOTE: The staining intensity was categorized into four grades as follows: –, no staining; +, a single cell and weak cells; ++, a few cells and diffuse plaques; +++, many and strong cells and diffuse plaques stained.

vealed advanced spongiosis leading to profound cavitation. Diffuse astrocytic proliferation in white and grey matter was observed.

Amyloid Precursor Protein Examination

Ischemic brains demonstrated widespread and multifocal diffuse APP/Aβ plaques predominantly in the hippocampus, cerebral and entorhinal cortex, and corpus callosum or around the lateral ventricles (FIGS. 2A,B,C and 3A). Multiple, abundant, extracellular APP/Aβ deposits embraced or adjoined the blood vessels, mainly capillaries spreading multifocally outward into the parenchyma. Perivascular deposits formed irregular, often asymmetric, well-delineated zones, which frequently encircled vessels, forming round, perivascular cuffs or halo. Diffuse, broad, but faintly positive perivascular areas were also seen. Endothelial, pericyte, ependymal, and neuronal cells were labeled also. Staining was seen mainly in undamaged cells. Animals with short survival manifested the strongest labeling to the Aβ and CAPP and weaker labeling to the NAPP (FIG. 2A,B,C, TABLE 1). Rats with long survival revealed increased brain staining to the CAPP as well as to the Aβ region (FIG. 3A,B, TABLE 1). In this group astrocytes exhibited strong reaction for CAPP and Aβ (FIG. 3B). Especially perivascular astrocytes showed very intense labeling of numerous very long, delicate, thin processes, which embraced or adjoined the capillaries.

Apolipoprotein E Examination

The immunoreactivity was observed not only intracellularly within neuronal cells (FIGS. 2D and 3D), less often, glial cells, but also extracellularly, in the perivascular areas (FIGS. 2E and 3C). Extracellular ApoE-positive zones were well delineated, irregular, and embraced or adjoined mainly the capillaries (FIG. 2E). Diffuse, broad, but faintly ApoE-positive perivascular or nonperivascular areas were also seen (FIG. 3C). Strong ApoE staining was noted also in irregular, spider-like, acellular necrotic foci. Staining was seen mainly in damaged cells, predominantly in neurons exhibiting signs of ischemic changes (FIG. 2D). Changes of ApoE expression

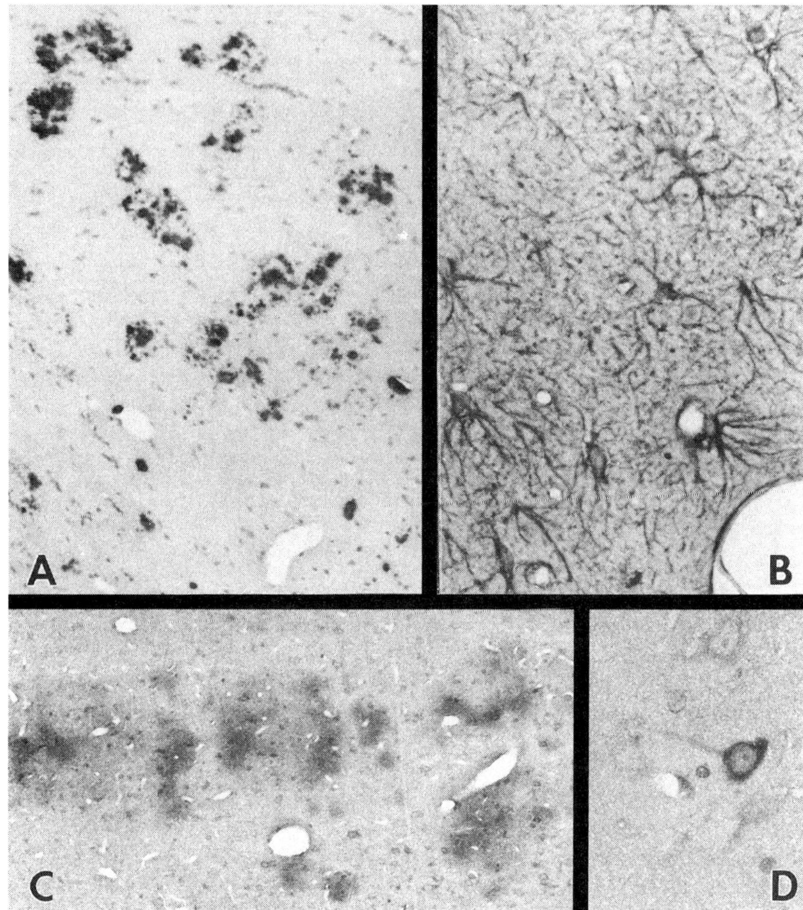

FIGURE 3. Extracellular deposits of Aβ (**A**, entorhinal cortex, 1 year survival; ×100) and immunostaining to Aβ in glial cells (**B**, hippocampus, 6 months survival; ×400) and extra- (**C**, cortex, 6 months survival; ×100) and intracellular (**D**, cortex, 1 year survival; ×400) expression of ApoE after ischemia.

appeared 2 days after CA and were present at all time intervals studied post-CA (FIGS. 2D,E and 3C,D, TABLE 1).

DISCUSSION

As a result of ischemia-reperfusion brain injury, the following neurodegenerative changes were observed: alterations in ApoE and biphasic nature of the APP expression, neuronal death, gliosis, and finally the brain atrophy. Our model provides neuropathological evidence which may mimic events which simulate early AD. Thus, this report emphasizes the usefulness of a unique method of evoking brain ischemia, which may have important applications in the human clinical arena with AD.

Neurodegenerative Changes during Ischemia-Reperfusion

Our studies indicate that transient brain ischemia in rats is followed by widespread neuronal damage, involving all brain structures, belonging or not to selectively vulnerable areas of the brain. In general the intensity of changes revealed marked individual variability. The extent and intensity of structural brain changes, as well as their nature, depended on the survival time after the ischemic episode. The postischemic brain alterations represent a gradually progressing process extending over a long period after the ischemic incident. The nature of the pathological processes is indicated by the pathological changes in the brain occurring during the whole experimental period, including one year of survival. They revealed characteristics of not only residual features resulting from early brain changes, but of an active pathological process even in the very late postichemic stage. The neurodegenerative process is characterized by specific dynamics consisting of early widespread pathological changes followed by localized neuronal loss, confined mostly to selectively vulnerable areas of the brain. The longer postischemic period displays nonspecific degeneration of the neurons. After one year of survival the process ended in generalized brain atrophy.[5,14,15] Brain atrophy occurring only in the ischemic rats, in contrast to their age-matched control not subjected to ischemic procedures, it permits one to reject an age-dependent origin of the atrophic processes. One more hallmark of late brain degeneration was manifested as diffuse white matter alterations taking the form of cavitation. This phenomenon may be explained by the increased expression of ApoE[11] and different fragments of APP[1,16] evoked by massive neuronal death with accompanying damage of the blood-brain barrier[17] occurring in the early and late stages after brain ischemia.

Amyloid Precursor Protein Changes during Ischemia-Reperfusion

We have found that ischemia in rats resulted in overexpression of either proteolytically cleaved fragments of the full-length APP or the entire APP molecule at times prior and during neuronal loss. Next increases in the extra- and intracellular space of the CAPP expression and the Aβ have been shown to occur during brain atrophy. The present study demonstrated that the duration of reperfusion is associated with differential extra- and intracellular alterations in APP domains, N-terminal and C-terminal. An initial response to ischemia was an increased intensity of staining to NAPP preceding evidence of neuronal loss. These early observations would probably support a neurotrophic function for NAPP. The disappearance in NAPP staining coincides with evidence of clear neuronal death and brain atrophy. However, loss of reactivity for NAPP was accompanied by the appearance of APP staining of proliferating astrocytes. A glial appearance of Aβ and CAPP staining occurred at a time when extensive neuronal loss was evident. The localization of some fragments of APP to astrocytes may be of significant relevance to AD in which chronic glial activation is thought to play a key role in the evolution of amyloid plaques.[18] In the present study the onset of brain atrophy was associated with the dominance of CAPP and Aβ staining and the appearance of this staining in glial cells. The localization of

CAPP within ischemic brain tissue underscores the likely importance of the CAPP in the pathogenesis of ischemia as in AD. These results suggest the possibility that the CAPP was modified, because the CAPP is critical for the seeding of amyloid plaque formation.[19]

Apolipoprotein E Changes during Ischemia-Reperfusion

In the present study increased neuronal staining was demonstrated to ApoE whose reactivity in brain is limited to astrocytes. Thus, the staining of neurons by ApoE observed here might be rather attributed to its internalization from the extracellular space. It is of interest in this respect that neuronal ApoE reactivity was already found in human brain with AD. Increased immunoreactivity of postischemic brain tissue to ApoE may have significant biological consequences for the evolution of postischemic outcome. In the present study ApoE reactivity was found in both slightly as well as markedly damaged neurons. We know that the hippocampal cholinergic terminals are vulnerable to ischemic insult and that presynaptic terminal destruction precedes postsynaptic CA1 cell death. Therefore, the accumulation of ApoE in pyramidal neurons after ischemia may be due to a large amount of cholesterol being mobilized during the terminal breakdown. The lipoprotein complexes may be transported to neurons through the lipid recycling mechanism described by Poirier *et al.*[20] In this connection it has been reported that brain ischemia induces cholesterol depletion. Since cholesterol is an important constituent in mammalian cells, the intense staining in neurons might reflect the requirements of cholesterol in wounded neurons. On the other hand, this accumulation of ApoE following ischemia may be a reflection of cholesterol leak from disappearing neurons. Perhaps the leak of cholesterol from neurons is a critical step leading to neuronal death. It is of interest to notice that perivascular deposits of ApoE colocalize with APP epitopes.[11] We suggest that the coincident distribution pattern for ApoE and Aβ reactivities implies formation of the insoluble and stable ApoE-Aβ complex which is known to exist in the brain of individuals with AD. It is, therefore, possible that ApoE and Aβ separately or in complexes adhere to the neuronal remnant after neuronal death and produce diffuse amyloid plaques. Interestingly, we found faint staining for ApoE remaining in the pyramidal cell layer even long after their disappearance. This finding suggested a deposition of proteins associated with ApoE which was resistant against scavenging processes, such as recycling, transport, and metabolism. These data suggest that ischemic damage including neuronal cell death may give rise to β-amyloidogenesis. This scheme of events could be interpreted as a neurotoxic response of ApoE to ischemic injury.[21] ApoE itself is toxic to neurons.[21] However, the fate of ApoE after ischemia remains to be determined, and the possibility remains that the continued presence of intra-/extracellular ApoE could contribute to the pathology.[21] *In vitro* ApoE binds to Aβ and promotes the formation of toxic complexes, and it has been suggested that immobilization of ApoE by Aβ may stop ApoE from fulfilling its role in compensatory mechanisms such as synaptic remodeling. Of particular significance in our study is the colocalization of ApoE and CAPP to degenerating neurons and extracellular space at a time when extensive neuronal necrosis and brain atrophy are apparent. Thus, it is of interest that generation of free radicals and lipid peroxidation after ischemia potentate the formation of Aβ aggregates via an interaction with ApoE. If membrane integrity is compromised in the

TABLE 2. Comparison of pathogenic cascade in two different neurodegenerative diseases of brain

Ischemia	Alzheimer's disease
Neurochemical Changes	
Ca movement	Ca movement
Excitatory amino acids	Excitatory amino acids
Free radicals	Free radicals
Cyclooxygenase activity	Cyclooxygenase activity
β-amyloid peptide	β-amyloid peptide
Apolipoprotein E	Apolipoprotein E
Apolipoprotein A1	Apolipoprotein A1
Apolipoprotein J	Apolipoprotein J
Presenilin	Presenilin
Cytokines	Cytokines
Blood-brain barrier	Blood-brain barrier
Pathological Changes	
Diffuse plaques	Diffuse plaques
Neuronal necrosis	Neuronal necrosis
Apoptosis	Apoptosis
Neuronal death	Neuronal death
Gliosis	Gliosis
Regional Changes	
Hippocampus	Hippocampus
Entorhinal cortex	Entorhinal cortex
Neocortex	Neocortex
Final Changes	
Atrophy	Atrophy
Dementia	Dementia

presence of ApoE-4, then neurons may be more susceptible to cell death.[21] Additionally, C-terminal domains of APP are purported to be potentially amyloidogenic, and the colocalization of ApoE and CAPP may be of significance in this respect. With regard to the possibility that ischemia-reperfusion injury may increase Aβ accumulation via an ApoE oxidation-driven mechanism, it is increasingly apparent that oxygen radicals and membrane lipid peroxidation play a significant role in mechanism(s) of neuronal death. It would suggest that the simultaneous induction of ApoE and APP/Aβ during brain ischemia-reperfusion injury might underlie the increased risk of development of AD in cases with chronic brain ischemia. The presented observation support a similarity of fundamental pathogenesis between brain ischemia and Alzheimer's disease (TABLE 2).

Brain Ischemia as Trigger of Alzheimer's Disease

Amyloid has been known for years to accumulate as fibers in AD brain. A long-lasting hypothesis states that Aβ fibers destroy neurons in brain and cause dementia. Dogma holds that Aβ fibrils cause AD. But we have found that even without Aβ fibrils only with soluble Aβ, there can be devastating consequences for neurons following brain ischemia. It may be that ischemic disease of brain and AD have to some extent a shared etiology (TABLE 2). Another possibility is that ischemic and/or anoxic disease of brain is a key factor in the etiology of AD. Finally, in AD etiology, it is looking like the association of disease with the vascular/ischemic component of the dementia syndromes is very important rather than with dogmatic AD pathology.

ACKNOWLEDGMENTS

This work was supported by CSR Grant 4.PO5A.091.12 and by PAS.

REFERENCES

1. PLUTA, R. *et al.* 1994. Complete cerebral ischemia with short-term survival in rats induced by cardiac arrest. I. Extracellular accumulation of Alzheimer's β-amyloid protein precursor in the brain. Brain Res. **649:** 323–328.
2. PLUTA, R. *et al.* 1996. Evidence of blood-brain barrier permeability/leakage for circulating human Alzheimer's β-amyloid-(1–42)-peptide. NeuroReport **7:** 1261–1265.
3. BRETELER, M.M.B. *et al.* 1998. Vascular disease and vascular risk factors and dementia. Alzheimer's Rep. **1:** S25–S28.
4. PLUTA, R. *et al.* 1991. Reassessment of a new model of complete cerebral ischemia in rats. Method of induction of clinical death, pathophysiology and cerebrovascular pathology. Acta Neuropathol. **83:** 1–11.
5. PLUTA, R. *et al.* 1997. Late extracellular deposits of β-amyloid precursor protein in ischaemic rat brain show different immunoreactivity to the N- and C-terminal. Alzheimer's Res. **3:** 51–57.
6. PLUTA, R. *et al.* 1994. Platelet occlusion phenomenon after short- and long-term survival following complete cerebral ischemia in rats produced by cardiac arrest. J. Brain Res. **35:** 466–471.
7. PLUTA, R. *et al.* 1997. Changes in amyloid precursor protein and apolipoprotein E immunoreactivity following ischemic brain injury in rat with long-term survival: influence of idebenone treatment. Neurosci. Lett. **232:** 95–98.
8. SAUNDERS, A.M. *et al.* 1993. Association of apolipoprotein E allele ε4 with late-onset familial and sporadic Alzheimer's disease. Proc. Natl. Acad. Sci. USA **90:** 8098–8102.
9. POIRIER, J. 1994. Apolipoprotein E in animal models of CNS injury and in Alzheimer's disease. TINS **17:** 525–530.
10. KOUNNAS, M.Z. *et al.* 1995. LDL receptor-related protein, a multifunctional apo E receptor binds secreted beta-amyloid precursor protein and mediates its degradation. Cell **82:** 331–340.
11. KIDA, E. *et al.* 1995. Complete cerebral ischemia with short-term survival in rat induced by cardiac arrest. II. Extracellular and intracellular accumulation of apolipoproteins E and J in the brain. Brain Res. **674:** 341–346.
12. HALL, E.D. *et al.* 1995. Increased amyloid protein precursor and apolipoprotein E immunoreactivity in the selectively vulnerable hippocampus following transient forebrain ischemia in gerbils. Exp. Neurol. **135:** 17–27.
13. ISHIMARU, H. *et al.* 1996. Accumulation of apolipoprotein E and β-amyloid-like protein in a trace of the hippocampal CA1 pyramidal cell layer after ischaemic delayed neuronal death. NeuroReport **7:** 3063–3067.
14. PLUTA, R. *et al.* 1998. Cerebral accumulation of β-amyloid following ischemic brain injury with long-term survival. Acta Neurochir. [Suppl.] **71:** 206–208.
15. HOSSMANN, K.A. *et al.* 1987. Recovery of integrative central nervous function after one hour global cerebro-circulatory arrest in normothermic cat. J. Neurol. Sci. **77:** 305–320.

16. KALARIA, R. *et al.* 1993. Accumulation of the beta amyloid precursor protein at sites of ischemic injury in rat brain. NeuroReport **4:** 211–214.
17. PLUTA, R. *et al.* 1994. Early blood-brain barrier changes in the rat following transient complete cerebral ischemia induced by cardiac arrest. Brain Res. **633:** 41–52.
18. WIŚNIEWSKI, H.M. *et al.* 1989. Ultrastructural studies of the cells forming amyloid fibers in classical plaques. Can. J. Neurol. Sci. **16:** 535–542.
19. ESTUS, S. *et al.* 1992. Potentially amyloidogenic, carboxyl-terminal derivatives of the amyloid protein precursor. Science **255:** 726–728.
20. POIRIER, J. *et al.* 1993. Cholesterol synthesis and lipoprotein reuptake during synaptic remodeling in hippocampus in adult rats. Neuroscience **55:** 81–90.
21. MOULDER, K.L. *et al.* 1999. Analysis of a novel mechanism of neuronal toxicity produced by an apolipoprotein E-derived peptide. J. Neurochem. **72:** 1069–1080.

Alterations of Alzheimer's Disease in the Cholesterol-fed Rabbit, Including Vascular Inflammation

Preliminary Observations

D. LARRY SPARKS,[a,c] YU-MIN KUO,[a] ALEX ROHER,[a] TIM MARTIN,[b] AND RONALD J. LUKAS[b]

[a]Sun Health Research Institute, Sun City, Arizona, USA

[b]Barrow Neurological Institute, Phoenix, Arizona, USA

ABSTRACT: We determined the levels of endothelial inflammation using MECA-32 antibody and α4 nicotinic receptor subunit densities employing [^{3}H]epibatidine binding in the brains of Alzheimer's disease (AD) patients, cholesterol-fed rabbits, and appropriate controls. We also assessed rabbit brain for β-amyloid levels and immunohistochemical localization, and for evidence of blood-brain barrier breach using normally-excluded Evans Blue dye. Dietary cholesterol induced a twofold increase in β-amyloid concentration in rabbit hippocampal cortex, which may be related to the appearance of β-amyloid immunoreactivity in the neuropil. Epibatidine binding was significantly decreased in AD superior frontal cortex, but unchanged in the superior frontal cortex of cholesterol-fed rabbits. Increased vascular MECA-32 immunoreactivity occurred in AD and cholesterol-fed rabbit brain. Evans Blue dye could be found in the parenchyma of cholesterol-fed rabbits only, and appeared as pockets of dye surrounding small blood vessels. The data suggest that vascular inflammation can lead to breach of the blood-brain barrier, which may produce biochemical derangements in surrounding brain tissue that are conducive to production of β-amyloid.

INTRODUCTION

We first reported and others have confirmed a link between cardiovascular disorder and the presence of Alzheimer-like neuropathology.[1–4] Pathological studies suggest that cardiovascular disorder and/or hypertension is a common occurrence in Alzheimer's disease (AD).[2] Clinical studies indicate a relationship between cardiovascular disease,[5] hypertension,[6] and circulating cholesterol levels[7–10] as risk factors for AD.

Based on the foregoing, we investigated brains of the best characterized animal model of human coronary heart disease, the cholesterol-fed rabbit, for Alzheimer-like neuropathology.[4,11–16] We found that feeding rabbits 2% cholesterol for 8 weeks causes the neuronal accumulation of β-amyloid immunoreactivity,[11,15] apo-

[c]Address for correspondence to: D. Larry Sparks, 10515 Santa Fe Drive, Sun City, AZ 85351. Tel.: (602) 876-5463; fax: (602) 876-5461.
e-mail: Lsparks@mail.sunhealth.org

lipoprotein E immunoreactivity,[13] cathepsin D immunoreactivity,[14] and superoxide dismutase immunoreactivity.[15] The experimental cholesterol diet also induces occasional parenchymal accumulations of β-amyloid immunoreactivity,[11,15] microgliosis,[16] apoptosis,[16] and vascular activation of superoxide dismutase.[4] Similar activation of vascular superoxide dismutase is also observed in AD brain.[4] In addition, feeding rabbits control diet for two weeks after 8 weeks of cholesterol diet causes a significant reduction in the levels of β-amyloid immunoreactivity.[12] Furthermore, it is reported that cholesterol fed to apolipoprotein E-deficient mice causes a significant increase in β-amyloid concentration in the brain,[17] and spontaneously hypercholesterolemic Watanabe rabbits exhibit a pattern of accumulation of neuronal β-amyloid immunoreactivity similar to that found in cholesterol-fed rabbit brain (personal communication, Ralph Martins, Perth Australia).

In the current studies we investigated the cholesterol-fed rabbit brain for 1) β-amyloid immunoreactivity, 2) concentrations of β-amyloid, 3) levels of nicotinic binding, 4) immunohistochemical evidence of vascular inflammation with MECA-32 antibody,[18,19] and 5) evidence of breakdown of the blood-brain barrier after infusion with Evans Blue dye. In AD and age-matched control subjects we investigated the hippocampal formation for evidence of vascular inflammation and the frontal cortex for levels of nicotinic binding.

METHODS

New Zealand white rabbits were fed a 2% cholesterol diet (plus 0.5% cholic acid) or control diet for 8 weeks ($n = 4$ in each group) or 12 weeks ($n = 8$ in each group). The rabbits fed control or cholesterol diet for 8 weeks were perfusion-fixed with 4% buffered paraformaldehyde, and the brains were stored in perfusate for nearly four years before being investigated for MECA-32 immunoreactivity only. Two pairs of rabbits fed cholesterol or control diet for 12 weeks were infused with Evans Blue dye (2% at 1 ml/kg body weight) 60 minutes prior to sacrifice and perfusion of the brain with 2% buffered paraformaldehyde. The hippocampus and hippocampal cortex were viewed blind to group designation for passage of the Evans Blue dye across cerebral blood vessels in hippocampus and hippocampal cortex. The remaining 6 pairs of rabbits were sacrificed by exsanguination, and the fresh brain was removed. Half of the brain was immerse-fixed in 4% buffered paraformaldehyde until use (within 3 months), and the other half was stored fresh-frozen at $-70°C$ until use. Immunohistochemistry and chemical quantification of β-amyloid were performed on frontal cortex and hippocampal cortex. Nicotinic binding studies were performed on superior frontal cortex.

Samples of human brain were obtained from the Sun Health Research Institute brain bank. Fixed sections of hippocampus and hippocampal cortex from AD patients ($n = 7$; 76.5 ± 3.3 years; 3.2 ± 0.4 hours postmortem interval) and nondemented controls ($n = 6$; 80.3 ± 2.6 years; 2.7 ± 0.2 hours postmortem interval) were processed for MECA-32 immunohistochemistry. MECA-32 antibody interacts exclusively with endothelial cells in the central nervous system (CNS) that are undergoing inflammation in multiple sclerosis and an accepted animal model of multiple sclerosis (MS), experimental allergic encephalitis (EAE).[18,19] Fresh-frozen samples of superior frontal cortex binding from 6 AD patients, 7 low pathology controls (minimal number of senile plaques (SP) and rare or no neurofibrillary tangles (NFT)) and 5 high pathology controls (moderate numbers of SP and few NFT) were investigated for nicotinic binding.

MECA-32 Immunohistochemical Studies

MECA-32 immunohistochemical studies utilized 50-μm vibratome sections processed by free-floating methods that do not use H_2O_2 to inhibit endogenous peroxidase activity, as H_2O_2 has deleterious effects on the endothelial cell layer. After removal from cryoprotectant or buffered paraformaldehyde, the sections were washed in dilution media for one hour at room temperature (dilution media = 0.01 M phosphate-buffered saline (PBS), pH 7.4 with 0.5 ml/liter Triton X-100 added). The sections were transferred to 0.1 M sodium periodate in 0.01 M PBS, pH 7.4, for 20 minutes to remove remaining endogenous peroxidase activity. The sections were washed in dilution media, and incubated for an hour in dilution medium with 3% horse serum. Following incubation at 24°C for 48 hours in primary antibody (1:3 dilution with 0.01 M PBS with 1% normal horse serum and 0.4% Triton X-100), sections were washed three times for 10 minutes in dilution media and incubated in secondary antibody (rat anti-IgG H&L; Vector) as per the ABC protocol using TBS with 0.2% Triton X-100 and 1% horse serum as the solvent. The sections were then washed twice with TRIS buffer (0.05 M, pH 7.6) for 10 minutes, and twice with 1.0 M sodium acetate/0.2 M imidazole (pH 7.4) for 10 minutes. The antibody reaction was developed with diaminobenzidine (DAB) in sodium acetate/imidazole buffer containing 2.5% nickel ammonium sulfate and 0.005% H_2O_2. The reaction was terminated by three washes in TRIS buffer (three minutes each). Sections were then dehydrated and coverslipped. Analysis of sections was done blind to group designations.

Characterization of nAChR Ligand Binding Sites

Fresh-frozen tissue was processed into membrane fractions as described.[20,21] High-affinity nicotinic binding to the α4 nicotinic receptor subunit sites was detected and quantified using [^{3}H]epibatidine (EBDN) as the probe. EBDN binding assays were terminated by GF/C filtration after 1–3 hours incubation at 37°C.[22] Assay samples containing membranes plus EBDN were used to define total binding. Samples supplemented with unlabeled and membrane-permeant nicotine (10 μM) or epibatidine (100 nM) were used to define nonspecific binding.

Evans Blue Microscopic Analysis

Evans Blue microscopic analysis was performed on 50-μm vibratome sections without further histologic preparation. Samples of brain perfused first with Evans Blue dye and then buffered paraformaldehyde (4%) were sectioned, mounted on gelatin coated slides, coverslipped, and viewed and photographed blind to group-designation.

Europium Immunoassay for Quantitation of β-Amyloid Peptides

Europium immunoassay (EuIA) for quantitation of β-amyloid peptides was modified according to the previously published techniques.[23,24] Cortex (0.2 g) was rinsed twice with 3 ml PBS and finely minced with a razor blade. The tissue was thoroughly disrupted in 4 ml of 98% formic acid using a Dounce glass homogenizer. The specimens were loaded into 5-ml polyallomer tubes and centrifuged for 30 minutes at 250,000 $\times$ g in a Sorvall TH-650 rotor at 5°C. An aliquot of 500 ml was carefully taken from the middle of the tube and loaded onto a FPLC equipped with a Superose 12 size-exclusion column. The column was equilibrated and the chromatography developed with 80% glass distilled formic acid. Fractions corresponding to the retention time of 4.5 kDa (defined by the synthetic β-amyloid1–42 ($A\beta_{1-42}$)) were collected and pooled, and the acid was eliminated by vacuum centrifugation. The dried specimens were dissolved in 50 ml of 80% formic acid, diluted with 500 ml of 0.25 M Tris-HCl, pH 7.4 with 30% acetonitrile, neutralized with 10 N NaOH and the pH adjusted to 7.4.[23] The final volume was brought to 5 ml by the addition of TTBS (0.05% Tween 20 in 20 mM Tris-HCl and 0.5 M NaCl, pH 7.4). For β-amyloid quantitation, polyclonal antibodies R163 or R165 (10 mg/ml in 10 mM Na_2CO_3, pH 9.6) were coated to the wells of microtiter plates and used as the capture antibodies.[24] Bovine serum albumin (1%) in TTBS was used as blocking solution for 1 hour. One hundred μl of the specimens or of the $A\beta_{40}$ and $A\beta_{42}$ standards were applied to the wells and allowed to stand at room temperature for 2 hours on a rocking platform. The unbound materials were removed by washing the plate three times with TTBS. Europium-labeled 4G8 antibody (4 mg/ml) was added to the wells and incubated for 2 hours, followed by four washes with TTBS and three washes with double distilled deionized water. Finally, the Eu-enhancement solution (Wallac Inc., Gaithersburg, MD) was added to each well, and the plates were read in a fluorimeter using excitation and emission wavelengths of 320 and 615 nm, respectively.[24] The values, obtained from quadruplicate wells, were calculated based on standard curves generated on each plate.

RESULTS

As previously reported in 8-μm paraffin embedded sections,[11,15] we observed enhanced neuronal β-amyloid immunoreactivity in 50-μm vibratome sections of each cholesterol-fed rabbit compared to control (FIG. 1). In contrast to our previous reports, β-amyloid immunoreactivity filled entire neurons in thicker vibratome sections. Two of the six cholesterol-fed animals exhibited apparent extracellular plaque-like structures; an example from each animal is seen in FIGURES 1C and 1D.

Concentration of β-amyloid was measured in fresh-frozen frontal and hippocampal cortex from each control and cholesterol-fed rabbit. Total β-amyloid concentration was doubled in the hippocampal cortex of the cholesterol-fed rabbits (TABLE 1; trend $p = 0.08$) and was not different in the frontal cortex. It should be noted that the highest levels of β-amyloid observed in the cholesterol-fed rabbits occurred in the two animals exhibiting extracellular plaque-like structures.

Binding to α4 nicotinic receptor subunits was significantly reduced in AD superior frontal cortex compared to high pathology controls (TABLE 2). There was no dif-

TABLE 1. Concentrations of total β–amyloid (combined 40 and 42 amino acid length) in the frontal cortex and hippocampal cortex of New Zealand white rabbits fed control or 2% cholesterol diet for 12 weeks (means ± SEM in pg/mg cortex)

Group	n	Frontal Cortex	Hippocampal Cortex
Control	6	19.2 ± 7.7	14.9 ± 7.4
Cholesterol	6	15.0 ± 6.7	30.8 ± 7.2*

* Trend $p = 0.08$.

TABLE 2. [³H]Epibatidine binding to α4 nicotinic receptor subunits in the frontal cortex of Alzheimer's disease patients, and high and low pathology age-matched controls (means ± SEM, and epibatidine binding is in fmol/mg protein)

Group	n	Age (years)	Epibatidine	PMI (hrs)
Low path C	7	85.5 ± 1.2	19.2 ± 3.7	2.8 ± 0.4
High path C	5	81.4 ± 2.9	18.5 ± 1.0*	2.7 ± 0.2
AD	6	79.3 ± 3.5	12.6 ± 1.5	2.7 ± 0.3

ABBREVIATIONS: Low path C, low pathology control; high path C, high pathology control; AD, Alzheimer's disease; PMI, postmortem interval.
* $p < 0.05$ compared to AD.

TABLE 3. [³H]Epibatidine binding in frontal cortex from rabbits fed cholesterol or control diet for 12 weeks (means ± SEM, and binding values are in fmol/mg protein)

Group	n	Epibatidine
Control	6	34.3 ± 3.0
Cholesterol	6	34.5 ± 4.0

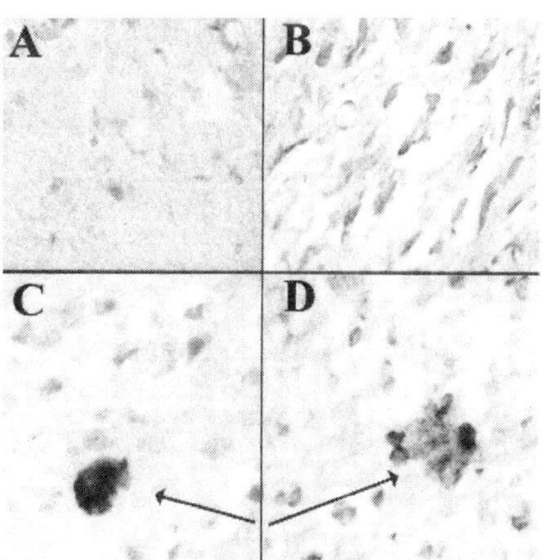

FIGURE 1. β–Amyloid immunoreactivity in hippocampal cortex of New Zealand white rabbits fed control or 2% cholesterol diet for 12 weeks. Fifty-micron vibratome sections were reacted with 10D5 antibody recognizing the N-terminal 1–16 of β-amyloid. Neuronal immunoreactivity is pronounced in the cholesterol-fed rabbits (**B–D**) compared to control (**A**), and extracellular deposits plaque-like were observed in two of six cholesterol-fed animals (D) and in no control.

ference in the level of α4 nicotinic binding between high and low pathology controls (TABLE 2). Similarly there was no difference in α4 nicotinic binding of the superior frontal cortex between control-fed and cholesterol-fed rabbits (TABLE 3).

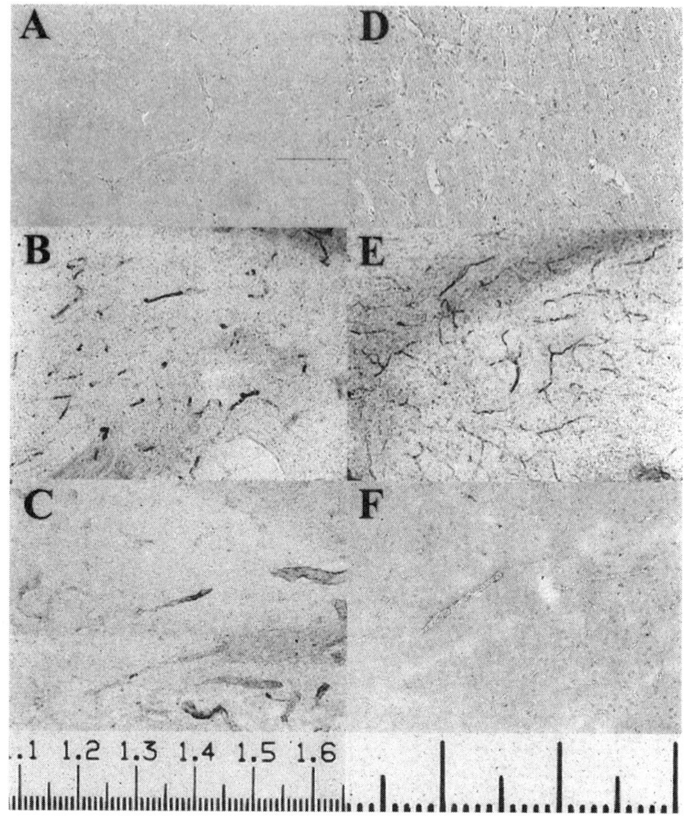

FIGURE 2. MECA-32 immunoreactivity in human and rabbit brain. The antibody MECA-32 highlights endothelial cells undergoing inflammation.[18,19] **(A)** No MECA-32 immunoreactivity was observed in five of six control subjects investigated; one control individual did exhibit slight vascular staining similar to that observed in the least affected cholesterol-fed rabbit (F) (40×). **(B,C)** Each Alzheimer's disease subject exhibited pockets of vascular MECA-32 immunoreactivity varying in extent and intensity. The highest level of immunoreactivity was similar to that seen in (E), a high mid-level of immunoreactivity in AD is seen in (B) (20×), and the low mid-level of immunoreactivity is seen in (C) (40×). The lowest level of immunoreactivity was comparable to that seen in the least affected rabbit (F). **(D)** No rabbit fed control diet exhibited MECA-32 immunoreactivity (40×). **(E,F)** All cholesterol-fed rabbits exhibited degrees of cerebrovascular MECA-32 immunoreactivity. Such immunoreactivity occurred in isolated patches rather than throughout a section. The highest level of immunoreactivity observed is shown in (E) (20×), and the lowest level is shown in (F) (40×). 20×, lower left grid; 40×, lower right grid.

MECA-32 immunoreactivity highlights endothelial cells undergoing inflammation.[18,19] We applied MECA-32 antibody to sections of AD and age-matched control brain tissue and control-fed and cholesterol-fed rabbit brain tissue; no immunoreactivity was observed in any sample if the primary antibody was omitted. Only one of the six human controls showed any discernable vascular MECA-32 immunoreactivity (not

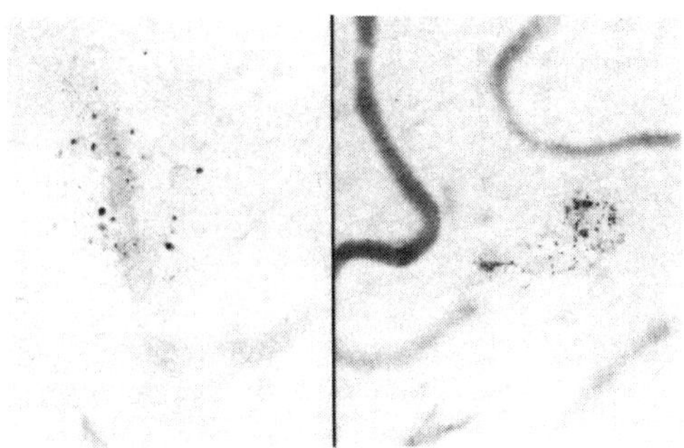

FIGURE 3. Evans Blue dye seepage through the cerebrovasculature in cholesterol-fed rabbit brain. Only isolated pockets of Evans Blue dye were observed in cholesterol-fed rabbits, and no such pockets of Evans Blue were observed in any section of control-fed rabbit brain (not shown).

shown); this immunoreactivity was similar to that observed in the least affected cholesterol-fed rabbit (FIG. 2F). All other age-matched human controls showed no MECA-32 immunoreactivity (FIG. 2A). All AD subjects exhibited pockets of cerebrovascular MECA-32 immunoreactivity (FIGS. 2B and 2C). The highest and lowest levels of vascular MECA-32 immunoreactivity (not shown) were comparable to that observed in the brains of cholesterol-fed rabbits (FIGS. 2E and 2F, respectively).

Vascular MECA-32 immunoreactivity could not be identified in any control rabbit brain, whether from archival tissue (8 weeks of diet) or shortly-stored tissue (12 weeks of diet; FIG. 2D). Each of the archival cholesterol-fed rabbit brains (8 weeks of diet) exhibited faint vascular MECA-32 immunoreactivity (not shown, but comparable to FIG. 2F). All of the cholesterol-fed rabbits investigated within months of sacrifice showed cerebrovascular MECA-32 immunoreactivity (FIGS. 2E and 2F). Most showed pockets of vascular immunoreactivity similar to that seen in FIGURE 2E or as shown for AD in FIGURE 2B. Only one of the animals fed cholesterol for 12 weeks showed weak vascular MECA-32 immunoreactivity (FIG. 2F).

Four 50-micron vibratome sections of each rabbit brain perfused with Evans Blue dye after 12 weeks of control ($n = 2$) or cholesterol diet ($n = 2$) were mounted and coverslipped without further histologic preparation. Every section of hippocampus and hippocampal cortex from both cholesterol-fed rabbits exhibited isolated pockets of Evans Blue dye surrounding capillaries (FIG. 3). No such pockets of Evans Blue dye were observed in any section of either control-fed rabbit brain (not shown). The number of pockets of Evans Blue identified in the cholesterol-fed rabbits was considerably less than the number of vessels exhibiting MECA-32 immunoreactivity.

DISCUSSION

We confirm here that dietary cholesterol induces accumulation of intraneuronal β–amyloid immunoreactivity. We previously reported that most of the intraneuronal β–amyloid immunoreactivity is likely the C-100 fragment of β-amyloid precursor protein (βAPP) after beta metabolism.[4] Here, a nearly significant twofold increase in the concentration of β–amyloid in the hippocampal cortex was observed in rabbits fed cholesterol for 12 weeks. The methods to determine the concentration of β-amyloid excluded the C-100 fragment, perhaps explaining the disparity between an 8–10-fold increase in the number of neurons expressing β–amyloid immunoreactivity in the hippocampal cortex and only a twofold increase in β-amyloid levels. These data also suggest that most intraneuronal β-amyloid is the C-100 fragment. It is noteworthy that the highest concentrations of β-amyloid among the cholesterol-fed rabbits occurred in the two animals exhibiting extracellular deposits. This may suggest that it is not until β-amyloid immunoreactivity is observable in the parenchyma that elevated levels of β-amyloid can be identified. In other words, significant increases in β-amyloid concentration may occur only after β-amyloid is immunohistochemically demonstrable in the neuropil.

Consistent with previous reports,[25–27] we found that α4 nicotinic receptor subunit binding identified with [³H]epibatidine is reduced in AD superior frontal cortex. Reduced epibatidine binding has been consistently demonstrated in temporal cortex of AD patients,[25,26] but does not seem to correlate with β-amyloid load on a regional basis in the brain.[27] This could be viewed as consistent with our observation of no difference in epibatidine binding between high and low pathology controls. The major difference between our high and low pathology controls is senile plaque burden, and the major difference between our controls and our AD population is the level of NFT pathology. Similarly, we found no difference in epibatidine binding between control-fed and cholesterol-fed rabbits. This may be consistent with finding no difference between our human control groups, because cholesterol diet seems to induce β-amyloid pathology without producing alterations consistent with NFT pathology.

We report for the first time that there is increased vessel MECA-32 immunoreactivity, and therefore vascular inflammation, in AD. Six of the 7 AD subjects investigated had vessels that were intensely-to-moderately immunoreactive with MECA-32 antibody and only 1 of 6 nondemented controls showed faint vascular immunoreactivity. MECA-32 antibody interacts exclusively with endothelial cells in the CNS that are undergoing inflammation in multiple sclerosis and an accepted animal model of MS, experimental allergic encephalitis (EAE).[18,19] Such vascular inflammation is widespread in MS and EAE. In the case of AD, increased vascular MECA-32 immunoreactivity occurs only in isolated pockets. This could suggest a microenvironmental alteration or attack of blood vessels in AD rather than a generalized disorder of the vasculature. Previous reports do suggest a reactive process is occurring in the AD vasculature,[28] which may be related to endothelial degeneration and localized breaches of the blood-brain barrier in the disorder.[29,30] We would suggest that localized endothelial inflammation in AD is part of the above-noted reactive process leading to proposed breaches of the blood-brain barrier.

We report that isolated pockets of cerebrovascular MECA-32 immunoreactivity are produced by dietary cholesterol in the rabbit. No control-fed rabbit exhibited vascular MECA-32 immunoreactivity, and each cholesterol-fed rabbit exhibited MECA-32 immunoreactivity. These observations are similar to findings in AD, but different in that there was considerably more variability in the intensity of the immunoreactivity and number of vessels affected in the cholesterol-fed rabbit. Nevertheless, it would seem that increased circulating cholesterol levels might be able to induce vascular inflammation in rabbit brain.

Increased circulating cholesterol also seems to be able to produce isolated breaches of the blood-brain barrier, identified as isolated pockets of Evans Blue surrounding capillaries. Such pockets of Evans Blue dye were not observable in control-fed rabbits. Although we have not yet identified the anatomic coincidence of MECA-32 immunoreactivity and pockets of Evans Blue dye, we would hypothesize that the processes may be linked. Because consistently more capillaries exhibit MECA-32 immunoreactivity than exhibit pockets of Evans Blue dye in cholesterol-fed rabbit brain, it is possible that increasingly severe endothelial inflammation can lead to breach of the blood-brain barrier. This would be consistent with a previously proposed mechanism of vascular dysfunction in AD.[28–30]

We suggest that excess cholesterol in the blood in rabbits induces change at the surface of the endothelial cell leading to isolated patches of inflammation, degeneration, and breach of the blood-brain barrier. In turn, this process may set in motion a cascade of biochemical derangement in the underlying brain tissue leading to β-amyloidogenesis in the rabbit brain. We would further suggest that it might be increased circulating concentrations of free radicals caused by increased levels of cholesterol that initiates endothelial inflammation, and that a similar mechanism could be active in AD.[4]

REFERENCES

1. SPARKS, D.L. *et al.* 1990. Cortical senile plaques in coronary artery disease, aging and Alzheimer's disease. Neurobiol. Aging **11:** 601–607.
2. SPARKS, D.L. *et al.* 1995. Increased density of neurofibrillary tangles (NFT) in non-demented individuals with hypertension. J. Neurol. Sci. **131:** 162–169.
3. SONEIRA, C.F. & T.M. SCOTT. 1996. Severe cardiovascular disease and Alzheimer's disease: senile plaque formation in cortical areas. Clin. Anat. **9:** 118–127.
4. SPARKS, D.L. 1999. Neuropathologic links between Alzheimer's disease and vascular disease. *In* Alzheimer's Disease and Related Disorders. K. Iqbal, D.F. Swaab, B. Winblad & H.M. Wisniewski, Eds. Vol. 6: 153–163. John Wiley & Sons Ltd. New York.
5. MARTINS, C. *et al.* 1990. Effect of age and dementia on the prevalence of cardiovascular disease. Age **13:** 9–11.
6. SKOOG, I. *et al.* 1996. 15-year longitudinal study of blood pressure and dementia. Lancet **347:** 1141–1145.
7. JARVIK, G.P. *et al.* 1995. Interactions of apolipoprotein E genotype, total cholesterol level, age, sex in prediction of Alzheimer's disease: a case-control study. Neurology **45:** 1092–1096.
8. GRANT, W.B. 1997. Dietary links to Alzheimer's disease. Alzheimer's Dis. Rev. **2:** 42–55.
9. KALMIJN, S. *et al.* 1997. Dietary fat intake and the risk of incident dementia in the Rotterdam study. Ann. Neurol. **42:** 776–782.
10. NOTKOLA, I.-L. *et al.* 1998. Serum total cholesterol, apolipoprotein E epsilon 4 allele, and Alzheimer's disease. Neuroepidemiology **17:** 14–20.
11. SPARKS, D.L. *et al.* 1994. Induction of Alzheimer-like β-amyloid immunoreactivity in the brains of rabbits with dietary cholesterol. Exp. Neurol. **126:** 88–94.
12. SPARKS, D.L. 1996. Intraneuronal β-amyloid immunoreactivity in the CNS. Neurobiol. Aging **17:** 291–299.
13. SPARKS, D.L. *et al.* 1995. Increased density of cortical apolipoprotein E immunoreactive neurons in rabbit brain after dietary administration of cholesterol. Neurosci. Lett. **187:** 142–144.
14. HAAS, U. & D.L. SPARKS. 1996. Cathepsin D: activity and immunocytochemical localization in Alzheimer's disease and aging. Mol. Chem. Neuropathol. **29:** 1–14.

15. SPARKS, D.L. 1997. Dietary cholesterol induces Alzheimer-like β-amyloid immunoreactivity in rabbit brain. Nutr. Metab. Cardiovasc. Dis. **7:** 255–266.

16. STREIT, W.J. & D.L. SPARKS. 1997. Activation of microglia in the brains of humans with heart disease and hypercholesterolemic rabbits. J. Mol. Med. **75:** 130–138.

17. DURHAM, R.A. *et al.* 1998. Effect of age and diet on the expression of beta-amyloid 1–40 and 1–42 in the brains of apolipoprotein-E-deficient mice. Neurobiol. Aging **19:** S281.

18. DOPP, J.M. *et al.* 1994. Expression of ICAM-1, VCAM-1, L-selectin, and leukosialin in the mouse central nervous system during the induction and remission stages of experimental allergic encephalomyelitis. J. Neuroimmunol. **54:** 129–144.

19. ENGELHARDT, B. *et al.* 1994. Cell adhesion molecules on vessels during inflammation in the mouse central nervous system. J. Neuroimmunol. **51:** 199–208.

20. LUKAS, R.J. 1984. Properties of curaremimetic neurotoxin binding sites in the rat central nervous system. Biochemistry **23:** 1152–1160.

21. LUKAS, R.J. 1990. Heterogeneity of high affinity nicotinic [^{3}H]acetylcholine binding sites. J. Pharmacol. Exp. Ther. **253:** 51–57.

22. HOUGHTLING, R.A. *et al.* 1994. [^{3}H]Epibatidine binding to nicotinic cholinergic receptors in brain. Med. Chem. Res. **4:** 538–546.

23. KUO, Y.-M. *et al.* 1998. Elevated low-density lipoprotein in Alzheimer's disease correlates with brain A-beta 1–42 levels. BBRC **252:** 711–715.

24. KUO, Y.-M. *et al.* 1999. High Levels of circulating Aβ$_{42}$ are sequestered by plasma proteins in Alzheimer's disease. BBRC **257:** 787–791.

25. WARPMAN, U. & A. NORDBERG. 1995. Epibatidine and ABT 418 reveal selective losses of alpha4 beta2 nicotinic receptors in Alzheimer brains. Neuroreport **6:** 2419–2423.

26. HELLSTROM-LINDAHL, E. *et al.* 1999. Regional distribution of nicotinic receptor subunit mRNAs in human brain: comparison between Alzheimer and normal brain. Brain Res. Mol. Brain Res. **66:** 94–103.

27. MARUTLE, A. *et al.* 1999. Neuronal nicotinic receptor deficits in Alzheimer patients with the Swedish amyloid precursor protein 670/671 mutation. J. Neurochem. **72:** 1161–1169.

28. KALARIA, R.N. & S.N. KROON. 1992. Expression of leukocyte antigen CD34 by brain capillaries in Alzheimer's disease and neurologically normal subjects. Acta Neuropathol. (Berl.) **82:** 606–612.

29. KALARIA, R.N. & P. HEDERA. 1995. Differential degeneration of the cerebral microvasculature in Alzheimer's disease. Neuroreport **6:** 477–480.

30. KALARIA, R.N. 1996. Cerebral vessels in ageing and Alzheimer's disease. Pharmacol. Ther. **72:** 193–214.

Animal Model of Alzheimer-like Vascular Pathology and Inflammatory Reaction

J. RHODIN,[a,d] T. THOMAS,[a,c] M. BRYANT,[a] AND E.T. SUTTON[b]

Departments of [a]Anatomy and [b]Physiology and Biophysics, College of Medicine, University of South Florida, Tampa, Florida, 33612, USA

[c]Woodlands Medical and Research Center, Oldsmar, Florida 34677, USA

ABSTRACT: This *in vivo* animal model of vascular inflammatory reaction facilitates morphologic and hemodynamic analyses of leukocyte-endothelial interaction and can be monitored by video microscopy and electron microscopy. The model has served as a rapid means to explore the deleterious vascular actions and inflammatory response to the cytokines tumor necrosis factor, interleukin-1 and amyloid-β, as well as the protective effects of superoxide dismutase, estrogen, and cytokine antagonists.

INTRODUCTION

There is substantial evidence that inflammatory mechanisms are involved in several pathological conditions ranging from atherosclerosis, arthritis, cancer, and neurodegenerative diseases such as Alzheimer's disease.[1-4] Significant research has gone into the development of animal models that exhibit characteristic neuropathological features of Alzheimer's disease (AD). However, most of these animal models, including transgenic mice overexpressing mutant amyloid precursor protein (APP)[5] or presenelin genes,[6] do not show the characteristic neuropathological or cognitive features of AD. Increasing evidence of vascular dysfunction contributing to the pathology of AD[7] prompted us to develop an animal model of AD-like vascular pathology.[3]

MATERIALS AND METHODS

General

The transparent, thin mesenteric membrane of rodents contains a 2-dimensional network of microvessels, which makes it possible to observe blood flow and interaction between formed elements of the blood and the vascular wall. The live preparation was observed and recorded by video microscopic techniques. The same segments were subsequently fixed and retrieved for analysis by transmission electron microscopy.

[d]Address for correspondence: J. Rhodin, Department of Anatomy, University of South Florida College of Medicine, 12901 Bruce B. Downs Blvd., Tampa, Florida 33612. Tel.: (813) 974-9390; fax: (813) 974-2052.

e-mail: jrhodin@com1.med.usf.edu

TABLE 1. Agents tested at the indicated concentrations

Saline (control)	0.25 ml — 2 minutes
Amyloid-β (Aβ$_{1-40}$)	
(fresh; nonaggregated)	100 ng/g b.w.
Superoxide dismutase (SOD)	150 units/ml
Aβ	100 ng/g b.w.
SOD	300 units — 60 minutes
TNF-α	2 ng/100 g b.w.
IL-1β	2 ng/100 g b.w.
TNF-binding protein (TNF-bp)	2 mg/kg b.w. — wait 10 minutes
Aβ	100 ng/g b.w.
IL-1 receptor antagonist (IL-1ra)	2 mg/kg b.w. — wait 10 minutes
Aβ	100 ng/g b.w.

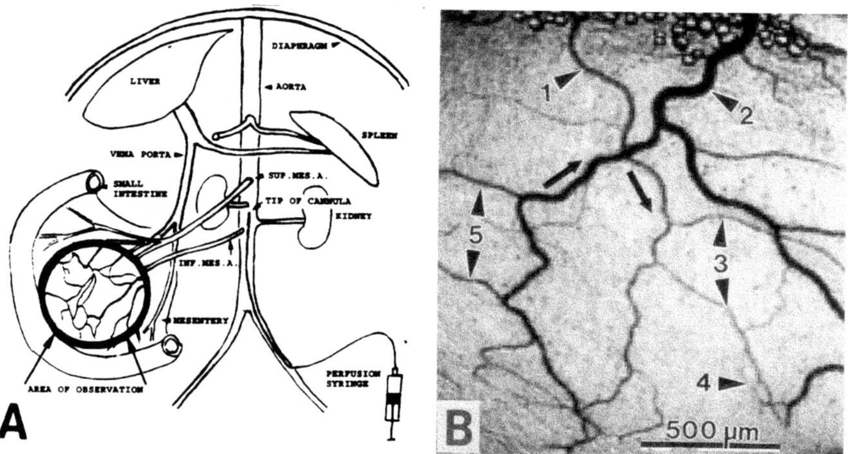

FIGURE 1. (A) Schematic drawing of the mesenteric preparation. **(B)** Video recording of an area similar to the circle in (A). Arterioles (1) are *lightly shaded*. Venules (2) appear *darker*. Precapillary arterioles (3), capillaries (4), postcapillary venules (5). *Arrows* indicate direction of blood flow. Mag. 40×.

Animals

Adult male Sprague-Dawley rats were anesthetized intraperitoneally with 60 mg/kg pentobarbital. An aortic cannula was introduced and its tip positioned near the exit of a mesenteric artery (FIG. 1). Part of the small intestine was exteriorized and draped over a lucite pedestal in a cradle and mounted on the stage of a light microscope.

Agents Tested

All agents were infused via the aortic cannula in amounts of 0.25 ml for 2 minutes (TABLE 1).

RESULTS

The results of infusing Aβ, TNF-α, and IL-1β were quite similar, as were the results of infusing SOD, TNF-bp, and IL-1ra. Therefore, we will account for these results collectively.

Infusion of Aβ, TNF-α, and IL-1β

In Vivo *Observations*

About 30 minutes after the initial infusion, leukocytes became attached to arterioles and precapillary arterioles. At the end of the 60-minute observation time of a 1000-μ stretch of arterioles, an average of 15–20 leukocytes were attached and about 5–10 leukocytes had transmigrated the arteriolar wall, which often had become considerably thickened. Platelets became marginated and/or tumbled along the arteriolar endothelium, and some reached the subendothelial space. In the postcapillary venules and muscular venules, there was an increase in leukocyte and platelet margination and migration into the subendothelial space. In the perivascular space, mast cells became activated, as judged by degranulation, and macrophages were actively moving about, often circling mast cells in an apparent cell-to-cell signaling. The severity of the above reactions was most pronounced after administration of Aβ and TNF, and less so after exposure to IL-1.

Electron Microscope Observations

The arteriolar endothelium was severely damaged, but to varying degrees. Cytoplasmic organelles such as mitochondria and endoplasmic reticulum became dilated, and vacuoles of varying sizes appeared (FIG. 2A & B). The endothelial cells developed a gap of up to 1 μ wide, exposing the endothelial basal lamina. Platelets often filled these gaps. At times, the entire endothelium was detached, floating freely in the arteriolar lumen (FIG. 3B). The endothelial cell nucleus was then pyknotic. The smooth muscle cells were distorted by the leakage of plasma, and often pyknotic. In the bay-like areas between the smooth muscle cells, fibrillar material (FIG. 2C) appeared at times, presumably amyloid. Several of the marginated leukocytes were actually monocytes (FIG. 3A). Although several leukocytes were recorded to transmigrate, only a few were retrieved in the electron microscope analysis. Platelets and erythrocytes were found in the subendothelial space between the distorted smooth muscle cells. The cytological alterations of the postcapillary venules and muscular venules closely mimicked those described for arterioles (FIG. 3C). One exception was the postcapillary venules after exposure to IL-1β. There was a very large number of leukocytes transmigrating, and many were lodged in the subendothelial space. Another exception was the reactivity of the arterioles, which was modest (FIG. 3A).

Infusion of SOD, TNF-bp, and IL-1ra followed by Aβ Infusion

In Vivo *Observations*

In all three experiments, there was only a very limited degree of leukocyte margination, both in arterioles and in venules. At the end of the 60-minute observation time of a 1000-μ stretch of arterioles, an average of 2–4 leukocytes were attached. None transmigrated, and all became detached. There was no platelet margination or

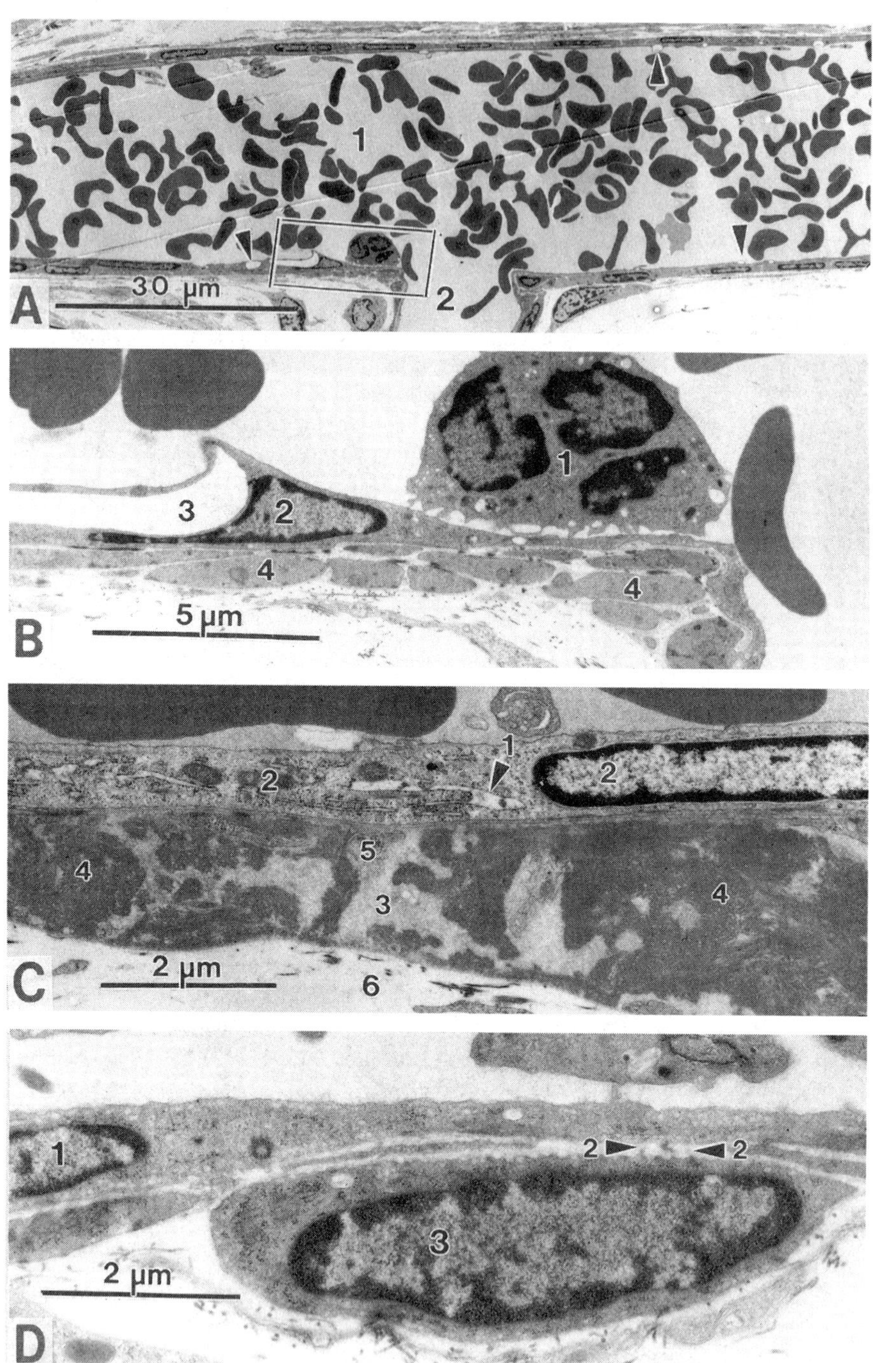

FIGURE 2. *Caption on following page.*

tumbling in the arterioles. In the venules, there was only the usual, modest margination and rolling of leukocytes. Platelets were not marginating. Mast cells were not activated, judged by the absence of degranulation. And macrophages displayed only a limited degree of activity. These observations correspond to a normal, control situation.

Electron Microscope Observations

Similarly, in all three experiments, the ultrastructural appearance of the walls of the arterioles and the venules were completely normal (FIGS. 2D & 3D). The endothelial cells were undamaged, the smooth muscle cells were not distorted, and there was no leakage of plasma into the subendothelial space.

DISCUSSION

Our *in vivo* observations and the follow-up of electron microscope analyses, often of the identical areas observed and recorded *in vivo*, indicate and confirm our previous observations[3] related to the role of Aβ in the induction of vascular damage. Furthermore, we also confirmed the vascular response to TNF-α and IL-1β. In all three experiments, we observed the classic inflammatory response with margination and transmigration of leukocytes in postcapillary venules and muscular venules.[8,9] The unusual aspect of this response was that it also occurred in arterioles and precapillary arterioles. This is a rare event observed in cases of traumatic injury.[10] Also, these vascular segments are usually involved in monocyte transmigration in a situation of an inflammatory response in the development of atherosclerosis.[1]

TNF-α is a key mediator in an inflammatory response and acts as a pleiotropic peptide to elicit the production of other cytokines, among them IL-1β. Our *in vivo* and electron microscope observations after introduction of TNF-α and IL-1β are almost identical to those observed after Aβ administration, confirming our hypothesis[3] that Aβ triggers the release of these cytokines from monocytes, macrophages, and endothelial cells by interacting with receptor cites, resulting in the generation of reactive oxygen species (ROS), which in turn also activate mast cells to release histamine, TNF-α, and IL-1β.

FIGURE 2. (A) Aβ alone. This is a 30-μ wide arteriole (1) and the exit of a 20-μ precapillary arteriole (2) sectioned parallel to their long axes. There are many vacuoles (*arrows*) in the endothelial cells. Images like this can easily be correlated with the live video recordings of the same vascular segment. Mag 950×. **(B)** Aβ alone. Enlargement of rectangle in (A). There is a marginated leukocyte (1) adhering to the endothelial lining near the precapillary exit. The cytoplasm of the endothelial cell (2) is damaged by large vacuoles (3). At this point in time, there is no plasma leakage that would distort the smooth muscle cells (4). Mag. 5700×. **(C)** Aβ alone. Wall of a 30-μ arteriole. Dilated profiles of endoplasmic reticulum (1) in the endothelial cell (2) are an indication of damage caused by the Aβ. The subendothelial space, normally occupied by smooth muscle cells, is filled with plasma (3) and fibrillar amyloid (4), leaving only remnants (5) of smooth muscle cells. There are no fibrillar deposits in the perivascular space (6). Mag. 10,800×. **(D)** SOD + Aβ. Wall of a 25-μ precapillary arteriole. This is a completely normal appearance. The endothelial cell (1) is not damaged. The subendothelial space is narrow (2) and not occupied by plasma or fibrillar amyloid. The smooth muscle cells (3) have a normal shape. Mag. 13,500×.

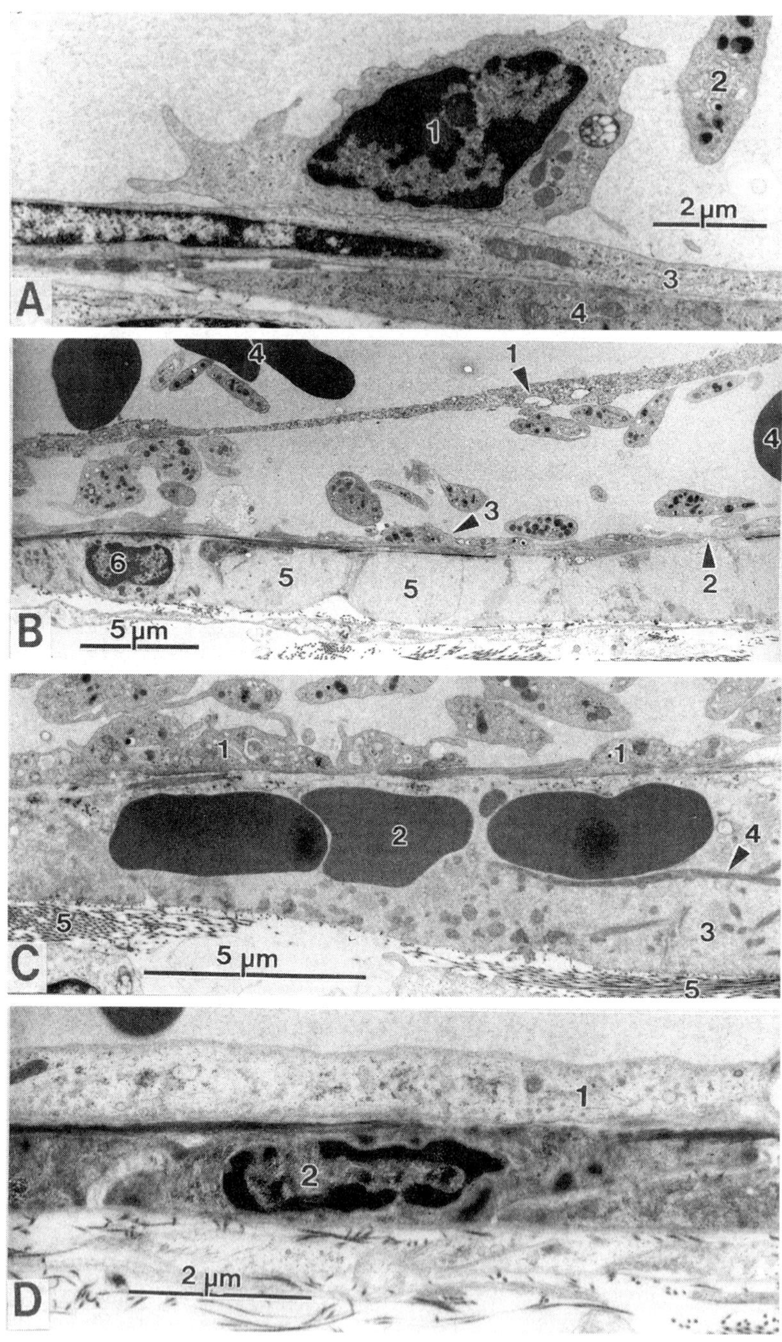

FIGURE 3. *Caption on following page.*

Thus, an increase of Aβ begins a cascade of events including an upregulation of cytokines and adhesion molecules, leukocyte and platelet margination and transmigration along with endothelial damage. Furthermore, leukocytes, erythrocytes and platelets along with fibrin and Aβ can pass into or across the vessel wall. One must also consider the role of the platelets, since reactive oxygen species (ROS) stimulate the tumbling and margination of platelets on the endothelium, mediated by P-selectin.[11] Platelets carry more than 90% of the circulating amyloid.[12] Activated platelets have been implicated as origins of the β-amyloid peptide fragment of APP (Aβ)[13–15] and during degranulation of the platelets would deposit the Aβ in walls of arterioles, a characteristic of Alzheimer's disease.

Further support for our hypothesis that Aβ triggers the release of cytokines is gained through our *in vivo* and electron microscope observations that inhibition of the oxygen radicals by the free radical scavenger SOD, and by blocking the effects of TNF and Il-1 through introduction of TNF-bp and IL-1ra greatly diminishes or eliminates the vascular inflammatory response.

REFERENCES

1. Ross, R. 1999. Atherosclerosis—an inflammatory disease. N. Engl. J. Med. **340:** 115–125.
2. Luster, A.D. 1998. Chemokines—chemotactic cytokines that mediate inflammation. N. Engl. J. Med. **338:** 436–445.
3. Thomas, T. *et al.* 1997. *In vivo* vascular damage, leukocyte activation and inflammatory response induced by β-amyloid. J. Submicrosc. Cytol. Pathol. **29:** 293–304.
4. Ghiso, J. *et al.* 1994. Unifying features of systemic and cerebral amyloidosis. Neuropathol. Exp. Neurol. **54:** 276–281.
5. Andersen, K. *et al.* 1995. Do nonsteroidal anti-inflammatory drugs decrease the risk for Alzheimer's disease? Neurology **45:** 1441–1445.
6. Duff, K. *et al.* 1996. Increased amyloid-β-42(43) in brains of mice expressing mutant presenilin 1. Nature **383:** 710–713.
7. Kalaria, R.N. 1996. Cerebral vessels in aging and Alzheimer's disease. Pharmacol. Ther. **72:** 193–214.
8. Marchesi, V.T. & H.W. Florey. 1960. Electron micrographic observations on the emigration of leucocytes. Q. J. Exp. Physiol. **45:** 343–348.

FIGURE 3. (A) IL-1β alone. Wall of a 25-μ arteriole. There is a leukocyte (monocyte) attached to the endothelial lining (1), a sign of activation of adhesion molecules. The nearby platelet (2) is freely suspended. The endothelial cytoplasm (3) and the smooth muscle cell (4) are not damaged. Mag. 7,800×. (B) TNF-α alone. Wall of a severely damaged 30-μ arteriole. The endothelial cell (1) is detached from its basal lamina (2), which is now covered by an incomplete layer of platelets (3). The endothelial cytoplasm (1) is vacuolated, and its nucleus (not shown) pyknotic. Erythrocytes (4) appear in the lumen as well as in the subendothelial space. The space normally occupied by smooth muscle cells is filled with plasma (5), and only one fairly intact smooth muscle cell (6) is present. Mag. 3300×. (C) TNF-α alone. Wall of a severely damaged 50-μ muscular venule. The endothelial lining is gone, and is replaced by numerous platelets (1) adhering to the endothelial basal lamina. The subendothelial space, normally occupied by smooth muscle cells contains erythrocytes (2), plasma (3), and fibrin (4). The perivascular space contains collagen fibrils (6) but no plasma. Mag. 6500×. (D) TNF-bp + Aβ. Wall of a 50-μ arteriole. This is completely normal. The endothelial cytoplasm (1) does not show signs of damage. The smooth muscle cells (2) are not distorted, and there is no leakage of plasma. Mag. 13,000×.

9. MARCHESI, V.T. 1961. The site of leucocyte emigration during inflammation. Q. J. Exp. Physiol. **46:** 115–118.
10. MAYROVITZ, H.N. *et al.* 1980. Leukocyte adherence in arterioles following extravascular tissue trauma. Microvasc. Res. **20:** 264–274.
11. FRENETTI, P.S. *et al.* 1995. Platelets roll on stimulated endothelium *in vivo*: an interaction mediated by endothelial P-selectin. Proc. Natl. Acad. Sci. USA **92:** 7450–7454.
12. DAVIES, T.A. *et al.* 1997. Stimulus responses and amyloid precursor protein processing in DAMI megakaryocytes. J. Lab. Clin. Med. **130:** 21–32.
13. BUSH, A.I. *et al.* 1990. The amyloid precursor protein of Alzheimer's disease is released by human platelets. J. Biol. Chem. **265:** 15977–15983.
14. VAN NOSTRAND, W.E. *et al.* 1990. Protease nexin II (amyloid precursor protein): a platelet alpha-granule protein. Science **248:** 745–748.
15. SCHMAIER, A.L. *et al.* 1993. Protease nexin-2/amyloid β protein precursor. J. Clin. Invest. **92:** 2540–2545.

Vascular Endothelium Is a Site of Free Radical Production and Inflammation in Areas of Neuronal Loss in Thiamine-deficient Brain

NOEL Y. CALINGASAN AND GARY E. GIBSON[a]

Weill Medical College of Cornell University at Burke Medical Research Institute, White Plains, New York 10605, USA

INTRODUCTION

Deficits in oxidative metabolism are central to the pathogenesis of many neurodegenerative diseases including Alzheimer's disease (AD).[1] Thiamine (vitamin B_1) deficiency (TD) is a classic animal model of impaired oxidative metabolism and selective neuronal death. As in AD, the neuron- and region-specific vulnerability in TD is associated with reduced activities of thiamine-dependent enzymes,[2] cholinergic deficits,[3] and memory loss.[4] Furthermore, in both TD and AD, neurons die while other cell types such as microglia, astrocytes, and endothelial cells do not. Although the precise mechanism responsible for selective vulnerability remains unclear for TD or any neurodegenerative disease, accumulating evidence supports the importance of cerebrovascular abnormalities. TD provides an animal model to study the mechanisms underlying the interaction between vascular changes, oxidative stress, and selective neuronal death. TD produces region-specific immunoglobulin G (IgG) accumulation, indicative of increased blood-brain barrier (BBB) permeability, in areas where neurons are destined to die.[5,6] Ultrastructurally, TD increases the number of vesicular profiles in BBB endothelial cells without altering the interendothelial tight junctions in the regions susceptible to TD-induced damage.[5] These results have stimulated interest in vascular factors as crucial elements in the pathogenesis of oxidative stress-mediated brain damage during TD. The cellular and molecular mechanisms of TD-induced death of select neuronal populations appear relevant to the selective vulnerability in neurodegenerative diseases associated with oxidative deficits.

NITRIC OXIDE SYNTHASE INDUCTION IN VASCULAR AND PERIVASCULAR CELLS IN VULNERABLE REGIONS DURING THIAMINE DEFICIENCY

Nitric oxide (NO) is a biological messenger and neurotransmitter, as well as a potential mediator of neurotoxicity. NO is formed from arginine by NO synthase

[a]Address for correspondence: G. E. Gibson, Weill Medical College of Cornell University at Burke Medical Research Institute, 785 Mamaroneck Avenue, White Plains, New York 10605. Tel.: (914) 597-2291; fax: (914) 597-2757.
e-mail: ggibson@med.cornell.edu

(NOS). Excessive NO is capable of disrupting the BBB permeability. During TD, enhanced expression of endothelial NOS (eNOS) immunoreactivity and nicotinamide adenine dinucleotide phosphate (NADPH) diaphorase reactivity (a general indicator of NOS activity) in microvessels accompany the region-specific increases in IgG extravasation.[7] IgG and other extraneuronal proteins may contribute to neuronal damage.

Induction of NOS also occurs in nonvascular cells after thiamine deprivation. TD increases inducible NOS (iNOS) immunoreactivity in microglia/macrophages in the thalamus, one of the vulnerable areas.[7] Many of these iNOS-immunoreactive cells surround blood vessels.

NOS induction likely plays an important role in the TD pathology, because nitrotyrosine formation increases in axons within areas of damage.[7] Nitrotyrosine is a specific nitration product of peroxynitrite, a potent oxidant generated by reaction of NO with superoxide, a free radical that accumulates in the thalamus.[8] Peroxynitrite can diffuse from its vascular or nonvascular origin such as microglia, and damage neurons by impairing the mitochondrial respiratory chain or mitochondrial calcium metabolism, by damaging DNA, or by inhibiting key enzymes of glucose metabolism,[9] including the α-ketoglutarate dehydrogenase complex.[10] Widespread peroxynitrite-mediated damage occurs in AD, as evidenced by the presence of intense nitrotyrosine immunoreactivity in neurons, including those bearing neurofibrillary tangles, one of the key pathological lesions in AD.[11]

The contribution of eNOS induction to TD-induced neurodegeneration appears more important than iNOS. Gene-targeted deletion of iNOS does not attenuate neuronal death induced by TD.[12] In contrast, preliminary studies revealed that absolute inactivation of eNOS mitigated the neuronal damage in TD brain.[13] Thus, iNOS is not a prerequisite for the TD-induced oxidative stress and neuronal demise.

ANTIOXIDANT AND INFLAMMATORY RESPONSES ARE ASSOCIATED WITH REGION-SPECIFIC MICROVESSELS DURING THIAMINE DEFICIENCY

Induction of the iron-sequestering protein, ferritin, as well as the oxidative stress marker, heme oxygenase-1 (HO-1) provides evidence of oxidative stress in blood vessels and microglia during TD. TD increases ferritin immunoreactivity in the walls of capillaries and larger blood vessels within the areas of neuronal damage and BBB breakdown but not in nonvulnerable areas.[7] In addition, numerous microglia with robust ferritin immunoreactivity occur in vulnerable regions. The ferritin-immunoreactive microglia display plump bodies with ramified processes, typical of the ferritin-positive activated microglia found in pathological brain tissues as in AD. Numerous activated microglia cluster along the periphery of microvessels. Iron histochemistry reveals that these activated microglia are also loaded with redox active iron, supporting the role of oxidative damage in TD pathology. The iron in TD may have originated from blood heme. Consistent with this idea is the detection in microglia of the oxidative stress marker, HO-1,[12] the rate-limiting enzyme that cleaves heme producing iron, biliverdin, and carbon monoxide. The pattern of HO-1 induction in microglia parallels the neuronal loss in the thalamus. Light HO-1 immunoreactivity also occurs in microvessel walls in the thalamus during TD. Superoxide dismutase, another indicator of oxidative stress accumulates in microglia of TD vulnerable regions.[8] In AD, iron accumulation could be an important source of oxidative damage, as evidenced by the detection of redox active iron and HO-1 in neurofibrillary tangles.[14,15]

OXIDATIVE STRESS IN NEURONS DURING THIAMINE DEFICIENCY

The submedial nucleus is the site of the earliest neuronal dropout in the thalamus. Although there is no evidence of neuronal oxidative stress in the submedial nucleus prior to the initial neuronal demise, oxidative stress appears to play a role in subsequent neurodegeneration during TD.[12] In neurons, TD increases the immunoreactivity for nitrotyrosine,[7] a specific nitration product of peroxynitrite, and for 4-hydroxynonenal,[12] a cytotoxic aldehyde that is produced during lipid peroxidation. These oxidative stress markers also accumulate in senile plaques and/or neurofibrillary tangles in brains of Alzheimer patients.[11,16] Reactive oxygen intermediates are known to activate the transcription factor, nuclear factor-κB (NF-κB). During late stages of TD, NF-κB immunoreactivity increases in the nuclei of neurons within the thalamus (unpublished results), consistent with the involvement of oxidative stress in the TD model.

SUMMARY AND CONCLUSION

Free radical production in vascular endothelial cells and inflammatory responses in perivascular microglia accompany the selective neuronal death induced by TD. Lipid peroxidation and tyrosine nitration occur in neurons within susceptible areas. Thus, region- and cell-specific oxidative stress contributes to selective neurodegeneration during TD. These data are consistent with the hypothesis that in TD, vascular factors constitute a critical part of a cascade of events leading to increases in bloodbrain barrier permeability to nonneuronal proteins and iron, leading to inflammation and oxidative stress. Inflammatory cells may release deleterious compounds or cytokines that exacerbate the oxidative damage to metabolically compromised neurons. Similar mechanisms may operate in the pathophysiology of neurodegenerative diseases in which vascular factors, inflammation and oxidative stress are implicated including AD.

REFERENCES

1. BLASS, J.P. & G.E. GIBSON. 1991. The role of oxidative abnormalities in the pathophysiology of Alzheimer's disease. Rev. Neurol. **147:** 513–525.
2. GIBSON, G.E., H. KSIEZAK-REDING, K.-F.R. SHEU, V. MYKYTYN & J.P. BLASS. 1984. Correlation of enzymatic, metabolic and behavioral deficits in thiamine deficiency and its reversal. Neurochem. Res. **9:** 803–814.
3. VORHEES, C.V., D.E. SCHMIDT & R.J. BARRETT. 1978. Effects of pyrithiamin and oxythiamin on acetylcholine levels and utilization in rat brain. Brain Res. Bull. **3:** 493–496.

4. LANGLAIS, P.J. & L.M. SAVAGE. 1995. Thiamine deficiency in rats produces cognitive and memory deficits on spatial tasks that correlate with tissue loss in diencephalon, cortex and white matter. Behav. Brain Res. **68:** 75–89.

5. CALINGASAN, N.Y., H. BAKER, K.-F.R. SHEU & G.E. GIBSON. 1995. Blood-brain barrier abnormalities in vulnerable brain regions during thiamine deficiency. Exp. Neurol. **134:** 64–72.

6. HARATA, N. & Y. IWASAKI. 1995. Evidence for early blood-brain barrier breakdown in experimental thiamine deficiency in the mouse. Metab. Brain Dis. **10:** 159–174.

7. CALINGASAN, N.Y., L.C.H. PARK, L.L. CALO, R.R. TRIFILETTI, S.E. GANDY & G.E. GIBSON. 1998. Induction of nitric oxide synthase and microglial responses precede selective cell death induced by chronic impairment of oxidative metabolism. Am. J. Pathol. **153:** 1381–1398.

8. TODD, K.G. & R.F. BUTTERWORTH. 1997. Evidence that oxidative stress plays a role in neuronal cell death due to thiamine deficiency [abstract]. J. Neurochem. **69:** S136.

9. BOLAÑOS, J.P., A. ALMEIDA, V. STEWART, S. PEUCHEN, J.M. LAND, J.B. CLARK & S.J.R. HEALES. 1997. Nitric oxide-mediated mitochondrial damage in the brain: mechanisms and implications for neurodegenerative diseases. J. Neurochem. **68:** 2227–2240.

10. PARK, L.C.H., H. ZHANG, K.-F.R. SHEU, N.Y. CALINGASAN, B.S. KRISTAL, J.G. LINDSAY & G.E. GIBSON. 1999. Metabolic impairment induces oxidative stress, compromises inflammatory responses, and inactivates a key mitochondrial enzyme in microglia. J. Neurochem. **72:** 1948–1958.

11. SMITH, M.A., P.L.R. HARRIS, L.M. SAYRE, J.S. BECKMAN & G. PERRY. 1997. Widespread peroxynitrite-mediated damage in Alzheimer's disease. J. Neurosci. **17:** 2653–2657.

12. CALINGASAN, N.Y., W.J. CHUN, L.C.H. PARK, K. UCHIDA & G.E. GIBSON. 1999. Oxidative stress is associated with region-specific neuronal death during thiamine deficiency. J. Neuropathol. Exp. Neurol. **58:** 946–958.

13. CALINGASAN, N.Y., P.L. HUANG, H.S. CHUN & G.E. GIBSON. 1999. Vascular factors are critical in the selective neuronal death in an animal model of impaired oxidative metabolism. Soc. Neurosci. Abstr. [abstract] **25:** 323.

14. SMITH, M.A., S. TANEDA, P.L. RICHEY, S. MIYATA, S.D. YAN, D. STERN, L.M. SAYRE, V.M. MONNIER & G. PERRY. 1994. Heme oxygenase-1 is associated with the neurofibrillary pathology of Alzheimer's disease. Am. J. Pathol. **145:** 42–47.

15. SMITH, M.A. & G. PERRY. 1995. Free radical damage, iron, and Alzheimer's disease. J. Neurol. Sci. **134:** 92–94.

16. SAYRE, L.M., D.A. ZOLAESQUE, P.L. HARRIS, G. PERRY, R.K. SALOMON & M.A. SMITH. 1997. 4-Hydroxynonenal-derived advanced lipid peroxidation end products are increased in Alzheimer's disease. J. Neurochem. **68:** 2092–2097.

Marked Hippocampal Neuronal Damage without Motor Deficits after Mild Concussive-like Brain Injury in Apolipoprotein E-deficient Mice

SEOL-HEUI HAN,[a,c] AND SEUNG-YUN CHUNG[b]

[a]Department of Neurology, Chungbuk National University Hospital, 62 Gaeshin-dong, Chungbuk 361-711, Korea

[b]Department of Pediatrics, Our Lady of Mercy Hospital, Catholic University Medical College, Bupyong-dong, Bupyong-ku, Inchon 403-016, Korea

ABSTRACT: Of various biological factors, only allele ε4 of apolipoprotein E (apoE, protein; APOE4, gene) has been thus far suggested as a major determinant of genetic risk for sporadic and late-onset familial Alzheimer's disease (AD). Environmental influences such as lack of education, traumatic brain injury, oxidative stress, environmental toxins, hormonal imbalances, and alterations in immune or inflammatory responses may also contribute to the pathogenesis of AD. Thus genetic susceptibility and environmental risk factors may have synergistic effects on the development of AD. The purpose of present report was to assess whether the gene (APOE) and the environmental risk factor (traumatic brain injury) could interact in hippocampal neuronal degeneration. We investigated the histopathological changes of hipoccampal regions after mild concussive-like brain injury without motor deficits in apoE-deficient mice using the recently described novel weight-drop device. Control mice revealed minimal neurodegenerative changes limited to CA2 and CA3, while apoE-deficient mice showed widespread neuronal degeneration throughout hippocampal subfields and part of dentate gyrus. We also observed widespread glial fibrillary acidic protein (GFAP) immunoreactivity throughout the hippocampus, which was more intense in apoE-deficient mice. The results of this study indicate that even very mild traumatic brain injury could result in widespread hippocampal damage in apoE-deficient mice. This again supports the hypothesis that apoE might play a neurotrophic or neuroprotective function in the central nervous system.

INTRODUCTION

Although the underlying pathogenic mechanism of Alzheimer's disease (AD) is still evasive, recent molecular genetic studies have identified several causative and/or susceptibility genes of it, such as the amyloid precursor protein, presenilin 1, presenilin 2, and allele ε4 of apolipoprotein E (apoE, protein; APOE4, gene) genes.[1–6]

[c]Address for correspondence: Seol-Heui Han, M.D., Department of Neurology, Chungbuk National University Hospital, 62 Gaeshin-dong, Chungbuk, Korea 361-711. Tel.: +82-431-2696372; fax: +82-431-2768929.

e-mail: shhan@med.chungbuk.ac.kr

Environmental influences such as lack of education, traumatic brain injury, oxidative stress, environmental toxins, and hormonal imbalances, and alterations in immune or inflammatory responses may also contribute to the pathogenesis of AD.[7] Of various biological factors, only the APOE4 has been thus far suggested as a major determinant of genetic risk factor for sporadic and late-onset familial AD.[4–6] Head trauma has been implicated as a possible environmental trigger for AD. Thus genetic susceptibility and environmental risk factors may have synergistic effects on the development of AD.[8,9] In this study, we investigated the histopathological changes of hipoccampal regions after mild concussive-like brain injury without motor deficits in apoE-deficient (apoE-KO) mice using the recently described novel weight-drop device.[10] While wild-type (WT) mice showed minimal neurodegenerative changes limited to CA2 and CA3, apoE-deficient mice showed widespread neuronal degeneration throughout hippocampal subfields and part of dentate gyrus. We also observed widespread glial fibrillary acidic protein (GFAP) immunoreactivity throughout the hippocampus, which was more intense in apoE-deficient mice. Regarding the function of different isoforms, early studies demonstrated isoform-specific effects of apoE on neurite outgrowth such that the E3 isoform promotes outgrowth, whereas the E4 isoform inhibits outgrowth, leading to the hypothesis that E4 may not provide effective neuronal repair or protection. Current data suggest interactions among the various possible biological and environmental influences that result in a common pathway leading to the development of AD.

MATERIALS AND METHODS

Animals

All apoE-deficient and their wild-type control mice (C57BL/6J, 22–25 g) were purchased from The Jackson Laboratory (Bar Harbor, ME). The animals were housed in groups of four per cage under standard condition ($23 \pm 1°C$, $50 \pm 5\%$ humidity) with a 12:12 h light-dark cycle (lights on at 09:00), fed with regular mouse chow and water *ad libitum*, and allowed 2 weeks of adaptation after arrival.

Induction of Concussive-like Brain Injury (CLBI)

We produced traumatic brain impact using Tang's method with minor modification.[10] Briefly, mice were anesthetized with halothane (about 3% in air, 40 ml/min for 50 sec) using a Small Animal Anesthetizer, which was confirmed by testing loss of corneal reflex. The weight drop device consists of a cylindrical-shaped acrylic weight (diameter 1 cm, length 20 cm, weight 21 g), a Plexiglas tube (inner diameter 14 mm), and a silicon rubber platform. The tube is held in place with a ring stand. A midline incision was performed, exposing the skull surface, then quickly placed in a prone position on the rubber platform so that the central region between the coronal and the lambdoid sutures was centered beneath the Plexiglas tube. The head was manually fixed at the bottom plane of the impact device. When a desired impacting height was determined, the weight was allowed to free-fall, striking the intended skull area. Following recovery from anesthesia, the mice were returned to their home cages with free access to food and water. In this study, height of 20 cm was found suitable to produce CLBI without any acute neurologic deficits. We evaluated the motor function and righting reflex response of traumatized mice at different time points (1, 24, and 72 h). All experiments were conducted in compliance with an animal protocol approved by the Chungbuk National University Hospital Animal Care and Use Committee.

Histology and Immunohistochemistry

Seventy-two hours after CLBI, animals were sacrificed under pentothal sodium anesthesia (5 mg/kg i.p.). They were perfused transcardially with ice-cold heparinized physiological saline followed by 4% paraformaldehyde (in 0.1 M phosphate buffer, PB) for 10–15 minutes. The brains were carefully removed, post-fixed in the same fixative at 4°C overnight, and then embedded in paraffin. Serial 6-μm coronal sections were cut and stained with hematoxylin and eosin (H&E). Adjacent sections were immunostained with a polyclonal antibody against glial fibrillary acidic protein (GFAP, 1:250, Boehringer-Mannheim).

Evaluation of Neuronal Damage

The extent of neuronal damage was assessed by one of us (SYC), who, blinded to the injury status and genotype of the mice and using a light microscope (Olympus, ×400), counted the number of pink acidophilic dead neurons, as described by Kaku *et al.*[11] Two consecutive sections at the level of dorsal hippocampus are expressed semiquantitatively, i.e., +, mild neuronal damage, ++, moderate neuronal damage, +++, severe neuronal damage.

RESULTS

Neurological Evaluation

The neurological status of the injured mice was evaluated by measuring motor function tasks, i.e., balancing on a round stick (20 cm long, diameter 0.5 cm, height 15 cm) and beam walking. None of the injured mice showed any motor deficits 1, 24, and 72 h after CLBI.

Histolopathological Observations (Table 1, Figs. 1–3)

Histological examination was focused on the hippocampal sectors, CA1, CA2, and CA3/4, and dentate gyri. Examinations of the brain sections 72 h after CLBI revealed that there were no contusions in the cerebrum, the cerebellum, or the brain-

TABLE 1. The degree of neuronal damage of hippocampal regions 72 hrs after CLBI

Mice	CA1	CA2	CA3	Hilus	DG
WT	0	+	+++	+	0
K-O	++	++	+++	++	++

ABBREVIATIONS: CLBI, concussive-like brain injury; WT, wild-type mice; DG, dentate gyrus; K-O, ApoE-deficient mice.

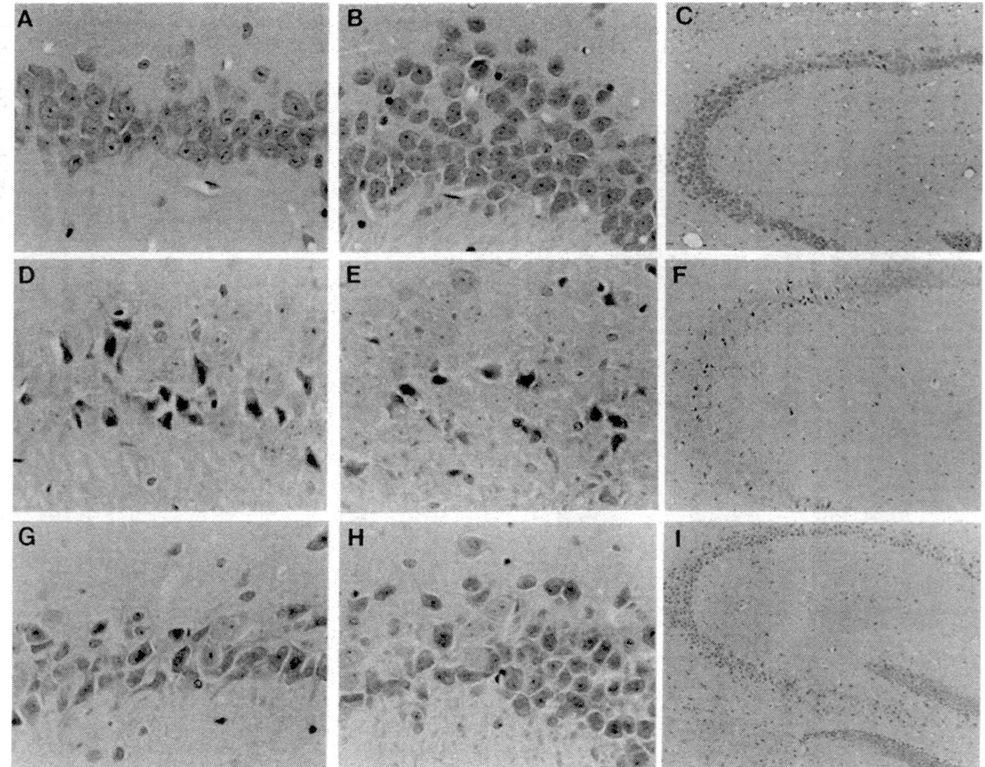

FIGURE 1. Hippocampal neurodegeneration after concussive-like brain injury (CLBI). Representative H&E-stained coronal sections illustrating acidophilic, shrunken dead neurons 72 h after CLBI (**A,D,G**, CA2; **B,E,H**, CA3). Note the difference in severity of neuronal damage between WT (**D,E,F**) and apoE-deficient mice (**G,H,I**). The *uppermost panel* shows no neuronal damage (A,B,C, sham-operated apoE-KO mice). (Original magnifications: A,B,D,E,G,H, ×400; C,F,I, ×100.)

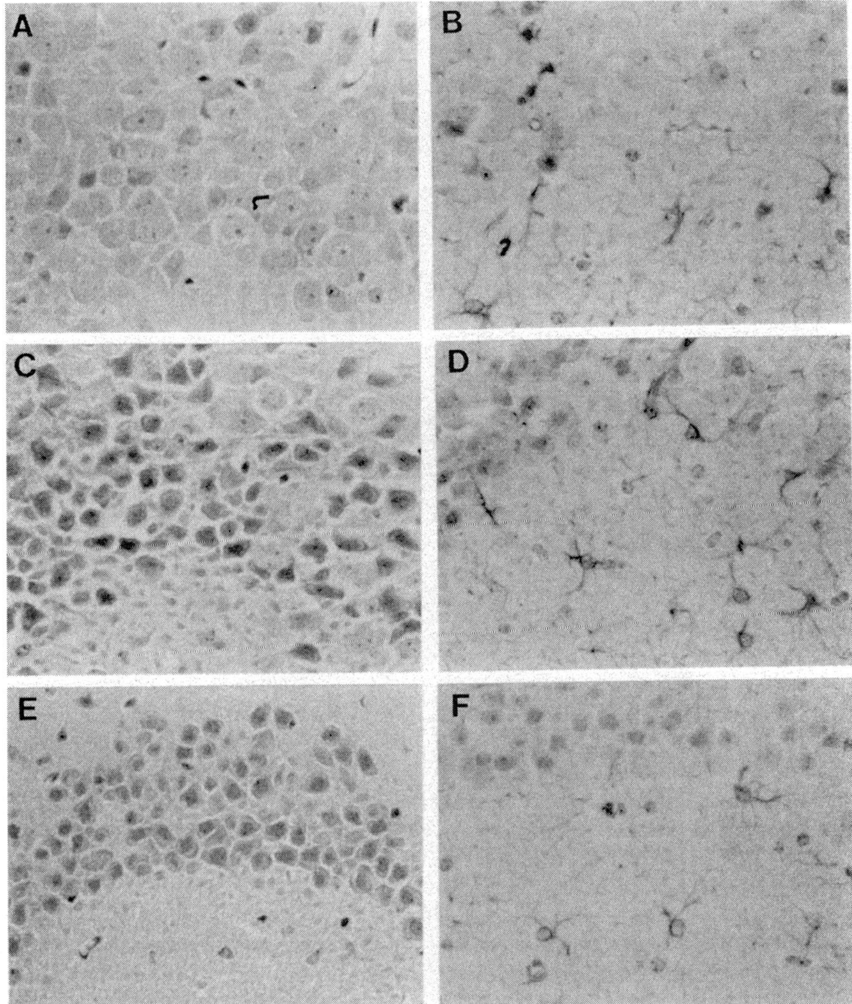

FIGURE 2. Hippocampal neurodegeneration and reactive astrogliosis. Representative H&E stained **(A,C,E)** and GFAP-immunostained **(B,D,F)** sections of CA3 hippocampal subfields. (A,B: WT mice, height injury level, 20 cm; C,D: WT mice, height of injury level, 35 cm; D,E: apoE-deficient mice, height of injury level, 20 cm). Note that the severity and GFAP immunoreactivity of apoE-deficient mice is comparable to more intensely injured WT animals. (All original magnifications, ×400.)

stem (data not shown). Pink acidophilic neurons with shrunken morphology were counted at a magnification of 400×. At the height of 20 cm, wild-type mice showed mild neuronal degeneration limited to the hippocampal subfields CA1 and CA2 (FIG. 1D,E,F), while apoE-deficient animals revealed severe degenerative changes in CA1, CA2, and CA3 and mildly damaged neurons in dentate gyrus at the same

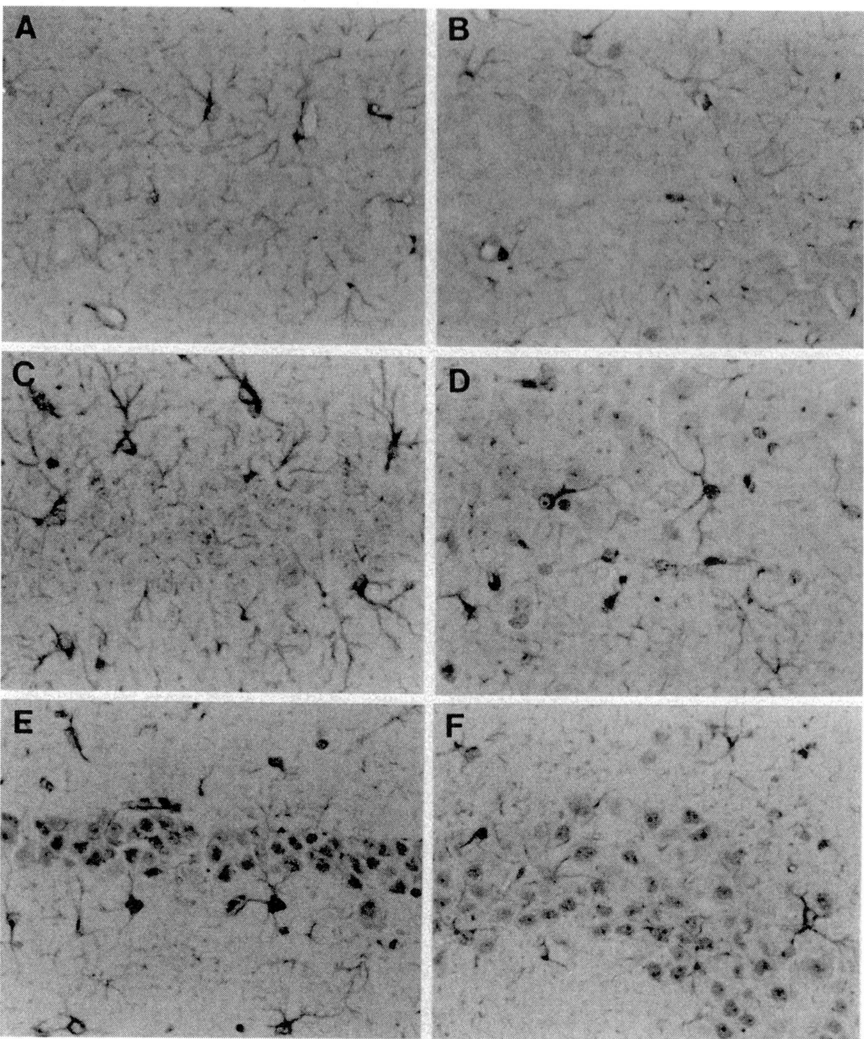

FIGURE 3. GFAP immunohistochemistry counterstained with hematoxylin coronal sections of CA2 (**A,C,E**) and CA3 (**B,D,F**) hippocampal subfields. Resting astrocytes are seen in sham-operated apoE-deficient mice (A,B). Activated astrocytes showing hypertrophied cell bodies and thick, long cytoplasmic processes with stronger immunoreactivity are seen in injured WT (C,D) and apo-E deficient (E,F) mice. Neuronal degeneration is also evident in this hematoxylin counter-stained sections (E,F). (All original magnifications, ×400.)

height (FIG. 1G,H,I). The severity of neuronal damage and degree of astrocytic activation seemed to be related to the intensity of the injury. At the height of 20 cm, the neuronal damage and GFAP immunoreactivity was minimal to mild (FIG. 2A,B), whereas neuronal damage was severe and GFAP immunogenecity was robust at the height of 35 cm (FIG. 2C,D). In the case with the apoE-KO animal, the degree of neuronal damage at the height of 20 cm was comparable to 35 cm-WT injury (FIG. 2E,F). While sham-operated apoE-deficient animals showed minimal GFAP immunoreactivity (FIG. 3A,B), both the WT (FIG. 3C,D) and apoE-KO (FIG. 3E,F) animals indicated robust astrocytic reactions. The difference of neuronal damage is also evident in the hematoxylin-counterstained GFAP immunohistochemistry (FIG. 3E,F).

DISCUSSION

Recent studies suggest that ApoE plays a neurotrophic role in the central nervous system (CNS) and that aberrant function of this molecule might result in genetic susceptibility to the effects of variety of CNS disorders. Moreover, these effects appear to be isoform-specific. The APOE4 is a well-documented risk factor for sporadic and late-onset familial Alzheimer's disease,[4] and has also been associated with poor outcome from intracerebral hemorrhage,[12] closed head injury,[13] dementia pugilistica,[16] stroke,[17] and cardiopulmonary bypass.[18] Thus apoE-deficient mice provide a useful system for studying the role of apoE in neuronal maintenance and repair. The present study has shown that mice deficient in apoE have an increased vulnerability even to the effects of the mildest form of brain injury when compared with wild-type littermate controls.

Our results are consistent with a number of other studies which have illustrated that apoE-KO mice have a worse outcome following various acute brain insults. A recent animal model study using apoE-deficient mice has shown that apoE-deficient animals had increased neuronal damage which paralleled motor and cognitive deficits and thus revealed that they recovered from closed head injury less adequately than the control mice.[19] In contrast to the previous model system, neither gross anatomical local lesion, contusion in the brain nor functional motor deficits, were observed in our CLBI model. This recently described novel weight-drop device could deliver very mild concussive-like brain injury, in which the damage to the brain is diffuse, the surgical preparation of animals is simple, and no other complicating factors such as infection are involved,[10] hence it is more likely to produce a condition mimicking human head concussion syndrome. In the present study, as with Chen *et al.*'s original description, the damaged neurons were located in the subfields of CA2 and CA3, and the hilar region in wild-type mice, while more extensive neuronal damage, i.e., entire hippocampal subfields and part of dentate gyrus, were found in apoE-deficient groups (FIG. 1). In control mice, the extent of neuronal damage was dependent upon the height of weight delivery. Minimal to mild neuronal injury was observed at the height of 20 cm, while severe neuronal damages were noted at the height of 35 cm. Interestingly, but as might to be expected, apoE-deficient mice showed comparable neuronal damage at the height of 20 cm. Differential immunoreactivity to GFAP antibody was evident with similar magnitude (FIG. 2). Even with mild CLBI, robust astrocytic reactions were noted in both apoE-deficient and wild-type mice (FIG. 3). Astrocytic activation or reactive gliosis is a characteristic response of the CNS to destructive tissue injury. Reactive astrocytes had a distinct morphology characterized by an enlarged cell body and long intertwined processes. Our findings were consistent with Bodjarian *et al.*'s study, in that they demonstrated increased GFAP mRNA expression after closed head injury where more intense and rapid expression was noted in the hippocampus.[20]

Although it has been suggested that apoE plays an important role in the response to acute brain injury, the mechanisms as yet remain unknown. One most plausible mechanism is a role of apoE is protection against oxidative insults and the ensuing lipid peroxidation, as suggested by a recent report that concentrations of 3-nitroxy-rosine, a marker for nitration of proteins produced by peroxynitrite, were significantly increased in the cerebral cortex, hippocampus, brainstem and cerebellum of apoE-deficient mice.[21] Moreover, the diminished recovery of apoE-deficient mice from head injury has been shown to be associated with a reduction in their ability to counteract oxidative damage.[22] ApoE , a protein produced by glial cells, is responsible for maintenance of the structural integrity of the microtubules within the axon of the neuron. It also has been suggested that apoE plays an important role in neuronal developmental processes including neurite outgrowth.[23] ApoE mRNA expression is upregulated during the neuroregenerative process and after brain injury.[24] Another possibility is that apoE exerts a neurotrophic effect on injured neurons as shown by *in vitro* evidence of promoting neuronal survival and neurite outgrowth[23,25] and *in vivo* experiment in an isoform-specific manner.[26] Consistent with previous observations, the present study showed that an ApoE-deficit results in severe hippocampal neuronal damage even in very mild CLBI compared with wild-type control. Thus alterations in apoE may impose deleterious effects on neuronal survival.

ACKNOWLEDGMENT

This work was supported by the Korea Science and Engineering Foundation (KOSEF) through the Brain Disease Research Center.

REFERENCES

1. VAN DUIJN, C.M., L. HENDRIKS, M. CRUTS, J.A. HARDY, A. HOFMAN & C. VAN BROECKHOVEN. 1991. Amyloid precursor protein gene mutation in early-onset Alzheimer's disease. Lancet **20:** 337–978.
2. LEVY-LAHAD, E., E.M. WIJSMAN, E. NEMENS, L. ANDERSON, K.A. GODDARD, J.L. WEBER, T.D. BIRD & G.D. SCHELLENBERG. 1995. A familial Alzheimer's disease locus on chromosome 1. Science **269:** 970–973.
3. SHERRINGTON, R., E.I. ROGAEV, Y. LIANG, E.A. ROGAEV, G. LEVESQUE, M. IKEDA, H. CHI, C. LIN, G. LI, K. HOLMAN, T. TSUDA, L. MAR, J.F. FONCIN, A.C. BRUNI, M.P. MONTESI, S. SROBI, I. RAINERO, L. PINESSI, L. NEE, I. CHUMAKOV, D. POLLEN, A. BROOKS, P. SANSEAU, R.J. POLINSKY, R.J. WASCO, H.A.R. DASILVA, J.L. HAINES, M.A. PERIKAK-VANCE, R.E. TANZI, A.D. ROSES, P.E. FRASER, J.M. ROMMMENS & P.H. ST. GEORGE-HYSLOP. 1995. Cloning of a gene bearing missense mutations in early-onset familial Alzheimer's disease. Nature **375:** 754–760.
4. STRITTMATTER, W.J., A.M. SAUNDERS, D. SCHMECHEL, M. PERICAK-VANCE, J. ENGHILD, G.S. SALVESON & A.D. ROSES. 1993. Apolipoprotein E: high avidity binding to β-amyloid and increased frequency of type 4 allele in late-onset familial Alzheimer's disease. Proc. Natl. Acad. Sci. USA **90:** 1977–1981.
5. CORDER, E.H., A.M. SAUNDERS, W.J. STRITTMATTER, D.E. SCHMECHEL, P.C. GASKELL, G.W. SMALL, A.D. ROSES, J.L. HAINES & M.A. PERICAK-VANCE. 1993. Gene dose of apolipoprotein E type 4 allele and the risk of Alzheimer's disease in late onset families. Science **261:** 921–923.

6. MAYEUX, R., Y. STERN, R. OTTMAN, T.K. TATEMICHI, M.-X. TANG, G. MAESTRE, C. NAGI, B. TYCKO & H. GINSBERG. 1993. The apolipoprotein ε4 allele in patients with Alzheimer's disease. Ann. Neurol. **34:** 752–754.

7. SMALL, G.W. 1998. The pathogenesis of Alzheimer's disease. Clin. Psychiatry **59**(Suppl. 9): 7–14 .

8. GENTLEMAN, S.M., D.I. GRAHAM & G.W. ROBERTS. 1993. Molecular pathology of head trauma: altered βAPP metabolism and the aetiology of Alzheimer's disease. Prog. Brain Res. **96:** 237–246.

9. MAYEUX, R., R. OTTMAN, G. MAESTRE, C. NAGI, M.-X. TANG, H. GINSBERG, M. CHUN, B. TYCKO & M. SHELANSKI. 1995. Synergistic effects of traumatic head injury and apolipoprotein-ε4 in patients with Alzheimer's disease. Neurology **45:** 555–557.

10. TANG. Y.P., Y. NODA, T. HASEGAWA & T. NABESHIMA. 1997. A concussive-like brain injury model in mice (I): impairment in learning and memory. J. Neurotrauma **14:** 851–862.

11. KAKU, Y., Y. YONEKAWA, T. TSUKAHARA, N. OGATA, T. KIMURA & T. TANIGUCHI. 1993. Alterations of a 200 kDa neurofilament in the rat hippocampus after forebrain ischemia. J. Cereb. Blood Flow Metab. **13:** 402–408.

12. ALBERTS, M.J., J.C. GRAFFAGNINO, C. MCCLENNY, D. DELONG, W. STRITTMATTER, A.M. SAUNDERS & A.D. ROSES. 1995. ApoE genotype and survival from intracerebral hemorrhage. Lancet **346:** 575.

13. NICOLL, J.A.R., G.W. ROBERTS & D.I. GRAHAM. 1995. ApoE4 allele is associated with deposition of amyloid-beta protein following head injury. Nat. Med. **1:** 135–137.

14. ROSES, A.D. & A.M. SAUNDERS. 1995. Head injury, amyloid beta and Alzheimer's disease (letter). Nat. Med. **1:** 603–604.

15. TEASDALE, M.C.G., J.A.R. NICOLL, G. MURRAY & M. FIDDES. 1977. Association of apolipoprotein E polymorphism with outcome after head injury. Lancet **350:** 1069–1071.

16. JORDAN, B.D., N.R. RELKIN, L.D. RAVDIN, A.R. JACOBS, A. BENNETT & S. GANDY. 1997. Apolipoprotein E epsilon4 associated with chronic traumatic brain injury in boxing. JAMA **278:** 136–140.

17. SLOOTER, A.J., M.X. TANG, C.M. VAN DUIJN, Y. STERN, A. OTT, K. BELL, M.M. BRETELER, C. VAN BROECKHOVEN, T.K. TATEMICHI, B. TYCKO, A. HOFMAN & R. MAYEUX. 1997. Apolipoprotein E epsilon4 and the risk of dementia with stroke. A population-based investigation. JAMA **277:** 818–821.

18. NEWMAN, M.F., N.D. CROUGHWELL, J.A. BLUMENTHAL, E. LOWRY, W.D. WHITE, W. SPILLANE, R.D. DAVIS, JR., D.D. GLOWER, L.R. SMITH & E.P. MAHANNA. 1995. Predictors of cognitive decline after cardiac operation. Ann. Thorac. Surg. **59:** 1326–1330.

19. CHEN, Y., L. LOMNITSKI, D.M. MICHAELSON & E. SHOHAMI. 1997. Motor and cognitive deficits in apolipoprotein E-deficient mice after closed head injury. Neuroscience **80:** 1255–1262.

20. BODJARIAN, N., S. JAMALI, N. BOISSET & M. TADIE. 1997. Strong expression of GFAP mRNA in rat hippocampus after a closed-head injury. Neuroreport **8:** 3951–3956.

21. MATTHEWS, R.T. & M.F. BEAL. 1996. Increased 3-nitrotyrosine in brains of Apo E-deficient mice. Brain Res. **718:** 181–184.

22. LOMNITSKI, L., R. KOHEN, Y. CHEN, E. SHOHAMI, V. TREMBOVLER, T. VOGEL & D.M. MICHAELSON. 1997. Reduced levels of antioxidants in brains of apolipoprotein E-deficient mice following closed head injury. Pharmacol. Biochem. Behav. **56:** 669–673.

23. HOLZMAN, D.M., R.E. PITAS, J. KILBRIDGE, B. NATHAN, R.W. MAJLEY, G. BU & A.L. SCHWAARTZ. 1995. Low density lipoprotein receptor-related protein mediates apolipoprotein E-dependent neurite outgrowth in a central nervous system-derived neuronal cell line. Proc. Natl. Acad. Sci. USA **92:** 9480–9484.

24. LASKOWITZ, D.T., K. HORSBURGH & A.D. ROSES. 1998. Apolipoprotein E and the CNS response to injury. J. Cereb. Blood Flow Metab. **18:** 465–471.

25. NATHAN, B.P., S. BELLOSTA, D.A. SANAN, K.H. WEISGRABER, R.W. MAHLEY & R.E. PITAS. 1994. Differential effects of apolipoprotein E3 and E4 on neuronal growth *in vitro*. Science **264:** 850–852.

26. VEINBERGS, I., M. MALLORY, M. MANTE, E. ROCKENSTEIN, J.R. GILBERT & E. MASLIAH. 1999. Differential neurotrophic effects of apolipoprotein E in aged transgenic mice. Neurosci. Lett. **265:** 218–222.

Cortical Cholinergic Denervation Elicits Vascular Aβ Deposition

ALEX E. ROHER,[a,d] YU-MIN KUO,[a] PAMELA E. POTTER,[a]
MARK R. EMMERLING,[b] ROBERT A. DURHAM,[b] DOUGLAS G. WALKER,[a]
LUCIA I. SUE,[a] WILLIAM G. HONER,[c] AND THOMAS G. BEACH[a]

[a]*Sun Health Research Institute, Sun City, Arizona 85351, USA*

[b]*Parke-Davis Pharmaceutical Research Division, Warner-Lambert Company,
Ann Arbor, Michigan 48105, USA*

[c]*Department of Psychiatry, University of British Columbia, Vancouver,
British Columbia, Canada*

ABSTRACT: Selective destruction of the cholinergic nucleus basalis magnocellularis (nbm) in the rabbit by the p75 neurotrophin receptor (NTR) immunoglobulin G (IgG) complexed to the toxin saporin leads to the deposition of amyloid-beta (Aβ) in and around cerebral blood vessels. In some instances, the perivascular Aβ resemble the diffuse deposits observed in Alzheimer's disease (AD). We propose that cortical cholinergic deprivation results, among other perturbations, in the loss of vasodilation mediated by acetylcholine. In addition to a dysfunctional cerebral blood flow, alterations in vascular chemistry affecting endothelial and smooth muscle cells may result in cerebral hypoperfusion and a breached blood-brain barrier (BBB). The selective removal of the rabbit nbm and Aβ accumulation may serve as an important nontransgenic, and more physiological, model for the testing of pharmacological and immunological agents designed to control the deposition and the deleterious effects of Aβ in AD.

INTRODUCTION

The neuropathology of Alzheimer's disease (AD) is characterized by the abundant accumulation of amyloid in cortical neuritic plaques and vascular walls, and by the intraneuronal deposition of neurofibrillary tangles.[1,2] The neuritic plaques represent a collection of dystrophic neurites and reactive glial cells that surround a core of fibrillar amyloid-beta (Aβ) peptide.[1] The neurofibrillary tangles are mainly composed of the microtubule-associated protein tau and membrane-derived glycolipids.[3,4] In addition to these lesions, there is an extensive vascular pathology affecting the microcirculation of the brain and leptomeninges.[5,6] The capillary and arteriolar tree in AD is extensively damaged, far beyond the anatomical changes observed during normal aging.[7] There are important changes in the blood-brain barrier (BBB) endothelium associated with AD such as basement membrane fenestration and duplication, loss of perivascular plexus, loss of endothelial cells, decrease in glu-

[d]Address for correspondence: Dr. Alex E Roher, Sun Health Research Institute, 10515 West Santa Fe Dr., Sun City, Arizona, 85351. Tel.: (602) 876-5465; fax: (602) 876-5698.
e-mail: aroher@mail.sunhealth.org

cose transporter activity, decrease in α-adrenergic receptors, decrease in protein kinase C (PKC) activity, increase in cyclic adenosine-5′,3′-monophosphate (cAMP) and increased nitric oxide levels.[7–14] In AD, the presence of Aβ deposits around cortical vessels appears to obliterate capillaries and arterioles causing vascular stenosis resulting in focal hypoxia and ischemia.[6,15,16] These perivascular deposits are dramatically exacerbated in those AD individuals carrying the apolipoprotein E (ApoE) ε4 allele.[17–19] Aβ deposition in larger cerebral and leptomeningeal vessels results in the destruction of the myocytes of the tunica media leading to failure in the control of cerebral blood flow (CBF).[7,16] The cerebral blood vessels are innervated by the cholinergic neurons of the nucleus basalis of Meynert (nbM) which effect vasodilation and by the noradrenergic locus ceruleous and serotonergic dorsal raphe nucleus which mediate vasoconstriction.[20,21] The neurons in these nuclei are extensively damaged in AD.[22,23] There are decreased neuronal numbers, and the remaining cells contain heavy deposits of paired helical filaments (PHF). Injury to these nuclei results in vascular denervation causing alterations in cerebral perfusion and disturbances in BBB integrity.

We hypothesized that during normal senescence, and more critically during the early, preclinical stages of AD, cholinergic denervation among other cellular perturbations may lead to vascular deposition of Aβ. To test this hypothesis we induced selective cholinergic denervation in the rabbit's brain using the ribosomal toxin saporin conjugated to an antibody raised against the p75 neurotrophin receptor (NTR). We chose the rabbit as a model because its nucleus basalis magnocellularis (nbm), which is equivalent to nbM in the human, is well developed and because the rabbit's Aβ amino acid sequence is 100% homologous to that of the human species.

METHODS

A specific hybridoma line expressing the monoclonal antibody ME20.2 recognizing the p75 NTR was obtained from the American Type Culture Collection (Rockville, MD). The immunoglobulin G (IgG) was produced, purified and tagged with saporin by Advanced Targeting Systems (Carlsbad, CA). In the following experiments eleven 12-week-old New Zealand white rabbits were utilized. Six rabbits, weighing from 2.09 to 2.27 kg, received a unilateral intracerebroventricular injection of 12 μl immunotoxin in sterile saline at a concentration of 2.7 μg/μl. Five rabbits serving as control animals received 12 μl sterile saline alone. The stereotactic coordinates used in both groups of animals were relative to bregma: $AP = 0$, $L = 2.2$ mm, and $D = 7.5$ mm. Six months after surgery, the rabbits were killed and brain slices (4 mm) ipsilateral and immediate to the site of injection were fixed in 4% paraformaldehyde and used for immunohistological studies. The remaining of the brain slices were immediately frozen at $-85°C$ for biochemical studies.

Aβ was detected using the antibodies 10D5, raised against Aβ residues 1–16 (Athena Neurosciences, South San Francisco, CA) and 4G8 raised against Aβ residues 17–24 (Senetek PLC, Maryland Heights, MO). The antibody ME20.4 (Advanced Targeting Systems, San Diego, CA) was used for the detection of p75 NTR. Forty-μm sections were cut on a freezing microtome and reacted with the antibodies, and the color reaction was developed using 3,3′-diaminobenzidine as the substrate.[24] Acetylcholinesterase enzyme histochemistry was performed following the method of Tago *et al.*[25] Cortical choline acetyltransferase (ChAT) was determined on frontal pole cerebral cortex ipsilateral to the injection site, using the method of Fonnum.[26] For the detection of microglia, the lectin Griffonia simplicifolia (Sigma, St. Louis, MO) was utilized as previously described.[27]

For Aβ quantification, cerebral cortex (100 mg) from rabbit brain was homogenized in 10 volumes of 2% diethylamine prepared in 0.9% NaCl and centrifuged at 12,000 × g for 20 min. The supernatant was neutralized with an equal volume of 0.5 M Tris-HCl, pH 7.5. The levels of Aβ peptides were measured by enzyme-linked immunosorbent assay (ELISA) using the C-terminal specific polyclonal antibodies R163 and R165, raised against $A\beta_{40}$ and $A\beta_{42}$, respectively, as capture antibodies. Antibody 4G8, recognizing $A\beta_{17-24}$, was used as reporter antibody.[28] Amyloid-β precursor protein (AβPP) was quantified by Western blotting using the monoclonal antiboby 22C11 (Roche Molecular Biochemical, Indianapolis, IN). In the 6-month-old control and immunotoxin-treated rabbits the levels of two synaptic proteins were determined by ELISA.[29] In this study we employed the polyclonal antibodies EP10 and SP15 (raised against synaptophysin) and SP12 (raised against SNAP-25).

RESULTS

Intraventricular injection of the IgG-saporin complex resulted in the selective ablation of the cholinergic neurons of the nucleus basalis magnocellularis (FIGS. 1A and 1B), with the concomitant loss of their cortical afferents (FIGS. 1C and 1D). The demise of the cholinergic neurons was determined by p75 NTR immunohistochemistry and acetylcholinesterase histochemistry.

In the immunotoxin-treated rabbits, there were abundant small and large cortical vessels with immunopositive Aβ deposits (FIGS. 2A, 2B, 2C, and 2D), which were not present in the control animals. In addition, there were diffuse deposits of immunopositive Aβ around some blood vessels (FIGS. 2E and 2F) and along the subpial region of the cortex (data not shown). Congo red and thioflavine-*S* staining were negative suggesting that the deposited Aβ peptide is not in the β-sheet conformation.

ELISA revealed that the immunotoxin-treated animals contained 2.5 and 8 times more $A\beta_{40}$ and $A\beta_{42}$, respectively, than the control rabbits (TABLE 1). These differences were statistically significant: $A\beta_{40}$, $p = 0.020$; $A\beta_{42}$, $p = 0.033$ (Student *t*-test, 2 tailed). In reference to the levels of soluble and full-length AβPP, no significant statistical differences were found between the immunotoxin-treated and the control rabbits.

TABLE 1. Choline acetyltransferase (ChAT) enzyme activity, synaptophysin and Aβ (N-40, N-42) in cerebral cortex of immunotoxin- and saline-injected animals

Treatment	ChAT (pmol/mg protein/min)	Synaptophysin[a]	N-40 (pmol/g)	N-42 (pmol/g)
Immunotoxin	0.21 ± 0.05*	0.485 ± 0.060	13.14 ± 6.32	12.65 ± 9.72
Saline	0.68 ± 0.08*	0.421 ± 0.029	5.09 ± 0.64	1.58 ± 1.15

[a]Values represent the amount of protein in μg required to generate an optical density value of 0.50.

* Value represents mean ± standard deviations.

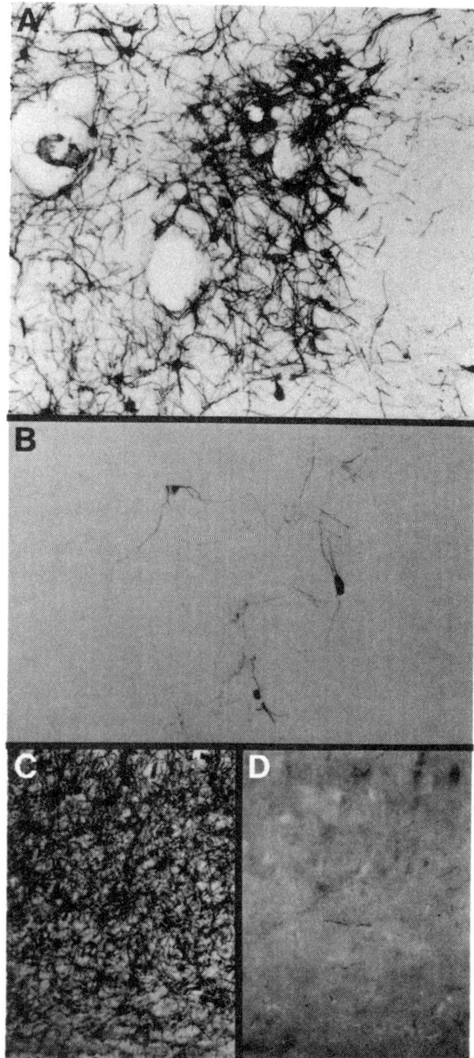

FIGURE 1. Selective immunotoxic elimination of cholinergic neurons. (**A**) The rabbit nucleus basalis magnocellularis (nbM) stained by p75 NTR immunohistochemistry. (**B**) The cholinergic neurons of the nbm annihilated by the p75 NTR IgG-saporin complex. Only a few scattered neurons remain in the nbm area. (**C**) Acetylcholinesterase staining of the cholinergic terminals in the cortical area of the rabbit brain. (**D**) Acetylcholinesterase histochemistry shows the complete demise of the cholinergic cortical afferents after treatment with the IgG-saporin complex.

In the immunotoxin-treated rabbits, there was a significant reduction in cortical cholinergic innervation, since the average levels of ChAT represented only 31% of the values observed in the control rabbits (TABLE 1). As expected, there was a modest decrease in the amount of synaptic proteins. In the immunotoxin-treated rabbits, synaptophysin was reduced by an average of 10% (TABLE 1) and SNAP-25 decreased by 13% when compared to the control values (not shown).

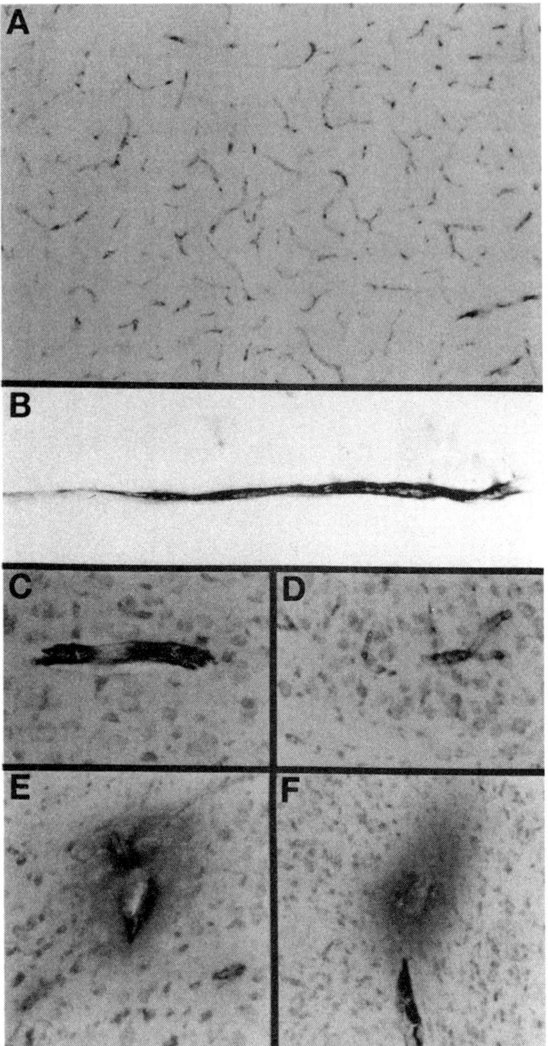

FIGURE 2. Vascular deposition of Aβ peptide immunostained by the 10D5 antibody. **(A)** A large number of cortical microvessels immunopositive for Aβ peptide. **(B, C and D)** Other cortical vessels immunopositive for the Aβ peptide. **(E and F)** Condensed and diffused Aβ deposition around cortical blood vessels in the immunotoxin treated rabbits.

DISCUSSION

The present study demonstrates for the first time that ablation of the cholinergic neurons of the nbm in the rabbit causes Aβ deposition around cerebral blood vessels and in the pia limitans. Aβ deposition was not observed in the sham-operated rabbits, nor in studies on aged rabbits.[27]

The loss of the cholinergic innervation from the nbm may be a seminal event in AD pathogenesis. In a recent study our group demonstrated that in the nondemented elderly population the presence of neurofibrillary degeneration is common in the nbM.[30] In this study, all individuals ($n = 31$; average age 79.0 years) exhibited neurofibrillary tangles (NFT) as detected by thioflavine-*S*, PHF immunochemistry, and double staining by PHF-1 and acetylcholinesterase. This observation suggests that degeneration of the nbM is the most probable cause of the cortical cholinergic denervation seen in the elderly and may be an important preclinical event in the pathogenesis of AD. In line with this hypothesis, it has been shown that cholinergic deficits antedate the emergence of senile plaques in normal aging,[31] and that there is an elevation in Aβ levels starting at age 50, as detected by Western blots.[32]

The elimination of cholinergic afferents may be the traumatic event that stimulates the production of Aβ in cortical neurons. In this scenario, the chronic reduction of m_1 and m_3 muscarinic receptor activation may reduce the nonamyloidogenic processing of AβPP and thereby increase the production of Aβ.[33] In the absence of AβPP overproduction, which in the present study appears not to differ from the control animals at least at 6 months postlesion, an alteration of AβPP processing needs to be contemplated. However, more AβPP and Aβ estimations are necessary in the immunotoxin-treated rabbits at earlier dates to distinguish between these possibilities.

The loss of cholinergic innervation of the nbm may also promote the sequestration of Aβ around blood vessels due to compromised vasomotor activity. Damage to the vasoactive neurons of the nbM would have serious repercussions. Endothelial cells and vascular myocytes have muscarinic receptors that on acetylcholine stimulation result in vasodilation possibly mediated by nitric oxide release. Perturbations in this chain of chemical events are likely to produce alterations in the control of CBF, and cerebral perfusion as well as changes in the integrity of the BBB. In a similar experiment, rats receiving intraventricular injections of 192 IgG-saporin, to elicit cortical cholinergic denervation, exhibited a marked decrease in CBF.[34] In the rat the most affected areas were the temporal and parietal cortices, which are also the most affected in terms of CBF failure in AD, especially in those patients who are ApoE ε4. Those who are ApoE ε4 may be more at risk for the vascular pathology seen in AD, since they appear to be hypocholinergic naturally.[35] One would also expect that the vasomotor dysfunction resulting from cholinergic deprivation of the brain vasculature would be exacerbated by factors such as: hypertension, hypercholesterolemia, hyperhomocysteinemia, and estrogen loss, all of which decrease vasomotor function and increase the risk for AD.[36–39] Vascular Aβ may also lead to decreased responsiveness of cerebral vessels by cholinergic stimulation as recently shown by Mullan's group.[40]

It has been recently demonstrated that antibodies against the human Aβ_{42} peptide produced in the human AβPP transgenic mice apparently prevent the amyloid deposition and toxicity, and perhaps facilitate the clearance of Aβ peptide from the brain.[41] The rabbit cholinergic model of Aβ deposition presented here thus becomes a very useful system to test the effectiveness of these antibodies in animals possessing an Aβ amino acid sequence identical to the human species.

ACKNOWLEDGMENTS

This work was partially supported by the State of Arizona Center for Alzheimer's Disease Research and by the Alzheimer's Association. This paper is dedicated to the memory of our colleague W. Harold Civin, M.D.

REFERENCES

1. KIDD, M. 1964. Alzheimer's disease: an electron microscopical study. Brain **87:** 307–320.
2. TERRY, R.D., N.K. GONATAS & M. WEISS. 1964. Ultrastructural studies in Alzheimer's presenile dementia. Am. J. Pathol. **44:** 269–297.
3. LEE, V.M., B.J. BALIN, L.J. OTVOS, & J.Q. TROJANOWSKI. 1991. A68: a major subunit of paired helical filaments and derivatized forms of normal Tau. Science **251:** 675–678.
4. GOUX, W.J., S. RODRIGUEZ & D.R. SPARKMAN. 1996. Characterization of the glycolipid associated with Alzheimer paired helical filaments. J. Neurochem. **67:** 723–733.
5. VINTERS, H.V., D.L. SECOR, S.L. READ, J.G. FRAZEE, U. TOMIYASU, T.M. STANLEY, J.A. FERREIRO & M.A. AKERS. 1994. Microvasculature in brain biopsy specimens from patients with Alzheimer's disease: an immunohistochemical and ultrastructural study. Ultrastruct. Pathol. **18:** 333–348.
6. MIYAKAWA, T. & R. KURAMOTO. 1989. Ultrastructural study of senile plaques and microvessels in the brain with Alzheimer's disease and Down's syndrome. Ann. Med. **21:** 99–102.
7. KAWAI, M., R.N. KALARIA, P. CRAS, S.L. SIEDLAK, M.E. VELASCO, E.R. SHELTON, H.W. CHAN, B.D. GREENBERG & G. PERRY. 1993. Degeneration of vascular muscle cells in cerebral amyloid angiopathy of Alzheimer disease. Brain Res. **623:** 142–146.
8. ZAROW, C., E. BARRON, H.C. CHUI & L.S. PERLMUTTER. 1997. Vascular basement membrane pathology and Alzheimer's disease. Ann. N.Y. Acad. Sci. **826:** 147–160.
9. GRAMMAS, P., A.E. ROHER & M.J. BALL. 1994. Increased accumulation of cAMP in cerebral microvessels in Alzheimer's disease. Neurobiol. Aging **15:** 113–116.
10. GRAMMAS, P., P. MOORE, T. BOTCHLET, O. HANSON-PAINTON, D.R. COOPER, M.J. BALL & A. ROHER. 1995. Cerebral microvessels in Alzheimer's have reduced protein kinase C activity. Neurobiol. Aging **16:** 563–569.
11. SIMPSON, I.A., K.R. CHUNDU, T. DAVIES-HILL, W.G. HONER & P. DAVIES. 1994. Decreased concentrations of GLUT1 and GLUT3 glucose transporters in the brains of patients with Alzheimer's disease. Ann. Neurol. **35:** 546–551.
12. SHIMOHAMA, S., T. TANIGUCHI, M. FUJIWARA & M. KAMEYAMA. 1986. Biochemical characterization of alpha-adrenergic receptors in human brain and changes in Alzheimer-type dementia. J. Neurochem. **47:** 1295–1301.
13. BRUEL, A., G. CHERQUI, S. COLUMELLI, D. MARGELIN, M. ROUDIER, P.M. SINET, M. PRIEUR, J.L. PERIGNON & J. DELABAR. 1991. Reduced protein kinase C activity in sporadic Alzheimer's disease fibroblasts. Neurosci. Lett. **133:** 89–92.
14. DORHEIM, M.A., W.R. TRACEY, J.S. POLLOCK & P. GRAMMAS. 1994. Nitric oxide synthase activity is elevated in brain microvessels in Alzheimer's disease. Biochem. Biophys. Res. Commun. **205:** 659–665.
15. WISNIEWSKI, H.M., A.W. VORBRODT & J. WEGIEL. 1997. Amyloid angiopathy and blood-brain barrier changes in Alzheimer's disease. Ann. N.Y. Acad. Sci. **826:** 161–172.
16. ROHER, A.E., J.D. LOWENSON, S. CLARKE, A.S. WOODS, R.J. COTTER, E. GOWING & M.J. BALL. 1993. β-Amyloid-(1–42) is a major component of cerebrovascular amyloid deposits: implications for the pathology of Alzheimer disease. Proc. Natl. Acad. Sci. USA **90:** 10836–10840.
17. GREENBERG, S.M., G.W. REBECK, J.P. VONSATTEL, T. GOMEZ-ISLA & B.T. HYMAN. 1995. Apolipoprotein E ε4 and cerebral hemorrhage associated with amyloid angiopathy. Ann. Neurol. **38:** 254–259.
18. PREMKUMAR, D.R., D.L. COHEN, P. HEDERA, R.P. FRIEDLAND & R.N. KALARIA. 1996. Apolipoprotein E-ε4 alleles in cerebral amyloid angiopathy and cerebrovascular pathology associated with Alzheimer's disease. Am. J. Pathol. **148:** 2083–2095.
19. LUE, L.-F., Y.M. KUO, A.E. ROHER, L. BRACHOVA, Y. SHEN, L. SUE, T. BEACH, J.H. KURTH, R. RYDEL & J. ROGERS. 1999. Soluble amyloid peptide concentration as a predictor of synaptic change in Alzheimer's disease. Am. J. Pathol. **155:** 853–862.
20. SATO, A. & Y. SATO. 1992. Regulation of regional cerebral blood flow by cholinergic fibers originating in the basal forebrain. Neurosci. Res. **14:** 242–274.
21. EDVINSSON, L., E.T. MACKENZIE & J. MCCULLOCH. 1993. Cerebral Blood Flow and Metabolism. Raven Press. New York.

22. ICHIMIYA, Y., H. ARAI, K. KOSAKA & R. IIZUKA. 1986. Morphological and biochemical changes in the cholinergic and monoaminergic systems in Alzheimer-type dementia. Acta Neuropathol. (Berl.) **70:** 112–116.

23. ZWEIG, R.M., C.A. ROSS, J.C. HEDREEN, C. STEELE, J.E. CARDILLO, P.J. WHITEHOUSE, M.F. FOLSTEIN & D.L. PRICE. 1988. The neuropathology of aminergic nuclei in Alzheimer's disease. Ann. Neurol. **24:** 233–242.

24. BEACH, T.G., H. TAGO, T. NAGAI, H. KIMURA, P.L. MCGEER & E.G. MCGEER. 1987. Perfusion-fixation of the human brain for immunohistochemistry: comparison with immersion-fixation. J. Neurosci. Methods **19:** 183–192.

25. TAGO, H., H. KIMURA & T. MAEDA. 1986. Visualization of detailed acetylcholinesterase fiber and neuron staining in rat brain by a sensitive histochemical procedure. J. Histochem. Cytochem. **34:** 1431–1438.

26. FONNUM, F. 1975. A rapid radiochemical method for the determination of choline acetyltransferase. J. Neurochem. **24:** 407–409.

27. STREIT, W.J. 1990. An improved staining method for rat microglial cells using the lectin from Griffonia simplicifolia (GSA I-B4). J. Histochem. Cytochem. **38:** 1683–1686.

28. RABY, C.A., M.C. MORGANTI-KOSSMANN, T. KOSSMANN, P.F. STAHEL, M.D. WATSON, L.M. EVANS, P.D. MEHTA, K. SPIEGEL, Y.M. KUO, A.E. ROHER & M.R. EMMERLING. 1998. Traumatic brain injury increases beta-amyloid peptide 1–42 in cerebrospinal fluid. J. Neurochem. **71:** 2505–2509.

29. HONER, W.G., P. FALKAI, C. YOUNG, T. WANG, J. XIE, J. BONNER, L. HU, G.L.BOULIANNE, Z. LUO & W.S. TRIMBLE. 1997. Cingulate cortex synaptic terminal proteins and neural cell adhesion molecule in schizophrenia. Neuroscience **78:** 99–110.

30. BEACH, T.G., L.I. SUE, S. SCOTT & D.L. SPARKS. 1998. Neurofibrillary tangles are constant in aging human nucleus basalis. Alzheimer's Reports **1:** 375–380.

31. DAVIES, P. & A.J. MALONEY. 1976. Selective loss of central cholinergic neurons in Alzheimer's disease. Lancet **2:** 1403.

32. FUNATO, H., M. YOSHIMURA, K. KUSUI, A. TAMAOKA, K. ISHIKAWA, N. OHKOSHI, K. NAMEKATA, R. OKEDA & Y. IHARA. 1998. Quantitation of amyloid β-protein (Aβ) in the cortex during aging and in Alzheimer's disease. Am. J. Pathol. **152:** 1633–1640.

33. NITSCH, R.M., B.E. SLACK, R.J. WURTMAN & J.H. GROWDON. 1992. Release of Alzheimer amyloid precursor derivatives stimulated by activation of muscarinic acetylcholine receptors. Science **258:** 304–307.

34. WAITE, J.J., D.P. HOLSCHNEIDER & O.U. SCREMIN. 1999. Selective immunotoxin-induced cholinergic deafferentation alters blood flow distribution in the cerebral cortex. Brain Res. **818:** 1–11.

35. ARENDT, T., C. SCHINDLER, M.K. BRUCKNER, K. ESCHRICH, V. BIGL, D. ZEDLICK & L. MARCOVA. 1997. Plastic neuronal remodeling is impaired in patients with Alzheimer's disease carrying apolipoprotein ε4 allele. J. Neurosci. **17:** 516–529.

36. SKOOG, I., B. LERNFELT, S. LANDAHL, B. PALMERTZ, L.A. ANDREASSON, L. NILSSON, G. PERSSON, A. ODEN & A. SVANBORG. 1996. 15-year longitudinal study of blood pressure and dementia. Lancet **347:** 1141–1145.

37. KALMIJN, S., L.J. LAUNER, A. OTT, J.C. WITTEMAN, A. HOFMAN & M.M. BRETELER. 1997. Dietary fat intake and the risk of incident dementia in the Rotterdam Study. Ann. Neurol. **42:** 776–782.

38. MILLER, J.W. 1999. Homocysteine and Alzheimer's disease. Nutr. Rev. **57:** 126–129.

39. BIRGE, S.J. & K.F. MORTEL. 1997. Estrogen and the treatment of Alzheimer's disease. Am. J. Med. **103:** 36S–45S.

40. CRAWFORD, F., Z. SUO, C. FANG & M. MULLAN. 1998. Characteristics of the *in vitro* vasoactivity of beta-amyloid peptides. Exp. Neurol. **150:** 159–168.

41. SCHENK, D., R. BARBOUR, W. DUNN, G. GORDON, H. GRAJEDA, T. GUIDO, K. HU, J. HUANG, K. JOHNSON-WOOD, K. KHAN, D. KHOLODENKO, M. LEE, Z. LIAO, I. LIEBERBURG, R. MOTTER, L. MUTTER, F. SORIANO, G. SHOPP, N. VASQUEZ, C. VANDEVERT, S. WALKER, M. WOGULIS, T. YEDNOCK, D. GAMES & P. SEUBERT. 1999. Immunization with amyloid-β attenuates Alzheimer-disease-like pathology in the PDAPP mouse. Nature **400:** 173–177.

β-Amyloid Excitotoxicity in Rat Magnocellular Nucleus Basalis

Effect of Cortical Deafferentation on Cerebral Blood Flow Regulation and Implications for Alzheimer's Disease

TIBOR HARKANY,[a,c] BOTOND PENKE,[b] AND PAUL G.M. LUITEN[a]

[a]*Department of Animal Physiology, University of Groningen, Haren, the Netherlands*

[b]*Department of Medical Chemistry, Szent-Györgyi Albert Medical University, Szeged, Hungary*

ABSTRACT: Alzheimer's disease is the most common type of dementia with a still largely unclear etiopathology. One of the factors that may directly contribute to the development and progression of the disorder is the abundant accumulation of β-amyloid peptides (Aβ) in senile plaques. In the present account we review coherent *in vivo* experimental evidence that Aβ infusion into the rat magnocellular nucleus basalis (MBN) induces abrupt and persistent behavioral dysfunctions, perturbations of sensory information processing, storage, and retrieval. These substantial behavioral changes are due to the loss of cholinergic neurons in the MBN and their ascending projections to the frontoparietal cortex. Both neuroanatomical and neurochemical observations pinpoint that infusion of Aβ into the rat basal forebrain significantly decreases choline-acetyltransferase and acetylcholinesterase activities and the population of—probably—M2 muscarinic acetylcholine receptors in the cerebral cortex. Neuropharmacological data indicate that Aβ toxicity is mediated by an excitotoxic cascade involving blockade of astroglial glutamate uptake, sustained activation of N-methyl-D-aspartate receptors and an overt intracellular Ca^{2+} influx. These changes are associated with increased nitric oxide synthase activity in cortical target areas that may directly lead to the generation of free radicals. Besides, as microvessels of the neocortex receive direct input from the MBN we assume that the loss of cholinergic innervation and hence that of tonic cholinergic vasoregulation ultimately leads to disturbances of vascular (endothelial) function and nutrient supply that may directly enhance neuronal vulnerability during aging and in Alzheimer's disease.

INTRODUCTION

One of the striking neuropathological hallmarks of Alzheimer's disease (AD) is the abundant accumulation of a 39–42 amino acid residue-containing peptide, termed β-amyloid protein (Aβ), in brain regions associated with memory formation.

[c]Address for correspondence: Dr. Tibor Harkany, Department of Animal Physiology, University of Groningen, Kerklaan 30, P.O. Box 14, NL-9750 AA Haren, the Netherlands. Tel.: +31 50 3632 353; fax: +31 50 3635 205.
e-mail: harkanyt@biol.rug.nl

Appearance of senile plaques with Aβ as their major constituent has long been regarded as a causal factor of AD. During the past decade a multitude of both *in vitro*[1–3] and *in vivo*[4–10,12–15] studies demonstrated the direct toxicity of Aβ or its derivatives, such as Aβ$_{25-35}$. Initially, Yankner *et al.*[1] demonstrated that Aβ is a neuroactive substance with a bimodal action profile. Whereas low (pM–nM) Aβ concentrations promote neural differentiation and growth, above a threshold level Aβ is toxic to nerve cells. As Aβ aggregates rapidly in aqueous solutions a critical role for the assembly state of the peptide was proposed to act as a pivotal determinant of its toxic effects.[2] Further, characterization of a molecular cascade mediating the neurotoxicity of Aβ on neurons has became a primary focus of *in vitro* studies and the involvement of Ca^{2+}-mediated excitotoxicity[3] and excess generation of free radicals emerged.[11]

Soon after the pioneering *in vitro* investigations on Aβ neurotoxicity Kowall *et al.*[12] reported toxic properties of Aβ in rat brain. During the past few years a broad spectrum of *in vivo* models were implicated in Aβ neurotoxicity research, each however with several limitations, like (I) substantially different concentrations and aggregation states of Aβ fragments, (II) a variety of peptide infusion protocols such as (i) acute local injections,[4–10,12,15] (ii) chronic Aβ infusion,[13] or (iii) intravascular perfusion of Aβ derivatives;[14] (III) differences of target brain areas (e.g., the hippocampus, the cerebral cortex, or basal forebrain nuclei), and (IV) different animal species.[15]

In the present account we report evidence for an excitotoxic nature of Aβ in an *in vivo* animal model of Aβ neurotoxicity which is based on amyloid peptide infusions in the magnocellular nucleus basalis (MBN). Furthermore, we will elaborate on the consequences of Aβ-induced cholinergic damage for cortical cerebral blood flow regulation and neuronal viability.

THE MAGNOCELLULAR NUCLEUS BASALIS MODEL
OF Aβ NEUROTOXICITY: BASIC OBSERVATIONS

Cholinergic neurons of the MBN provide the majority of cholinergic input to neocortical structures, particularly to the more frontal and parietal cortical areas.[16] Ascending cholinergic projections from distinct sub-regions of the MBN exhibit a topologically defined unilateral cortical innervation pattern, such that cholinergic projection fibers originating in the intermediate MBN (iMBN) invade the frontoparietal somatosensory cortex.[16] Lesions to the iMBN have long been used to study the anatomical and functional consequences of neurotoxin infusion, such as that of kainic acid,[17] or *N*-methyl-D-aspatrate (NMDA).[18] Damage to the cholinergic neurons of the MBN elicits profound disturbances of both spontaneous animal behaviors and memory formation.[6,7]

To investigate any direct cholinotoxic effect of Aβ or Aβ-related peptides like Aβ(Phe(SO$_3$H)^{24})25–35, Aβ was infused into the iMBN in a 200 μM concentration (0.2 nmol/μl). Aβ-induced lesions in the iMBN resulted in a broad range of behavioral dysfunctions, such as pronounced anxiety in the elevated plus maze (FIG. 1A), immobility in the small "open-field" (FIG. 1B) and in an "open-field."[6] Loss of memory acquisition became apparent in a one-way step-through passive avoidance paradigm (FIG. 1C), but not in the Morris water maze (FIG. 1D). The latter observation

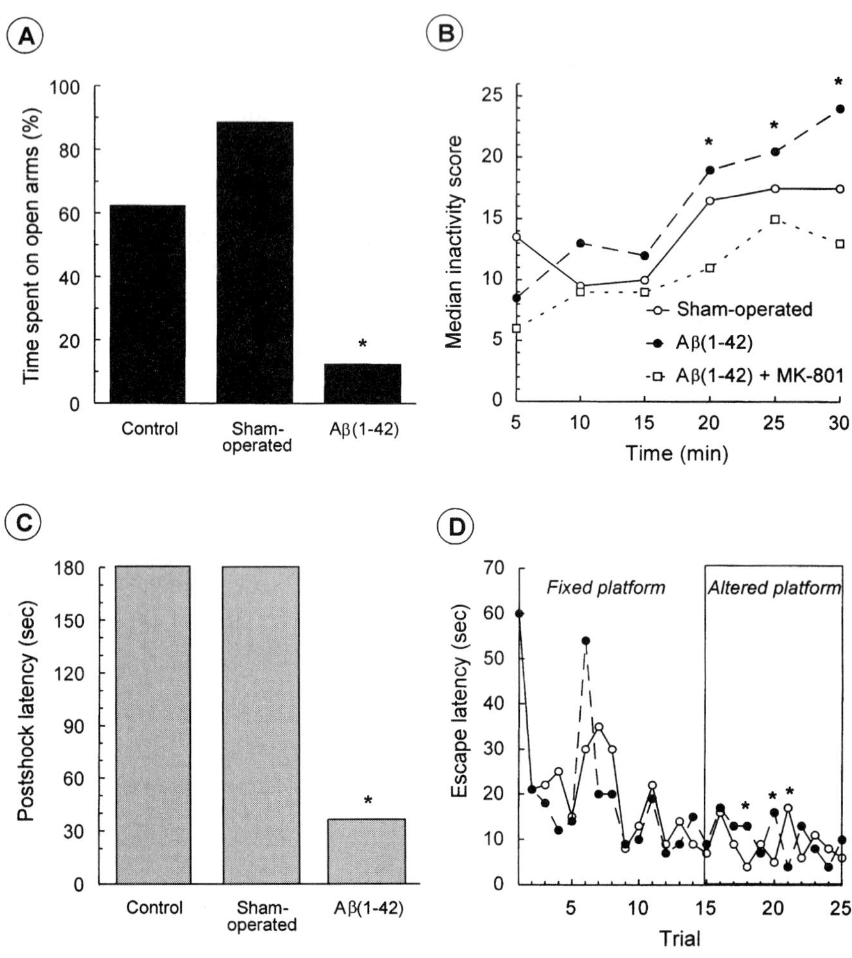

FIGURE 1. Behavioral consequences of $A\beta_{1-42}$ infusion into the rat MBN in four paradigms for the assessment of spontaneous behaviors (**A:** elevated plus maze, **B:** small "open-field") and learning and memory performance (**C:** one-way step-through passive avoidance, **D:** Morris water maze). Note the significant decrease of open arm entries in the elevated plus maze (A), the increased immobility (resting) frequency (B), and the loss of short-term memory in the postshock latency trial (24 h) of the passive avoidance test (C). Spatial learning capacity of $A\beta_{25-35}$-lesioned rats was not altered, relative to sham-operated animals (D). $A\beta_{1-42}$-induced behavioral dysfunctions were antagonized by acute pretreatment with the NMDA receptor blocker MK-801 (5 mg/kg of body weight, B). *p <0.05 (Mann-Whitney test); data are presented as medians.

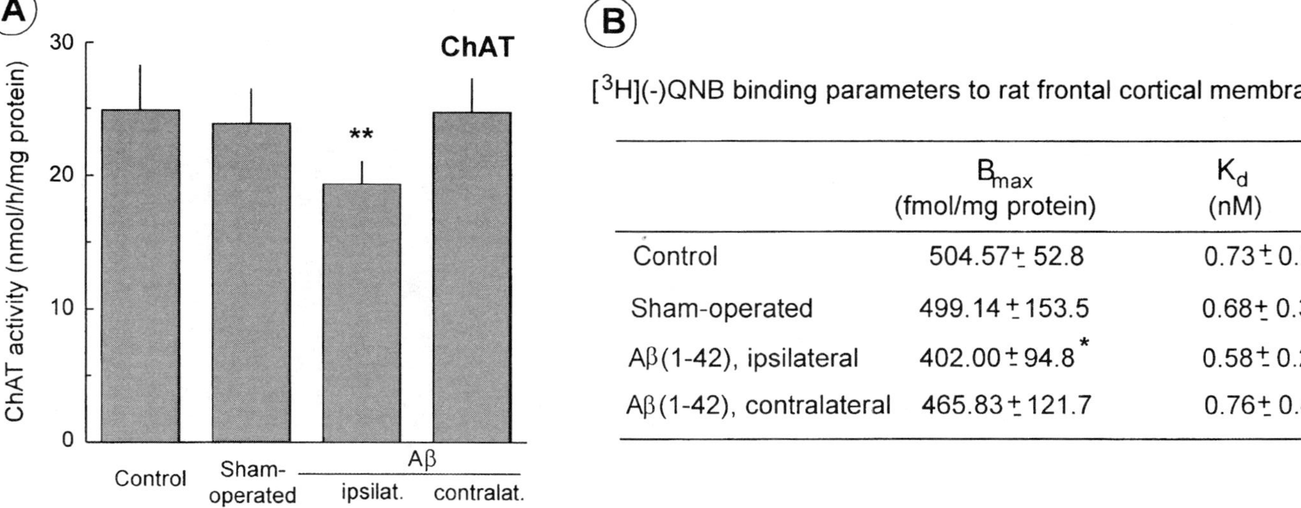

	B_{max} (fmol/mg protein)	K_d (nM)
Control	504.57 ± 52.8	0.73 ± 0.2
Sham-operated	499.14 ± 153.5	0.68 ± 0.3
Aβ(1-42), ipsilateral	402.00 ± 94.8 *	0.58 ± 0.2
Aβ(1-42), contralateral	465.83 ± 121.7	0.76 ± 0.4

FIGURE 2. *Caption on following page.*

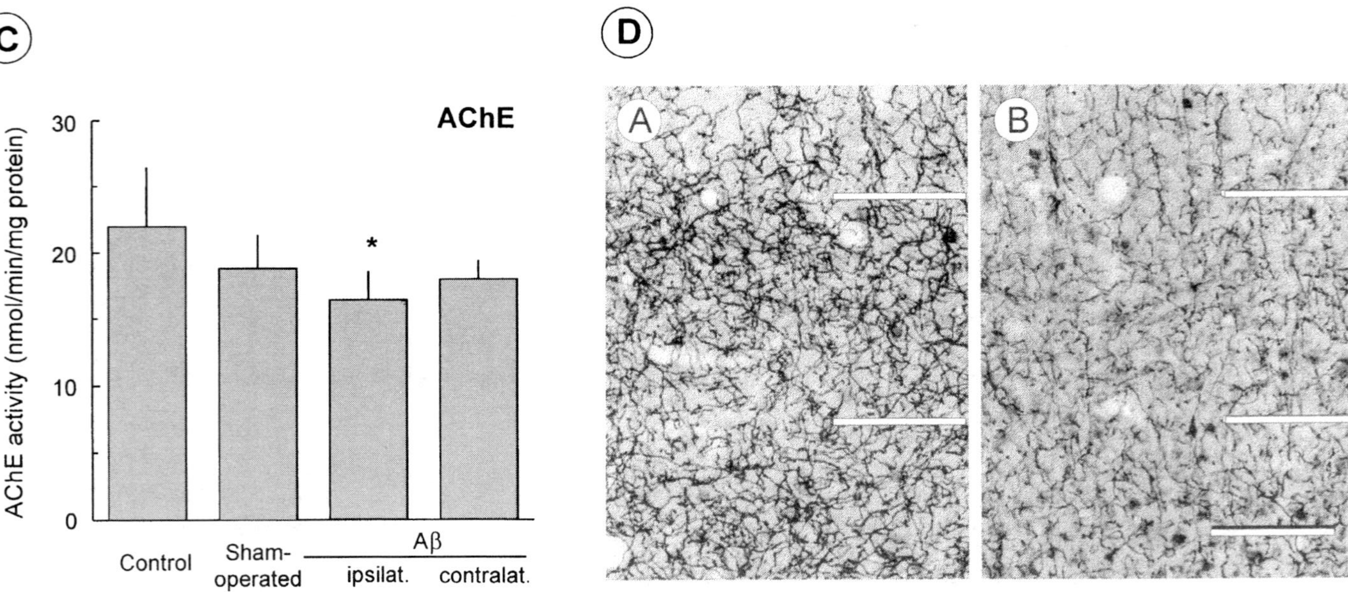

FIGURE 2. ChAT (**A**) and AChE (**C**) activities, and changes in receptor binding density (B_{max}) and dissociation constant (K_d) for [^{3}H](−)QNB binding in frontal cortical regions (**B**) of control, sham-operated and $A\beta_{1-42}$-treated animals. $A\beta_{1-42}$ injections into the MBN resulted in a significantly decreased ChAT activity (A) in the frontal cortices ipsilateral to the MBN injection as compared to all other groups examined, while AChE activity (C) in the ipsilateral frontal cortices was significantly reduced as compared to the control group. Note the extensive changes in the B_{max} value after $A\beta_{1-42}$ infusion into the MBN, while K_d remained unchanged. (**D**) Distribution of AChE-positive cortical cholinergic fibers originating in the damaged MBN subdivision. D/A represents a sham-lesioned, while D/B a $A\beta_{1-42}$-injected animal. **p <0.01, *p <0.05 (Student's t-test); data are reported as means ± SD. *Horizontal bars* in (D) depict layer V of the somatosensory cortex; *scale bar* = 150 μm.

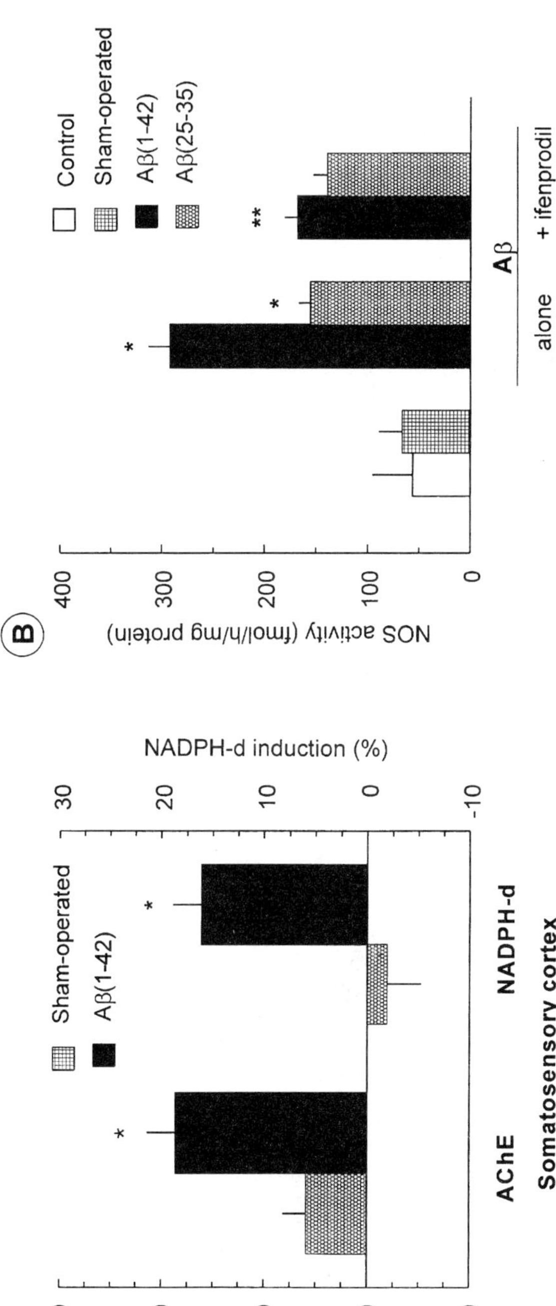

FIGURE 3. Loss of cholinergic (AChE-positive) projection fibers and activation of cortical NOS (**A**) 7 days postsurgery as a consequence of $A\beta_{1-42}$ infusion into the MBN. Injections of $A\beta_{1-42}$ elicited a significant loss of cholinergic projection fibers, whereas peptide infusion resulted in a marked activity increase of NOS as compared to sham-operated animals. (**B**) Cortical NOS activity and the effects of chronic ifenprodil (10 mg/kg of body weight, from 24 h postsurgery on) posttreatment following $A\beta_{1-42}$ or $A\beta_{25-35}$ infusions into the MBN. *$p<0.05$ vs. both naive and sham-control animals, while **$p<0.01$ vs. $A\beta_{1-42}$ (one-way analysis of variance). Data were expressed as percentages of the value of the contralateral side (A) and represent means ± SEM (A,B).

indicates target specificity of Aβ lesion, as hippocampus-related spatial learning performances were not altered. Neurochemical[4,7–9,19] and neuroanatomical[5,10,20] studies showed that detrimental effects of Aβ on cholinergic MBN function contribute to the behavioral disturbances. Altered cholinergic function involves significantly decreased choline-acetyltransferase (ChAT, FIG. 2A) and acetylcholinesterase (AChE, FIG. 2C,D) activities and the loss of M2, but not M1 muscarinic acetylcholine receptor (mAChR) binding sites (FIG. 2B[4]) in the fronto-parietal neocortex. These observations were further substantiated by histochemical experiments showing the loss of AChE-positive projection fibers to the somatosensory cortex (FIG. 2D).[6,8–10]

Aβ CHOLINOTOXICITY IS MEDIATED BY AN EXCITOTOXIC CASCADE

Whereas concentration- and amino acid sequence-dependent cholinotoxic properties of Aβ fragments could be firmly established, the identification of the cellular cascade by which Aβ elicits neurodegeneration is still largely unclear. Neuropharmacological data point to the involvement of a sustained NMDA receptor activation

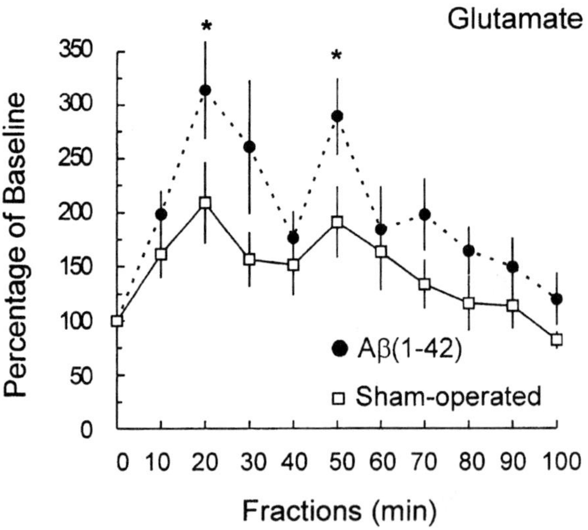

FIGURE 4. Time-profile of the extracellular glutamate concentration in the MBN of the rat following continuous microdialysis infusion of Aβ$_{1-42}$ in a 200 μM concentration. Extracellular concentration of glutamate exhibited rapid increases and reached its peak 20 min after the start of Aβ$_{1-42}$ infusion. Moreover, subsequent to the initial peak of the extracellular levels of glutamate, a second transient increase occurred at 50 min followed by a gradually decrementing profile of the extracellular amino acid content. *p <0.05 vs. sham-operated (one-way analysis of variance). Data are expressed as percentages of the baseline (means ± SEM).

in Aβ-induced pathological cellular signaling,[7–10] which is supportive to the leading hypothesis that an intracellular Ca^{2+} overload concomitant with an excess production of free radicals mediates Aβ toxicity on cultured neurons.[3,11] In this regard, both acute and chronic blockade of NMDA receptor function was proved to be highly effective in antagonizing Aβ toxicity *in vivo*[7,9,10] (FIG. 3B). Moreover, the fact that nitric oxide synthase (NOS) is activated in the neocortex upon infusion of Aβ into the MBN suggests a critical role for Ca^{2+}-triggered free radical generation (FIG. 3A). As such, vitamin E has recently been proven to be effective in the prevention of Aβ neurotoxicity,[7,21] which also points towards a role for free radicals in cascades mediating Aβ toxicity.

In vitro and *in vivo* data on Aβ neurotoxicity[9] together with the determination of excitotoxin-like properties of Aβ upon microdialysis infusion of the peptide into the MBN[8] revealed that Aβ initiates an excitotoxic cascade in the rat brain. Peptide infusion results (i) in the blockade of glutamate uptake by astrocytes that leads to (ii) a rapid and sustained increase of the extracellular concentrations of excitatory amino acid (EAA) neurotransmitters, such as aspartate and glutamate (FIG. 4). (iii) EAAs exert their effects by overt stimulation of their respective receptors including the NMDA receptor resulting in (iv) an intracellular Ca^{2+} ($[Ca^{2+}]_i$) overload. Sustained pathological concentrations of $[Ca^{2+}]_i$ may influence not only NOS activity, but also the function of intracellular Ca^{2+} pools, such as the mitochondria. Uncontrolled Ca^{2+} transients in mitochondria elicit uncoupling of the terminal oxidation cascade and lead to the generation of free radicals. Generally speaking, Ca^{2+}-mediated pathological Aβ signaling therefore ultimately leads to a subsequent formation of free radicals, and the two pathways converge to activation of "death signal" genes and fragmentation of DNA.

CHOLINERGIC DENERVATION OF CORTICAL MICROVESSELS: IMPLICATIONS FOR THE PATHOLOGY OF ALZHEIMER'S DISEASE

Besides the modulation of learning and memory formation in neocortical areas, cholinergic fibers originating in the basal forebrain influence vascular function and regional cerebral blood flow.[17] Ascending cholinergic fibers establish close but not direct contacts with endothelial cells of microvessels in the fronto-parietal neocortex.[22,23] Cholinergic end-feet were localized exclusively on mAChR-positive astroglial soma or leaflets (FIG. 5A–D) surrounding microvessels in a close (<30 μm) proximity to endothelial cells.[22,23] This feature enables direct regulation of regional blood flow and blood-brain barrier function if volume transmission of acetylcholine is considered.[17,22] These recent results indicate that interactions of the structural triads of ChAT-positive cholinergic perivascular terminals, mAChR-positive cholinoceptive astroglia, and endothelial cells are a key element in the neurogenic control of the intracortical microcirculation.

From a functional but also a pharmacological point of view cholinergic denervation profoundly influences local blood microcirculation, nutrient supply, and NOS activation.[10,17] Enhanced NO generation[10] can be postulated to modulate endothelial function in a bimodal manner. Increased NO production during the acute phase of Aβ-induced degeneration of cholinergic perivascular terminals results in transient

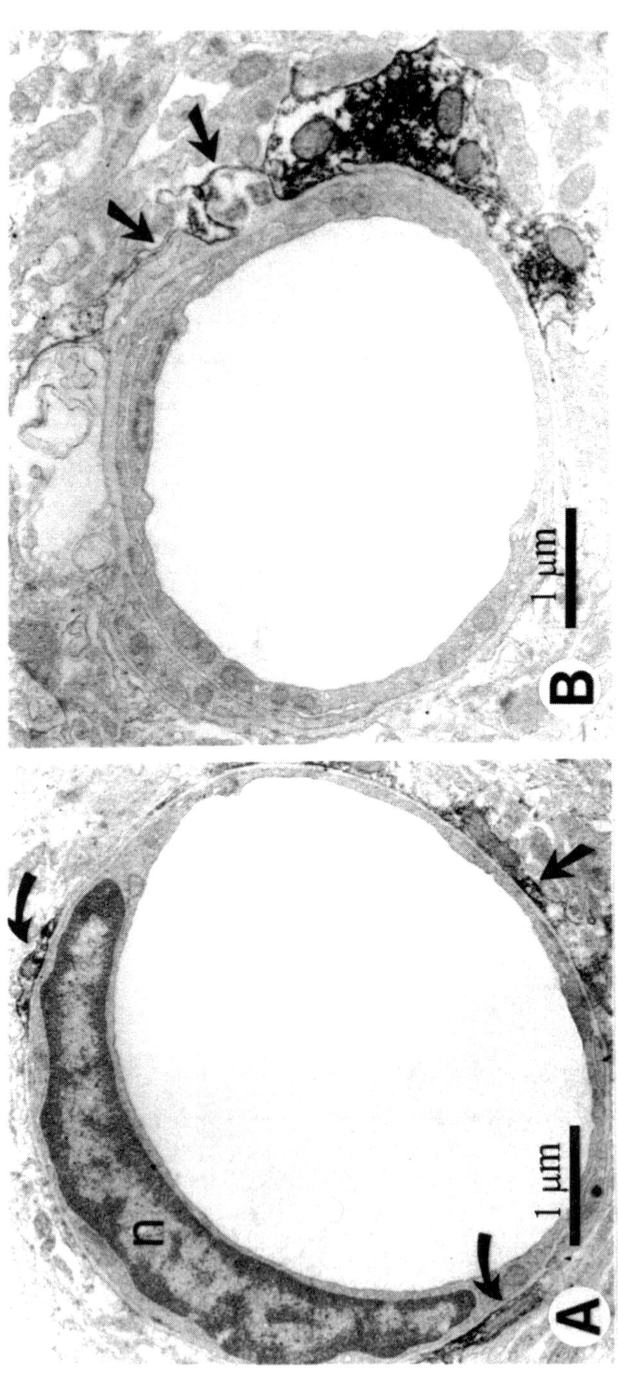

FIGURE 5. *Caption on following page.*

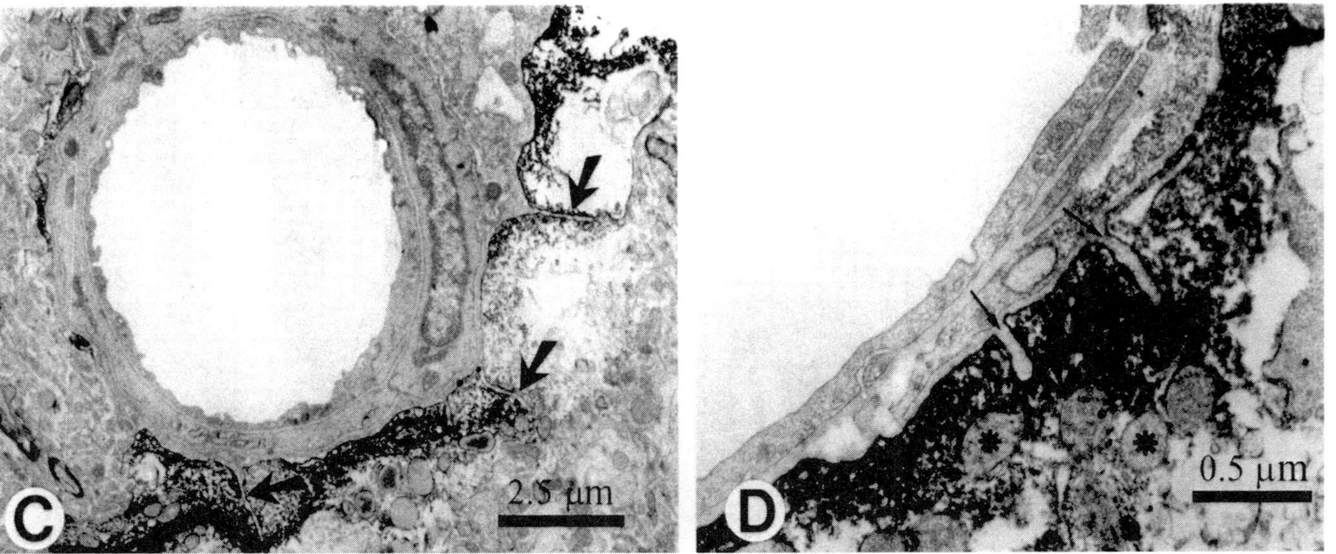

FIGURE 5. (**A**) Survey of a cortical capillary with a smooth and thin layer of cytoplasm in which several mitochondria and a large flattened nucleus can be identified. The endothelium is surrounded by a thin basement membrane. Several immunolabeled astrocytic processes are present in apposition to the basement membrane (*large arrows*). (**B**) Astrocyte immunoreactive for muscarinic receptor protein. A large, darkly labeled endfeet is connected by fine processes (*arrows*) to extensions protruding into the neuropil. (**C**) Large astrocytic complex with separate mAChR immunostained components in direct contact with the perivascular basement membrane. The compartments are separated by fingershape extensions of the basement membrane (*arrows*). (**D**) The basement membrane extensions as in (C) are indicated here at a higher magnification. Mitochondria are marked with an *asterisk*.

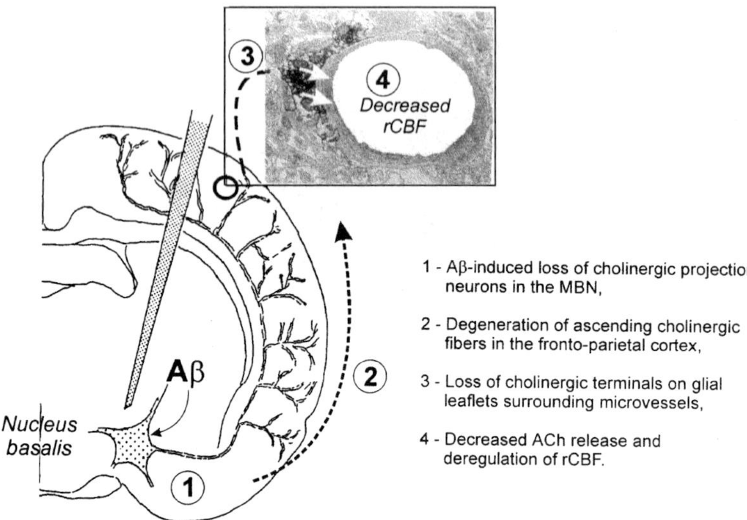

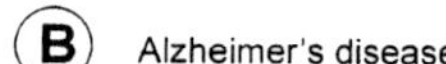

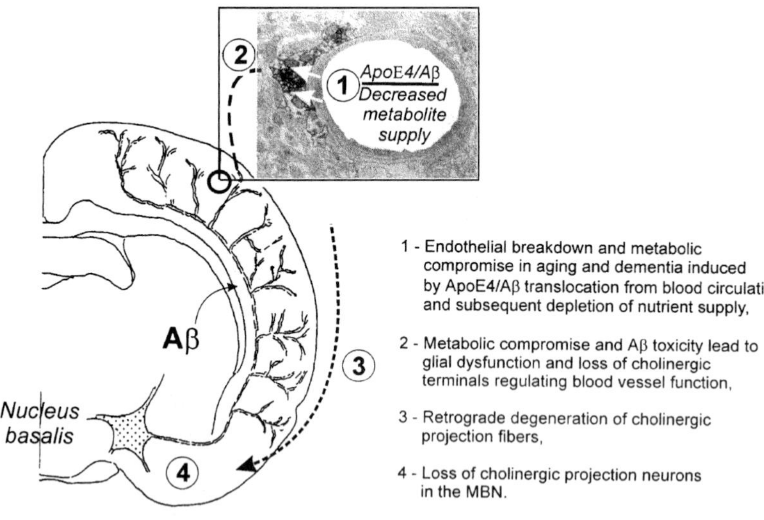

FIGURE 6. Comparison of successive steps of the neurotoxic cascades in the MBN lesion model of Aβ toxicity and during aging and Alzheimer's disease. Note the reversed sequence of events.

vasodilatation, whereas the permanent loss of cholinergic end-feet deregulates perivascular astroglial function and will lead to a reduced regional blood flow in the cerebral cortex. As aging is frequently associated with significantly decreased pO_2 and a metabolic compromise,[24] disturbances of cerebral blood flow regulation and endothelial function may render neurons vulnerable to excitotoxic (e.g., Aβ-induced) damage.

DISCUSSION

In conclusion, the data presented here provide compelling experimental evidence that Aβ and its derivatives exert cholinotoxicity[5] in the rat MBN. The neurotoxic action of Aβ is mediated by an excitotoxic cascade involving sustained activation of NMDA receptors and subsequent induction of NOS and generation of free radicals. Aβ-induced lesions to the MBN may deregulate cerebral blood flow and blood-brain barrier characteristics via the perturbation of both NO- and acetylcholine-mediated control of microvascular function. It is worth noting that exposure of MBN cells to Aβ induces a neurotoxic cascade that may affect cholinergic neuron integrity during aging and in AD in two ways (FIG. 6). First, Aβ triggers damage to cholinergic projection neurons, and second, this cholinergic neuron injury is the primary signal in the MBN reducing vasomotility and cerebral blood flow. As a result, such a chronic condition of hypoperfusion and impaired nutrient supply accompanied by the translocation of apolipoprotein E4/Aβ complexes from the blood circulation to brain parenchyma[25] will be a threat to intracortical cholinergic nerve terminals and by retrograde mechanisms can accelerate degeneration of cholinergic fibers and an ultimate loss of cholinergic MBN neurons in Alzheimer's disease.

REFERENCES

1. YANKNER, B.A. *et al.* 1990. Neurotrophic and neurotoxic effects of amyloid-β protein: reversal by tachykinin neuropeptides. Science **250:** 279–282.
2. PIKE, C. *et al.* 1993. Neurodegeneration induced by β-amyloid peptides *in vitro*: the role of peptide assembly state. J. Neurosci. **13:** 1676–1687.
3. MATTSON, M.P. *et al.* 1992. β-Amyloid peptides destabilize calcium homeostasis and render human cortical neurons vulnerable to excitotoxicity. J. Neurosci. **12:** 376–389.
4. HARKANY, T. *et al.* 1995. Cholinotoxic effects of β-amyloid(1–42) peptide on cortical projections of the rat nucleus basalis magnocellularis. Brain Res. **695:** 71–75.
5. HARKANY, T. *et al.* 1995. β-Amyloid(1–42) affects cholinergic but not parvalbumin-containing neurons in the septal complex of the rat. Brain Res. **698:** 270–274.
6. HARKANY, T. *et al.* 1998. β-Amyloid(Phe(SO$_3$H)^{24})25–35 in rat nucleus basalis induces behavioral dysfunctions, impairs learning and memory and disrupts cortical cholinergic innervation. Behav. Brain. Res. **90:** 133–145.
7. HARKANY, T. *et al.* 1999. N-Methyl-D-aspartate receptor antagonist MK-801 and radical scavengers protect cholinergic nucleus basalis neurons against β-amyloid neurotoxicity. Neurobiol. Dis. **6:** 109–121.
8. HARKANY, T. *et al.* 1999. Propionyl-IIGL tetrapeptide antagonizes β-amyloid excitotoxicity in rat nucleus basalis. NeuroReport **10:** 1693–1698.
9. HARKANY, T. *et al.* 1999. *In vivo* β-amyloid neurotoxicity is mediated by glutamate and calcium. Neuroscience. Submitted.
10. O'MAHONY, S. *et al.* 1998. β-Amyloid-induced cholinergic denervation correlates with enhanced nitric oxide synthase activity in rat cerebral cortex: reversal by NMDA receptor blockade. Brain Res. Bull. **45:** 405–411.

11. KELLER, J.N. & M.P. MATTSON. 1998. Roles of lipid peroxidation in modulation of cellular signaling pathways, cell dysfunction, and death in the nervous system. Rev. Neurosci. **9:** 105–116.
12. KOWALL, N.W. *et al.* 1991. An *in vivo* model for the neurodegenerative effects of β–amyloid and protection by substance P. Proc. Natl. Acad. Sci. USA **88:** 7247–7251.
13. NITTA, A. *et al.* 1994. β-Amyloid protein-induced Alzheimer's disease animal model. Neurosci. Lett. **170:** 63–66.
14. JANCSÓ, G. *et al.* 1998. β-Amyloid (1–42) peptide impairs blood-brain barrier function after intracarotid infusion in rats. Neurosci. Lett. **253:** 139–141.
15. GEULA, C. *et al.* 1998. Aging renders the brain vulnerable to amyloid β-protein neurotoxicity. Nat. Med. **4:** 827–831.
16. LUITEN, P.G.M. *et al.* 1985. The pattern of cortical projections from the intermediate parts of the magnocellular nucleus basalis in the rat demonstrated by tracing with *Phaseolus vulgaris*-leucoagglutinin. Neurosci. Lett. **57:** 137–142.
17. SATO, A. & Y. SATO. 1992. Regulation of cerebral blood flow by cholinergic fibers originating in the basal forebrain. Neurosci. Res. **14:** 242–274.
18. STUIVER, B.T. *et al.* 1996. *In vivo* protection against NMDA-induced neurodegeneration by MK-801 and nimodipine: combined therapy and temporal course of protection. Neurodegeneration **5:** 153–159.
19. ABE, E. *et al.* 1994. Administration of amyloid β-peptides into the medial septum of rats decreases acetylcholine release from hippocampus *in vivo*. Brain Res. **636:** 162–164.
20. GIOVANNELLI, L. *et al.* 1995. Differential effects of amyloid peptides β-(1–40) and β-(25–35) injections into the rat nucleus basalis. Neuroscience **66:** 781–792.
21. YAMADA, K. *et al.* 1999. Protective effects of idebenone and α-tocopherol on β-amyloid-(1–42)-induced learning and memory deficits in rats: implication of oxidative stress in β-amyloid-induced neurotoxicity *in vivo*. Eur. J. Neurosci. **11:** 83–90.
22. CHÉDOTAL, A. *et al.* 1994. Light and electron microscopic immunocytochemical analysis of the neurovascular relationships of choline acetyltransferase and vasoactive intestinal polipeptide nerve terminals in the rat cerebral cortex. J. Comp. Neurol. **343:** 57–71.
23. LUITEN, P.G.M. *et al.* 1996. Ultrastructural localization of cholinergic muscarinic receptors in rat brain cortical capillaries. Brain Res. **720:** 225–229.
24. DE JONG, G.I. *et al.* 1999. Cerebral hypoperfusion yields capillary damage in the hippocampal CA1 area that correlates with spatial memory impairment. Neuroscience **91:** 203–310.
25. MACKIC, J.B. *et al.* 1998. Human blood-brain barrier receptors for Alzheimer's amyloid-β 1–40. Asymmetrical binding, endocytosis, and transcytosis at the apical side of brain microvascular endothelial cell monolayer. J. Clin. Invest. **102:** 734–743.

Effect of a Memory-Enhancing Drug, AIT-082, on the Level of Synaptophysin

D.K LAHIRI,[a] Y.-W. GE, AND M.R. FARLOW

Institute of Psychiatric Research, Departments of Psychiatry and Neurology, Indiana University School of Medicine, Indianapolis, Indiana 46202, USA

ABSTRACT: Our objective is to study the effect of AIT-082 on the level of synaptophysin in cultured pheochromocytoma (PC12) cells. The drug AIT-082, a unique purine hypoxanthine derivative, is under development for the treatment of Alzheimer's disease (AD). We analyzed synaptophysin protein as an index of synaptic numbers and density and indirectly neuronal transmission. PC12 cells were treated with nerve growth factor (NGF) (50 ng/ml) and/or different doses of AIT-082 (5–50 ng/ml) obtained from NeoTherapeutics, CA. In the western immunoblots of conditioned media and cell lysates, we detected synaptophysin as 36–40 kDa protein bands. When PC12 cells were treated with NGF and samples were analyzed at 24 or 48 hours after treatment, the secretion of synaptophysin was drastically reduced in the conditioned medium. A significant reduction in the intracellular level of synaptophysin in NGF-treated samples was also noted. By contrast, when PC12 cells were treated with AIT-082, the secretion of synaptophysin was increased in the conditioned medium as compared to the control. There was also a significant increase in the intracellular levels of synaptophysin in AIT-082–treated cultures. NGF treatment resulted in sympathetic neuronal phenotypes in PC12 cells. As it is known that the immunoreactivity of the synaptophysin protein correlates with the density of the synaptic terminal, our results suggest that treatment by AIT-082 could enhance neurotransmitter release at the presynaptic terminal, which may play a role in the improvement of cognition seen in AD subjects.

INTRODUCTION

Alzheimer's disease (AD) is characterized by a severe loss of presynaptic cholinergic neurons and decreased levels of acetylcholine and choline acetyltransferase in the cortex.[1] Inhibition of cholinergic activity in the central nervous system (CNS) of patients with AD correlates with deterioration in scores on dementia rating scales. Currently, cholinesterase inhibition is the most widely studied and developed approach for treating symptoms of AD. Because anticholinesterase drugs such as tacrine, donepezil, and rivastigmine only moderately improve symptoms in AD, an alternative cholinergic approach that is not entirely based on cholinesterase inhibition but that improves other known biochemical abnormalities associated with the disease should be tried.

[a]Address for correspondence: Dr. D.K. Lahiri, Institute of Psychiatric Research, Indiana University School of Medicine, Room No.: PR-313, 791 Union Drive, Indianapolis, Indiana 46202–4887, USA. Tel.: (317) 274-2706; fax: (317) 274–1365.
e-mail: dlahiri@iupui.edu

One of the major neurochemical changes in AD is the cortical extracellular and vascular deposition of the amyloid beta-peptide (Aβ) which is derived from a large glycosylated membrane-bound beta-amyloid precursor protein (βAPP).[2] A constitutively expressed putative α–secretase enzyme bisects the Aβ domain within βAPP to release carboxyl-truncated soluble derivatives (sAPP) in conditioned media of cells.[2] In addition, there are a loss of presynaptic markers such as synaptophysin in Alzheimer's disease. Synaptophysin (i) is a synaptic vesicle-associated integral membrane protein (Mw~ 38), (ii) acts as a specific marker for presynaptic terminal, and (iii) is involved in neuronal transmission.[3] Our goal is to determine whether the drug AIT-082 can regulate the levels of βAPP and/or presynaptic protein markers. AIT-082 (Neotrofin), a unique purine hypoxanthine derivative, is currently being investigated in clinical trials for the treatment of AD. The present work is based on a previous report showing that AIT-082 can induce the expression of three neurotrophins, nerve growth factor (NGF), neurotrophin-3, and basic fibroblast growth factor (bFGF).[4] A combination of factors has been most effective in producing optimal trophic support for compromised neuron functions.[4] However, the effects of AIT-082 and trophic factors on the regulation of βAPP and presynaptic proteins have not been clearly explored. It is reasonable to hypothesize that multiple trophic factors may synergistically regulate the processing of βAPP and/or synaptophysin in a way that can lead to lowered levels of Aβ and/or increased neurotransmission. Here we investigate the level of synaptophysin in PC12 cells that were treated with NGF or AIT-082 and observed a differential effect of these agents on the level of synapotophysin.

EXPERIMENTAL PROCEDURES

Materials. AIT-082 was obtained from NeoTherapeutics (Irvine, CA). Nerve growth factor (NGF) and basic fibroblast growth factor (bFGF) were procured from Life Technologies (Gaithersburg, MD). Other chemicals were of high purity and purchased from Sigma (St. Louis, MO).

Cells and Culture Conditions. PC12 cells were cultured in RPMI 1640 medium containing 10% horse serum and 5% fetal bovine serum (FBS) in the presence of 5% CO_2 as per the ATCC's instructions. Media and sera were obtained from Life Technologies.

Treatment of Cells and Preparation of Cell Extract. Five to seven million PC12 cells were cultured to confluence in the regular medium. Before adding the drug, cells were fed with medium containing only 0.5% FBS (low serum). Cells were then allowed to differentiate in the presence of either NGF (50 ng/ml) or bFGF (50 ng/ml) for several days, as described previously.[5] In parallel, cells were also incubated with different doses of AIT-082 (10 nM–100 mM). Following incubation for a certain period of time, as indicated in FIGURE 1, the conditioned medium from each plate was collected, and the cells were centrifuged at 800 *g* for 10 minutes and lysed in the IP buffer as described.[6] Cells were sonicated and centrifuged at 11,000 *g* for 20 minutes at 4°C, and proteins of the supernatant (cell lysate) were measured.

PAGE and Western Immunoblotting. Thirty micrograns of proteins from the total cell lysate or 50 µg of conditioned media were separated on a 12% polyacrylamide

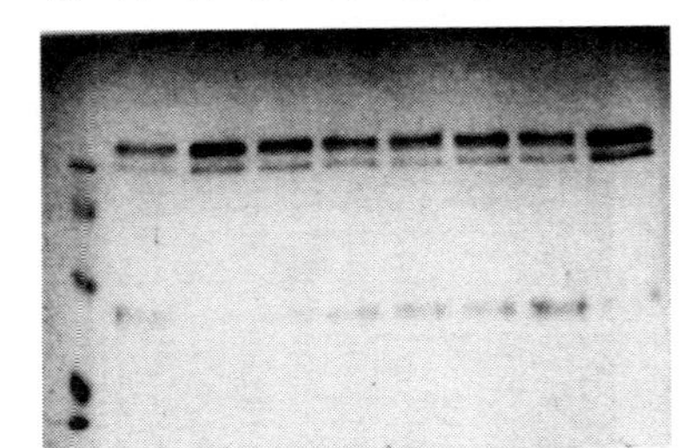
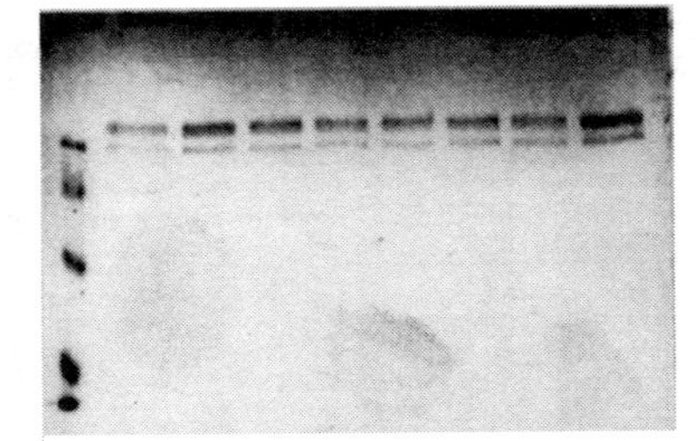
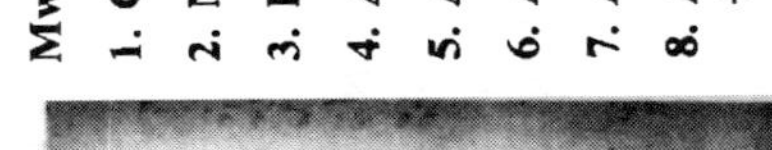

FIGURE 1. Detection of sAPP and synaptophysin proteins with a low dose of AIT-082. **(A)** Eight plates of PC12 cells in duplicate were cultured in regular RPMI medium to ~6 × 10^6 cells per plate. On the day of the experiment, cells were fed with the RPMI 1640 medium containing 0.5% serum either in the absence of any drug (lane 1), NGF (lane 2), or bFGF (lane 3) or in the presence of different doses of AIT-082 as indicated (lanes 4–8). After 48 hours of incubation, 50 μg samples of conditioned media were subjected to SDS-PAGE (12%), transferred to a nitrocellulose membrane, and stained with Ponceau stain (Sigma). Protein size markers shown on the left of the blot from *top to bottom* are: 107, 74, 49.3, 36.4, and 28.5 kDa. **(B)** The transferred proteins in the blot shown in FIGURE 1A were probed with anti-APP antibody (22C11), and immunodetection was carried out by the enzymatic color method as described previously.[6] **(C)** The blot that was used in FIGURE 1B was reprobed with antisynaptophysin antibody, and the immunochemical detection was similarly carried out. Since the membrane in FIGURE 1B was not stripped, the signal from the APP antibody remained.

gel containing SDS (SDS-PAGE).[6] Immunoblot analysis was performed in the Mini-PROTEAN II system of Bio-Rad, CA, and immunodetection of specific bands was performed as described previously.[6] The same filter was probed with multiple antibodies, which recognize different proteins in the blot, in a sequential manner after testing that these antibodies do not react with the same antigen.

Antibodies. The monoclonal antibody against the synaptophysin protein, which was procured from Boehringer Mannheim (Indianapolis, IN), reacts with vesicles of adrenal medulla and islet cells. The antibody also stains neurosecretory vesicles of PC12 cells. The epitome region of the monoclonal antibody 22C11 (Boehringer Mannheim) has been assigned to APP66-81 in the ectoplasmic cysteine-containing domain. The 22C11 clone recognizes all mature forms of βAPP found in cell membranes as well as the carboxyl-truncated, soluble forms secreted into the conditioned media and the APP-like proteins (APLP). The antibody against other presynaptic proteins, such as synaptotagmin, rSec8, and SNAP-25, were purchased from Transduction Labs (Lexington, KY). The biotinylated secondary antibodies, horse anti-mouse (Boehringer Mann-heim), were also used.

RESULTS

Treatment of NGF or bFGF results in a substantial increase in sAPP secretion in PC12 cells. NGF or bFGF treatment resulted in neuronal differentiation. In denaturing polyacrylamide gel, an equal amount of total protein was loaded from each of the conditioned medium samples, and the efficiency of transfer was verified by staining the membrane with Ponceau stain (FIG. 1A). When the immunoblot was probed with an antibody against N-terminal epitope of βAPP (22C11 clone), we detected distinct bands of 110 and 95 kDa, which correspond to soluble APP derivatives (sAPP) arising from different alternate forms of βAPP and/or their posttranslationally modified derivatives. With the NGF treatment, a significant increase in secretion of sAPP was observed (FIG. 1B, lane 2 vs. lane 1). With the bFGF treatment, a slight increase in secretion of sAPP was observed from the control (FIG. 1B, lane 3 vs. lane 1). NGF was previously shown to induce the release of sAPP from PC12 cultures.[7]

Treatment of AIT-082 results in a moderate increase in sAPP secretion in PC12 cells. When the PC12 cells were incubated with different doses of AIT-082, an increase in sAPP similar to that with bFGF treatment was observed from the control (FIG. 1B, lanes 4–7 vs. lane 1). When the cells were simultaneously treated with AIT-082 and NGF, a significant increase in sAPP release was observed (FIG. 1B, lane 8 vs. lane 1), which was more than that in cells treated with either NGF or AIT-082 alone (lanes 2, 6, and 8 vs. lane 1). A similar but smaller synergistic effect of bFGF and AIT-082 treatment was observed (data not shown). Thus, the level of soluble sAPP in the conditioned medium of PC12 cells with different agents used follows this order: NGF + AIT-082 > NGF > bFGF > AIT-082.

Treatment of NGF or bFGF results in a drastic reduction in synaptophysin release in PC12 cells. In the western immunoblot of conditioned media, we detected synaptophysin as 38 kDa protein bands (FIG. 1C). Thus, synaptophysin is a secretory protein of PC12 cells. When PC12 cells were treated with either NGF or bFGF, the secretion of synaptophysin was drastically reduced (~80–90%) in the conditioned medium from the control (FIG. 1C, lanes 2 and 3 vs. lane 1). This is evident when samples were analyzed after 24 and 48 hours of drug treatment under the condition in which an equal amount of protein was separated by SDS-PAGE. There was also a significant reduction in the intracellular level of synaptophysin in the NGF-treated cell lysates as compared to the control sample (data not shown). The basal level of secretion of the synaptophysin protein in the conditioned medium was less (~20%) than the level of total intracellular synaptophysin protein in PC12 cells (data not shown).

Treatment of AIT-082 results in a substantial increase in synaptophysin release in PC12 cells. In contrast, when PC12 cells were treated with AIT-082, secretion of synaptophysin was increased in the conditioned medium from the control sample in a dose-dependent manner (FIG. 1C, lanes 4–7 vs. lane 1). There was also a significant increase in the intracellular level of synatophysin in AIT-082–treated cultures as compared to the control sample (data not shown). We also studied other presynpatic terminal proteins. For example, whereas NGF treatment did not change the level of intracellular SNAP-25, AIT-082 treatment of PC12 cells resulted in an increase in the level of SNAP-25 protein (data not shown). AIT-082 treatment caused no significant change in other synaptic proteins such as rSec8 (110 kDa), synaptotagmin (65 kDa), and synapsin II a (74 kDa) (data not shown). Thus, treating PC12 cells with NGF resulted in decreased levels of synaptophysin, whereas under the same conditions, treating similar cells with AIT-082 caused a significant increase in the level of this protein.

DISCUSSION

Neurotransmitters are released from synaptic nerve terminals by exocytosis of synaptic vesicles, which are organelles situated at the distal terminus of the presynaptic neuron. The exocytotic process involves vesicle docking at the plasma membrane, priming, and fusion.[3,8,9] The fusion complex consists of several proteins such as syntaxins and SNAP-25 (synaptosomal-associated protein of 25 kDa). Other proteins such as synaptotagmin and rSec8 have regulatory roles in the synaptic vesicle pathway. Synaptophysin is used as a specific protein marker for presynaptic terminal. SNAP-25 and syntaxins are plasmalemmal proteins, whereas synaptophysin, a synaptic vesicle-associated protein, is a vesicular protein.[3] We analyzed the level of synaptophysin protein as an index of synaptic numbers and density and indirectly neuronal transmission. Using the PC12 cultures, we have shown here that the secretion of synaptophysin was increased in conditioned media and that there was also a significant increase in the intracellular levels of synaptophysin in AIT-082–treated cultures as compared to the control. NGF treatment of PC12 cells resulted in a substantial increase in sAPP release in conditioned medium, and AIT-082 treatment resulted in a mild increase in sAPP release under the dose used here.

We propose the following three reasons for the reduction in the level of synaptophysin observed with NGF treatment. First, the synthesis of synaptophysin may be reduced during synaptogenesis or neurite formation with NGF treatment through yet unknown mechanisms. Second, the synthesis rate of the protein may be unchanged, but synaptophysin may undergo posttransnational modifications so that it is inaccessible to antibody detection. Third, synaptophysin may be complexed with some other synaptic vesicle proteins, and this interaction may make synaptophysin unreactive to the antibody. For example, a recent report suggests a complex formation between synaptophysin and synaptobrevin, which is a hallmark of synaptic vesicle maturation.[10]

Unlike that of NGF, the effect of AIT-082 on synaptophysin is different, and we propose the following mechanisms to explain the effects of AIT-082 treatment in PC12 cells. First, there may be an overall increase in biogenesis (transcription) of synaptophysin message during drug treatment. But how this happens selectively without a change in other synaptic proteins remains to be investigated. An increase in RNA synthesis is suggested by an intracellular accumulation of the protein and its subsequent release into the medium. Second, drug treatment may alter the posttranslational modification of this integral membrane protein to an extent that results in an increased immunoreactivity in the western blot, without actually increasing its level. This can be verified by using different antibodies and treating the samples with various agents before running the gel. Third, synaptophysin may be complexed with other proteins inside the cell, but it is released as a consequence of drug treatment and is thus available for its detection. If that is the case, there should be greater formation of the complex between synatophysin and synaptobrevin and increased formation of different intermediate complexes such as 7s and 12s as proposed by Scheller.[3] These protein complexes are involved in the final release of neurotransmitters. It will be interesting to detect and characterize such complexes of synaptophysin with other protein markers.

The interaction of βAPP and synaptic vesicle protein is interesting. It is shown that βAPP is present in presynaptic clathirin-coated vesicles purified from bovine brain, along with the recycling synaptic vesicle integral membrane proteins such as synaptophysin and synaptotagmin.[11] Although βAPP is endocytosed together with recycling synaptic vesicle membrane proteins, it is subsequently sorted out from synaptic vesicles for retrograde transport to neuronal soma. [11] How AIT-082 drug treatment affects the trafficking of cell surface βAPP remains to be seen. These cell culture experiments provide a compelling reason to analyze the levels of pre synaptic proteins in CSF samples from AD patients who are treated with the drug. These findings have broad implications for AD. For example, the immunoreactivity of the synaptophysin protein correlates with the density of synaptic terminal; our results indicate that treatment with AIT-082 could enhance neurotransmitter release at the presynaptic terminal, which may be involved in the improvement of the cognitive impairment seen in AD subjects.

ACKNOWLEDGMENTS

We sincerely thank the support from the National Institutes of Health and Dr. M. Glasky, NeoTherapeutics, Irvine, CA.

REFERENCES

1. BECKER, R. *et al.* 1996. Alzheimer's Disease: Molecular Biology to Therapy. Birkhauser. Boston.
2. SELKOE, D.J. 1997. Alzheimer's disease: genotypes, phenotype, and treatment. Science **275**: 630–631.
3. SCHELLER, R.H. 1995. Membrane trafficking in the presynaptic nerve terminal. Neuron **14**: 893–897.
4. RATHBONE, M.P. *et al.* 1999. AIT-082 as a potential neuroprotective and regenerative agent in stroke and central nervous system injury. Exp. Opin. Invest. Drugs **8**: 1255–1262.
5. LAHIRI, D.K. *et al.* 1994. Tacrine alters the processing of beta-amyloid precursor protein in different cell lines. J. Neurosci. Res. **37**: 777–787.
6. LAHIRI, D.K. & M.R. FARLOW. 1996. Differential effect of tacrine and physostigmine on the secretion of the beta-amyloid precursor protein in cell lines. J. Mol. Neurosci. **7**: 41–49.
7. REFOLO, L.M. *et al.* 1989. Nerve and epidermal growth factors induce the release of the Alzheimer amyloid precursor from PC12 cell cultures. Biochem. Biophys. Res. Commun. **164**: 664–670.
8. KEE, Y. *et al.* 1995. Distinct domains of syntaxin are required for synaptic vesicle fusion complex formation and dissociation. Neuron **14**: 991–998.
9. PEVSNER, J. *et al.* 1994. Specificity and regulation of a synaptic vesicle docking complex. Neuron **13**: 353–361.
10. BECHER, A. *et al.* 1999. The synaptophysin — synaptobrevin complex: a hallmark of synaptic vesicle maturation. J. Neurosci. **19**: 1922–1931.
11. MARQUEZ-STERLING, N.R. *et al.* 1997. Trafficking of cell surface — amyloid precursor protein: evidence that a sorting intermediate participates in synaptic vesicle recycling. J. Neurosci. **17**: 140–151.

Differentiated Cerebrovascular Effects of Physostigmine and Tacrine in Cortical Areas Deafferented from the Nucleus Basalis Magnocellularis Suggest Involvement of Basalocortical Projections to Microvessels

PHILIPPE PERUZZI, DOMINIQUE VON EUW, AND PIERRE LACOMBE[a]

Laboratoire de Recherches Cérébrovasculaires, CNRS UPR 646, Université Paris 7, IFR 6, Circulation-Lariboisière, Faculté Lariboisière-Saint Louis, 10 avenue de Verdun, 75010 Paris, France

ABSTRACT: Cholinesterase inhibitors used to treat Alzheimer's disease according to the principle of cholinergic replacement therapy have proved to be less beneficial than expected. The present study was designed to investigate the cerebrovascular response to physostigmine and tacrine in the experimental model of lesioning of the nucleus basalis magnocellularis (NBM), a model involving a cholinergic deficit. Regional cerebral blood flow was measured by the [^{14}C]iodoantipyrine tissue sampling technique in conscious rats infused with i.v. physostigmine (0.2 mg/kg/h), tacrine (8 mg/kg/h), or saline, 3–5 weeks after unilateral lesion of the NBM with ibotenic acid. Physostigmine and tacrine dose-dependently increased blood flow in most cortical and subcortical regions compared to the control group. However, physostigmine caused smaller blood flow increases in several areas, mostly cortical, of the lesioned compared to the intact hemisphere. The converse was observed with tacrine. A facilitated circulatory response appeared in cortical areas deafferented from the NBM, especially in the frontal cortex. These results provide evidence for distinct NBM-dependent components of the cortical cerebrovascular effects of physostigmine and tacrine. They suggest the involvement of different cellular postsynaptic targets of the NBM. The physostigmine-type effects could involve direct projections onto an inhibitory cortical interneuron supersensitized by deafferentation. This arrangement may explain why physostigmine and perhaps other cholinergic agonists are unable to specifically compensate for a deficit in NBM functioning. The tacrine-type effects presumably involve projections to the microvasculature, including perivascular astrocytes. The neurovascular junction would be sensitized by deafferentation from the NBM. Our data suggest that the regulatory mechanisms of blood flow originating in the NBM might constitute a target of neurodegenerative processes of Alzheimer's disease.

[a]Address for correspondence: Pierre Lacombe, Laboratoire de Recherches Cérébrovasculaires, CNRS UPR 646, Faculté Lariboisière-Saint-Louis, 10 avenue de Verdun, 75010 Paris, France. Tel: 33 1 44 89 77 35; fax: 33 1 44 89 78 25.
e-mail: lacombe@ext.jussieu.fr

INTRODUCTION

Experimental studies conducted in rats bearing a lesion of the nucleus basalis magnocellularis (NBM), the equivalent of Meynert's nucleus in primates, have led to data that seem incompatible with the therapeutic strategy of Alzheimer's disease based on the use of cholinergic agents. Because cholinesterase inhibitors strongly increase cerebral blood flow, cerebrovascular investigations were conducted in an experimental model of cholinergic deficit. These experiments failed to confirm that cholinesterase inhibitors can enhance the functioning of the basalocortical system.[1–3] Thus, no evidence has been provided for NBM lesion-related cerebrovascular changes in the effects of indirect cholinergic agonists. This is intriguing in view of the clearly demonstrated denervation supersensitivity in the deafferented projection areas of the NBM.[4,5]

The present study was designed to determine if the cerebrovascular responses to physostigmine and tacrine were altered 3–5 weeks after lesioning of the NBM, thereby testing whether denervation supersensitivity alters the functioning of the basalocortical system. The results were compared with those previously obtained 1–2 weeks post-lesion.[2,3] Cerebral blood flow (CBF) was measured in various brain regions during i.v. infusion of the two drugs in conscious rats bearing a unilateral lesion of the NBM by ibotenic acid. This investigation helps to clarify how cholinesterase inhibitors functionally compensate for a chronic cholinergic deficit originating in the basalocortical system and suggests the existence of NBM postsynaptic targets of different cell type.

MATERIALS AND METHODS

Twenty-eight male Sprague-Dawley rats were used in this study according to a two-step procedure. First, the NBM was lesioned in the anesthetized animals and then CBF was measured in conscious, locally anesthetized rats during an intravenous infusion of tacrine, physostigmine, or saline. The experimental protocol was conducted in accordance with the French legislation on animal experimentation (Ministère de l'Agriculture, Bureau de la Protection Animale) and the European Community's Directives.

Unilateral Lesion of the Nucleus Basilis Magnocellularis

Lesioning of the NBM was undertaken 3–5 weeks before measurement of CBF. Four series of 10 rats weighing 260–310 g were anesthetized with chloral hydrate (400 mg/kg i.p.), and a stainless steel cannula was stereotaxically inserted into the NBM so that the tip was: 7.20 mm anterior to the interaural axis, 2.90 mm lateral, and +2.60 mm horizontal. Ibotenic acid (6 μg dissolved in 600 nl of sodium hydroxide-buffered saline) or saline was infused at a rate of 100 nl/min. The lesion efficacy was verified in 2–4 rats from each series, on 20 μm cryostat-cut brain sections stained for acetylcholinesterase. This lesioning procedure was previously shown to reduce ipsilateral choline acetyltransferase activity by 27–59% depending on the cortical areas considered.[2]

Experimental Protocols

Three to five weeks postlesion, rats (380–420 g) were anesthetized with halothane (1.0%) and catheterized in the two femoral veins for infusion of agents and radiotracer and in the two arteries for arterial pressure recording and serial arterial blood sampling. The rats were then installed in a prone position in a hammock and allowed to recover from anesthesia for 2 hours until CBF measurement. Arterial blood pressure and heart rate were continuously recorded. Rectal temperature was maintained at 37.5°C, especially during drug injection, because cholinesterase inhibitors reduced body temperature. Intravenous infusions of physostigmine (Sigma, E8500) at 0.2 mg/kg/h, or tacrine (Parke-Davis) at 8 mg/kg/h, or saline were started 20–30 minutes before CBF measurement. Arterial blood gases and pH were measured before drug infusion and just before CBF measurement.

Cerebral Blood Flow Measurement, Experimental Groups, and Statistics

The [^{14}C]iodoantipyrine technique was used to measure CBF as previously described.[2] The tracer solution (100 µCi/kg b.w.) was infused while a series of arterial blood samples were collected. The rat was then sacrificed and its brain rapidly dissected into 24 regions. Radioactivity in the arterial plasma and brain samples was counted by scintillation to calculate blood flow in each region.

Rats from each lesion series were randomly assigned to one of the four experimental groups for CBF measurement: sham-lesioned ($n = 7$), lesioned infused with i.v. saline ($n = 6$), lesioned infused with i.v. physostigmine at 0.2 mg/kg/h ($n = 6$), or i.v. tacrine at 8 mg/kg/h ($n = 9$). The significance of the effects of physostigmine and tacrine was assessed by an Anova followed by Dunnett's test for multiple-range analysis. Blood flow in homotopic regions of the two hemispheres (side-to-side differences) was compared using Student's paired t test.

RESULTS

Effects of the Nucleus Basilis Magnocellularis Lesion under Resting Conditions

The NBM lesion did not significantly alter the systemic variables (data not shown), but it significantly reduced blood flow in the parietal and occipital cortical areas ipsilateral to the lesion (FIG. 1). This result extends to a longer time scale, up to 5 weeks, that obtained 1–2 weeks after the lesion,[3] although less substantially.

Effects of Infusion of Physostigmine and Tacrine

Intravenous infusion of physostigmine and tacrine rapidly caused hypertension, less pronounced with physostigmine (13%) than with tacrine (23%), when compared to saline-infused rats. The highest MABP values during infusion remained below the upper limit of CBF autoregulation. Both agents elicited moderate hyperventilation and behavioral changes consisting of vibrissal vibrations, chewing, head rotations, and occasional limb and body movements.

Comparison of the cerebrovascular responsiveness to the drugs in the intact hemibrains with respect to the control group shows that 3–5 weeks after the lesion,

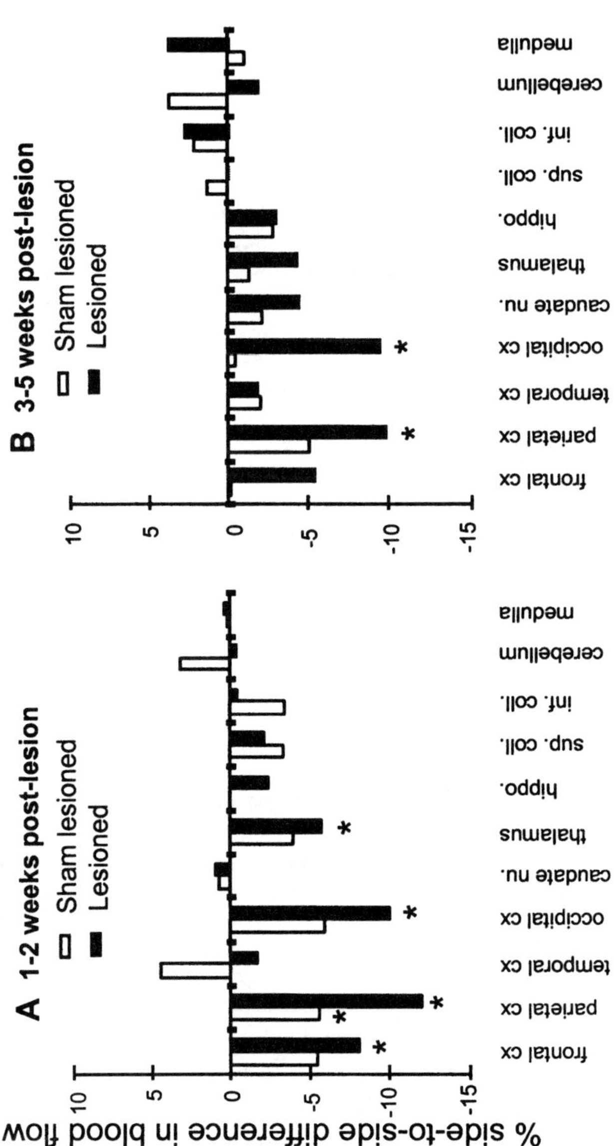

FIGURE 1. Side-to-side differences in blood flow (with respect to the intact side) induced by NBM lesion in various brain regions either 1–2 weeks (*left panel*) or 3–5 weeks postlesion (*right panel*). The 1–2–week data are derived from Ref. 3. *Significantly different from the intact side (p <0.05, paired t test).

physostigmine significantly enhanced blood flow in three cortical and two subcortical areas (FIG. 2A, empty bars). The greatest change was observed in a subcortical region (superior colliculus +38%) followed by the parietal cortex (+35%). Tacrine significantly enhanced blood flow in most regions (FIG. 2B, empty bars). In contrast to physostigmine, the greatest change was observed in the cortex (parietal area +163%) followed by subcortical regions (hippocampus +70%).

Effects of the Nucleus Basilis Magnocellularis Lesion on the Responses to Physostigmine and Tacrine

In the deafferented hemisphere, the cerebrovascular effects of physostigmine were significant only in the frontal cortex and in two subcortical regions (FIG. 2A, filled bars). The responses were smaller in several regions, except the frontal cortex. Side-to-side (ipsilateral versus contralateral) comparison (FIG. 3A), which displays the lesion-dependent component of the response, corroborates this finding by showing significant, negative differences in two cortical areas and in the thalamus. Unlike physostigmine, the responses to tacrine were more pronounced in the deafferented versus the intact hemisphere (FIG. 2B, filled bars) and presented a similar distribution in both hemibrains. FIGURE 3B shows an NBM-dependent "facilitated circulation" notably restricted to the frontal cortex at 3–5 weeks postlesion. Comparison between the patterns of regional responses reported in FIGURE 3 suggests that the NBM-dependent component of the responses to physostigmine in the frontal cortex (FIG. 3A) is inverted by a tacrine-type effect (FIG. 3B). Conversely for tacrine, the facilitated circulation seems limited to the frontal cortex due to the physostigmine-type effect.

DISCUSSION

This study provides evidence for distinct actions of the two cholinesterase inhibitors used. Lower cerebrovascular reactivity to physostigmine was observed in several areas of the deafferented hemisphere 3–5 weeks after the lesion, whereas the converse occurred with tacrine. These unexpected findings led us to question the mechanism of action of cholinesterase inhibitors. The magnitude and distribution of the cerebrovascular effects of NBM lesion, alone or in association with acutely administered physostigmine or tacrine, are analyzed in order to clarify the targets of the NBM projections that mediate the differential actions of these drugs.

Expected Cerebrovascular Effects of Nucleus Basilis Magnocellularis Lesion and of Cholinesterase Inhibitors

We presently report that the blood flow reduction previously observed 1–2 weeks after lesioning of the NBM[3] is still present at 5 weeks postlesion. This result shows that the NBM induces a tonic influence on the cortical circulation, which is not compensated after deafferentation. This is at variance with what was observed for the metabolic functioning of the cortex after the NBM lesion, because the rate of glucose use recovered in less than 2 weeks,[6] indicating a functional reorganization. Thus, NBM impairment may be chronically detrimental to brain circulatory function.

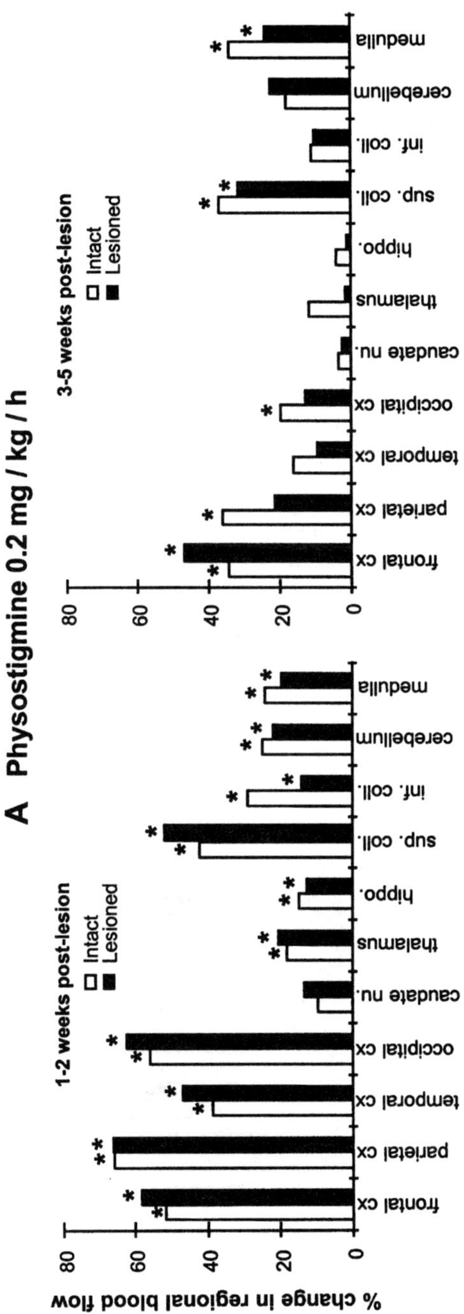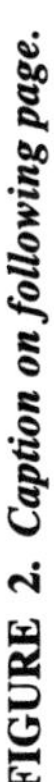

FIGURE 2. *Caption on following page.*

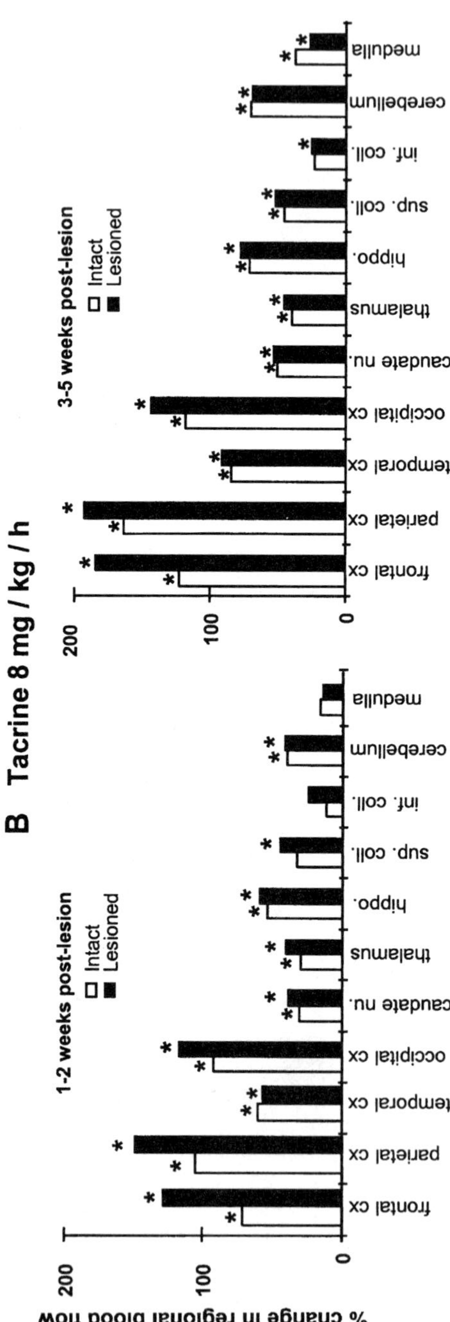

FIGURE 2. Changes in blood flow induced by i.v. infusion of physostigmine (**A**) or tacrine (**B**) 3–5 weeks after NBM lesion in brain regions of the intact and lesioned hemispheres compared to the control group. The 1–2–week physostigmine data are derived from Ref. 2 and the 1–2–week tacrine data from Ref. 3. *Significant difference in blood flow compared to the homotopic regions of the control group ($p < 0.05$, Anova plus Tukey's test).

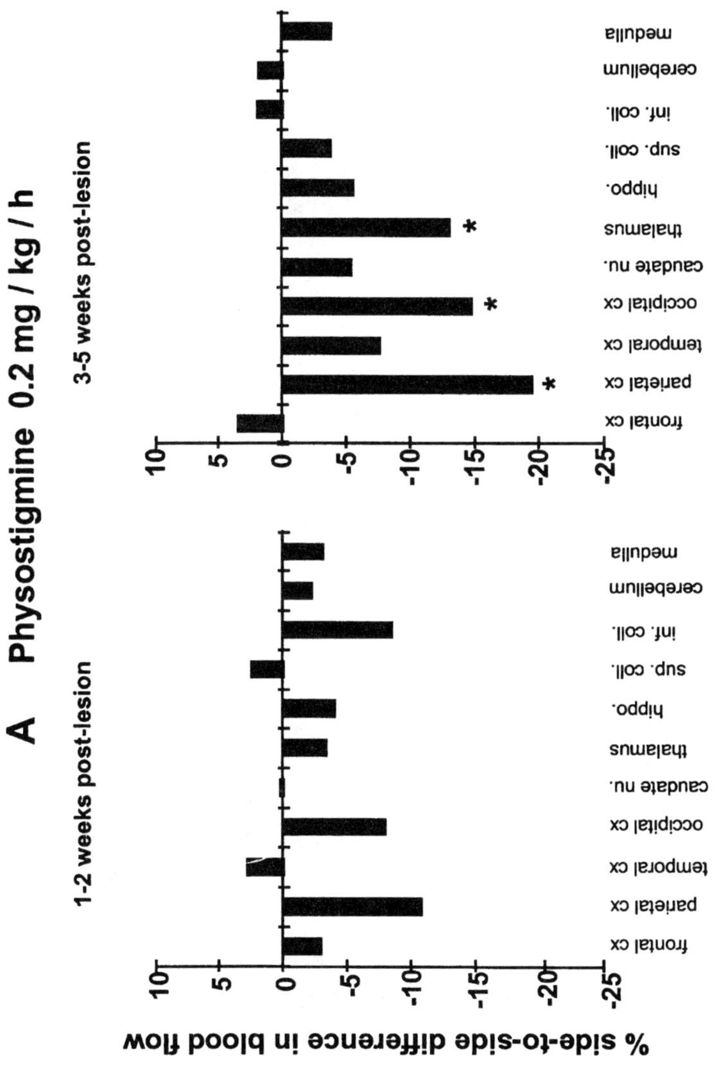

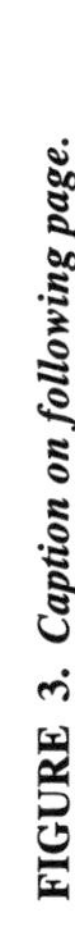

FIGURE 3. *Caption on following page.*

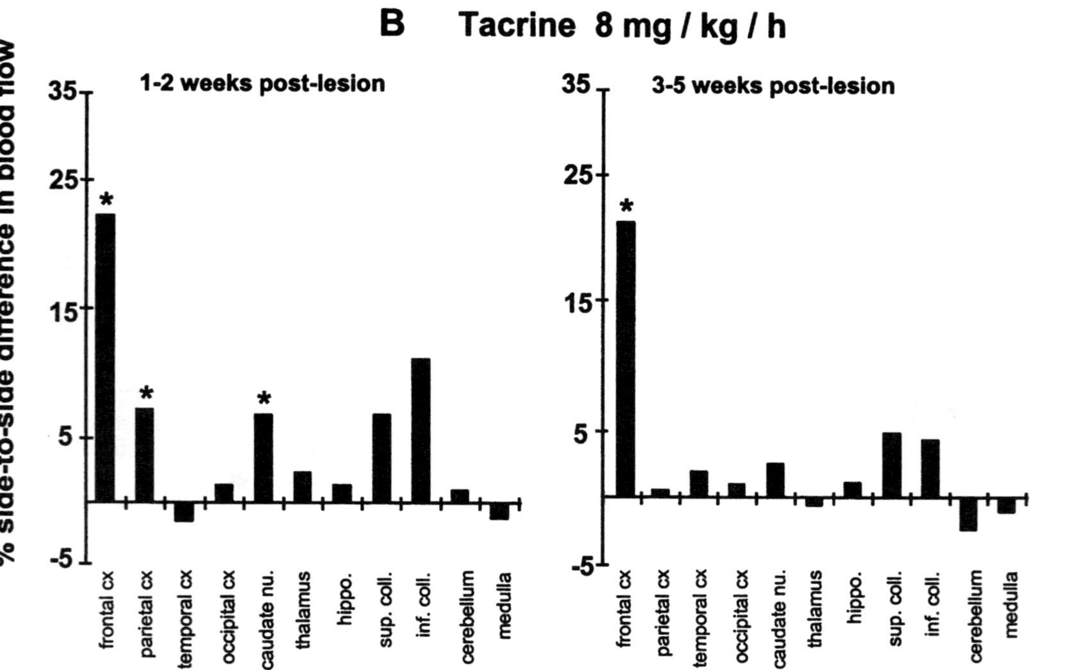

FIGURE 3. Side-to-side differences in blood flow (with respect to the intact side) induced by physostigmine (**A**) and tacrine (**B**) in various brain regions either 1–2 weeks (*left panels*) or 3–5 weeks postlesion (*right panels*). Comparison of **A** and **B** suggests both common and distinct properties of physostigmine and tacrine, differently expressed among the regions. The 1–2–week physostigmine data are derived from Ref. 2 and the 1–2–week tacrine data from Ref. 3. *Significantly different from the intact side ($p < 0.05$, paired t test).

Several experimental arguments support the finding that the cholinergic deficit is prominently involved in the hypoperfusion resulting from lesioning the NBM. The time course of the blood flow decreases is concordant with that in cortical choline acetyltransferase activity.[7] Considering the vasodilatory activity of ACh (see Ref. 8 for references), these blood flow reductions can be ascribed to impairment of cholinergic NBM projections. Such a contention is consistent with the concomitant increases in blood flow and ACh release elicited by NBM stimulation[9] and with the fact that this cerebrovascular response is doubled by physostigmine.[10] Hence, the well known vasodilatory effect of cholinesterase inhibitors[1] can be related to an increased extracellular concentration of ACh.[11] This effect should be less in the deafferented than in the intact hemisphere 1–2 weeks after NBM lesion, when the projection fibers are degenerated. Later, if denervation supersensitivity occurs, ipsilateral versus contralateral differences in the drug-induced cerebrovascular effects should diminish in the projection areas of the cholinergic NBM neurons. In fact, a completely different picture was observed. Our results can be explained by at least two mechanisms: (1) an inhibition that prevents blood flow from increasing more in the intact hemisphere in response to both agents, and (2) a facilitation of the response to tacrine in the deafferented cortex.

Nucleus Basilis Magnocellularis Lesion Reveals Inhibition Elicited by Physostigmine and Tacrine

Paradoxically, reduced responsiveness to physostigmine in the lesioned hemibrain did not appear at 1–2 weeks, but at 3–5 weeks postlesion, which is a sufficient time for denervation supersensitivity to occur.[4,5] This result can most likely be ascribed to an inhibitory cortical interneuron that receives cholinergic NBM fibers and becomes supersensitized after deafferentation. A cholinoceptive inhibitory cortical interneuron has already been hypothesized,[12] but it is not known if it receives NBM projections. Such an interneuron can account for (1) the absence of a lesion-dependent reduced responsiveness to cholinesterase inhibitors at 1–2 weeks postlesion (FIG. 1, left panel), (2) the trend to smaller effects of the lesion after 3–5 weeks (FIG. 1, right panel), and (3) the smaller responsiveness to physostigmine in cortical compared to subcortical regions at 3–5 weeks postlesion (FIG. 2A).

Comparison of the patterns of regional distribution of the various cerebrovascular effects observed provides evidence for the arrangement of NBM projections in the cortical circuitry. Analogy between the distribution of the cortical effects of the NBM lesion (FIG. 1), which is mirrored by the responses to cholinesterase inhibitors (FIG. 2), indicates that both effects are mediated by the same neuron. This neuron might correspond to the cholinergic bipolar neuron contacting cortical microvessels[8] or that presented as a "vasodilator intracortical neuron"[13] and eventually that expressing M2-muscarinic receptors.[14] The additional analogy with the cortical distribution of the NBM-dependent antagonistic effect of physostigmine, except for the frontal cortex (FIG. 3A), leads to the postulate that the inhibitory interneuron projects to the "vasodilator neuron."

In subcortical regions, the NBM-dependent effects of physostigmine and tacrine are modest compared with their NBM-independent effects, and they are mostly of the physostigmine type. That found in the thalamus under physostigmine is nonetheless probably great enough to be of functional significance. The cerebrovascular effects observed presumably reflect the respective influence of the two cholinesterase inhibitors on the functioning of neuronal systems and suggest their potentialities on NBM-related cognitive functions. Altogether, our results substantiate the fact that the basalocortical system becomes silent when treated with physostigmine or tacrine.

Lesion-Induced Change in Reactivity to Tacrine

The enhanced cortical blood flow responsiveness to tacrine found in the deafferented hemibrain 3–5 weeks after lesioning the NBM again suggests denervation supersensitivity. However, this facilitated circulation was already present after 1–2 weeks (FIG. 3B) and remained stable for at least 5 weeks. This phenomenon would therefore not primarily implicate neuronal elements. A major feature of the facilitation is its marked frontal predominance, a distribution that is also observed in the cortical blood flow responses to NBM stimulation.[15] Anatomic studies have shown that cortical microvessels receive cholinergic innervation directly originating in the NBM and that most of these fibers abut perivascular astrocytes.[16] These data designate the neurovascular junction of basalocortical terminals, including the astrocyte, as the main unit involved in the facilitation. Arguments support this statement. First, a large fraction of astrocytes possesses perivascular endfeet, suggesting a cerebrovascular function.[17,18] Second, astrocytes undergo prolonged morphologic changes to remote deafferentation soon after neuronal lesion.[19] Moreover, tacrine might intervene in areas deafferented from cholinergic terminals through some nonclassical mechanisms of cholinesterases[20] as well as through an increase in the synthesis of amyloid precursor proteins, reported to be rapid and persistent after NBM lesioning.[7] The latter phenomenon is sensitive to tacrine[21] and modulated by muscarinic receptors.[22,23]

In conclusion, our results provide evidence for dual properties of cholinesterase inhibitors. One is responsible for inhibition of the basalocortical system. This action implies that cholinesterase inhibitors cannot properly fulfill the principle of cholinergic replacement therapy for Alzheimer's disease, because they fail to specifically compensate for a chronic deficit of NBM functioning. However, another property represented here by tacrine is responsible for a circulatory facilitation in a cortical area deafferented from the NBM, an effect that might be of importance with respect to brain perfusion in Alzheimer's disease. This is corroborated by studies showing that (1) cortical blood flow is highly sensitive to NBM activation,[15] an effect that is strongly age dependent,[24] (2) brain microvessels are the site of pathophysiologic changes in Alzheimer's disease,[25,26] primarily involving perivascular astrocytes,[27] and (3) enhancement of the circulation is beneficial in Alzheimer's disease.[28,29] Thus, our results support the idea that impairment of the mechanisms of blood flow regulation might constitute a link between a cholinergic deficit and neurodegenerative processes. An insufficient nutrient blood supply may impair metabolic functioning, especially during functional activation. Conversely, circulatory improvement as obtained by prolonged tacrine treatment[28] might lead to clinical benefits.

ACKNOWLEDGMENTS

This work was supported by grants from the Centre National de la Recherche Scientifique (UPR 646 and UMR 6551) and the Université Paris 7-Denis Diderot. The authors thank Dr. G. Bitan, Parke-Davis Laboratory (France), for generously providing the tacrine.

REFERENCES

1. SCREMIN, O.U., C. TORRES, A.M.E. SCREMIN, M. O'NEAL, D. HEUSER & K.S. BLISARD. 1991. Role of nucleus basalis in cholinergic control of cortical blood flow. J. Neurosci. Res. **28:** 382–390.

2. PERUZZI, P., P. LACOMBE, V. MORO, E. VAUCHER, F. LEVY & J. SEYLAZ. 1993. The cerebrovascular effects of physostigmine are not mediated through the substantia innominata. Exp. Neurol. **122:** 319–326.

3. PERUZZI, P., J. BORREDON, J. SEYLAZ & P. LACOMBE. 1996. Tacrine overcompensates for the decreased blood flow induced by basal forebrain lesion in the rat. NeuroReport **8:** 103–108.

4. LAMOUR, Y., P. DUTAR & A. JOBERT. 1982. Spread of acetylcholine sensitivity in the neocortex following lesion of the nucleus basalis. Brain Res. **252:** 377–381.

5. BRONZETTI, E., M.G. CAPORALI, L. FELICI, T. NIGLIO, A. SCOTTI DE CAROLIS & F. AMENTA. 1993. Muscarinic cholinoceptor subtypes in the rat frontoparietal cortex after ipsilateral lesions of the nucleus basalis magnocellularis. Pharmacology **46:** 301–307.

6. LAMOUR, Y.A., H.W. HOLLOWAY, D.M. LARSON & T.T. SONCRANT. 1993. The effect of lesion of the nucleus basalis magnocellularis on local glucose utilization in the rat: time course. Neurodegeneration **2:** 41–50.

7. WALLACE, W.C., S.T. AHLERS, J. GOTLIB, V. BRAGIN, J. SUGAR, R. GLUCK, P.A. SHEA, K.D. DAVIS & V. HAROUTUNIAN. 1993. Amyloid precursor protein in the cerebral cortex is rapidly and persistently induced by loss of subcortical innervation. Proc. Natl. Acad. Sci. USA **90:** 8712–8716.

8. CHÉDOTAL, A., C. COZZARI, M.-P. FAURE, B.K. HARTMAN & E. HAMEL. 1994. Distinct choline acetyltranferase (ChAT) and vasoactive intestinal polypeptide (VIP) bipolar neurons project to local blood vessels in the rat cerebral cortex. Brain Res. **646:** 181–193.

9. SATO, A. & Y. SATO. 1995. Cholinergic neural regulation of regional cerebral blood flow. Alzheimer Dis. Assoc. Disord. **9:** 28–38.

10. DAUPHIN, F., P. LACOMBE, R. SERCOMBE, E. HAMEL & J. SEYLAZ. 1991. Hypercapnia and stimulation of the substantia innominata increase rat frontal cortical blood flow by different cholinergic mechanisms. Brain Res. **553:** 75–83.

11. MESSAMORE, E., U. WARPMAN, N. OGANE & E. GIACOBINI. 1993. Cholinesterase inhibitor effects on extracellular acetylcholine in rat cortex. Neuropharmacology **32:** 745–750.

12. DUTAR, P., M.-H. BASSANT & Y. LAMOUR. 1990. Effects of tetrahydro-9-aminoacridine on cortical and hippocampal neurons in the rat: an *in vivo* and *in vitro* study. Brain Res. **527:** 32–40.

13. GOLANOV, E.V. & D.J. REIS. 1995. Vasodilation evoked from medulla and cerebellum is coupled to bursts of cortical EEG activity in rats. Am. J. Physiol. **268:** R454–R467.

14. SMILEY, J.F., A.I. LEVEY & M.-M. MESULAM. 1998. Infracortical interstitial cells concurrently expressing M2-muscarinic receptors, acetylcholinesterase and nicotinamide adenine dinucleotide phosphate-diaphorase in the human and monkey cerebral cortex. Neuroscience **84:** 755–769.

15. VAUCHER, E., J. BORREDON, G. BONVENTO, J. SEYLAZ & P. LACOMBE. 1997. Autoradiographic evidence for flow-metabolism uncoupling during stimulation of the nucleus basalis of Meynert in the conscious rat. J. Cereb. Blood Flow Metab. **17:** 686–694.

16. VAUCHER, E. & E. HAMEL. 1995. Cholinergic basal forebrain neurons project to cortical microvessels in the rat: electron microscopic study with anterogradely transported Phaseolus vulgaris Leucoagglutinin and choline acetyltransferase immunocytochemistry. J. Neurosci. **15:** 7427–7441.

17. MORO, V., K. KACEM, V. SPRINGHETTI, J. SEYLAZ & F. LASBENNES. 1995. Microvessels isolated from brain: localization of muscarinic sites by radioligand binding and immunofluorescent techniques. J. Cereb. Blood Flow Metab. **15:** 1082–1092.

18. KACEM, K., P. LACOMBE, J. SEYLAZ & G. BONVENTO. 1998. Structural organization of the perivascular astrocyte endfeet and their relationship with the endothelial glucose transporter: a confocal microscopy study. Glia **23:** 1–10.
19. HAJOS, F. & A. CSILLAG. 1995. The remote astroglial response (RAR): a holistic approach for evaluating the effects of lesions of the central nervous system. Neurochem Res. **20:** 571–577.
20. LAYER, P.G. 1995. Nonclassical roles of cholinesterases in the embryonic brain and possible links to Alzheimer Disease. Alzheimer Dis. Assoc. Disord. **9:** 29–36.
21. MORI, F., C.C. LAI, F. FUSI & E. GIACOBINI. 1995. Cholinesterase inhibitors increase secretion of APPs in rat brain cortex. NeuroReport **6:** 633–636.
22. NITSCH, R.M. 1996. From acetylcholine to amyloid: neurotransmitters and the pathology of Alzheimer's disease. Neurodegeneration **5:** 477–482.
23. ROBERSON, M.R. & L.E. HARRELL. 1997. Cholinergic activity and amyloid precursor protein metabolism. Brain Res. Rev. **25:** 50–69.
24. SERCOMBE, R., P. LACOMBE, C. VERRECCHIA, V. SPRINGHETTI, E.T. MACKENZIE & J. SEYLAZ. 1994. Basal forebrain control of cortical blood flow and tissue gases in conscious aged rat. Brain Res **662:** 155–164
25. DE LA TORRE, J.C. 1994. Impaired brain microcirculation may trigger Alzheimer's disease. Neurosci. Biobehav. Rev. **18:** 397–401.
26. KALARIA, R.N. 1996. Cerebral vessels in ageing and Alzheimer's disease. Pharmacol. Ther. **72:** 193–214.
27. WYSS-CORAY, T., E. MASLIAH, M. MALLORY, L. MCCONLOGUE, K. JOHNSON-WOOD, C. LIN & L. MUCKE. 1997. Amyloidogenic role of cytokine TGF-β1 in transgenic mice and in Alzheimer's disease. Nature **389:** 603–606.
28. MINTHON, L., K. NILSSON, S.P. EDVINSSON, P.E. WENDT & L. GUSTAFSON. 1995. Long term effects of tacrine on regional cerebral blood flow changes in Alzheimer's disease. Dementia **36:** 245–251.
29. PROHOVNIK, I., S.E. ARNOLD, G. SMITH & L.R. LUCAS. 1997. Physostigmine reversal of scopolamine-induced hypofrontality. J. Cereb. Blood Flow Metab. **17:** 220–228.

Plasma Total Homocysteine and Cognitive Performance in a Volunteer Elderly Population

M. BUDGE,[a] C. JOHNSTON, E. HOGERVORST, C. DE JAGER, E. MILWAIN, S.D. IVERSEN, L. BARNETSON, E. KING, AND A.D. SMITH

OPTIMA (Oxford Project To Investigate Memory and Ageing), Department of Pharmacology, University of Oxford and Radcliffe Infirmary, Woodstock Road, Oxford OX2 6HE , UK

BACKGROUND

Case-control studies have demonstrated associations between moderately elevated blood levels of total homocysteine (tHcy) and cerebrovascular disease,[1] vascular dementia,[2–4] and Alzheimer's disease.[3–5] Clarke *et al.*[3] showed an association between elevated tHcy, low levels of folate and vitamin B12, and histopathologically confirmed Alzheimer's disease. However, the influence of elevated tHcy levels or its biologic determinants on cognitive performance in the normal elderly and on the development of cognitive impairment or its progression to dementia is not well established. Riggs *et al.*[6] and La Rue *et al.*[7] have suggested that levels of plasma homocysteine, vitamin B12, and folate may exert differential effects on cognitive abilities. Recently, Jensen *et al.*[8] reported negative relationships between elevated tHcy levels (>15 μmol/L) and a broad range of cognitive, quality of life, and psychologic variables in 80-year-old subjects. However, these studies could not assess whether these associations were independent of differences in age, gender, IQ, and depression. Furthermore, it is important to explore the relationship between tHcy and cognitive performance as continuous variables, rather than as dichotomous variables.

The aim of this study was to examine the influence of plasma tHcy levels on global cognitive performance in 156 elderly community volunteers.

METHODS

Subjects. One hundred fifty-six community-dwelling, self-caring volunteers over 60 years of age (range 60–91 years) were recruited for a new, three-year (annual visits) longitudinal study aimed at further defining early markers or predictors of cognitive impairment and their relationship to the subsequent development of dementia. Participants were excluded if they: (1) scored $\leq$ 80 on the CAMCOG[9] or $\leq$ 24 on the Mini-Mental State Examination (MMSE) at the initial screening visit, (2) reported significant progressive subjective memory complaints, (3) lived in institutional care,

[a]Address for correspondence: Dr. Marc Budge, OPTIMA (Oxford Project To Investigate Memory and Ageing), Department of Pharmacology, University of Oxford, Radcliffe Infirmary, Woodstock Road, Oxford OX2 6HE, UK. Tel: 44-1865-224356; fax: 44-1865-224099.
e-mail: marc.budge@pharm.ox.ac.uk

TABLE 1. Baseline characteristics of the population ($n = 156$)

Variable	Mean (SD)	Range
Age (y)	74.1 (6.2)	61–91
Gender	51% females	
Smokers	52% ever	6% current
BMI	26 (4)	19–37
CAMCOG	98 (4)	84–105
MMSE	29 (1)	24–30
GDS (0–30)	5 (4)	0–16
IQ (NART)	118 (9)	92–131
TSH (mU/L)	2 (2)	0.1–12
Vitamin B12 (pmol/l)	433 (246)	130–2000
Serum folate (μg/l)	12 (4)	5–20
Serum creatinine (mmol/l)	105 (17)	66–172
tHcy (μmol/l)	12.6 (3.8)	6–26

or (4) were unable to complete the CAMDEX[9] examination. Concomitant physical disease such as diabetes mellitus, coronary artery disease, hypertension, or prior transient ischemic attack/minor cerebrovascular accident (>1 year previously) were not reasons for exclusion. Ethical approval was granted by the Central Oxford Research Ethics Committee. Informed consent was obtained from all participants for all testing.

Assessment. At enrollment, a CAMDEX[9] examination, Nelson Adult Reading Test (NART), and the 30-point Geriatric Depression Scale (GDS) were administered. CAMCOG and MMSE scores were derived from the CAMDEX, whilst a full-scale IQ score was generated from the NART. Medical history, medication, smoking, alcohol and beverage intake, and use of vitamin supplements were documented. Physical examination concentrating on cardiovascular and neurologic systems was performed.

Blood Sampling. Nonfasting blood samples were taken for estimation of tHcy, serum vitamin B12, RBC/serum folate, thyroid stimulating hormone (TSH), and serum creatinine levels. Blood samples for tHcy were collected into EDTA tubes, immediately refrigerated at 4°C, and subsequently centrifuged and plasma aliquotted for storage at −70°C. Total time from blood sampling to storage at −70°C was always less than 2 hours. For tHcy, the Abbott-Axis Imx immunoassay was used;[10] folate and vitamin B12 were measured by Abbott Imx binding assay and immunoassay procedures, respectively.

Statistical Analysis. Linear regression analysis was used to determine the relationship between tHcy and age and gender, and CAMCOG score and age, gender, and tHcy. Thereafter, multiple regression analysis was used to explore the interrelationship between the variables entered into the primary model. Variables entered were CAMCOG (dependent variable), tHcy, age, gender, full-scale IQ (NART), and GDS score. An analysis of variance with CAMCOG score by tHcy quintile group was performed to check the linearity of the tHcy – CAMCOG score association.

TABLE 2. Multiple regression analysis of the influence of total plasma homocysteine (tHcy) on the CAMCOG score

Determinants of the CAMCOG Score	Coefficient for a 10 µm Change in tHcy	SE	p
tHcy alone	−3.59	0.88	<0.001
tHcy plus gender	−3.73	0.90	<0.001
tHcy plus gender, age, IQ	−2.47	0.79	0.002
tHcy plus gender, age, IQ, GDS	−2.40	0.80	0.002

RESULTS

Selected characteristics of the study population are outlined in TABLE 1. The CAMCOG scores were inversely related to tHcy levels ($p = 0.002$, $r^2 = 0.11$; FIG. 1), and this association was independent of age, gender, full-scale IQ (NART), and depression (GDS score), as shown in TABLE 2. The association of CAMCOG with tHcy levels was linear across all tHcy quintiles (F ratio 9.7, F_{prob} 0.002). A significant difference in CAMCOG scores ($p < 0.05$) was present between the lowest and highest tHcy quintiles. If we assume a conservative self-correlation for nonfasting serial plasma tHcy values of 0.78,[11] the association between plasma tHcy and overall CAMCOG score remained significant ($p = 0.009$) independent of age, gender, GDS score, and full-scale IQ (NART). The results of a single measurement of tHcy indicate that a 10 µmol/L increase in the tHcy level may be associated with a 3-point decrease in the CAMCOG score. We found no association between tHcy levels and the MMSE score, but this result may be due to insufficient numbers of study participants.

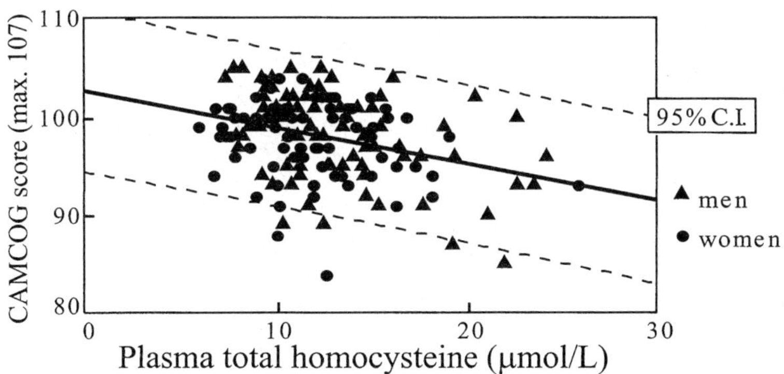

FIGURE 1. Relationship between total plasma homocysteine level and the CAMCOG score. The results are for 156 elderly community volunteers, none of whom had a CAMCOG score below the cut-off for dementia of 79. The correlation $p = 0.002$, $r^2 = 0.11$ has not been corrected for the influence of other confounders. C.I., predicted interval for simple observations.

DISCUSSION

The level of tHcy appears to determine about 11% of the variance of the CAM-COG score in this screened, elderly, community volunteer population, with higher tHcy levels being associated with a lower CAMCOG score. In view of this association, it will be important to establish whether blood tHcy levels or its biologic determinants (folate and/or vitamin B12) in the normal elderly, either in their own right or as a marker, may contribute to the development of cognitive impairment or dementia. Further longitudinal investigation of this relationship will establish the mechanism and strength of homocysteine's influence and help decide whether consideration of intervention studies is warranted.

ACKNOWLEDGMENTS

This work was supported by grants from the Medical Research Council, Bristol-Myers Squibb, and the European Biomed programme.

REFERENCES

1. Perry, I.J., H. Refsum *et al.* 1995. Prospective study of serum total homocysteine concentration and risk of stroke in middle-aged British men. Lancet **346:** 1395–1398.
2. Nilsson, K., L. Gustafson *et al.* 1996. Hyperhomocysteinaemia: a common finding in a psychogeriatric population. Eur. J. Clin. Invest. **26:** 853–859.
3. Clarke, R., A.D. Smith *et al.* 1998. Folate, vitamin B12, and serum total homocysteine levels in confirmed Alzheimer disease. Arch. Neurol. **55:** 1449–1455.
4. Lehmann, M., C.G. Gottfries *et al.* 1999. Identification of cognitive impairment in the elderly: homocysteine is an early marker. Dement. Geriatr. Cogn. Disord. **10:** 12–20.
5. McCaddon, A., G. Davies *et al.* 1998. Total serum homocysteine in senile dementia of Alzheimer type. Int. J. Geriatr. Psychiatry **13:** 235–239.
6. Riggs, K.M., A. Spiro *et al.* 1996. Relations of vitamin B-12, vitamin B-6, folate, and homocysteine to cognitive performance in the Normative Aging Study. Am. J. Clin. Nutr. **63:** 306–314.
7. La Rue, A., K.M. Koehler *et al.* 1997. Nutritional status and cognitive functioning in a normally aging sample: A 6-y reassessment. Am. J. Clin. Nutr. **65:** 20–29.
8. Jensen, E., O. Dehlin *et al.* 1998. Plasma homocysteine in 80-year-olds: relationships to medical, psychological and social variables. Arch. Gerontol. Geriatr. **26:** 215–226.
9. Roth, M., F.A. Huppert *et al.* 1988. CAMDEX: The Cambridge examination for mental disorders of the elderly. :72pp. Cambridge University Press. Cambridge.
10. Frantzen, F., A.L. Faaren *et al.* 1998. Enzyme conversion immunoassay for determining total homocysteine in plasma or serum. Clin. Chem. **44:** 311–316.
11. Clarke, R., P. Woodhouse *et al.* 1998. Variability and determinants of total homocysteine concentrations in plasma in an elderly population. Clin. Chem. **44:** 102–107.
12. Clarke, R., C. Frost *et al.* 1998. Lowering blood homocysteine with folic acid based supplements: meta-analysis of randomised trials. Br. Med. J. **316:** 894–898.

Cardiovascular and Other Risk Factors for Alzheimer's Disease and Vascular Dementia

JOHN S. MEYER,[b] GAIANE M. RAUCH, RONALD A. RAUCH,[a] ANWARUL HAQUE, AND KATE CRAWFORD

Cerebral Blood Flow Laboratory and [a]Radiology Service, Veterans Administration Medical Center, and Departments of Neurology and [a]Radiology, Baylor College of Medicine, Houston, Texas 77030, USA

ABSTRACT: Factors accelerating cerebral degenerative changes represent potentially modifiable risks for cognitive decline. Putative risks accelerating subtle cognitive decline and dementia were correlated with repeated measures of cerebral atrophy, CT densitometry, perfusions, and cognitive testing among 224 neurologically and cognitively normative aging volunteers. After age 60, cerebral atrophy, ventricular enlargement, polioaraiosis, and leukoaraiosis geometrically increased as perfusions declined. Risks accelerating perfusional decline, cerebral atrophy, polioaraiosis, and leukoaraiosis were: transient ischemic attacks (TIAs), hypertension, smoking, hyperlipidemia, male gender. At age 71.5 ± 11.9, subtle cognitive decline began, accelerated by TIAs, hypertension, and heart disease. Leukoaraiosis began before cognitive decline. TIAs, hypertension, and hyperlipidemia correlated with vasciular dementias. Excessive cortical perfusional decreases and cerebral atrophy correlated with cognitive decline. Family history of neurodegenerative disease correlated with Alzheimer's disease. We concluded that TIAs, hypertension, hyperlipidemia, smoking, and male gender accelerate cerebral degenerative changes, cognitive decline, and dementia.

INTRODUCTION

Epidemiologic, longitudinal studies of elderly subjects have identified risk factors for cerebral degenerative changes and dementias.[1–7] Risks predisposing to vascular dementias (VAD) and Alzheimer's (DAT) are primarily cardiovascular.[1,5,7,8] Cross-sequential analyses of VAD indicate that control of stroke risk factors delay or prevent strokes and cognitive decline.[9,10] Risk factor multiplicity geometrically increase strokes and cognitive impairments.

As a result, a multifactorial pathogenesis of VAD has evolved.[5,6,11] Risks multiply in frequency and severity during aging and complicate DAT, increasing the prevalence of DAT among elderly with heart disease[1] and those with hypertension.[8] Similar risks probably contribute to more subtle cognitive impairments. Identification of risks for subtle cognitive decline require longitudinal studies among normative populations at entry, followed with serial cognitive testing.

[b]Address for correspondence: John Stirling Meyer, M.D., Director, Cerebrovascular Research Laboratories, Bldg. 110, Room 225, VAMC, 2002 Holcombe Boulevard – 151A, Houston, Texas 77030, USA. Tel: (713) 794-7814; fax (713) 794-7583.

TABLE 1. Significant influences of risk factors after follow-up on cerebral atrophic measures, leukoaraiosis and polioaraiosis, and perfusional declines among 224 originally normative aging subjects at study entry

	Cerebral Atrophy	Ventricular Enlargement	Leuko-Araiosis	Polio-Araiosis	Perfusional Declines		White matter
					Cortex	Subcortex	
Male gender					Male*	Male*	Male*
Low education						Hypertension*	
Hypertension	Hypertension*	Hypertension*					
Heart disease							
Hyperlipidemia			Hypertension*				
Diabetes mellitus							
Smoking				Smoking*	Smoking*	Smoking*	
Alcohol							
FHx of CVD							
FHx of ND							
History of TIAS							TIAs*
Lack of ERT							

ABBREVIATIONS: FHx, family history; CVD, cerebrovascular diseases; ND, neurodegenerative diseases; TIA, transient ischemic attack; ERT, estrogen replacement therapy.

*Significant association.

METHODS

Two hundred twenty-four cognitively and neurologically normative subjects (mean age 59.5 ± 15.8, 22–89 years) have been followed for 4.3 ± 3.1 years. Subjects were recruited from friends, relatives, and caregivers of patients with dementia.[3] The likelihood of "normative" volunteers developing dementia was high because family histories of DAT or VAD were present among many. Protocols were approved by Institutional Review Boards of Baylor College of Medicine. After signing informed consent, subjects completed questionnaires, returning at least once annually for serial medical, neurologic, CT, and mental status examinations.

Cognitive status was measured by Cognitive Capacity Screening Examinations (CCSE). CCSE correlates well with more detailed neuropsychologic testing.[12,13] CCSE shows statistically significant test–retest reproducibility of ± 2 points among normal volunteers.[2,3,6,7,10,14,15] To identify subtle cognitive decline, sustained decreases of three or more points below baseline scores at entry were significant.

Cerebral CT volumes, tissue densities, and perfusions were measured by 26% xenon-enhanced CT-CBF methodology.[16] Results were correlated with personal and familial risk factors. Those showing unchanged CCSE (Group U) were compared with those showing subtle decline or dementia (Group S+D). There were 22 patients in Groups S (CCSE ≥ 3). There were 19 patients in Group D, developing dementia, 8 with VAD, 11 with DAT. Dementia types were classified according to pathologically verified clinical criteria.[6,17] Associated risk factors were analyzed to determine which accelerated cerebral degenerative changes. Risk factors analyzed (TABLES 1 and 2) included: (1) age, (2) gender, (3) educational status dichotomized above or

 413

TABLE 2. Risk factors among cognitively and neurologically "normative" volunteers at study entry comparing those developing cognitive decline (Group S+D) with those who were unchanged (Group U)

	Group U		Group S+D		Total		Group U vs Group S+D
n	183		41		224		
Mean age (SD)	55.2	(14.9)	68.9	(13.6)	59.5	(15.8)	$p < 0.002$
TIA (%)	19	(10.3)	11	(26.8)	30	(13.4)	$p < 0.050$
Educational status							
Less than high school graduate (%)	12	(6.5)	4	(9.7)	16	(7.1)	
High school graduate+ (%)	171	(93.5)	37	(90.3)	208	(92.9)	
Hypertension (%)	65	(35.5)	32	(78.0)	93	(41.5)	$p < 0.010$
Heart disease (%)	45	(24.5)	23	(56.1)	68	(30.4)	$p < 0.010$
Hyperlipidemia (%)	68	(37.1)	29	(70.7)	97	(43.3)	$p < 0.050$
Diabetes mellitus (%)	8	(4.4)	7	(17.1)	15	(6.7)	$p < 0.050$
Smoking (%)	96	(52.5)	31	(75.6)	127	(56.6)	
Alcohol consumption (%)	68	(37.1)	13	(31.7)	81	(36.2)	
Family history of cerebrovascular disease (%)	45	(24.5)	10	(24.3)	55	(24.5)	
Family history of neurodegenerative disease(%)	20	(10.9)	7	(17.1)	26	(11.6)	
Estrogen replacement therapy (%)	57	(31.1)	12	(29.3)	69	(30.8)	

Group U: Normal volunteers with unchanged cognition.
Group S+D: Normal volunteers with cognitive decline.

below high school graduation, (4) hypertension, (5) heart disease, (6) hyperlipidemia, (7) diabetes mellitus, (8) cigarette smoking, (9) alcohol consumption, (10) family history of cerebrovascular and Alzheimer diseases, and (11) absence of estrogen replacement therapy among postmenopausal women. Risk factors were treated.

Annual rates of change were calculated from plain CT scans providing changes in regional cerebral atrophy and tissue densities within gray and white matter. CT scans were contrasted by 8 minutes of inhalation of 26% xenon for measuring regional perfusions.[2,3,7,10,14–16,18]

Cerebral CT (global and local) densities were determined at first (CTD1) and final (CTD2) visits. Annual percentage changes in CT densities were adjusted according to time intervals between evaluations as follows:

Annual percentage changes in CT densities = [(CTD2-CTD1/CTD1]/Time interval × 100.

Volume ratios for reduced densities in white matter (leukoaraiosis) as well as volume ratios for reduced densities in gray matter (polioaraiosis) were calculated.[2,3,7,10,14,15]

Atrophic changes and ventricular and subarachnoidal space enlargement were calculated as:

ATI (%) = (cerebrospinal fluid volume/intracranial volume) × 100;

Subarachnoid spaces volume ratio (%) =
$$\text{subarachnoid spaces volume/intracranial volume} \times 100;$$

Ventricular space volume ratio = ventricular space volume/intracranial volume $\times$ 100.

Global and local values for cerebral blood flow at first and final visits were calculated.[19] LCBFs were determined at first (LCBF1) and final (LCBF2) visits. Annual percentage changes for cerebral perfusion (%/year) were calculated as follows:

Annual percentage changes in LCBF =
$$[(\text{LCBF2-LCBF1})/\text{LCBF1}]/\text{Time interval} \times 100.$$

Influences of individual risk factors on cerebral atrophy, leukoaraiosis, and polioaraiosis were evaluated at study entry utilizing analysis of covariance (ANCOVA) adjusting for age effects (TABLE 1). Pearson's r correlated CCSE scores with age at entry and final visits. Student' s t test evaluated age at entry and between Groups U and S+D. Chi square analysis evaluated risk factor distributions between subjects age 60 or less compared to those 60 or over. Student's t test compared: annual changes of volumetric measures, densitometric measures, and cerebral perfusion. Polynomial regression analyzed cross-sectional data for age at study entry with cerebral atrophy (atrophic indices), decreased cortical tissue densities (polioaraiosis and leukoaraiosis). Logistic regression analysis determined combinations of risk factors contributing to cognitive decline.

RESULTS

FIGURE 1 displays declining mean CCSE scores among cognitively intact subjects at entry with advancing age ($r = -0.20$, $p <0.004$) and at final visits ($r = -0.39$, $p <0.001$). Subjects in Group S+D ($n = 41$, open circles) developed significant cognitive decline after mean interval of 3.9 ($\pm$ 3.0) years. Most remained cognitively unchanged (Group U, $n = 183$, filled circles). Cognitive decline occurred predominantly after age 60 (86%); however, 58% of Group U were over age 60 ($x^2 = 11.5$, $p <0.001$).

FIGURE 2 illustrates regression analyses correlating age at entry with changes in atrophy and CT tissue densities. Cerebral atrophy ($r = 0.56$, $p <0.001$), ventricular enlargement ($r = 0.58$, $p <0.001$), leukoaraiosis ($r = 0.36$, $p <0.001$) and polioaraiosis ($r = 0.48$, $p <0.001$) increased during normal aging, with geometric progression after age 60. Basal ganglia volume ratios decreased with advancing age ($r = -0.22$, $p <0.004$). Regression analysis revealed that cortical and subcortical perfusions declined together during aging.

Parenchymal atrophy, leukoaraiosis and polioaraiosis, and ventricular enlargement correlated with cortical and subcortical perfusional declines, particularly in frontal, temporal, parietal cortex, and putamen.

ANCOVA (TABLE 1) revealed that cerebral atrophy and ventricular enlargement ($p <0.006$) are accelerated by hypertension, polioaraiosis, and smoking ($p <0.030$). Leukoaraiosis was influenced by hyperlipidemia ($p <0.020$). Perfusional declines in cortex and subcortex were associated with both male gender ($p <0.001$) and smoking ($p <0.020$). Decreased subcortical perfusion was associated with hypertension ($p <0.050$). TIAs were associated with decreased white matter perfusion ($p <0.050$).

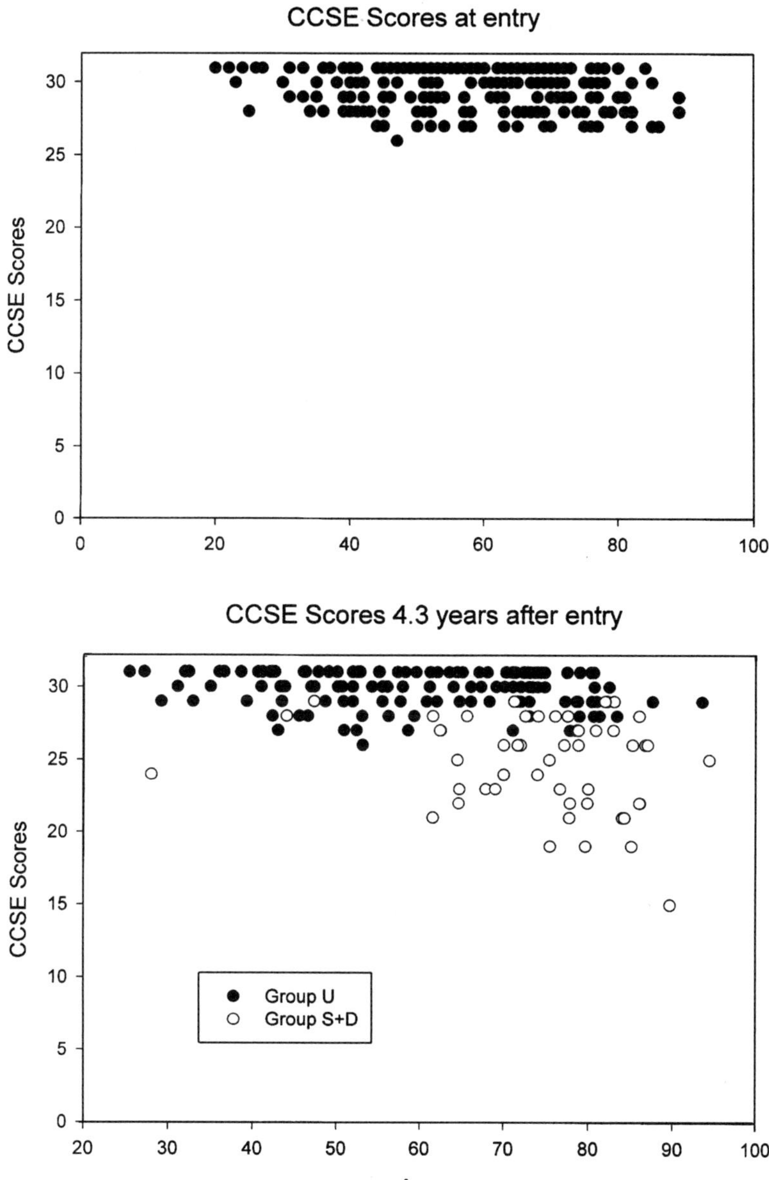

FIGURE 1. Plots of CCSE scores at entry and final visits, with age at visits, among 218 volunteers. After mean interval of 4.3 (± 3.1) years, some developed cognitive decline (Group S+D, *n* = 41, *empty circles*), but the majority remained cognitively unchanged (Group U, *n* = 183, *filled circles*). As shown, cognitive decline occurred after 60 years of age. There is unavoidable overlapping of some circles representing individual cases.

TABLE 3. Comparisons of annual changes of cerebral volumetric, densitometric, and perfusional measures among Group S+D and Group U subjects over age 60

	Group U		Group S+D		
n	69		30		
Age at entry (SD)	70.1	(6.6)	70.6	(5.9)	
Years Followed (SD)	3.2	(1.7)	4.8	(4.2)	
Annual Changes of Volumetric Measures (%/year)					
Atrophic index (ATI)	11.7	(13.2)	28.0	(23.9)	*p* <0.010
Ventricular enlargement	10.9	(17.1)	36.0	(47.1)	*p* <0.050
Subarachnoid space Enlargement	28.5	(75.0)	26.5	(34.6)	
Leuko-araiosis	14.9	(23.1)	19.3	(9.4)	*p* <0.050
Polio-araiosis	18.2	(33.2)	33.8	(53.0)	*p* <0.050
Global cortical volume	−1.3	(6.6)	−1.6	(5.0)	
Global subcortical volume	2.8	(22.7)	2.1	(10.3)	
Global white matter volume	−0.3	(4.4)	−3.7	(4.6)	*p* <0.010
Annual Changes of Densitometric Measures (%/year)					
Global cerebral density	−0.9	(1.9)	−1.5	(2.4)	
Global cortical density	−1.0	(2.5)	−1.5	(2.7)	
Frontal cortex	−0.8	(2.3)	−1.8	(3.4)	
Temporal cortex	−1.1	(2.0)	−1.3	(3.2)	
Parietal cortex	−1.1	(2.2)	−1.9	(2.7)	
Occipital cortex	−1.3	(3.4)	−1.7	(4.3)	
Global subcortical density	−0.9	(2.3)	−1.4	(3.2)	
Caudate nucleus	−0.9	(2.5)	−1.6	(3.8)	
Putamen	−0.8	(2.2)	−1.2	(3.5)	
Thalamus	−0.7	(2.5)	−1.5	(2.8)	
Global white matter density	−0.9	(1.6)	−1.7	(1.6)	*p* <0.050
Frontal white matter	−0.8	(2.7)	−2.0	(2.3)	
Internal capsule	−0.7	(2.6)	−1.7	(3.6)	
Occipital white matter	−1.4	(4.8)	−1.4	(1.7)	
Annual Changes of Perfusional Measures (%/year)					
Global cerebral blood flow (CBF)	−2.3	(5.0)	−6.2	(7.1)	*p* <0.050
Global cortical CBF	−3.5	(7.1)	−6.6	(7.5)	
Frontal cortex	−2.7	(9.2)	−8.6	(14.6)	*p* <0.050
Temporal cortex	−4.0	(9.6)	−7.4	(8.4)	
Parietal cortex	−2.6	(9.0)	−8.1	(15.1)	
Occipital cortex	−2.7	(12.0)	−1.5	(14.6)	
Global subcortical CBF	−2.0	(7.7)	−5.1	(19.9)	
Caudate nucleus	−0.7	(11.5)	−3.6	(32.3)	
Putamen	−1.4	(10.2)	−1.1	(32.7)	
Thalamus	−2.5	(10.1)	−0.4	(17.6)	
Global white matter CBF	1.0	(7.9)	1.1	(10.0)	
Frontal white matter	−1.3	(7.6)	−0.2	(8.9)	
Internal capsule	−0.8	(4.5)	−0.9	(9.4)	
Occipital white matter	0.8	(7.5)	−0.6	(10.1)	

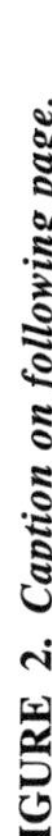

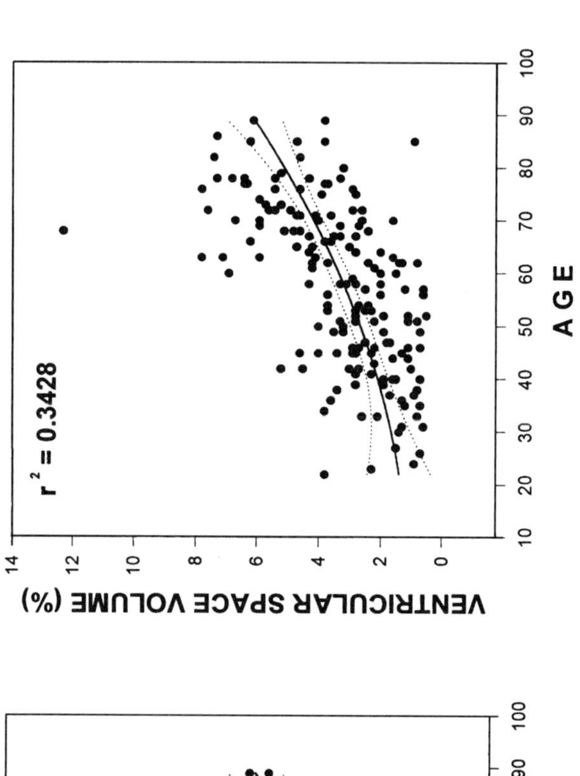

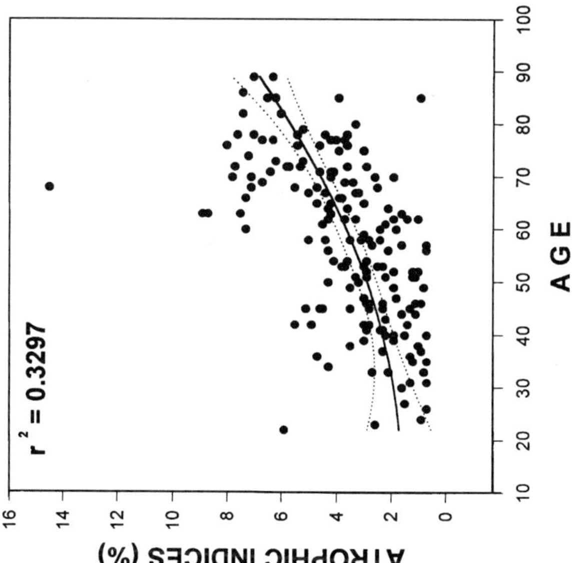

FIGURE 2. *Caption on following page.*

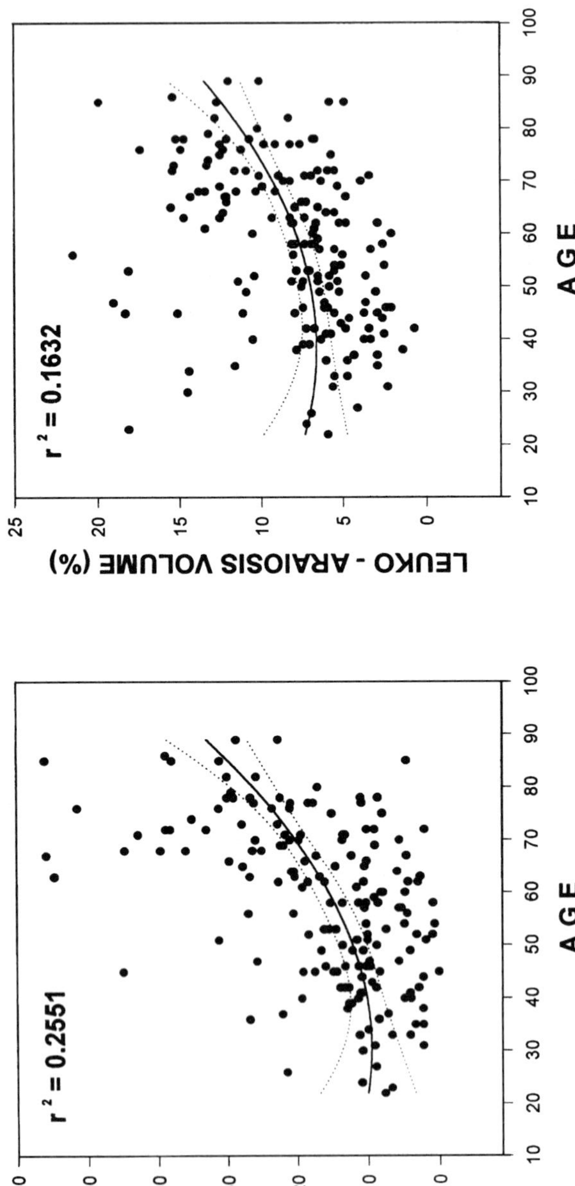

FIGURE 2. Polynomial regression analyses with 95% confidence intervals showing increased cerebral atrophy (atrophic indices) and decreased cortical tissue densities (ventricular volume ratios, polioaraiosis, and leukoaraiosis) with advancing age. All slopes are significant at $p < 0.001$.

TABLE 2 summarizes risk factors among normative volunteers at entry. During follow-up, 41 showed declines in cognition (Group S+D), starting mean age 71.5 (±11.9) years. Contrasted with Group U, cognitive declines were associated with TIAs (26.8%), hypertension (78.0%), heart disease (56.1%), hyperlipidemia (70.7%), and diabetes mellitus (17.1%).

Logistic regression analysis indicated hypertension (OR = 2.9, 95% CI = 1.4–6.1) as the primary predictor of cognitive decline. TIAs (OR = 2.0, 0.2–6.1), hyperlipidemia (OR = 1.9, 95% CI = 0.8–5.6), heart disease (OR = 1.1, 95% CI = 0.7–4.2), and diabetes mellitus (OR = 1.1, 95% CI = 0.1–9.2) independently did not predict cognitive decline.

TABLE 3 contrasts annual percentage changes between Group U and Group S+D, after age 60, for cerebral atrophic, degenerative, and perfusional measures. Among Group S+D, cerebral atrophy (ATI, p <0.010), ventricular enlargement (p <0.050), leukoaraiosis (p <0.050), polioaraiosis (p <0.050), global white matter volume (p <0.010), and global white matter densities (p <0.050) exceeded those among Group U. Shrinkage of white matter volumes associated with low density changes in both cortex and white matter were associated with cognitive decline. Global cerebral (p <0.050) and frontal cortical perfusions (p <0.050) accelerated with cognitive decline.

FIGURE 3 compares Group S+D with Group U 4.3 years before onset of cognitive decline. Leukoaraiosis and white matter perfusional decreases were already present, so that degenerative changes in white matter density precede cerebral atrophy as a marker among those destined for cognitive decline.

In Group S+D, 8 developed VAD and 11 developed DAT. Six VAD developed silent lacunar infarctions and two hemiparetic cerebral infarctions determined by CT scanning. Those destined to develop VAD had more frequent TIAs (p <0.050), hypertension (p <0.050), and hyperlipidemia (p <0.050) compared with Group U. Subjects developing DAT had more family histories of DAT compared to Group U (p <0.010) or VAD (p <0.050).

DAT showed the greatest rates of cerebral atrophy (29.1%/year, p <0.010) and ventricular enlargement (15.1%/year, p <0.050). VAD showed greater cortical perfusional declines (−2.6%/year, p <0.050), with cerebral atrophy (14.3%/year, p <0.050) and greater ventricular enlargement (27.9%/year, p <0.050) than Group U. Annual percentages for cerebral atrophy among both VAD and DAT exceeded that of 11.7%/year in Group U.

DISCUSSION

Age-related cerebral degenerative changes are coupled with decreased perfusion, known to be secondary to decreased cerebral metabolic demands.[2,14,20,21] During aging, declines in cerebral tissue densities in gray (polioaraiosis) and white matter (leuko-araiosis) reflect neuronal degenerative changes, which progress concurrently with cerebral perfusional declines. Rates of polio- and leukoaraiosis accelerate geometrically after age 60, correlating with cortical and subcortical atrophy and ventricular enlargement. Hypertension, smoking, TIAs, hyperlipidemia, and male gender accelerate cerebral perfusional declines, leukoaraiosis, and cerebral atrophy.

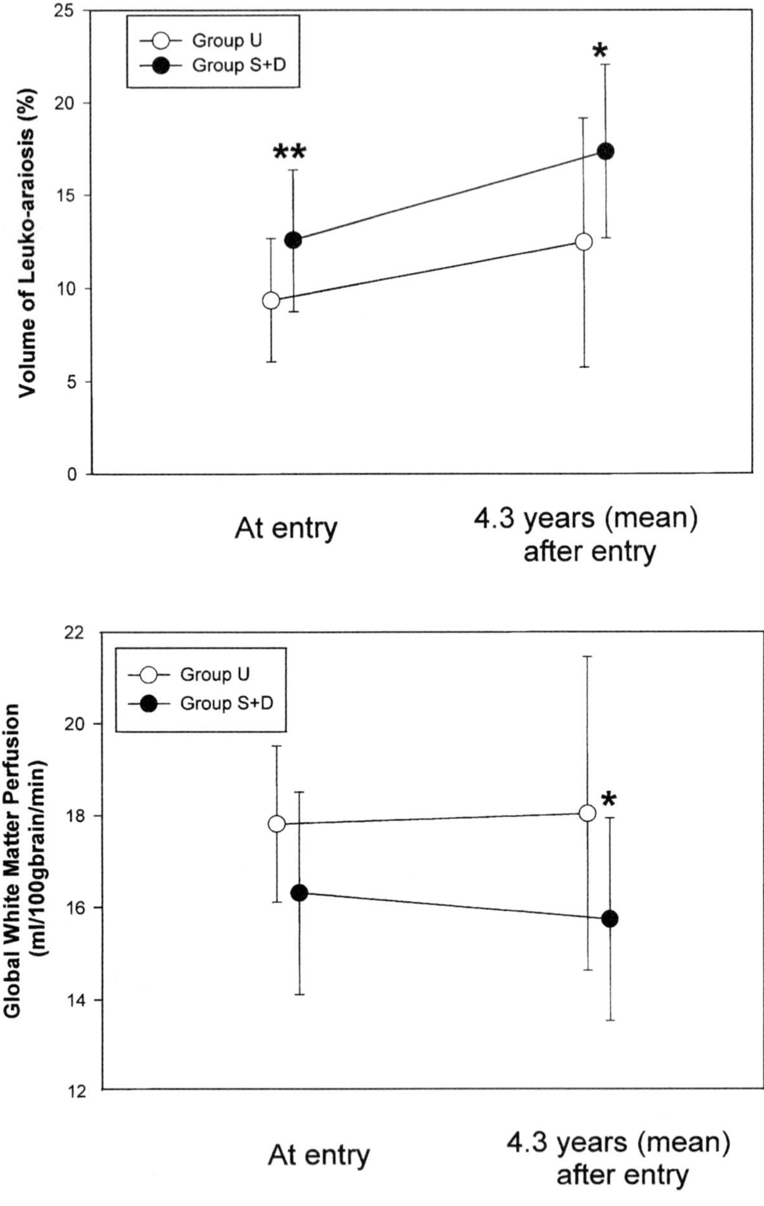

FIGURE 3. Changes of volume (leukoaraiosis) and global white matter perfusion at time of study entry and at time of last visit (after 4.3 [± 3.1] years). Before cognitive decline appeared in Group S+D, volumes of leukoaraiosis were significantly increased, and white matter perfusions were decreased compared to Group U. *p <0.050 compared to Group U; **p <0.010 compared to Group U.

The incidence of dementia starting after a mean age of 60 was about 1.5% per year, which is admittedly high for a "normative" cohort, but attributable to recruitment of "normative" subjects with family histories of DAT and VAD.

CT observations are consonant with neuropathologic evidences of decreased synaptic density during aging into neuronal shrinkage or loss being exacerbated by Alzheimer's disease[22] and cerebral ischemia.[23] Cerebral cortical atrophy, polioaraiosis, and leukoaraiosis are associated with cerebral perfusional decline and correlate with known progression of neuronal and synaptic degeneration during aging [2,22,24,25]

Reported evidence shows that hypertension exacerbates cerebral degenerative changes during aging,[26] particularly in temporo-occipital regions. Exacerbations of cerebral degenerative changes by stroke risk factors clarify why some individuals become demented after strokes, whereas others do not,[6,26] and how long-standing hypertension, atherosclerosis, and heart disease predispose and accelerate both VAD and DAT.[1,2,5,6,8,9,14,15,27]

Annual rates of cerebral atrophy, ventricular enlargement, and leukoaraiosis accelerate geometrically after age 60, with marked individual variations.[7] Individual differences are accounted for by accompanying risk factors. CSF volumes in subarachnoid and ventricular spaces increase with advancing age among normal individuals, especially after age 60.[2,7,20,21] "Normal" age-related cerebrocortical atrophy has been attributed to neuronal shrinkage and/or loss with decreased cortical synaptic densities[22,28] probably related to neuronal apoptosis aggravated by ischemia and genetic factors.[24,26] Experimental studies of cognitive decline during aging among rhesus monkeys correlate at autopsy with thinning of prefrontal cortex and myelin breakdown (leukoaraiosis) with reduced white matter volumes.[29]

Leukoaraiosis is detectable in 9–19% of older "normal" subjects,[2,14,30–35] and virtually always present in VAD[14] and in 30–60% of DAT patients.[30,31] Leukoaraiosis is age related[2,14,30–35] and accelerated by hypertension,[31] episodic hypotension,[35] heart disease, diabetes mellitus, heavy alcohol consumption, and strokes, particularly of the lacunar type.[23,34] Leukoaraiosis correlates with advancing age, cerebral atrophy, hypoperfusion of white matter, and cognitive impairments.[14] Tissue densities decrease in both gray and white matter during human aging, correlating with perfusional declines. Shrinkage and atrophy of the brain are generally considered to be risk factorz for cognitive decline.[6,36]

Optimal preservation of cognition during "normal" aging should include identification and control of risk factors, because many patients developing DAT and VAD show subtle cognitive decline preceding overt dementia. Reported beneficial effects for preventing VAD include control of stroke risk factors,[9,37] and probably this applies among DAT patients with remediable cardiovascular risk factors.[1,6,8,9,11] Optimal cognitive maintenance includes control of multiple cardiovascular risk factors,[9] including TIAs, hyperlipidemia,[9,37,38] smoking,[9,10,39] hypertension,[8,9,40] cardiovascular disorders, [40] and diabetes mellitus.[41]

REFERENCES

1. KATZMAN, R. *et al.* 1989. Development of dementing illnesses in an 80-year-old volunteer cohort. Ann. Neurol. **25:** 317–324.

2. MEYER, J.S. *et al.* 1994. CT changes associated with normal aging of the human brain. J. Neurol. Sci. **123:** 200–208.

3. MEYER, J.S. *et al.* 1994. Problems encountered with longitudinal neurological, psychometric and cerebral CT imaging among stroke data bank patients with dementia. Neuroepidemiology **13:** 340–344.

4. PERSSON, G. *et al.* 1996. A prospective population study of psychosocial risk factors for late onset dementia. Intern. J. Geriat. Psychiat. **11:** 15–22.

5. DESMOND, D.W. 1996. Vascular dementia: a construct in evolution. Cerebrovas. Brain Metab. Rev. **8:** 296–325.

6. LOEB, C. *et al.* 1996. Vascular dementia: still a debatable entity? J. Neurol. Sci. **143:** 31–40.

7. AKIYAMA, H. *et al.* 1997. Normal human aging: factors contributing to cerebral atrophy. J. Neurol. Sci. **152:** 39–49.

8. SKOOG, I. *et al.* 1996. 15-year longitudinal study of blood pressure and dementia. Lancet **347:** 1141–1145.

9. KONNO, S. *et al.* 1997. Classification, diagnosis and treatment of vascular dementia. Drugs & Aging **5:** 361–373.

10. MEYER, J.S. *et al.* 1995. Effects of chronic cigarette smoking and abstention on cerebral perfusion among neurologically normal volunteers. *In* Brain Imaging of Nicotine and Tobacco Smoking. E. F. Domino, Ed. NPP Books. Michigan.

11. LANCET CONFERENCE WRITING COMMITTEE. 1996. The challenge of the dementias. Lancet **347:** 1303–1307.

12. FOLSTEIN, M.F. *et al.* 1975. "Mini-Mental State": a practical method for grading the cognitive state of patients for the clinician. J. Psychiat. Res. **12:** 189–198.

13. HERSHEY, L.A. *et al.* 1987. Validation of cognitive and functional assessment instruments in vascular dementia. Int. J. Psychiatry Med. **17:** 183–192.

14. MEYER, J.S. *et al.* 1995. Prospective CT confirms differences between vascular and Alzheimer's dementia. Stroke **26:** 735–742.

15. MEYER, J.S. *et al.* 1995. Computed tomography cerebral blood flow values compared in normal aging, ischemic vascular dementia and Alzheimer's disease. *In* Quantitative Cerebral Blood Flow Measurements Using Stable Xenon/CT: Clinical Applications. M. Tomonaga, A. Tanaka & H. Yonas, Eds. Futura Publishing Co., Inc. New York.

16. MEYER, J.S. *et al.* 1988. Imaging local cerebral blood flow by xenon-enhanced computed tomography – technical optimization procedures. Neuroradiology **30:** 283–292.

17. GOLD, G. *et al.* 1997. Sensitivity and specificity of newly proposed clinical criteria for possible vascular dementia. Neurology **49:** 690–694.

18. TERAYAMA, Y. *et al.* 1993. Comparison of polio-araiosis and leuko-araiosis in dementias of ischemic vascular and Alzheimer types. J. Stroke Cerebrovasc. Dis. **3:** 267–275.

19. KETY, S.S. 1956. Human cerebral blood flow and oxygen consumption as related to aging. J. Chron. Dis. **3:** 478–486.

20. SHEAR, P.K. *et al.* 1995. Longitudinal volumetric computed tomographic analysis of regional brain changes in normal aging and Alzheimer's disease. Arch. Neurol. **52:** 392–402.

21. WALDEMAR, G. 1995. Functional brain imaging with SPECT in normal aging and dementia. Cereb. Brain Metab. Rev. **7:** 89–130.

22. MASLIAH, E. *et al.* 1993. Quantitative synaptic alterations in the human neocortex during normal aging. Neurology **43:** 192–197.

23. VAN ZAGTEN, M. *et al.* 1996. Significant progression of white matter lesions and small deep (lacunar) infarcts in patients with stroke. Arch. Neurol. **53:** 650–655.

24. BREDESEN, D.E. 1995. Neural apoptosis. Ann. Neurol. **38:** 839–851.

25. CHARRIAUT-MARLANGUE, C. *et al.* 1996. Apoptosis and necrosis after reversible focal ischemia: an in situ DNA fragmentation analysis. J. Cereb. Blood Flow Metab. **16:** 186–194.

26. STRASSBURGER, T.L. *et al.* 1997. Interactive effects of age and hypertension on volumes of brain structures. Stroke **28:** 1410–1417.

27. TAKEDA, S. *et al.* 1986. Association of atherosclerosis with increased atrophy of brain matter in the elderly. J. Am. Geriatr. Soc. **34:** 259–262.
28. ANDERSON, J.M. *et al.* 1983. The effect of advanced old age on the neurone content of the cerebral cortex. Observations with an automatic image analyzer point counting method. J. Neurol. Sci. **58:** 235–246.
29. PETERS, A. *et al.* 1996. Neurobiological bases of age-related cognitive decline in the rhesus monkey. J. Neuropathol. Exp. Neurol. **55:** 861–874.
30. GEORGE, A.E. *et al.* 1986. Leukoencephalopathy in normal and pathologic aging: 1. CT of brain lucencies. Am. J. Neuroradiol. **7:** 561–566.
31. AWAD, I.A. *et al.* 1986. Incidental subcortical lesions identified on magnetic resonance imaging in the elderly. I. Correlation with age and cerebrovascular risk factors. Stroke **17:** 1084–1089.
32. HACHINSKI, V.C. *et al.* 1987. Leuko-araiosis. Arch. Neurol. **44:** 21–23.
33. STEINGART, A. *et al.* 1987. Cognitive and neurologic findings in demented patients with diffuse white matter lucencies on computed tomographic scan (leuko-araiosis). Arch. Neurol. **44:** 36–39.
34. SULLIVAN, P. *et al.* 1990. Risk factors for white matter changes detected by magnetic resonance imaging in elderly. Stroke **21:** 1424–1428.
35. RAIHA, I. *et al.* 1993. Relationship between vascular factors and white matter low attenuation of the brain. Acta. Neurol. Scand. **87:** 286–289.
36. DE LEON, M.J. *et al.* 1989. Alzheimer's disease: longitudinal CT studies of ventricular change. Am. J. Neuroradiol. **10:** 371–376.
37. HEBERT, P.R. *et al.* 1997. Cholesterol lowering with statin drugs, risk of stroke, and total mortality. J.A.M.A. **278:** 313–321.
38. SKOOG, I. 1994. Risk factors for vascular dementia: a review. Dementia **5:** 137–144.
39. BRENNER, D.E. *et al.* 1993. Relationship between cigarette smoking and Alzheimer's disease in a population-based case-control study. Neurology **43:** 293–300.
40. KOKMEN, E. *et al.* 1991. Clinical risk factors for Alzheimer's disease: a population-based case-control study. Neurology **41:** 1393–1397.
41. LANDIN, K. *et al.* 1993. Low blood pressure and blood glucose levels in Alzheimer's disease: evidence for a hypometabolic disorder? J. Intern. Med. **233:** 357–362.

Critically Attained Threshold of Cerebral Hypoperfusion: Can It Cause Alzheimer's Disease?

J.C. DE LA TORRE[a]

Department of Neurosciences, University of California, San Diego, La Jolla, California 92093, USA

ABSTRACT: After nearly a century of inquiry, the cause of sporadic Alzheimer's disease (AD) remains to be found. On the subject of AD pathogenesis, recent basic and clinical evidence strongly argues in favor of the concept that AD is linked to brain circulatory pathology. This concept, when viewed from many different medical disciplines and from close pre-morbid similarities to vascular dementia, assembles and hypothetically explains most of the key pathologic events associated with the development of AD. These pathologic events are triggered in AD by impaired cerebral perfusion originating in the microvasculature which affects the optimal delivery of glucose and oxygen and results in an energy metabolic breakdown of brain cell biosynthetic and synaptic pathways. We propose that two factors converge to initiate cognitive dysfunction and neurodegeneration as expressed in AD brain: (1) advanced aging, and (2) the presence of a condition that lowers cerebral perfusion. The first factor introduces a normal but potentially deconstructing process that lowers cerebral blood flow in proportion to increased aging, whereas the second factor adds a crucial burden that further lowers brain perfusion to a *critical threshold* that triggers neuronal metabolic compromise. When age and a condition that lowers cerebral perfusion converge, *critically attained threshold of cerebral hypoperfusion* (CATCH) results. CATCH is a cyclical and progressive cerebrovascular insufficiency that will destabilize neurons, synapses, neurotransmission, and cognitive ability, eventually evolving into a neurodegenerative process characterized by the formation of senile plaques, neurofibrillary tangles, and amyloid angiopathy. The concept of impaired cerebral perfusion as the cause of this dementia also explains the heterogeneic profile observed in AD patients, because an extensive list of risk factors for AD are also reported to significantly diminish blood flow to the aging brain.

INTRODUCTION

We have proposed[13,14,18] and will attempt to briefly document here that Alzheimer's disease (AD) is caused by two converging factors that come together to create first, cognitive dysfunction and later, neurodegeneration. These factors are:

[a]Address for correspondence: J.C. de la Torre, MD, PhD, University of California, San Diego, Department of Neurosciences (MTF-0624), 9500 Gilman Drive, La Jolla, CA 92093. Tel.: (858) 822-3182; fax: (858) 822-3183.
e-mail: jdelator@ucsd.edu

(1) advanced aging, and (2) the presence of a condition that lowers cerebral perfusion. The first factor induces a normal but potentially pernicious process that lowers cerebral blood flow in proportion to increased aging. The second factor adds a crucial element that further burdens brain perfusion and can be described as "the straw that breaks the camel's back." Convergence of these two factors will lead to a *critically attained threshold of cerebral hypoperfusion* (CATCH), *initially in specific regions of the brain, such as the entorhinal cortex and hippocampal CA1.* CATCH is a sustained and progressive circulatory insufficiency that will metabolically destabilize vulnerable neurons, synaptic pathways, and neurotransmission. The end-point of impaired brain perfusion is a slowdown followed by meltdown of cognitive function and the expanding evolution of neurodegeneration and its associated formation of senile plaques, neurofibrillary tangles, and amyloid angiopathy.

Khachaturian[33] defined six essential parameters that should be met if a unifying hypothesis on the cause of AD is to be seriously considered. These parameters and a descriptive explanation for each parameter are presented in this review.

1. A UNIFYING HYPOTHESIS MUST PROVIDE A SIMPLE AND PLAUSIBLE EXPLANATION BASED ON ESTABLISHED BIOLOGIC PROCESSES

As stated in the introduction, CATCH is an abnormal process that ostensibly leads to regional capillary degeneration in AD brains.[8,12,35,36,46,50] Capillary degeneration has been shown to develop experimentally in selective regions of rat brain when chronic cerebral hypoperfusion is induced in aging animals for a year.[12,35] Regional brain capillary deformities set the stage for neuronoglial energy crisis. The reason for this is that "disturbed" rather than "laminar" microvascular blood flow results from the cylindrical deformation of capillaries. Consequently, glucose and oxygen fail to reach their neuronal targets in optimal concentrations, eventually creating an energy crisis at the mitochondrial level that ramifies into multiple systems affecting brain cells intrinsically and their external environment. Both rat and AD capillary changes consist of basement membrane thickening, collagen deposition, endothelial cell collapse, pericyte degeneration, and vessel lumen distortion. Although the capillary changes in AD are demonstrated in many different regions of the brain (we assume because most postmortem material is obtained during the late stage of AD), the capillary degeneration in rats is first noted in the CA1 hippocampal sector, the same region that, together with the entorhinal cortex, reveals the initial and severest pathologic damage seen in AD brains.[20,61] The rat capillary changes were also associated with spatial memory deficits, mimicking the visuospatial memory decline seen at the onset of AD.[12,35] These findings indicate that lowering cerebral blood flow experimentally in rats for 12 months results in region-specific capillary changes. In addition, because it is well known that the more we age, the less blood flow reaches specifc regions of the brain, such as the hippocampus,[17,38] a collective regional cerebral blood flow (rCBF) burden was probably produced in these animals.

2. THE HYPOTHESIS MUST EXPLAIN THE SPECIFICITY OF NEURONAL DYSFUNCTION, SYNAPTIC LOSS, AND NEURONAL DEATH

The metabolic and biochemical cascade initiated by reduced perfusion to the brain results from lowered delivery of glucose and oxygen to neurons and glia cells. Because brain metabolic energy is almost exclusively served by a steady supply of glucose, which together with oxygen generates ATP, chronic brain hypoperfusion initiates an alarm reaction characterized by increased hippocampal glial activation and oxidative stress.[5,51] This condition triggers energy pathologic pathways that involve lowered oxidation of glucose, reduced cytochrome oxidase, impaired aerobic glycolysis, and lowered ATP synthesis.[23,29,41] Energy metabolic compromise generates free radicals that contribute to excitotoxic build-up of glutamate in the extracellular space.[34] This occurs when free radicals inhibit glial cell uptake of glutamate by blocking membrane Na^+, K^+-ATPase transport of this amino acid.[59] The resulting extracellular glutamate build-up reaches excitotoxic levels, dispensing damage and death of neurons within its range. As the main energy fuel of the brain, lowered ATP production reduces Na^+, K^+-ATPase ion pumping, impairs acetylcholine synthesis, interferes with Ca^{2+} homeostasis, releases the protein kinase PK-40[erk], and promotes abnormal protein trafficking and posttranslational modifications within the faltering Golgi apparatus.[24,34,39,48,54] Persistent chronic brain ischemia leads to formation of reactive oxygen species, cytokine production, and inflammatory reactions.[21]

The third and final phase of this metabolic cascade occurs as follows: progressive Golgi apparatus damage[54] heralds neuronal structural collapse possibly beginning in CA1 hippocampus and the beginning of an apoptotic or necrotic pathway for the affected cells, which in turn enhance and extend cognitive deficits as neuronal damage spreads to other parts of the brain. It should be noted that abnormally processed amyloid precursor protein (APP) within the fragmented Golgi apparatus can produce amyloidogenic Aβ. Moreover, aberrations in energy-dependent motor protein synthesis linking microtubules with the Golgi complex[10] can further damage this organelle and contribute to posttranslational modification of tau from neuronal cytosol into the axon. Molecular structural modification of tau is believed to promote neurofibrillary tangles (NFTs).[5] Additionally, the release of the protein kinase PK 40[erk] induced by lowered synthesis of ATP can phosphorylate tau abnormally, leading to the production of paired helical filaments (PHF), as found in AD tissue.[48]

Thus, there appear to be a number of pathologic pathways that can lead to the deposition of Aβ and NFTs in the latter stages of AD. During this time of increased Aβ and NFT production, Na^+, K^+-ATPase is being downregulated as a result of ever-decreasing ATP activity. The Na^+, K^+-ATPase pump consumes about 60% of all ATP in the brain in order to maintain cellular ionic gradients, action potentials, synaptic transmission, and protein synthesis among others.[24] When this ionic pump begins to operate suboptimally, Ca^{2+} transport across cell membranes,[37] axoplasmic flow, and axodendritic synaptic function are affected adversely.[16] Eventually, synaptic neurotransmitter dysfunction and synaptic loss result from impaired axonal transport of vesicles, further corrupting the already compromised cognitive status more severely. The end stage of AD involves advanced regional neuronal loss, brain atrophy, and progressive cognitive meltdown.

3. THE HYPOTHESIS MUST ACCOUNT FOR THE
CLINICAL SYMPTOMS OF AD

A growing number of clinical studies in AD patients support the premise that AD is caused by chronic cerebral hypoperfusion that leads to microvascular failure. For example, (1) a consistent reduction in temporoparietal CBF is present in AD which correlates positively with cognitive decline;[3,4,51] (2) capillary changes involving basement membrane thickening, endothelial cell compression, pericyte degeneration, and luminal distortion occur in the majority of AD brains;[8,46,50] (3) glucose and oxygen brain metabolism is consistently depressed in AD and depressed values correlate positively with disease severity;[4,28,29] (4) glucose transporter 1, located in the compressed endothelial cells, is markedly deficient in AD brains, further reducing glucose availability to neurons and glia;[32,52] (5) regional "misery perfusion" develops in AD brains which is reflected by elevation of oxygen extraction factor (OEF) most notably in ischemic temporoparietal lobes where neuropathologic changes are most severe;[42,57] (6) lastly and most compellingly, regional hypometabolism found in AD brains does not appear to result from neurodegenerative changes but it actually precedes it.[22] Moreover, evidence shows that senile plaque formation does not contribute to lowered energy metabolism in AD.[29]

Additional data from several clinical reports support a cerebrovascular pathogenic role in AD. These reports[8,47,60] and a recent longitudinal study using SPECT measurements of rCBF in elderly individuals with "questionable" AD (i.e., subjects with memory trouble who did not meet NINDS/ADRDA criteria for *probable* AD) revealed that only those subjects with significant cerebral hypoperfusion in the hippocampal region *later* developed AD within a 2-year follow-up period.[31] The conclusion from this study is that SPECT rCBF analysis can accurately identify subjects with memory difficulties who will later develop AD.[31]

4. THE HYPOTHESIS MUST EXPLAIN THE HETEROGENEITY OF AD

We have stated that for AD to develop, advanced aging and a condition that further lowers CBF must be present. Because the list for such conditions is indeed long, and getting longer (TABLE 1), it seems evident that Alzheimer's dementia develops from an assault on the cerebral perfusion system of the aged individual by an assorted and distinctly different variety of blood flow–lowering conditions. When such a cerebral blood flow–lowering condition (which also happens to be an important risk factor for AD) is present during advanced aging, the clinical heterogeneic pattern characteristic of the AD syndrome is expressed.

5. THE HYPOTHESIS MUST DEMONSTRATE A RELATONSHIP
BETWEEN KNOWN RISK FACTORS FOR AD AND THE
NEUROBIOLOGY OF THE DISEASE

Many vascular-related disorders are known to reduce cerebral perfusion and, in the presence of progressive aging, will further contribute to lowering blood flow to the brain.[17] For example, the role between a number of cerebrovascular risk factors

TABLE 1. Direct and indirect risk factors for Alzheimer's disease and vascular dementia which have been reported to reduce or impair cerebral perfusion

Vascular Risk Factor	Dementia Affected
Ischemic stroke	Alzheimer's disease/vascular dementia
Diabetes mellitus	Alzheimer's disease/vascular dementia
Atrial fibrillation	Alzheimer's disease/vascular dementia
Atherosclerosis	Alzheimer's disease/vascular dementia
Thrombogenic factors	Alzheimer's disease/vascular dementia
Brain vessel wall pathology	Alzheimer's disease/vascular dementia
Hypertension/hypotension	Alzheimer's disease/vascular dementia
Amyloid angiopathy	Alzheimer's disease/vascular dementia
Blood-brain barrier dysfunction	Alzheimer's disease/vascular dementia
High serum fibrinogen levels	Alzheimer's disease/vascular dementia
Elevated serum viscosity	Alzheimer's disease/vascular dementia
Heart disease	Alzheimer's disease/vascular dementia
High homocysteine levels	Alzheimer's disease/vascular dementia
Oxidative stress	Alzheimer's disease/vascular dementia
Hyperlipidemia/HDL-cholesterol	Alzheimer's disease/vascular dementia
Smoking/alcoholism	Alzheimer's disease/vascular dementia
Apolipoprotein E_4	Alzheimer's disease/vascular dementia

whose primary effect is to lower blood flow to the brain and their association with the eventual development of AD has been strongly confirmed by the Rotterdam Study which examined a large series of AD patients and normal aging subjects.[7,11,26] More intriguing still, a list of vascular risk factors encountered in vascular dementia are also risk factors for AD (TABLE 1).

For example, ischemic stroke, diabetes mellitus, atherosclerosis, atrial fibrillation, mitral valve prolapse, thrombogenic factors, brain vessel wall pathology, amyloid angiopathy, blood-brain barrier dysfunction, high serum fibrinogen levels, elevated serum viscosity, cardiac disease, and hypotension/hypertension are common risk factors for AD and vascular dementia. Indirect vascular risk factors, such as smoking, alcoholism, hyperlipidemia, high homocysteine levels, and high LDL-cholesterol, are also shared by both dementias. All of these conditions have different pathologies but are linked by one common factor, reduction or impairment of cerebral perfusion. The Rotterdam Study also concluded from recent epidemiologic evidence that many of the risk factors listed above did not appear to constitute a separate disease entity but rather was part of the pathologic mosaic that characterizes AD.[26]

It is important to point out, however, that vascular-related disease need not be present to lower CBF during aging. Physiometabolic changes, such as menopause, can also reduce CBF and put female subjects at similar risk for AD as their male counterparts.[44] This CBF decline and potential risk for AD can be diminished with estrogen replacement therapy given during menopause.[44] Curiously, we know of no reports in which surgically induced menopause in premenopausal women (following bilateral oophorectomy) is a risk factor for AD even when patient noncompliance for estrogen replacement therapy is demonstrated. The reason may lie with the subject's age, because young, ovariectomized rats show no drop in CBF even when estrogen replacement therapy is withheld.[27] Consequently, physiometabolic changes such as menopause in the presence of aging removes women's hormonal protection from AD and exposes them to the same risk for this disorder as aging males.

6. THE HYPOTHESIS SHOULD CONNECT CELL DEATH AND DYSFUNCTION TO CLINICAL AD SYMPTOMS AND MOLECULAR LESIONS FOUND IN AD BRAIN

Experimental data from our laboratory and those of others show consistent molecular, behavioral, and cellular markers derived from chronic brain hypoperfusion in rats and those reported in AD. For example, mild chronic brain hypoperfusion for 1–4 weeks in aging rats induces a deficit in visuospatial memory acquisition, a reactive glial response predominantly in the hippocampus, lowered glucose utilization in brain, and a reduction in the levels of cytochrome oxidase in CA1.[15] Between 6 and 8 weeks of chronic brain hypoperfusion, MAP-2 loss appears in apical dendrites of CA1 neurons, but no structural changes are yet evident in the neuronal soma at the light microscopic level.[1] Subsequently, at 25 weeks, some neuronal damage is recorded in CA1,[45] and at 52 weeks, significant capillary degeneration is observed in CA1.[12,35] All during this time, spatial memory impairment continues and often worsens.

The main point to be condensed from these chronic hypoperfusion findings is that cognitive behavior, energy metabolism, and dendritic postsynaptic function affecting CA1 are impaired in these animals *in the absence of structural damage to neurons or to senile plaque and neurofibrillary tangle formation in this region* (FIG. 1). Despite a lack of neuronal structural damage, it is evident from these studies that experimentally hypoperfused CA1 neurons are metabolically dysfunctional, and this is reflected by the local glial reaction, cytochrome oxidase reduction, MAP-2 loss, reduced brain uptake of glucose and oxygen, and spatial memory deficits (FIG. 2).

If AD neurons react in a similar fashion as the aging rat model, therapy aimed at restoring neurometabolic function or blood flow during the early stages of AD is a promising research venue.

Clinical genetic data in AD patients reveal a pattern closely associated with reduced cerebral perfusion. Of the three genes that express mutant proteins that appear linked to AD (APP, PS1, and PS2) and the AD susceptibility gene (apoEε_4), all are related to reduced CBF. APP has been shown to be transported by fast anterograde transport, and disruption of this transport, for example by reduced ATP synthesis, can result in abnormal processing of Aβ in brain. Numerous studies have shown that APP accumulation in brain is associated with cerebral ischemia and infarction (for review see Refs. 62 and 63).

Reports that the presence of apoEε_4 increases the prevalence of atherosclerosis, coronary artery disease, and cerebrovascular ischemia are of interest in view of studies showing that these conditions are significant AD risk factors.[6,11] It is possible that carriers of ApoEε_4 express a greater risk factor for cerebrovascular disease and indirectly for AD than as a direct genetic risk factor for AD. ApoEε_4 can also accel-

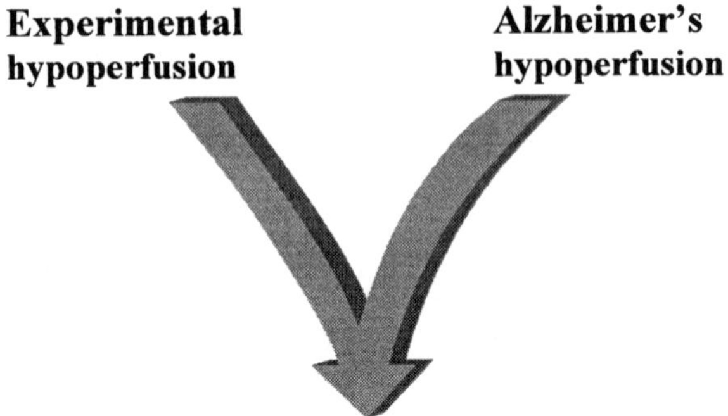

FIGURE 1. Outcome similarities between experimentally induced cerebral hypoperfusion in animals and cerebral hypoperfusion that develops in Alzheimer's disease. Both animals and humans evolve neuronal metabolic dysfunction, neuronal structural changes, and eventually neuronal atrophy.

erate the process that leads to amyloid angiopathy in AD brain vessels, a condition that often leads to cortical hemorrhage.[24] ApoEε4 is reported to be associated with cerebral hypoperfusion in temporoparietal brain regions of patients with AD,[53] a finding that, together with the foregoing data, suggests apoEε4 may contribute to the progressive CBF fall found in AD brains. Recently, it was shown that soluble Aβ peptide administered to rodents can reduce CBF by mechanisms not yet understood.[55] Aβ deposition in the cerebral microvasculature (amyloid angiopathy) could be an important contributing source of chronic hypoperfusion in AD, particularly in carriers of the apoEε4 allele.

Presenilins (PS1 and PS2) belong to a novel family of genes whose mutations, although rare, appear linked to early-onset familial Alzheimer's disease. PS1 genes are expressed by neurons throughout the brain, where they localize near the Golgi apparatus in the endoplasmic reticulum (ER).[40] PS1 mutation may render such neurons vulnerable to apoptosis or aberrant protein synthesis in the ER, and this abnormal gene expression can be triggered by different insults,[43] including cerebral ischemia.[56] The role of PS1 in brain is unknown, but radiolabeled HMPAO-SPECT studies have revealed reduced cerebral perfusion in temporoparietal cortex of *symptomatic* AD patients carrying the PS1 gene; alternatively, *asymptomatic* PS1 carriers showed similar regional cerebral hypoperfusion.[30] These intriguing findings indicate in a dramatic fashion that cerebral perfusion deficits are detectable in PS1 carriers who may later develop AD. Moreover, we speculate that brain hypoperfusion leading to neuronal energy crisis could contribute to presenilin mutation during packaging or transport of this protein in a compromised Golgi complex. Similarly, protein mutations in the Golgi may explain abnormal APP processing and produc-

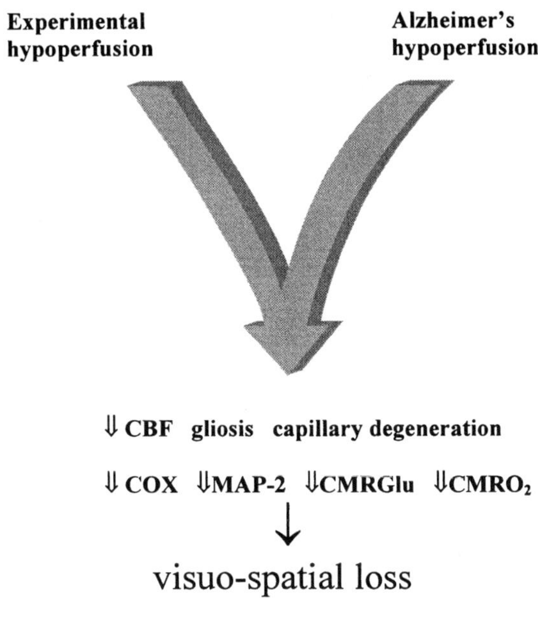

FIGURE 2. Specific changes seen after experimentally induced chronic brain hypoperfusion in animals and those developing in Alzheimer's disease. Note that significant decrease in cerebral blood flow (CBF) is accompanied by gliosis, capillary degeneration, and reductions in cytochrome oxidase (COX), microtubule-associated protein-2 (MAP-2), cerebral metabolic rate of glucose (CMRGlu), and cerebral metabolic rate of oxygen (CMRO₂). These cellular and metabolic changes may be responsible for the visuo-spatial loss, an early sign of cognitive impairment seen in both animals and Alzheimer patients. Parallel deficits to visuo-spatial loss are synapse loss, senile plaque formation (Alzheimer only), neurofibrillary tangle formation (Alzheimer only), and progressive neurodegeneration. The appearance of progressive neurodegeneration signals the rapid decline of cognitive function in Alzheimer patients.

tion of Aβ. It should be noted that the Golgi apparatus is smaller in size in Alzheimer neurons when apoEε₄ allele is present in these patients.[49] The foregoing data imply that APP, apoEε₄ and presenilin genes may actively contribute to cerebral hypoperfusion and complicate normal protein trafficking and posttranslational alterations induced by a degenerating Golgi apparatus and dysfunctional ER.

At this point, it would seem reasonable to add a seventh parameter to this review.

7. THE HYPOTHESIS MUST ADDRESS THE CLINICAL SYMPTOMS OF AD WITH SPECIFICALLY DESIGNED THERAPY THAT WILL IMPROVE OR REVERSE THIS DISORDER

Although no therapy has so far been shown to be effective, it should be noted that all drugs that have been reported to allay or delay the cognitive decline in AD, such as cholinesterase inhibitors, cholinomimetics, and estrogen, are known to increase brain perfusion.[19] Nonsteroidal antiinflammatory agents reported to reduce AD risk also improve blood flow through their platelet-deaggregating and antithrombotic effects.[9] Therapy designed to subtantially increase cerebral perfusion, such as omental transposition to brain or introducing vasoactive endothelial growth factor to brain tissue, could have substantial effects on outcome when early diagnosis of AD is made.

SUMMARY AND CONCLUSIONS

It is proposed that conditions that lower brain blood flow in the presence of aging will reach a critically attained threshold of cerebral hypoperfusion that will damage brain capillaries. Regional capillary degeneration may be one of the first anatomic abnormalities that is expressed by impaired delivery of essential nutrients to the brain, resulting in the development of metabolic energy compromise. In this context, it is noteworthy to point out that the vast majority of AD patients suffer from microvascular pathology in the form of capillary distortions with or without amyloid angiopathy.[7,18,46,50]

AD symptoms appear to begin following greatly persistent and reduced cerebral perfusion in direct relation to dwindling glucose and oxygen delivery; using reverse logic, it is highly unlikely that AD can occur when CBF is normal. Thus, when nutrient delivery to the brain falls below a suboptimal level, the metabolic cascade shown in FIGURES 1 and 2 will follow in a cyclical, persistent, and progressive order. Chronic subdelivery of glucose and oxygen to brain tissue would eventually have a disruptive effect on oxidative phosphorylation and mitochondrial production of ATP that fuels the dependent transport systems used by neurons and glial cells. This dependence on energy substrates to drive reactions within brain cells involving ion pumping, protein synthesis, axoplasmic flow, neurotransmission, and synaptic activity is absolute.

Consequently, the evidence that critical threshold cerebral hypoperfusion causes AD can be summarized as follows:

1. CBF declines progressively with advancing age and worsens with AD;

2. CBF reduction in AD patients is proportional to cognitive loss and lowered glucose metabolism;

3. Brain cells rely exclusively on energy (supplied mainly by glucose) for all their metabolic processes;

4. The majority of AD patients show microvascular abnormalities;

5. Most conditions that lower cerebral perfusion in the presence of aging are risk factors for AD;

6. Drugs that improve cerebral perfusion lower the risk for AD and may delay cognitive decline;

7. No evidence exists that metabolically dysfunctional or dying neurons can alter blood flow, either to decrease it or to increase it;

8. No evidence exists that capillaries shut down around dead neurons;

9. Brain hypometabolism in AD precedes neurodegenerative changes;

10. AD susceptibility genes apoEε_4 and PS1 are associated with cerebral hypoperfusion and, in the case of PS1, may herald AD symptoms.

In view of the foregoing findings, we propose that aging in the presence of a perfusion-lowering condition will in time lead to CATCH syndrome initially in specific brain regions, such as the entorhinal cortex and hippocampal CA1. Regional brain hypoperfusion will subsequently injure the architecture of the brain microvasculature to provoke suboptimal delivery of energy substrates to the brain. It is further proposed that an energy-deficient physiometabolic cascade follows critical threshold hypoperfusion and promotes neuronal dysfunction and onset of cognitive decline.

REFERENCES

1. ABDOLLAHIAN, N.P., A. CADA, F. GONZALEZ-LIMA & J.C. DE LA TORRE. 1998. Cytochrome oxidase: a predictive marker of neurodegeneration. *In* Cytochrome Oxidase in Neuronal Metabolism and Alzheimer's Disease. F. Gonzalez-Lima, Ed.: 233–261. Plenum Press. New York.

2. BARTENSTEIN, P., S. MINOSHIMA, C. HIRSCH & K. BUCH. 1997. Quantitative assessment of cerebral blood flow in patients with Alzheimer's disease. J. Nucl. Med. **38:** 1095–1101.

3. BENSON, D.F., D. KUHL, R. HAWKINS, M. PHELPS, F. CUMMINGS & Y. TSAI. 1983. The fluorodeoxyglucose 18F scan in Alzheimer's disease and multi-infarct dementia. Arch. Neurol. **40:** 711–714.

4. BLASS, J.P. 1993. Pathophysiology of the Alzheimer's syndrome. Neurology (Suppl. 4): S25–S38.

5. BOTET, J.P., M. SENTÍ, X. NOGUES, J. RUBIES-PRAT, J. ROQUER, L. DOLHABERRIAGUE & J. OLIVE. 1992. Lipoprotein and apolipoprotein profile in men with ischemic stroke. Stroke **23:** 1556–1562.

6. BRETELER, M.M. 1998. Epidemiological evidence of a connection between Alzheimer's disease and vascular dementia. Neurobiol. Aging **19:** S150.

7. BUÉE, L., P.R. HOF, C. BOURAS, A. DELACOURTE, D. PERL, J.H. NORRISON & H.M. FILLIT. 1994. Pathological alterations of the cerebral microvasculature in Alzheimer's disease and related demented disorders. Acta Neuropathol. **87:** 469–480.

8. CELSIS, P., A. AGNIEL, D. CARDEBAT, J.F. DEMONET, P. OUSSET & M. PUEL. 1997. Age related cognitive decline: a clinical entity? A longitudinal study of cerebral blood flow and memory performance. J. Neurol. Neurosurg. Psychiatry **62:** 601–608.

9. CHEMTOB, S., K. BEHARRY, T. BARNA, B.R. VARMA & J.V. ARANDA. 1991. Differences in the effects of newborn piglet of various non-steroidal anti-inflammatory drugs on cerebral blood flow but not on cerebrovascular prostaglandins. Ped. Res. **30:** 106–111.

10. CHEN, Y., S. WEII, Z. MOURELATOS, J. GONATAS, K. OKAMOTO & N.K. GONATAS. 1998. The fragmented neuronal Golgi apparatus in ALS includes the trans-Golgi-network: functional implications. Acta Neuropathol. **95:** 245–253.

11. DAVIGNON, J., R.E. GREGG & C.F. SING. 1988. Apolipoprotein E polymorphism and atherosclerosis. Atherosclerosis **8:** 1–21.

12. DE JONG, G.I., E. FARKAS, J. PLASS, J.N. KEIJSER, J.C. DE LA TORRE & P.G.M. LUITEN. 1999. Cerebral hypoperfusion yields capillary damage in hippocampus CA1 that correlates to spatial memory impairment. Neuroscience. In press.

13. DE LA TORRE, J.C. 1994. Impaired brain microcirculation may trigger Alzheimer's disease. Neurosci. Behav. Rev. **18:** 397–401.

14. DE LA TORRE, J.C. 1992. Does brain microvessel pathology provoke Alzheimer's disease? Soc. Neurosci. Abstr. **18:** 564.

15. DE LA TORRE, J.C., A. CADA, N. NELSON, R.J. SUTHERLAND & F. GONZALEZ-LIMA. 1997. Reduced cytochrome oxidase and memory dysfunction after chronic brain ischemia in aged rats. Neurosci. Lett. **223:**165–168.

16. DE LA TORRE, J.C. 1997. Cerebromicrovascular pathology in Alzheimer's disease compared to normal aging. Gerontology **43:** 26–43.

17. DE LA TORRE, J.C. 1997. Cerebrovascular changes in the aging brain. Adv. Cell Aging Gerontol. **2:** 77–107.

18. DE LA TORRE, J.C. & T. MUSSIVAND. 1993. Can disturbed brain microcirculation cause Alzheimer's disease? Neurol. Res. **15:** 146–153.

19. DE LA TORRE, J.C. 1997. Hemodynamic consequences of deformed microvesseles in the brain in Alzheimer's disease. Ann. N.Y. Acad. Sci. **826:** 75–91.

20. DE LEON, M.J., A. CONVIT, S. DESANTI & M. BOBINOSKI. 1997. Contribution of structural neuroimaging to the early diagnosis of Alzheimer's disease. Int. Psychogeriatrics **9:** 183–190.

21. DEL ZOPPO, G.J. 1997. Microvascular responses to cerebral ischemia/inflammation. Ann. N.Y. Acad. Sci. **823:** 132–147.

22. DUARA, R., W.W. BARKER, J. CHANG & F. YOSHII. 1992. Viability of neocortical function shown in behavioral activation state PET studies in Alzheimer's disease. J. Cerebr. Blood Flow Metab. **12:** 927–934.

23. ERECINSKA, M. & I. SILVER. 1989. ATP and brain function. J. Cerebr. Blood Flow Metab. **9:** 2–12.

24. GREENBERG, S.M., M.E. BRIGGS, B.J. HYMAN, G. KOKORIS & C. TAKIS. 1996. Apolipoprotein E_4 is associated with the presence and earlier onset of hemorrhage in cerebral amyloid angiopathy. Stroke **27:** 1333–1337.

25. HATANPAA, K., K. CHANDRASEKARAN, D.R. BRADY & S.I. RAPOPORT. 1998. No association between Alzheimer plaques and decreased levels of cytochrome oxidase unit mRNA, a marker of neuronal energy metabolism. Brain Res. Mol. Brain Res. **59:** 13–21.

26. HOFMAN, A., A. OTT, M. BRETELER, M. BOTS, A. SLOOTER & D. GROBBEE. 1997. Atherosclerosis, apolipoprotein E, and prevalence of dementia and Alzheimer's disease in the Rotterdam study. Lancet **349:**151–154.

27. HOLSCHNEIDER, D.P. & O.U. SCREMIN. 1998. Effects of ovariectomy on cerebral flow in rats. Neuroendocrinology **67:** 260–268.

28. HOYER, S. 1986. Senile dementia and Alzheimer's disease, brain blood flow and metabolism. Prog. Neuro-Psychopharmacol. Biol. Psychiatry **10:** 447–478.

29. HOYER, S. 1991. Brain energy metabolism and its significance for Alzheimer's disease; *In* Alzheimer's Disease: Basic Mechanisms, Diagnosis and Therapeutic Strategies. K. Iqbal, D.R.C. McLachlan, B. Winblad & H.M. Wisniewski, Eds. :53–57. Wiley. New York.

30. JOHNSON, K.A., F. LOPERA, K. JONES, A. BECKER & R.A. SPERLING. 1998. Presenilin 1-associated abnormalities in regional cerebral perfusion. Neurobiol. Aging **19:** S83.

31. JOHNSON, K.A., K. JONES, B.L. HOLMAN, J. BECKER, P.A. SPIERS, A.. SATLIN & M.S. ALBERT. 1998. Preclinical prediction of Alzheimer's disease using SPECT. Neurology **50:** 1563–1571.

32. KALARIA, R.N. & S.E. HARIK. 1989. Reduced glucose transporter at the blood brain barrier and in the cerebral cortex in Alzheimer's disease. J. Neurochem. **53:** 1083–1088.

33. KHACHATURIAN, Z.S. 1994. Calcium hypothesis of Alzheimer's disease and brain aging. Ann. N.Y. Acad. Sci. **747:**1–11.

34. KRISTIAN, T. & B.K. SIESJO. 1998. Calcium in ischemic cell death. Stroke **29:** 705–718.

35. LUITEN, P.G.M., G.I. DE JONG, E. FARKAS, J. PLASS, R. DE VOS & E.N. JANSEN. 1998. Cerebral microvascular breakdown in dementias and after experimental cerebral hypoperfusion. Neurobiol. Aging **19:** S290.

36. MANCARDI, G.L., F. PERDELLI, A. LEONARDI & O. BUGIANI. 1980. Thickening of the basement membrane of cortical capillaries in Alzheimer's disease. Acta Neuropathol. **49:** 79–83.

37. MARK, R.J., D.A. BUTTERFIELD & M.P. MATTSON. 1995. Amyloid beta-peptide ion motive ATPase activities: evidence for a role in neuronal Ca^{2+} homeostasis and cell death. J. Neurosci. **15:** 6239–6249.

38. MARTIN, A.J., K.J. FRISTON, J.G. COLEBATCH & R. FRACKOWIAK. 1991. Decreases in regional cerebral blood flow with normal aging. J. Cerebr. Blood Flow Metab. **11:** 684–689.

39. MATTSON, M.P. 1997. Central role of oxyradicals in the mechanism of amyloid β-peptide cytotoxicity. Alzheimer's Dis. Rev. **2:** 1–14.

40. MATTSON, M.P., Q. GUO, K. FURUKAWA & W.A. PEDERSEN. 1998. Presenilins, the endoplasmic reticulum and neuronal apoptosis in Alzheimer's disease. J. Neurochem. **70:** 1–14.

41. MEIER-RUGE, W. & C. BERTONI-FREDDARI. 1996. The significance of glucose turnover in the brain in the pathogenic mechanisms of Alzheimer's disease. Rev. Neurosci. **7:** 1–19.

42. NAGATA, K., R.J. BUCHAN, E. YOKOYAMA, Y. KONDOH & M. SATO. 1997. Misery perfusion with preserved vascular reactivity in Alzheimer's disease. Ann. N.Y. Acad. Sci. **826:** 272–281.

43. NEVE, R.L. & N.K. ROBAKIS. 1998. Alzheimer's disease: a re-examination of the amyloid hypothesis. Trends Neurosci. **21:** 15–19.

44. OHKURA, T., K. ISSE, K. AKAZAWA, M. HAMAMOTO, Y. YAOI & N. HAGINO. 1994. Evaluation of estrogen treatment in female patients with dementia of the Alzheimer type. Endocr. J. **41:** 361–371.

45. PAPPAS, B.A., J.C. DE LA TORRE, C. DAVIDSON, M. KEYES & T. FORTIN. 1996. Chronic reduction of cerebral blood flow in the adult rat: late emerging CA1 cell loss and memory function. Brain Res. **708:** 50–58.

46. PERLMUTTER, L.S., M.A. MYERS & E. BARRON. 1994. Vascular basement membrane components and the lesions of Alzheimer's disease. Micros. Res. Tech. **28:** 204–215.

47. PROHOVNIK, I., R. MAYEUX, H. SACKHEIM & G. SMITH. 1998. Cerebral perfusion as a diagnostic marker of early Alzheimer's disease. Neurology **38:** 931–937.

48. RODER, H.M., P.A. EDEN & V.M. INGRAM. 1993. Brain protein kinase PK40^{erk} converts tau into PHF-like form as found in Alzheimer's disease. Biochem. Biophys. Res. Commun. **193:** 639–647.

49. SALEHI, A. & D. SWAAB. 1998. Relationship between neuronal activity, neuropathological hallmarks and genetic background in Alzheimer's disease. Neurobiol. Aging **19:** S5.

50. SCHEIBEL, A.B., T. DUONG & O. TOMIYASU. 1986. Microvascular changes in Alzheimer's disease. *In* The Biological Substrates of Alzheimer's Disease.: 77–192. Academic Press. New York.

51. SIMARD, D., J. OLESEN, O.B. PAULSON, N.A. LASSEN & E. SKINHOJ. 1971. Regional cerebral blood flow and its regulation in dementia. Brain **94:** 273–287.

52. SIMPSON, I.A., K.R. CHUNDU, T. DAVIES-HILL, W. HONER & P. DAVIES. 1994. Decreased concentrations of GLUT1 and GLUT3 glucose transporters in the brains of patients with Alzheimer's disease. Ann. Neurol. **35:** 546–551.

53. SPERLING, R.A., K.J. JONES, D. RENTZ, M.S. ALBERT & D.L. HOLMAN. 1998. SPECT cerebral perfusion and apolipoprotein E genotype. Neurology **50:** A438–A439.

54. STIEBER, A., Z. MOURELATOS & N.D. GONATAS. 1996. In Alzheimer's disease the Golgi apparatus of a population of neurons without neurofibrillary tangles is fragmented and atrophic. Am. J. Pathol. **148:** 415–426.

55. SUO, Z., J. HUMPHREY, A. KUNDTZ, F. SETHI, F. CRAWFORD & M. MULLAN. 1998. Soluble Alzheimer's ß-amyloid constricts the cerebral vasculature *in vivo*. Neurosci. Lett. **257:** 77–80.

56. TANIMUKAI, K., M. IMAIZUMI, K. KUDO, M. TOHYAMA & M. TAKEDA. 1998. Alzheimer-associated presenilin-1 gene is induced in gerbil hippocampus after transient ischemia. Brain Res. Mol. Brain Res. **54:** 212–218.

57. TOHGI, H., H. YONEZAWA, S. TAKAHASHI & N. SATO. 1998. Cerebral blood flow and oxygen metabolism in senile dementia of Alzheimer's type and vascular dementia with deep white matter changes. Neuroradiology **40:** 131–137.

58. VIJAYAN, V.K., J. GEDDES, K. ANDERSON & H. CHAN-CHUI. 1980. Astrocyte hypertrophy in the Alzheimer's disease hippocampal formation. Exp. Neurol. **112:** 72–78.

59. VOLTERRA, A., D. TROTTI, C. TROMBA, S. FLORIDI & G. RACAGNI. 1994. Glutamate uptake inhibition by oxygen free radicals in rat cortical astrocytes. J. Neurosci. **14:** 2924–2932.

60. WALDEMAR, G., P. HOGH & O.B. PAULSON. 1997. Functional brain imaging with single-photon emission computed tomography in the diagnosis of Alzheimer's disease. Int Psychogeriatr. **9:** 223–227.
61. WEST, M.J., P.D. COLEMAN, D.G. FLOOD & J.C. TRONCOSO. 1994. Differences in the pattern of hippocampal neuronal loss in normal aging and Alzheimer's disease. Lancet **344:** 769–772.
62. YAM, P.S., J. PATTERSON, D.I. GRAHAM, T. TAKASAGO, D. DEWAR & J. MCCULLOCH. 1998. Topographical and quantitative assessment of white matter injury following focal ischemic lesion in the rat brain. Brain Res. Brain Res. Protoc. **4:** 315–322.
63. YAM, P.S., T. TAKASAGO, D. DEWAR, D.I. GRAHAM & J. MCCULLOCH. 1997. Amyloid precursor protein accumulates in white matter at the margin of a focal ischemic lesion. Brain Res. **760:** 150–157.

The Renin Angiotensin System and Alzheimer's Disease

PHILIPPE AMOUYEL,[a,d] FLORENCE RICHARD,[a] CLAUDINE BERR,[b]
ISABELLE DAVID-FROMENTIN,[c] AND NICOLE HELBECQUE[a]

[a]INSERM U508, Institut Pasteur de Lille, Lille, France

[b]INSERM U360, Hôpital de la Salpétrière, Paris, France

[c]Gérontologie Clinique, Centre Hospitalier Emile Roux, Limeil Brévannes, France

ABSTRACT: Recent reports sustain the hypothesis of tight links between vascular and neurodegenerative diseases: associations between atherosclerosis lesions and Alzheimer's disease (AD), increased risk of AD for hypertensive subjects, decreased risk of dementia for elderly treated with hypotensive drugs, and a major impact of apolipoprotein E polymorphism, a protein of the lipid metabolism, on the occurrence of AD. All these results suggest that vascular determinants, both environmental and genetic, may predispose to or speed up dementia. As a major player of vascular homeostasis, the renin angiotensin system (RAS) proteins constitute an interesting source of candidate genes. Among these, the angiotensin I–converting enzyme gene (*ACE*), a central enzyme of the RAS, presents in its sequence a deletion (D)/insertion (I) polymorphism associated with variations of plasma ACE levels and with the risk of myocardial infarction. We explored the impact of this genetic polymorphism on the risk of cognitive impairment and of dementia in several epidemiological studies. Physiopathological hypotheses suggest a possible involvement of the RAS proteins in the occurrence and evolution of AD. Moreover, although inconsistent, several results of case-control studies tend to suggest that the *ACE* I/D genetic polymorphism may constitute a genetic susceptibility factor for dementia, reinforcing the hypothesis of a major implication of vascular risk factors in the occurrence of dementia.

INTRODUCTION

During aging, vascular and Alzheimer's disease (AD) seem to be associated more frequently than previously expected: stroke and AD often coexist, and brains of patients with dementia frequently present pathological features of both AD and cerebrovascular diseases[1]; cerebrovascular disease was also reported to influence the severity of AD clinical symptoms[2]; and atherosclerotic risk was associated with AD,[3] suggesting that vascular risk factors may be potential determinants of AD. Reinforcing this hypothesis, necropsy studies showed that brains of nondemented patients, who died as a result of severe coronary artery disease, contained more senile plaques than brains of subjects without heart diseases.[4] Moreover, higher blood pres-

[d]Address for correspondence: Prof. Philippe Amouyel, INSERM U508, Institut Pasteur de Lille, 1 rue Calmette, F-59019 Lille, France. Tel.: +33 3 20 87 77 10; fax: +33 3 20 87 78 94.
e-mail: philippe.amouyel@pasteur-lille.fr

sure levels are frequently detected in subjects who developed dementia than in those who did not.[5]

Thus, AD and vascular factors could be associated in a causative way or at least share common environmental and genetic determinants. Among the genetic susceptibility factors of AD implicated in vascular risk, the polymorphism of the apolipoprotein E gene (*ApoE*) may be one of these shared determinants.[6] Indeed, in the nervous system, ApoE seems to be a cornerstone protein in the maintenance of brain. *ApoE* polymorphism is associated with variations of transport and clearance of hydrophobic compounds such as lipids or amyloid substances, with variations in neurite outgrowth and with Tau phosphorylations, antioxidant properties, inflammatory properties, acetylcholine production, and damaged cell repair processes. All these properties constitute potential biological links between AD risk and the ε4 allele of the *ApoE* polymorphism. Other attractive biological candidate links between AD and vascular risk are the components of the renin angiotensin system (RAS).

THE RAS AND THE CENTRAL NERVOUS SYSTEM

The RAS is a complex biochemical pathway (FIG. 1). One of its key enzymes is the angiotensin I–converting enzyme (ACE).[7] This enzyme (dipeptidyl carboxypeptidase 1 [DCP1]) promotes the transformation of angiotensin I into angiotensin II, a potent vasoconstrictor peptide, and the degradation of bradykinin, a vasodilator. ACE is detected both in the circulation and linked to the cell membrane. Although large variations exist in plasma ACE levels, these levels are very stable within individuals, suggesting a strong genetic determination. The *ACE* gene, located on chromosome 17, has an insertion (I allele)/deletion (D allele) genetic polymorphism in its noncoding region. The circulating and cellular levels of ACE are partly genetically determined through this polymorphism: subjects bearing the *ACE* D alleles have higher levels of enzyme than the I allele carriers.[7,8] At the beginning of the nineties, the *ACE* D allele was associated with cardiovascular diseases.[9] Subjects bearing the

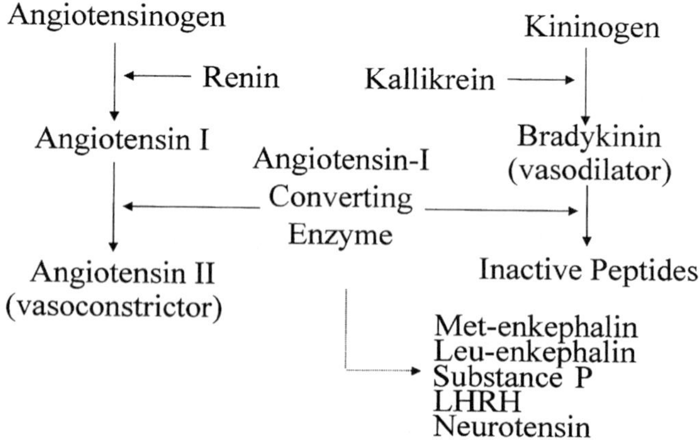

FIGURE 1. The renin angiotensin system.

TABLE 1. Association studies of *ACE* I/D polymorphism and Alzheimer's disease

ACE D Allele Frequencies (*n*)	Cases	Controls	*p*
Amouyel *et al.*, 1996[17]	0.59 (228)	0.51 (255)	<0.01
Tysoe *et al.*, 1997[19]	0.55 (110)	0.63 (110)	NS
Scacchi *et al.*, 1998[20]	0.62 (80)	0.63 (153)	NS
Chapman *et al.*, 1998[21]	0.66 (49)	0.66 (40)	NS
Kehoe *et al.*, 1999[18]	0.46 (542)	0.54 (386)	<0.0001

NS = nonsignificant.

ACE D allele seems to be at higher risk of myocardial infarction, of late coronary occlusion[10] and in-stent restenosis after angioplasty.[11] The impact of this *ACE* polymorphism on hypertension is less consistent.

The renin angiotensin system components are detected in the central nervous system.[12] ACE is located in the brain.[13] In animals, cognitive processing acquisition and recall of newly learned tasks are influenced by manipulation of brain angiotensin levels.[12] Increased levels of angiotensin II are suggested to induce an inhibitor influence on acquisition by reducing acetylcholine release; this reduction in central cholinergic functioning is deleterious to cognitive functions. Thus, ACE inhibitors reducing angiotensin II synthesis will remove an inhibitory influence upon acetylcholine release. In humans, the use of ACE inhibitor treatment in hypertensive subjects was associated after 6 months in general well-being, work performance, and improved cognitive function; conversely other hypotensive drugs did not exhibit such effects.[14] Altered brain densities of ACE were described in AD patients[15]: significant increases of ACE were reported in the hippocampus, parahippocampal gyrus, caudate nucleus, and temporal cortex of AD-affected subjects.[16]

EPIDEMIOLOGICAL EVIDENCE OF THE IMPLICATION OF THE RAS IN AD

In a sample of subjects over 60 years, the *ACE* D allele was associated with severe cognitive impairment (i.e., a Mini-Mental State Examination [MMSE] score less than 10 and/or a diagnosis of dementia).[17] The relative risk of an individual bearing the *ACE* DD genotype (approximated by the odds ratio in a case-control study) to be severely cognitively impaired was 1.60 (95% CI [1.04–2.36], $p<0.03$). This effect was more pronounced in men (3.25, 95% CI [1.40–7.58], $p<0.03$), suggesting, as often reported in the cardiovascular domain, an increased and earlier effect of vascular risk factor in that gender. Other authors analyzed the possible relationships between *ACE* I/D polymorphism and AD risk (TABLE 1). One study considered D as a risk factor,[17] one as a protective factor,[18] and three[19–21] did not detect any effect. The most recent one,[18] suggesting a protective effect of the *ACE* D allele, consisted of three UK populations (TABLE 2). If we compare the *ACE* D allele distributions in this study to the ones of other control groups, we can observe an almost balanced distribution of the D and I alleles. This distribution seems to be modified after 80. Except for the Belfast AD cases, the distribution in AD patients is also balanced between

TABLE 2. Association study of *ACE* I/D polymorphism and Alzheimer's disease in three UK populations

Population	n	*ACE* D	*ACE* I	Age (Years)	Reference
Belfast cases	209	0.43	0.57	77 ± 6	18
London cases	135	0.50	0.50	82 ± 7	18
Cardiff cases	198	0.49	0.51	70 ± 9	18
London controls	111	0.59	0.41	81 ± 5	18
Cardiff controls	77	0.60	0.40	74 ± 6	18
Belfast controls	198	0.49	0.51	77 ± 6	18
Belfast controls	180	0.50	0.50	53 ± 9	9
Copenhagen controls	7263	0.51	0.49	65 ± 2	22
French controls	255	0.51	0.49	79 ± 8	17
Cambridge controls	270	0.56	0.44	>80	23
French centenarians	310	0.62	0.38	>100	24

the D and I alleles. Most of the effects seems to be due to a depletion of the I allele at advanced ages.

Other ongoing epidemiological studies, cross sectional and prospective, will help to conclude whether the *ACE* D allele is a risk or protective factor for AD or, alternatively, if it has no relationship with AD risk.

CONCLUSION

The potential impact of *ACE* polymorphism on AD and of the RAS in general remains to be elucidated. The most consistent evidence for the hypothesis of a link between RAS and neurodegenerative processes comes from physiopathological studies. Conversely, the genetic epidemiological means of assessment, studying the association between *ACE* I/D polymorphism and AD occurrence, is controversial. Whether this association, whatever its sign, is due to a concomitant variation of the allele frequencies with age or reflects a causative association, remains an open question. Given the numerous means of therapeutic control of the RAS in humans, the hypothesis of a specific influence of the RAS on neurodegenerative process would be very attractive. Results from ongoing prospective studies will help to address these various issues.

REFERENCES

1. PASQUIER, F. & D. LEYS. 1997. Why are stroke patients prone to develop dementia? J. Neurol. **244:** 135–142.
2. SNOWDON, D.A., L.H. GREINER, J.A. MORTIMER *et al.* 1997. Brain infarction and the clinical expression of Alzheimer disease. The Nun Study. JAMA **277:** 813–817.
3. HOFMAN, A., A. OTT, M.M. BRETELER *et al.* 1997. Atherosclerosis, apolipoprotein E, and prevalence of dementia and Alzheimer's disease in the Rotterdam Study. Lancet **349:** 151–154.

4. SPARKS, D.L., J.C. HUNSAKER, S.W. SCHEFF *et al.* 1990. Cortical senile plaques in coronary artery disease, aging and Alzheimer's disease. Neurobiol. Aging **11:** 601–607.

5. SKOOG, I., B. LERNFELT, S. LANDAHL *et al.* 1996. Fifteen-year longitudinal study of blood pressure and dementia. Lancet **347:** 1141–1145.

6. WEISGRABER, K.H. & R.W. MAHLEY. 1996. Human apolipoprotein E: the Alzheimer's disease connection. FASEB J. **10:** 1485–1494.

7. RIGAT, B., C. HUBERT, F. ALHENC-GELAS *et al.* 1990. An insertion/deletion polymorphism in the angiotensin I–converting enzyme gene accounting for half the variance of serum enzyme levels. J. Clin. Invest. **86:** 1343–1346.

8. COSTEROUSSE, O., J. ALLEGRINI, M. LOPEZ & F. ALHENC-GELAS. 1993. Angiotensin I–converting enzyme in human circulating mononuclear cells: genetic polymorphism of expression in T-lymphocytes. Biochem. J. **290:** 33–40.

9. CAMBIEN, F., O. POIRIER, L. LECERF *et al.* 1992. Deletion polymorphism in the gene for angiotensin-converting enzyme is a potent risk factor for myocardial infarction. Nature **359:** 641–644.

10. HAMON, M., C. AMANT, C. BAUTERS *et al.* 1996. ACE polymorphism, a genetic predictor of occlusion after coronary angioplasty. Am. J. Cardiol. **78:** 679–681.

11. AMANT, C., C. BAUTERS, J.C. BODART *et al.* 1997. D allele of the angiotensin I–converting enzyme is a major risk factor for restenosis after coronary stenting. Circulation **96:** 56–60.

12. WRIGHT, J.W. & J.W. HARDING. 1994. Brain angiotensin receptor subtypes in the control of physiological and behavioral responses. Neurosci. Biobehav. Rev. **18:** 21–53.

13. ERDOS, E.G. & R. SKIDGEL. 1987. The angiotensin I–converting enzyme. Lab. Invest. **56:** 345–348.

14. CROOG, S.H., S. LEVINE, M. TESTA *et al.* 1986. The effects of antihypertensive therapy on the quality of life. N. Engl. J. Med. **314:** 1657–1664.

15. BARNES, N.M., C.H. CHENG, B. COSTALL *et al.* 1991. Angiotensin converting enzyme density is increased in temporal cortex from patients with Alzheimer's disease. Eur. J. Pharmacol. **200:** 289–292.

16. ARREGUI, A., E.K. PERRY, M. ROSSOR & B.E. TOMLINSON. 1982. Angiotensin converting enzyme in Alzheimer's disease increased activity in caudate nucleus and cortical areas. J. Neurochem. **38:** 1490–1492.

17. AMOUYEL, P., F. RICHARD, D. COTTEL *et al.* 1996. The deletion allele of the angiotensin I converting enzyme gene as a genetic susceptibility factor for cognitive impairment. Neurosci. Lett. **217:** 203–205.

18. KEHOE, P.G., C. RUSS, S. MCILORY *et al.* 1999. Variation in DCP1, encoding ACE, is associated with susceptibility to Alzheimer disease. Nat. Genet. **21:** 71–72.

19. TYSOE, C., D. GALINSKY, D. ROBINSON *et al.* 1997. Analysis of alpha-1 antichymotrypsin, presenilin-1, angiotensin-converting enzyme, and methylenetetrahydrofolate reductase loci as candidates for dementia. Am. J. Med. Genet. **74:** 207–212.

20. SCACCHI, R., L. DE BERNARDINI, E. MANTUANO *et al.* 1998. DNA polymorphisms of apolipoprotein B and angiotensin I–converting enzyme genes and relationships with lipid levels in Italian patients with vascular dementia or Alzheimer's disease. Dement. Geriatr. Cogn. Disord. **9:** 186–190.

21. CHAPMAN, J., N. WANG, T.A. TREVES *et al.* 1998. ACE, MTHFR, factor V Leiden, and APOE polymorphisms in patients with vascular and Alzheimer's dementia. Stroke **29:** 1401–1404.

22. AGERHOLM-LARSEN, B., B.G. NORDESTGAARD, R. STEFFENSEN *et al.* 1997. ACE gene polymorphism: ischemic heart disease and longevity in 10,150 individuals. A case-referent and retrospective cohort study based on the Copenhagen City Heart Study. Circulation **95:** 2358–2367.

23. GALINSKY, D., C. TYSOE, C.E. BRAYNE *et al.* 1997. Analysis of the apo E/apo C-I, angiotensin converting enzyme and methylenetetrahydrofolate reductase genes as candidates affecting human longevity. Atherosclerosis **129:** 177–183.

24. SCHACHTER, F., L. FAURE-DELANEF, F. GUENOT *et al.* 1994. Genetic associations with human longevity at the APOE and ACE loci. Nat. Genet. **6:** 29–32.

Neurocardiovascular Instability, Hypotensive Episodes, and MRI Lesions in Neurodegenerative Dementia

CLIVE BALLARD,[a,c] JOHN O'BRIEN,[a] BOB BARBER,[a] PHILIP SCHELTENS,[b] FIONA SHAW,[a] IAN MCKEITH,[a] AND ROSE ANNE KENNY[a]

[a]Institute for the Health of the Elderly, Wolfson Research Centre, Newcastle General Hospital, Westgate Road, Newcastle upon Tyne NE4 6BE, United Kingdom

[b]Academisch Ziekenhuis VU, Amsterdam, The Netherlands

ABSTRACT: We investigated whether carotid sinus hypersensitivity (CSH) and orthostatic hypotension (OH) were associated with a greater severity of hyperintensities on MRI scan in 30 patients with neurodegenerative dementia (17 dementia with Lewy bodies, 13 Alzheimer's disease), who had a detailed evaluation of OH and CSH during active standing and head-up tilt. Patients also underwent a 1.0 Tesla MRI scan, from which hyperintensities were rated on a standardized scale. A blood pressure (BP) drop >30 mm Hg during carotid sinus massage or active standing was significantly associated with the severity of MRI hyperintensities in the deep white matter (OR 10.0, 95%; CI 1.8–55.7) and in the basal ganglia (OR 11.0, 95%; CI 1.2–99.5) but not in periventricular areas (OR 1.4, 95%; CI 0.3–1.8). Patients with the cardio-inhibitory form of CSH with the largest BP drops were the most at risk. Further longitudinal studies need to investigate the direction of causality to determine whether CSH or OH predispose to MRI hyperintensities and accelerate cognitive decline.

INTRODUCTION

Hyperintense lesions detected using MRI imaging occur frequently in elderly patients, especially those with dementia.[1,2] They include periventricular (PVH), basal ganglia (BGH), and deep white matter hyperintensities (DWMH). Correlative neuropathological studies have suggested that DWMH are the result of microvascular pathology.[3] This is supported by evidence suggesting that hypertension is a key risk factor.[4] Although less studied, orthostatic hypotension (OH) may also be important,[5] particularly among patients with previous hypertension. The importance of microvascular pathology has been emphasized in recent reports.[6]

Orthostatic hypotension (OH) and carotid sinus hypersensitivity (CSH) occur in 15% and 4% of the healthy elderly population, respectively,[7] both manifesting as in-

[c]Institute for the Health of the Elderly, Wolfson Research Centre, Newcastle General Hospital, Westgate Road, Newcastle upon Tyne NE4 6BE, United Kingdom. Tel.: 0191 273 5251; fax: 0191 272 5291.
e-mail: c.g.ballard@ncl.ac.uk

termittent drops in blood pressure (BP), which tend to be more severe in CSH.[8] They increase with age[8] and hypertension[9] and are seen in up to 30% of patients with unexplained falls and syncope.[10] CSH and OH are markedly elevated in dementia sufferers, with a combined frequency of 40% in patients with Alzheimer's disease (AD) and 50% in patients suffering from dementia with Lewy bodies (DLB).[11]

We hypothesized that episodes of recurrent hypotension would be associated with BGH and DWMH in neurodegenerative dementia.

METHOD

Thirty patients from a representative clinical dementia case register, with an operationalized diagnosis of probable DLB (consensus criteria)[12] or probable AD (NINCDS ADRDA criteria)[13] from a standardized psychiatric assessment, were enrolled in the study. Fifty cases from the overall case register cohort have now come to postmortem with positive predictive values of 95% for DLB and 78% for AD against neuropathological diagnosis.

Patients also received an ECG, phasic blood pressure, and heart rate measurements during 2 min of active standing, carotid sinus massage (both supine and tilted/upright), and prolonged head-up tilt to 70° for 30 min. OH and CSH were diagnosed using standardized criteria.[14] The clinical and cardiovascular assessment procedures are described fully elsewhere.[11]

MRl scans were performed on a 1.0 Tesla Siemens MRI scanner. Axial whole-brain images of 5-mm thickness were obtained using proton density–weighted and T_2-weighted turbo/fast spin echo sequences to allow detailed visualization of white matter lesions, rated on the Scheltens scale by an expert rater (ps), blind to the results of the OH and CSH assessment. The associations of PVH, BGH, and DWMH with BP drops >30 mm Hg were evaluated with odds ratios and 95% confidence intervals.

RESULTS

Thirty patients were studied (mean age 75.7, SD 5.6, 57% female, mean CAM-COG 55.3, SD 20.7, 17 DLB, 13 AD). Ten (33%) of the patients had significant BGH, 19 (63%) had significant DWMH, and 11 (37%) had moderate or severe PVH. BP drop >30 mm Hg (either postural hypotension on active standing or BP drop during carotid sinus massage) was significantly associated with BGH (OR 11.0, 95% CI 1.2–99.5) and DWMH (OR 10.0, 95% CI 1.8–55.7), but not with PVH (OR 1.4, 95% CI 0.3–1,8) (details in TABLE 1). There was no evidence that age (mean age BGH, 76.7; DWMH, 75.6), systolic BP (mean BGH 124.7, mean no BGH 123.6; mean DWMH 126.2, mean no DWMH 119.9; Mann-Whitney U Test $z = 1.0$, $p = 0.31$) or diastolic BP (mean BGH 62.6, mean no BGH 63.8; mean DWMH 68.4, mean no DWMH 57.6; Mann-Whitney U Test $z = 1.54$, $p = 0.12$) were significant confounding factors. Correlations with BGH (Spearman's $r = +0.94$) and DWMH ($r = +0.65$) severity were, however, especially strong in the six patients with a past history of hypertension.

TABLE 1. Neurocardiovascular instability and MRI hyperintensities in neurodegenerative dementia

Largest BP Drop in mmHg (Carotid Sinus Massage or Active Standing)	Hyperintense Lesions					
	Periventricular		Basal Ganglia		Deep White Matter	
	Absent/ mild ($n = 19$)	Moderate/ severe ($n = 11$)	Yes ($n = 10$)	No ($n = 20$)	Yes ($n = 19$)	No ($n = 11$)
<20	2	2	0	4	0	4
20–29	5	3	1	7	4	4
30–39	4	2	2	4	5	1
40–49	1	2	1	2	3	0
50–59	3	0	2	1	2	1
60–69	3	1	2	2	3	1
70–79	0	1	1	0	1	0
80–89	1	0	1	0	1	0

NOTE: For 29/30 patients the largest BP drop occurred with carotid sinus massage. One patient had an orthostatic drop >50 mmHg on active standing.

DISCUSSION

Clearly the current cohort represents only a pilot study with a modest number of patients; nevertheless, a significant statistical relationship emerged suggesting BGH and DWMH were associated with BP drops >30 mm Hg during either carotid sinus massage or active standing. Severe hypotensive episodes are hence an important association of small vessel ischemic damage, the most likely neuropathological correlate of these lesions.

Autonomic failure in multisystem atrophy is associated with depletion of catecholaminergic neurons in the ventrolateral medulla,[15] and it is possible that the basal ganglion lesions identified in the current study either predisposed persons directly to CSH or acted as an indicator of lesions in the brain stem, which are more difficult to identify with MRI techniques. It seems, however, more likely that repeated hypotensive insults might be an important cause of small vessel ischemic damage.

CSH and OH are both common in dementia patients[11] and predispose them to disabling symptoms such as syncope and falls; these observations are hence important whatever the direction of causality. If, however, longitudinal studies suggest that hypotensive episodes do predispose persons to microvascular pathology, the implications for the prognosis and treatment of these dementia patients will be particularly important.

REFERENCES

1. ALMKVIST, O., L.O. WAHLUND, G. ANDERSSON-LUNDMAN *et al.* 1992. White matter hyperintensity and neuropsychological functions in dementia and healthy aging. Arch. Neurol. **49:** 626-632.

2. O'BRIEN, J.T., D. AMES & I. SCHWIETZER. 1996. White matter in depression and Alzheimer's disease: a review of magnetic resonance imaging studies. Int. J. Geriatr. Psychiatry. **11:** 681–694.

3. FAZEKAS, F., R. SCHMIDT & P. SCHELTENS. 1998. Pathophysiologic mechanisms in the development of age related white matter changes of the brain. Dementia **9:** 2–5.

4. SKOOG, I. 1998. A Review on Blood Pressure and Ischaemic White Matter Lesions. Dementia **9:** 13–17.

5. MATSUSHITA, K., Y. KURIYAMA, K. NAGATSUKA *et al.* 1994. Periventricular white matter lucency and cerebral blood flow autoregulation in hyperintensive patients. Hypertension **23:** 565–568.

6. ESIRI, M., G. WILCOCK & J.H. MORRIS. 1997. Neuropathological assessment of the lesions of significance in vascular dementia. J. Neurol. Neurosurg. Psychiatry **63:** 749–753.

7. CAMPBELL, A.J. & K.J. REIN. 1985. Postural hypotension in old age: prevalence, associations and prognosis. J. Clin. Gerontol. Exp. **7:** 163–175.

8. RICHARDSON, D.A., R.S. BEXTON & F.E. SHAW. 1997. Prevalence of cardioinhibitory carotid sinus hypersensitivity in patients 50 years or over presenting to the accident and emergency department with "unexplained" or "recurrent" falls. Pace **20:** 820–823.

9. STRASBERG, B., A. SAGIE, S. ERDMAN *et al.* 1989. Carotid sinus hypersensitivity and carotid sinus syndrome. Prog. Cardiovasc. Dis. **31:** 379–391.

10. McINTOSH, S., D. DA COSTA & R.A. KENNY. 1993. Outcome of an integrated approach to the investigation of dizziness, falls and syncope in elderly patients referred to a syncope clinic. Age Ageing **22:** 53–58.

11. BALLARD, C.G., F. SHAW & I. McKEITH. 1998. High prevalence of neurovascular instability in neurodegenerative dementias. Neurology **52:** 251–252.

12. McKEITH, I.G., D. GALASKO. K. KOSAKA *et al.* 1996. Consensus guidelines for the clinical and pathologic diagnosis of dementia with Lewy bodies (DLB). Neurology **47:** 1113–1124.

13. McKHANN, G., D. DRACHMAN, M. FOLSTEIN *et al.* 1984. Clinical diagnosis of Alzheimer's disease: report of the NINCDS-ADRDA Work Group under the auspices of Department of Health and Human Services Task Forces on Alzheimer's Disease. Neurology **44:** 939–944.

14. HUDSON, W.M., C.A. MORLEY, E.J. PERRIN *et al.* 1985. Is a hypersensitive carotid sinus reflex relevant? Clin. Prog. Electrophysiol. Pacing **3:** 155–159.

15. BENARROCH, E.E., I.L. SMITHSON & P.A. LOW. 1998. Depletion of catecholaminergic neurons of the rostral ventrolateral medulla in multiple systems atrophy with autonomic failure. Ann. Neurol. **43:** 156–163.

β–Amyloid Vasoactivity and Proinflammation in Microglia Can Be Blocked by cGMP-Elevating Agents

DANIEL PARIS,[a] TERRENCE TOWN, TIMOTHY PARKER, JAMES HUMPHREY, AND MICHAEL MULLAN

The Roskamp Institute, University of South Florida, Tampa, Florida 33613, USA

BACKGROUND

Vascular damage and reactive gliosis are often found colocalized with amyloid deposits in Alzheimer's disease (AD) brain,[1] suggesting that the cerebrovasculature may be a clinically relevant site of AD pathology and may contribute to the neuroinflammatory process in AD. Using intact rat aortae in a tissue bath system, we have previously shown that freshly solubilized β-amyloid (Aβ) peptides are able to impair relaxation in response to acetylcholine[2] or the nitric oxide (NO) donor sodium nitroprusside (SNP).[3] Furthermore, we have demonstrated that Aβ peptides are able to potentiate the vasoconstriction induced by endothelin-1 (ET-1),[4,5] which is one of the most potent cerebral vasoconstrictors in the brain.[6] Interestingly, Aβ's enhancement of ET-1-induced vasoconstriction has been shown to be mediated independently of the presence of an intact endothelium,[5] suggesting that the ability of vascular smooth muscle cells to determine the dynamic caliber of the blood vessel may be directly impacted by Aβ.

The molecular mechanism of Aβ vasoactivity has been suggested to be mediated via free radicals,[2] because superoxide dismutase appears to partially oppose Aβ's vasoconstrictive effect.[5] We have recently shown, however, that the pathway to Aβ vasoactivity is not impacted by the superoxide dismutase mimic and peroxynitrite scavenger MnTBAP,[4] catalase, or the water-soluble vitamin E analogue Trolox (data not shown). Furthermore, we have shown that Aβ vasoactivity is not due to an inhibition of nitric oxide synthase (NOS) activity, since inactivation of NOS does not mimic or modulate the vasoactive properties of Aβ.[3] Collectively, these results show that Aβ vasoactivity is not mediated by reactive oxygen species, and they prompted us to search for an alternative mechanism.

Soluble guanylyl cyclase (sGC) is responsible for the synthesis of cGMP, and NO stimulates sGC in underlying vascular smooth muscle cells, resulting in vasorelaxation. This effect is antagonized by ET-1, which has been shown to impede increases in cGMP levels in vessels stimulated with the NO donor SNP. This balance between NO and ET-1 provides one mechanism for control of cerebral vasotonus, and, since we showed that Aβ can oppose NO-induced vasorelaxation and enhance ET-1-induced vasoconstriction, we evaluated the possibility that Aβ may oppose the NO/

[a]Address for correspondence: Daniel Paris, The Roskamp Institute, University of South Florida, 3515 E. Fletcher Ave., Tampa, FL 33613.

cGMP pathway, thereby potentiating ET-1-induced vasoconstriction. Cyclic GMP levels are modulated essentially by two mechanisms: sGC stimulation leads to increased cGMP production, and activation of cGMP phosphodiesterases (cGMP-PDEs) results in degradation of cGMP. Our data show that, whereas Aβ does not mediate its vasoconstrictive effect via inhibition of sGC, activation of cGMP-PDE is involved, because a specific type V cGMP-PDE inhibitor (dipyridamole) is able to block Aβ's vasoactive effect in a statistically interactive manor.

We then asked the question whether the signal transduction pathway mediating Aβ's vasoconstrictive effect might generally mediate Aβ bioactivity in different cell types. To evaluate this possibility, we investigated Aβ's effect on cultured microglia, a cell type that has been implicated as a mediator of neuroinflammation in AD brain. We show that various cGMP-elevating agents are able to attenuate Aβ-induced leukotriene B4 (LTB4) (a proinflammatory eicosanoid) production in microglia. Taken together, our data show that Aβ's effects on both isolated vessels and cultured microglia can be modulated by cGMP, and suggest that Aβ's bioactivity can be brought about via a common signal transduction pathway in different systems.

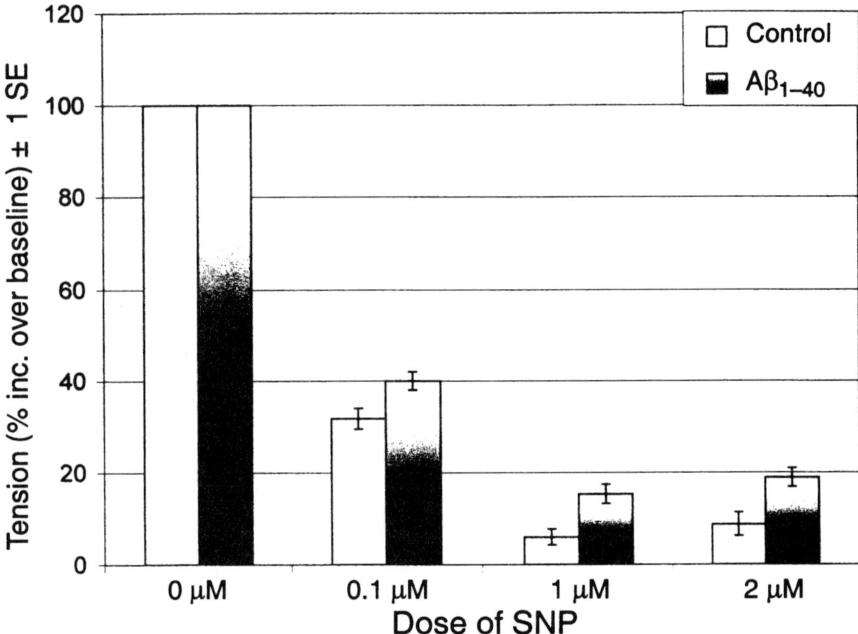

FIGURE 1. Effect of Aβ on SNP-induced relaxation. Control vessels and vessels pretreated with 1 mM of freshly solubilized Aβ$_{1-40}$ were constricted with 3.5 nM of PE. Further relaxation was induced with the doses of SNP shown. Data were then standardized such that the maximum value for PE-induced tension was 100% for both Aβ and control channels. Aβ ($p < 0.001$) and SNP ($p < 0.001$) were significant factors in the ANOVA, although there was no significant interaction between them ($p = 0.890$). Aβ decreases the induced relaxation at 0.1 mM SNP ($p < 0.02$), at 1 mM SNP ($p < 0.01$), and at 2 mM SNP ($p < 0.01$).

RESULTS AND DISCUSSION

Vessels were treated with phenylephrine (PE, 3.5 nM) to obtain a stable long-lasting constriction. We observed, in vessels co-treated with Aβ and PE, that the relaxation induced by SNP was reduced in comparison to the relaxation induced by the same amount of SNP in control vessels (FIG. 1). These data suggested two possibilities: either Aβ was able to inhibit the stimulation of soluble guanylyl cyclase (sGC) by NO, or it increased the degradation of cGMP. We investigated the role of sGC in the vasoactivity mediated by Aβ by using a highly selective inhibitor of sGC, 1H-[1,2,4]oxadiazolo[4,3,-a]quinoxalin-1-one (ODQ). These data showed that the vas-

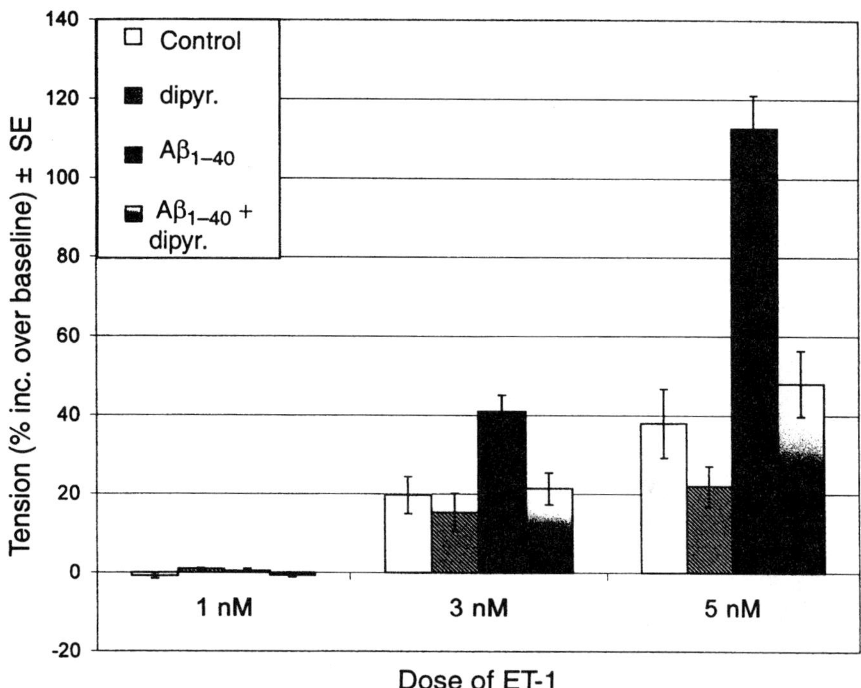

FIGURE 2. Effect of dipyridamole on Aβ-enhancement of ET-1-induced vasoconstriction. Certain aortic rings were treated with 1 μM of freshly solubilized Aβ_{1-40}, 10 μM of dipyridamole (dipyr.), or Aβ + dipyr 5 min before the addition of a dose range of ET-1. Results are expressed as the mean ± 1 SE of the percentage vasoconstriction increase over baseline. There were significant main effects of ET-1 ($p < 0.001$), Aβ ($p < 0.001$), and dipyr ($p < 0.001$), as well as significant interactive terms between ET-1 and either Aβ ($p < 0.001$) or dipyr ($p < 0.001$). Further, there was significant interaction among ET-1, Aβ, and dipyr ($p < 0.05$). One-way ANOVA revealed significant between-treatment group differences across all ET-1 doses ($p < 0.001$), and post-hoc comparison between control vessels and Aβ-treated vessels revealed a significant difference ($p < 0.01$), as did Aβ-treated vessels compared to Aβ + dipry-treated aortae ($p < 0.01$).

oconstriction induced by ET-1 was synergistically enhanced after ODQ treatment, but was only additive, as opposed to statistically interactive, with Aβ and ODQ co-treatment.[3] This result suggested that Aβ vasoactivity was not mediated via inhibition of sGC. In this same report, we demonstrated that stimulation of sGC with YC-1, a NO-independent activator of sGC, was only able to reduce Aβ-induced vasoconstriction in an additive manner, further supporting that Aβ vasoactivity was not due to modulation of sGC activity. Moreover, inhibition of NOS activity by L-NAME-enhanced ET-1 induced vasoconstriction, yet this effect was merely additive in conjunction with Aβ, showing that Aβ vasoactivity does not result from an alteration of NOS activity or NO production.

Having established that Aβ vasoactivity was not due to an alteration of the NO-mediated synthesis of cGMP, we went on to examine whether cGMP hydrolysis was involved. We used dipyridamole (dipyr), a specific inhibitor of type V cGMP-PDE, to test the possible involvement of cGMP-PDE in mediating Aβ vasoactivity. We observed that dipyridamole was able to interactively block Aβ-enhancement of ET-1-induced vasoconstriction, suggesting that Aβ stimulates cGMP degradation (FIG. 2).

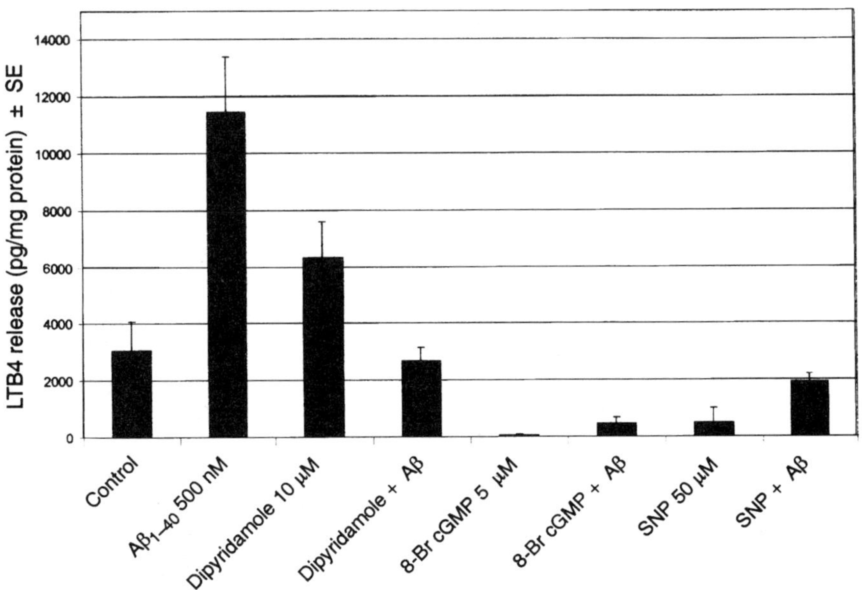

FIGURE 3. Effect of cGMP elevation on Aβ-induced microglial LTB4 release. For each condition presented, $n = 6$. ANOVA revealed significant main effects of Aβ ($p < 0.01$), dipyridamole (10 µM, $p = 0.01$), 8-Br cGMP ($p < 0.001$), and SNP ($p < 0.001$). Significant interactive terms were noted between Aβ and each drug used ($p < 0.01$). Post-hoc testing did not reveal significant differences between control and each drug used or control and drug + Aβ ($p > 0.05$). This shows that each drug used alone does not significantly affect constitutive LTB4 release, and administration of each drug in combination with Aβ results in total blockade of Aβ-induced microglial LTB4 release.

In order to further confirm this hypothesis, we measured cGMP levels in Aβ-treated aortae and found that cGMP levels were reduced in Aβ-treated vessels compared to untreated controls.[3] Data thus far had suggested that Aβ's vasoactivity is mediated through a specific signal transduction pathway impacting cGMP levels. We hypothesized that Aβ may exert its biological activity via similar mechanisms in various cell types. Thus, we investigated the effects of cGMP-elevating agents on Aβ's activation of a proinflammatory pathway in N9 microglial cells (kindly provided by Dr. Ricciardi-Castagnoli, Cellular Pharmacology Center, Milan, Italy).

We choose leukotriene B4 (LTB4), which is a proinflammatory eicosanoid end-product of the classical arachidonic acid/5-lipoxygenase pathway, as a marker of microglial proinflammation. Data showed that treatment of N9 microglia with Aβ resulted in marked LTB4 release. This effect was significantly attenuated by co-treatment of microglia with Aβ and the cGMP-elevating agents dipyridamole, SNP, or a cell-permeable analogue of cGMP, 8-bromo cGMP (8-Br cGMP, FIG. 3). Taken together, these data show that cGMP-elevating agents display antiinflammatory properties, and, specifically, are able to block Aβ vasoactivity and proinflammatory response in microglial cells. Furthermore, these results suggest that the intracellular signaling pathway triggered by Aβ is conserved across different cellular systems, because drugs that oppose Aβ vasoactivity also block Aβ-induced microglial inflammation.

ACKNOWLEDGMENTS

This work was supported by the generosity of Mr. and Mrs. Robert Roskamp. M. Mullan is the recipient of a Veteran's Administration Merit Award.

REFERENCES

1. ITAGAKI, S., P.L. MCGEER, H. AKIYAMA *et al.* 1989. Relationship of microglia and astrocytes to amyloid deposits of Alzheimer's disease. J. Neuroimmunol. **24:** 173–182.
2. THOMAS, T., G. THOMAS, C. MCLENDON *et al.* 1996. β-Amyloid mediated vasoactivity and vascular endothelial damage. Nature **380:** 168–171.
3. PARIS, D., T. TOWN, T.A. PARKER *et al.* 1999. Inhibition of Alzheimer's β-amyloid induced vasoactivity and pro-inflammatory response in microglia by a cGMP-dependent mechanism. Exp. Neurol. **157:** 211–221.
4. PARIS, D., T.A. PARKER, T. TOWN *et al.* 1998. Role of peroxynitrite in the vasoactive and cytotoxic effects of Alzheimer's β-amyloid peptide. Exp. Neurol. **152:** 116–122.
5. CRAWFORD, F., Z. SUO, C. FANG & M. MULLAN. 1998. Characteristics of the in vitro vasoactivity of beta-amyloid peptides. Exp. Neurol. **150:** 159–168.
6. EHRENREICH, H. & L. SCHILLING. 1995. New developments in the understanding of cerebral vasoregulation and vasospasm: the endothelin-nitric oxide network. Cleve. Clin. J. Med. **62:** 105–116.

β-Amyloid Fragment 25–35 Induces Changes in Cytosolic Free Calcium in Human Platelets

LUCIANO GALEAZZI,[a] TIZIANA CASOLI,[b,c] SERGIO GIUNTA,[a]
PATRIZIA FATTORETTI,[b] NATASCIA GRACCIOTTI,[b]
UGO CASELLI,[b] AND CARLO BERTONI-FREDDARI[b]

[a]*Clinical Laboratory, Geriatric Hospital "U. Sestilli" I.N.R.C.A.,
Via della Montagnola 164, 60100 Ancona, Italy*

[b]*Neurobiology of Aging Laboratory, "N. Masera" I.N.R.C.A. Research Department,
Via Birarelli 8, 60121 Ancona, Italy*

The beta-amyloid (βA) peptide has a central role in Alzheimer's disease (AD). Indeed, the major histopathologic hallmarks of AD include βA deposits in brain parenchima (senile plaques) and also around and within the walls of blood vessels (cerebral amyloid angiopathy).[1] βA deposits are the final result of an amyloidogenic process triggered by oxidative and conformational modifications and by cross-linking of βA.[2–4] βA is a peptide produced by the proteolysis of the amyloid precursor protein (APP). It has been reported that abnormalities of brain APP metabolism may be reflected in platelets, which also possess all the machinery to generate the amyloid β (Aβ)-fragment from APP; moreover, platelets are the primary source of Aβ-peptide in human blood.[5–7] In human cortical neurons β-amyloid peptides have been shown to destabilize calcium homeostasis and cause neurodegenerative effects.[8,9] Alteration in calcium homeostasis induced by Aβ have been reported also for nonneuronal cells.[10,11] Moreover, it has been demonstrated that $A\beta_{25-35}$ increases cellular APP by inhibiting its secretory processing in human extraneuronal cells.[12] The data reported above encourage further exploration about amyloid and platelets as a peripheral laboratory mirroring central amyloid metabolism and activity.[1] In the present paper we investigate the effects of neurotoxic $A\beta_{25-35}$ peptide on platelets and we show that this Aβ-fragment is able to induce dose-dependent changes of calcium concentration and degenerative effects in normal human platelets.

Blood samples were taken from male healthy donors aged between 31 and 50 years (mean age: 38 ± 7). Citrated blood was centrifuged for 10 min at 200 × g to obtain platelet-rich plasma (PRP). Platelets were separated from PRP by centrifugation at 2000 × g for 20 min and washed twice in phosphate-buffered saline (PBS) 0.1 M, pH 7.4. Platelets were resuspended at a density of 10^8/ml in Hepes buffer containing 145 mM NaCl, 5 mM KCl, 1 mM $CaCl_2$, 1 mM $MgCl_2$, 10 mM Hepes, 10 mM glucose, adjusted to pH 7.4. Ten μM prostaglandin E_1 (PGE_1) was added to prevent aggregation. The platelet suspension was incubated in 1 μM $A\beta_{25-35}$

[c]Address for correspondence: Dr. Tiziana Casoli, Neurobiology of Aging Laboratory, "N. Masera" I.N.R.C.A. Research Department, Via Birarelli 8, 60121 Ancona, Italy. Tel.: +71 8004203; fax: +71 206791.
e-mail: t.casoli@inrca.it

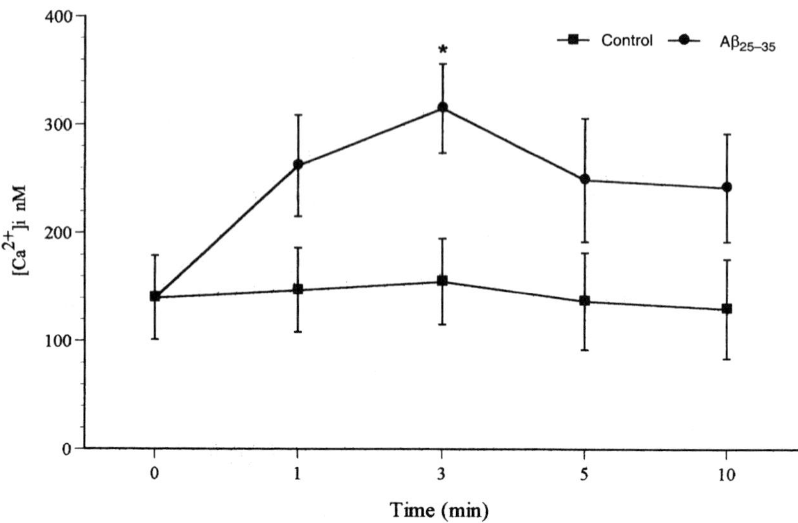

FIGURE 1. Time course of $[Ca^{2+}]_i$ in human platelets exposed to 1 μM Aβ_{25-35}. Values are means $\pm$ SEM of 6 individual experiments. *p <0.05 versus control.

at 37°C for 1, 3, 5, and 10 min. Other platelet samples were exposed to increasing concentration of Aβ_{25-35} (0, 0.1, 1, 10, and 20 μM) for 3 min at 37°C. The platelet suspensions were centrifuged at 2000 × g for 10 min, resuspended in Hepes buffer, and loaded with Fura-2 AM for 45 min at 37°C. Platelet pellets were either resuspended in Hepes buffer for fluorescence measurements or fixed overnight in 2.5% glutaraldehyde in 0.1 M sodium cacodylate buffer, pH 7.3 at 4°C for electron microscopy studies. Platelet suspensions were transferred to a Kontron SFM 25 spectrofluorometer for fluorescence measurements. Excitation wavelengths were 340 and 380 nm, and emission wavelength was 510 nm. $[Ca^{2+}]_i$ levels were calculated according to Grynkiewicz et al.[13] Data were expressed as means $\pm$ standard error of the mean (SEM). An analysis of variance (ANOVA) and the Student-Neuman-Keuls test were used to compare these means. Significance was assigned at p <0.05. Fixed platelets were washed twice with sodium cacodylate buffer, postfixed in 1% buffered osmium tetroxide, dehydrated in a graded series of ethanol and embedded in Durcupan ACM resin. Ultrathin sections were stained with uranyl acetate and lead citrate. Following 1 μM Aβ_{25-35} incubation, the maximum rise in $[Ca^{2+}]_i$ was reached at 3 min with an average increment of 50.8% above control values and of 55.6% above basal values. Following 5 and 10 min 1 μM Aβ_{25-35} incubation, intraplatelet free calcium concentration was not statistically different from basal levels (FIG. 1). Incubation of platelet suspension with Aβ_{25-35} up to 1 μM caused a statistically significant increase of $[Ca^{2+}]$ only for 1 μM Aβ_{25-35}. Platelet incubation with 10 and 20 μM of the β-amyloid active fragment (FIG. 2) caused a not significant decrease of $[Ca^{2+}]_i$.

FIGURE 3 shows representative ultrastructural pictures of platelets corresponding to three different steps in our experimental conditions. The first step (FIG. 3A)

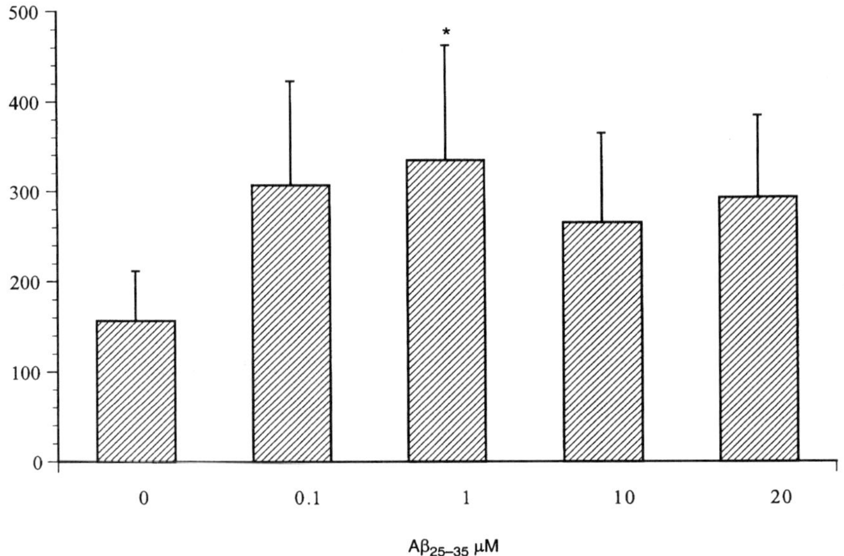

FIGURE 2. Concentration dependence of intraplatelet free calcium changes. Data are means ± SEM ($n = 5$). *$p < 0.05$ compared with Aβ$_{25-35}$ basal value.

represents platelets in the basal state. They appear discoid with some evaginations. The second step (FIG. 3B) corresponds to platelets exposed for 3 min to 0.1 and 1 μM Aβ$_{25-35}$ and for 1 and 3 min to 1 μM Aβ$_{25-35}$. There is an increased heterogeneity of platelet morphology: some maintain an ultrastructure similar to that of the basal state, others have a swollen cytoplasm with a disintegrated internal structure. The third step corresponds to the exposure for the longest times (5 and 10 min) and to the highest concentrations (10 and 20 μM) of βA (FIG. 3C). In this condition, the number of intact platelets is drastically reduced, and a substantial amount of microvesicles and platelet fragments are present, suggesting that most platelets are lysed.

The β-amyloid peptide (βA) is a major constituent of senile plaques, one of the characteristic pathological features of Alzheimer's disease (AD), and several lines of evidence suggest that βA has a causative role in AD. Loss of calcium regulation has been proposed as the mechanism of toxicity of βA.[8,9] Aβ$_{25-35}$ has been shown to increase the intracellular free calcium concentration in PC12 cells[14] and determine an amplification of the K$^+$-induced rise in [Ca^{2+}] in dissociated mouse brain cells.[15] Alterations in calcium homeostasis induced by βA have been reported also for nonneuronal cells. Eckert *et al.*[10] demonstrated that β-amyloid and its neurotoxic fragment Aβ$_{25-35}$ amplify calcium signal in circulating lymphocytes, supporting the hypothesis of a widespread effect of Ca^{2+}-mediated βA toxicity. Human platelets have often been used to investigate the neuronal metabolism in neuropsychiatric diseases. It has also been shown that platelets contain relatively large amounts of APP.[17] This study documents that neurotoxic Aβ$_{25-35}$ peptide is able to cause dose-

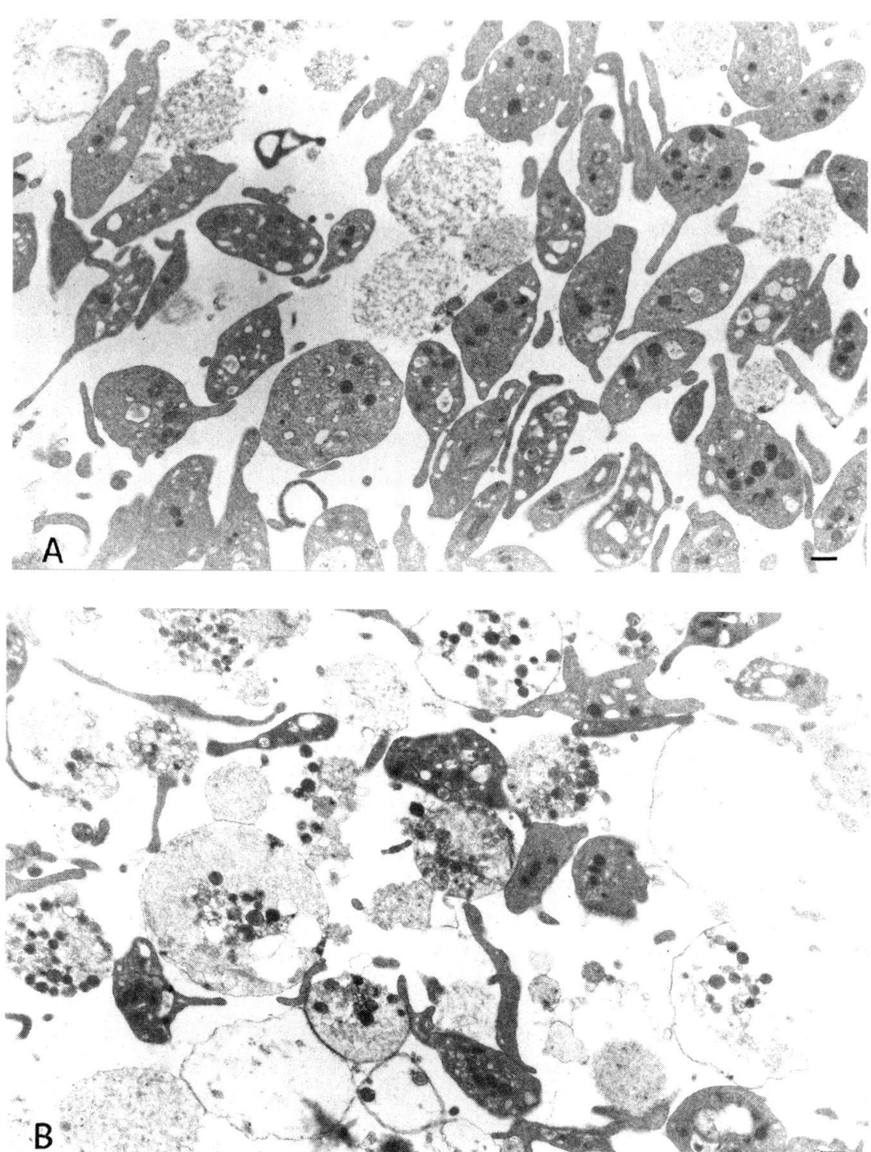

FIGURE 3. Platelet ultrastructure after exposure to Aβ$_{25-35}$. **(A)** Basal state: the cells have a characteristic discoid shape with some extending pseudopods. Their morphology reflects that of fresh platelets. **(B)** Cells incubated for 3 min with 0.1 and 1 μM Aβ$_{25-35}$ and for 1 min with 1 μM Aβ$_{25-35}$: platelets are swollen, and the cytoplasm appears diluted. Most of the cells are badly damaged. **(C)** Platelets incubated for 5 and 10 min in 1 μM Aβ$_{25-35}$ and for 3 min in 10 and 20 μM Aβ$_{25-35}$: numerous cell debris and microvesicles from lysed platelets can be identified. *Scale bar* = 0.5 μM.

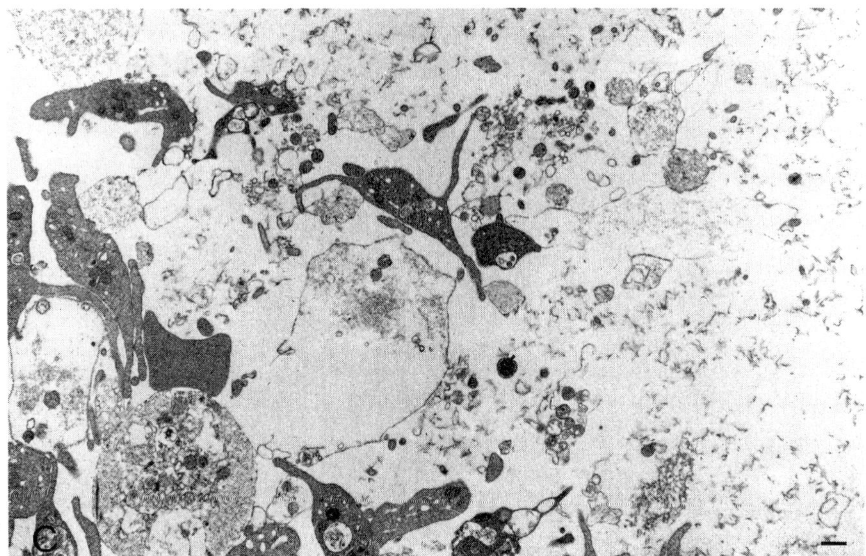

FIGURE 3. *Continued.*

dependent abnormalities in intracellular calcium control mechanisms and degenerative alterations in human platelets of healthy subjects. Therefore, the results reported in this paper, although in a different experimental model, exactly overlap those previously reported by Mattson *et al.*,[8] demonstrating that β-amyloid peptides induce changes in intracellular calcium and degenerative effects in cells. Our results confirm the possibility reported by Bush and Tanzi[5] that events and abnormalities of neuron metabolism may be reflected in platelets. $A\beta_{25-35}$ peptide destabilizes calcium homeostasis in human platelets, and elevations in intraplatelet free calcium concentration can be observed within minutes of incubation with $A\beta_{25-35}$, while the same effect was demonstrated in neuronal cell cultures after days of exposure.[8] In addition, the $[Ca^{2+}]_i$ changes observed occur upon the direct exposure of platelets to βA; while lymphocytes and neuronal cell cultures showed βA-induced amplification of the $[Ca^{2+}]$ response only after previous exposure of these cells to other stimuli.[10,8] Although our data cannot demonstrate the specific mechanism of action of β-amyloid, they do suggest some possibilities. The incubation of the platelet suspension in increasing concentrations of β-amyloid active fragment reveals a biphasic effect of βA fragment on cytosolic $[Ca^{2+}]_i$, with an increase at low doses and a decrease at higher concentrations of the peptide. Electron microscopy results strongly suggest that high doses of $A\beta_{25-35}$ are likely to determine toxic effects on platelets associated with a significant decrease of the fluorescence signal. $[Ca^{2+}]_i$ increment may determine a number of responses that include shape change, dense granule and α-granule secretion, and the activation of Ca^{2+}-dependent proteases, which finally leads to the disintegration of platelets.[18] Thus our data support that human platelets represent a good model to study the effect of β-amyloid, confirming that peripheral cells may be of help to get more insights into the mechanisms leading to the onset and progression of Alzheimer's disease.

REFERENCES

1. SHOULSON, I. 1998. Experimental therapeutics of neurodegenerative disorders: unmet needs. Science **282**: 1072–1074.
2. DYRKS, T., E. DYRKS, T. HARTMANN, C. MASTERS & K. BEYREUTHER. 1992. Amyloidogenicity of βA4-bearing amyloid protein precursor fragment by metal-catalyzed oxidation. J. Biol. Chem. **267**: 18210–18217.
3. DYRKS, T., E. DYRKS, C.L. MASTERS & K. BEYREUTHER. 1993. Amyloidogenicity of rodent and human βA4 sequences. FEBS Lett. **324**: 231–236.
4. GALEAZZI, L., P. RONCHI, C. FRANCESCHI & S. GIUNTA. 1999. *In vitro* peroxidase oxidation induces stable dimers of β-amyloid (1–42) through dityrosine bridge formation. Amyloid **6**: 7–13.
5. BUSH, A.I. & R. TANZI. 1998. Alzheimer disease-related abnormalities of amyloid β precursor protein isoforms in the platelet. Arch. Neurol. **55**: 1179–1180.
6. DI LUCA, M., L. PASTORINO, A. BIANCHETTI *et al.* 1998. Differential level of platelet amyloid β precursor protein isoforms: an early marker for Alzheimer disease. Arch. Neurol. **55**: 1195–1200.
7. CHEN, M., N.C. INESTROSA, G.S. ROSS & H.L. FERNANDEZ. 1995. Platelets are the primary source of amyloid β-peptide in human blood. Biochem. Biophys. Res. Commun. **213**: 96–103.
8. MATTSON, M.P., B. CHENG, D. DAVIS *et al.* 1992. β-Amyloid peptides destabilize calcium homeostasis and render human cortical neurons vulnerable to excitotoxicity. J. Neurosci. **12**: 376–389.
9. MATTSON, M.P., K.P. TOMASELLI & R.E. RYDEL. 1993. Calcium-destabilizing and neurodegenerative effects of aggregated β-amyloid peptide are attenuated by basic FGF. Brain Res. **621**: 35–49.
10. ECKERT, A., H. HARTMANN & W.E. MULLER. 1993. β-Amyloid protein enhances the mitogen-induced calcium response in circulating human lymphocytes. FEBS Lett. **330**: 49–52.
11. ECKERT, A., H. HARTMANN & W.E. MULLER. 1994. Alteration of intracellular calcium regulation during aging and Alzheimer's disease in nonneuronal cells. Life Sci. **55**: 2019–2029.
12. SCHMITT, T.L., E. STEINER, K. TRIEB *et al.* 1997. Amyloid beta-protein (25–35) increases cellular APP and inhibits the secretion of APPs in human extraneuronal cells. Exp. Cell Res. **234**: 336–340.
13. GRYNKIEWICZ, G., M. POENIE & R.Y. TSIEN. 1985. A new generation of Ca^{2+} indicators with greatly improved fluorescence properties. J. Biol. Chem. **260**: 3440–3450.
14. FUKUYAMA, R., K.C. WADHWANI, Z. GALDZICKI *et al.* 1994. β-Amyloid polypeptide increases calcium-uptake in PC12 cells: a possible mechanism for its cellular toxicity in Alzheimer's disease. Brain Res. **667**: 269–272.
15. HARTMANN, H., A. ECKERT & W.E. MULLER. 1993. Aging enhances the calcium sensitivity of central neurons of the mouse as an adaptive response to reduced free intracellular calcium. Biochem. Biophys. Res. Commun. **194**: 1216–1220.
16. BORN, G.V.R. 1988. Platelets and neurobiological research. Experientia **44**: 113–115.
17. VAN NOSTRAND, W.E., A.H. SCHMAIER, J.S. FARROW *et al.* 1990. Protease nexin II (amyloid β-protein precursor): a platelet α-granule protein. Science **248**: 745–748.
18. HOLMSEN, H. 1981. Energy metabolism and platelet responses. Vox Sang. **40**(Suppl. 1): 1–7.

Vascular Involvement in Cognitive Decline and Dementia

Epidemiologic Evidence from the Rotterdam Study and the Rotterdam Scan Study

MONIQUE M.B. BRETELER[a]

Department of Epidemiology and Biostatistics, Erasmus Medical Center Rotterdam, 3000 DR Rotterdam, the Netherlands

INTRODUCTION

Over the last decade evidence has been accumulating for an involvement of vascular mechanisms or vascular pathology in the etiology of cognitive impairment and Alzheimer's disease, in particular in elderly subjects. Epidemiological studies have largely contributed to these notions. In this paper the evidence from two such prospective population-based studies is summarized. In the Rotterdam Study we investigated the putative role of vascular risk factors and markers of vascular disease in the development of cognitive decline and (subtypes of) dementia, and performed an initial study on the determinants and clinical significance of cerebral white matter lesions. Based on these results, we then initiated the Rotterdam Scan, in which causes and consequences of degenerative and vascular brain changes are investigated prospectively. A discussion of potential underlying mechanisms and of related findings from other studies falls outside the scope of this paper, but has been the subject of several recently published reviews.[1,2]

STUDY DESIGN AND STUDY POPULATION

Rotterdam Study

The Rotterdam Study is a prospective population-based study aimed at investigating determinants of chronic and disabling diseases in the elderly.[3] The study started in 1990 when all inhabitants aged 55 years or over of Ommoord, a suburb of Rotterdam, were invited to participate. Subjects living in institutions were included in the study. Of 10,275 eligible subjects 7,983 (78%) agreed to participate. At baseline, participants were interviewed at home and subsequently clinically examined during two visits at a research center. Baseline examinations included assessment of medical history, medication, noninvasive measurements of atherosclerosis, and measurements of vascular risk factors. Serum and DNA was collected and stored for fu-

[a]Address for correspondence: Monique M.B. Breteler, M.D., Ph.D., Dept. of Epidemiology & Biostatistics, Erasmus Medical Center Rotterdam, PO Box 1738, 3000 DR Rotterdam, the Netherlands. Tel.: +31 10 408 7489; fax: +31 10 408 9382.
email: breteler@epib.fgg.eur.nl

ture use. A first follow-up survey was done 1993–1994, and a second follow-up survey 1997–1999. In addition, the total cohort is continuously being monitored for major morbidity and mortality, including onset of memory problems or dementia, through linkage of the general practitioners' (GPs') records and the municipality records with the study database, thereby ensuring complete follow-up. The study was approved by the Medical Ethics Committee of Erasmus University/Academic Hospital Rotterdam, and signed informed consent and permission to retrieve information from treating physicians and pharmacy databases was obtained from all participants.

Assessment of Dementia and Alzheimer's Disease

Assessment of dementia in the Rotterdam Study is done similarly in the baseline and follow-up examinations through a stepwise procedure.[4–6] All participants of the Rotterdam Study are screened for dementia with the Mini Mental State Examination (MMSE) and the Geriatric Mental Schedule (GMS). Screenpositives (MMSE <26 or GMS >0) are subsequently examined by a physician with the Cambridge Examination for Mental Disorders of the Elderly (CAMDEX). Those who are suspected for dementia are then referred for further examination by a neurologist, a neuropsychologist, and—if possible—neuroimaging. Of subjects who cannot be reexamined in person, information is obtained from the GPs and the regional institute for outpatient mental health care, which covers the entire study population. The final diagnosis is made by a consensus panel. A diagnosis of dementia is based on DSM-III-R criteria, a subdiagnosis of Alzheimer's disease is based on NINCDS-ADRDA criteria. At baseline, screening and examination for dementia was performed in 7,528 individuals, and 482 were diagnosed to be demented.[7] This resulted in a cohort of 7,046 subjects at risk for dementia.

MRI Study within the Rotterdam Study

In 1991, an age and gender stratified random sample was drawn from participants in the Rotterdam Study, and these people were invited for additional neuropsychological testing and brain MR imaging. Of 128 invited subjects 111 participated. Axial T2 weighted images were obtained on a 1.5 Tesla Philips Gyroscan. Overall severity of white matter lesions was rated as 0 (no or slight periventricular hyperintensity, less than 5 punctate lesions, no confluent lesions), 1 (moderate periventricular hyperintensity or more than 5 punctate lesions, no confluent lesions), or 2 (severe periventricular hyperintensity or confluent lesions).

Rotterdam Scan Study

The Rotterdam Scan Study is a prospective population-based study that was designed to investigate determinants and consequences of brain abnormalities in the elderly. To allow the investigation of long-term and short-term determinants of neurodegenerative changes, participants were randomly selected from two large ongoing prospective cohort studies, the Zoetermeer Study and the Rotterdam Study. The Rotterdam Study has been described above; the Zoetermeer Study is a population-based study among 10,361 subjects, aged between 5–91 years at baseline (1975–1978) of determinants of various chronic diseases.[8] Subjects were invited to the Rotterdam Scan Study in 1995–1996 by letter, and subsequently contacted by telephone. Upon agreement to participate eligibility was assessed. Not eligible were those with dementia, blindness, or MRI contraindications, including prosthetic valves, pacemaker, cerebral aneurysm clips, a history of intraocular metal fragment, cochlear implants, and claustrophobia. In total, 1904 subjects were invited, who were randomly selected in strata of age (5 years), gender, and study from a larger pool of subjects in the appropriate age groups from the two primary studies. Of these 1717 were eligible. Data collection included assessment of medical history, medication, noninvasive measurements of atherosclerosis, measurements of vascular risk factors, neuropsychological testing, and MRI scanning. Serum and DNA were collected and stored for future use. Complete information, including a cerebral MRI scan, was obtained from 1077 persons (63%): 563 from the Rotterdam Study and 514 from the Zoetermeer Study. The proportion who responded and had complete information declined from 73% among subjects aged between 60–70 years to 48% among participants aged between 80–90 years. Each participant signed an informed consent form. The Medical Ethics Committee of Erasmus University approved the study.

MRI Scanning Protocol

MRI scanning was performed on 1.5 Tesla machines (Gyroscan (Philips, Best, the Netherlands) for subjects recruited from the Zoetermeer Study, and a VISION (Siemens, Erlangen, Germany) for participants originating from the Rotterdam Study. The scanning protocol included a series of axial T1, T2, and Proton Density (PD) weighted images for the assessment of white matter lesions and 3-D (DIRE-HASTE) or IR sequences for the assessment of atrophy.

White Matter Lesions Rating Scale

White matter lesions (WML) were rated separately for the periventricular and deep subcortical region on hard copies (printed with a reduction factor of 2.7) and considered present if hyper-intense on both PD and T2 weighted images and not iso-intense with the liquor on T1 weighted images. Periventricular WML were rated semiquantitatively (range 0-9). For subcortical WML a total volume was approximated based on number and size of all lesions. The inter- and intra-rater studies showed a good to excellent agreement (weighted kappa's for periventricular white matter lesions 0.79–0.90, inter- and intra-rater intra-class correlation coefficients for subcortical white matter lesions 0.88 and 0.95).

RESULTS

Vascular Factors and Cognitive Function in the Rotterdam Study

Population Distribution of Cognitive Function according to Vascular Risk

On the premise that there is little evidence for a sharp distinction between demented and nondemented persons and that cognitive impairment is a quantitative rather than a qualitative characteristic, we evaluated the impact of overt or clinically silent vascular disease by comparing the age- and sex-matched population distributions of cognitive function of subjects with and without vascular pathology. For subjects with vascular disease the distributions were shifted toward lower values accompanied by an increased variability. Correspondingly, the proportion of subjects with low scores, in the "dementia range," increased.[9]

Homocysteine

Homocysteinemia is a well-recognized risk factor for cardiovascular disease. We assessed baseline homocysteine levels in a random sample of nondemented subjects who had participated in the baseline and first follow-up examination and related this to cognitive decline (defined as drop in MMSE score >1 point/year (approximately >1 SD). The analyses were based on 472 subjects. Subjects with higher homocysteine levels (upper tertile) had a 40% increased risk of cognitive decline; however, possibly due to lack of power, this failed to reach statistical significance.[10]

Vascular Factors and Dementia in the Rotterdam Study

Atherosclerosis

In a cross-sectional analysis on the baseline cohort, indicators of atherosclerosis of the carotid arteries (wall thickness and plaques as measured by ultrasonography) and the presence of atherosclerosis of the large vessels of the legs (assessed by the ratio of the ankle-to-brachial systolic blood pressure) were associated with Alzheimer's disease.[11] The prevalence of Alzheimer's disease increased with the degree of atherosclerosis. The odds ratio for Alzheimer's disease in those with severe atherosclerosis was 3.0 (95% CI 1.5–6.0) as compared to those without atherosclerosis. A strong interaction between apolipoprotein E (ApoE) ε4 allele and atherosclerosis was observed. Subjects with at least one ApoE ε4 allele and severe atherosclerosis had a nearly 20 times increased risk for Alzheimer's disease.[11] Since ApoE ε4 is not only associated with Alzheimer's disease but is also involved in atherosclerosis, we then evaluated whether ApoE genotype was associated with dementia through atherosclerosis. Since neither adjusting nor stratification for atherosclerosis altered the association of ApoE with dementia, atherosclerosis seems not to be an intermediate factor. We did however confirm a synergistic effect between ApoE ε4 and atherosclerosis on the risk of dementia, which fits the hypothesis that ApoE is involved in the response to cerebral damage.[12]

Smoking Risk

People who smoked cigarettes had a more than twofold increased risk to develop Alzheimer's disease.[13] This finding contrasted with results from earlier studies that reported a protective effect from smoking. A possible explanation is that the studies that showed a protective effect included much younger cases, and that the relation between smoking and Alzheimer's disease is age-dependent, for example, because of different genetic susceptibility. Some support for this comes from the observation among early onset patients that the inverse association between smoking and Alzheimer's disease was limited to carriers of the ApoE ε4 allele.[14] Smoking may exert different and opposite effects on the risk of Alzheimer's disease, being generally harmful through, for example, a vascular mechanism, but also partly beneficial in specific individuals, especially in those who carry an ApoE ε4 allele.[15] Our finding in the Rotterdam Study that the elevated relative risk was particularly present for smokers without the ApoE ε4 allele, is in line with this hypothesis.[13]

Diabetes Mellitus

We evaluated the relation between diabetes mellitus and dementia both cross-sectionally and prospectively. Subjects with diabetes mellitus had dementia more often than those without, in particular subjects with insulin-treated diabetes (odds ratio for dementia 3.2 (95% CI 1.4–7.5), odds ratio for Alzheimer's disease 2.8 (95% CI 1.0–8.0)).[16] Those with diabetes were also more likely to develop dementia and Alzheimer's disease during on average 2.1 years of followup (relative risk of Alzheimer's disease 1.9 (95% CI 1.2–3.1)).[17] The risk of Alzheimer's disease was again highest among subjects who were treated with insulin (RR 4.3; 95% CI 1.7–10.5).

Atrial Fibrillation

In the Rotterdam Study, atrial fibrillation as assessed in standard 12-lead ECGs, was significantly more frequent among subjects with dementia (age- and gender-adjusted odds ratio 2.3; 95% CI 1.4–3.7). The relation was slightly stronger for subjects with clinically diagnosed Alzheimer's disease than for subjects with vascular dementia, and could not be explained by a history of stroke. The associations were stronger in women than for men (age-adjusted odds ratio for dementia 3.1 (95% CI 1.7–5.5) and 1.3 (95% CI 0.5–3.1), respectively).[18]

Hemostasis

Thrombosis plays a central role in the pathogenesis of vascular disease. This raises the question whether hemostatic status is also of importance for the development of dementia. A low anticoagulant response of plasma to activated protein C (APC), or APC resistance, increases the risk of venous thrombosis as well as stroke.[19,20] A low APC response is frequently due to the factor V Leiden mutation;[21] however, no association between factor V Leiden and stroke has been found.[22,23] In a cross-sectional analysis based on prevalent cases of dementia of the Rotterdam Study, response to APC was not associated with dementia or its subtype Alzheimer's disease.[24] Carriers of the factor V Leiden mutation had a more than twofold increased probability of being demented than those without that mutation, which was borderline significant. Although the association seemed stronger for vascular dementia, it was present among Alzheimer patients as well.[24] Other abnormalities in the hemostatic and thrombotic systems, including hypercoagulability (as further assessed by thrombin/antithrombin complex (TAT); fibrinogen; prothrombin fragments 1+2) and abnormal endogeneous fibrinolytic activity (as measured through plasminogen activator inhibitor type 1 (PAI-1); tissue type plasminogen activator (t-PA) and D-dimer were assessed in the same study population. TAT and t-PA were associated with both Alzheimer's disease and vascular dementia, suggesting that predominantly increased thrombin generation was associated with dementia.[25]

Lipids

In the Rotterdam Study no relation was found between serum cholesterol levels and risk of dementia within 2 years (unpublished data). High dietary baseline intake of total fat, saturated fat, and cholesterol, which reflects habitual dietary intake, did however increase the risk of dementia and Alzheimer's disease (RR = 2.4, 95% CI 1.1–5.2; RR = 1.9, 95% CI 0.9–4.0; and RR = 1.7, 95% CI 0.9–3.2, respectively). Fish consumption on the other hand, an important source of n-3 polyunsaturated fatty acids, was inversely related to incident dementia (RR = 0.4, 95% CI 0.2–0.91), and in particular to Alzheimer's disease (RR = 0.3, 95% CI 0.1–0.9).[26]

Inflammation

There is increasing evidence that inflammatory processes may be involved in the etiology of dementia and Alzheimer's disease,[27–29] either through a local neuro-inflammatory response that contributes to cerebral amyloid deposition, or through the involvement of inflammation in the occurrence and progression of atherosclerosis. Studies that reported lower risks of Alzheimer's disease in subjects who used nonsteroidal antiinflammatory drugs (NSAIDs) have been interpreted as supporting this notion. In a cross-sectional analysis on the baseline cohort of the Rotterdam Study, prevalence of AD was significantly lower in users of NSAIDs as compared to the total cohort of nonexposed.[30] However, studies on NSAIDs are particularly vulnerable for misclassification of exposure, and confounding by contraindication. Therefore, we subsequently performed a matched case-control study, nested in the Rotterdam Study cohort, to study NSAID use in the 10 years prior to the onset of AD. In this study, which still had some potential for bias but in which at least case ascertainment was complete and data on drug use were obtained from GPs' medical records, we could not confirm our earlier findings.[31]

Vascular Factors, White Matter Lesions, and Cognition

Cerebral white matter lesions are considered to mainly reflect cerebrovascular pathology and are abundantly present in demented subjects.[32] The precise etiology of the cerebral white matter lesions remains to be elucidated, in particular in Alzheimer's disease, but small vessel disease, on the basis of longstanding hypertension, chronic or acute hypoperfusion, or endothelial damage, seems to play an important role.

In a random subsample of 111 participants of the Rotterdam Study, several vascular risk factors and indicators of vascular disease were associated with presence and severity of cerebral white matter lesions, including several noninvasive indicators of atherosclerosis, history of stroke or myocardial infarction, factor VIIc actitivity, and fibrinogen level.[7,33] Blood pressure level, hypertension, and plasma cholesterol were significantly associated with white matter lesions in younger subjects (aged 65–74 years) only. Nondemented persons with white matter lesions performed significantly worse on tests of cognitive function, in particular those assessing executive control and mental speed.[34]

To investigate these associations in more depth, we then initiated the Rotterdam Scan Study. In this cohort of 1077 persons we found that diastolic and systolic blood pressure levels were associated with both subcortical and periventricular cerebral white matter lesions.[35] However, since the actual blood pressure level is the resultant of a lifelong exposure to factors that have influenced it and does not provide information on previous blood pressure level, we investigated the relation between change in blood pressure and white matter lesions. We found a J-shaped relation between change of diastolic blood pressure over a period of 20 years and both types of white matter lesions, which could in part be attributed to subjects with a history of myocardial infarction. A possible explanation for this J-shape is that among persons with advanced vascular pathology, possibly because of longstanding hypertension, cerebral autoregulation is impaired. When we investigated several noninvasive indicators of atherosclerosis, including intima-media wall thickness of the carotid arteries, plaques in the carotid arteries, and aortic calcifications, in relation to white matter lesions we found significant associations with severe periventricular white matter lesions but not with subcortical white matter lesions. This suggests that different pathophysiological events underlie periventricular and subcortical white matter lesions, possibly related to vascularization. This finding was of particular interest in the light of the relation that we observed between white matter lesions and cognitive function: when periventricular lesions were analyzed conditional on subcortical lesions and vice versa, the periventricular lesions were associated with worse cognitive function, but the subcortical lesions were not.[36]

CONCLUSION

There is a considerable evidence now from our studies in Rotterdam that consistently points to an increased risk of dementia, including Alzheimer's disease, for persons with vascular risk factors and vascular disease. Other epidemiologic studies corroborate our findings. It is as yet unclear whether the association between vascular risk factors and Alzheimer's disease reflects a direct etiologic relation, a triggering effect of vascular disease on Alzheimer pathology, a shared etiology, or diagnostic misclassification due to overdiagnosing Alzheimer's disease in subjects with mixed pathology. However, it seems that what we clinically call Alzheimer's disease is a multifactorial disorder, in particular at older age; and that vascular pathology causes or contributes to the dementia syndrome in a substantial proportion of all demented patients. Future epidemiologic studies will have to confirm and quantify these associations also over longer periods of followup and help identify specific mechanisms.

REFERENCES

1. SKOOG, I., R.N. KALARIA & M.M.B. BRETELER. 1999. Vascular factors and Alzheimer's disease. Alzheimer Dis. Assoc. Disord. **13** (Suppl. 3): S106–S114.
2. BRETELER, M.M.B. Vascular risk factors for Alzheimer's disease: an epidemiologic perspective. *In* Cerebrovascular Amyloidosis in Alzheimer's Disease and Related Disorders. M.M. Verbeek, H.V. Vinters & R.M. de Waal, Eds. Kluwer Academic Publishers. Dordrecht, the Netherlands. In press.
3. HOFMAN, A., D.E. GROBBEE, P.T.V.M. DE JONG, P.T.V.M. & F.A. VAN DEN OUWELAND. 1991. Determinants of disease and disability in the elderly: the Rotterdam elderly study. Eur. J. Epidemiol. **7**: 403–422.
4. BRETELER, M.M.B., F.A. VAN DEN OUWELAND, D.E. GROBBEE & A. HOFMAN. 1992. A community-based study of dementia: the Rotterdam elderly study. Neuroepidemiology **11** (Suppl. 1): 23–28.
5. OTT, A., M.M.B. BRETELER, F. VAN HARSKAMP, J.J. CLAUS, T.J.M. VAN DER CAMMEN, D.E. GROBBEE & A. HOFMAN. 1995. Prevalence of Alzheimer's disease and vascular dementia: association with education: the Rotterdam Study. BMJ **310**: 970–973.

6. OTT, A., M.M.B. BRETELER, F. VAN HARSKAMP, T. STIJNEN & A. HOFMAN. 1998. Incidence and risk of dementia: the Rotterdam Study. Am. J. Epidemiol. **147:** 574–580.

7. BRETELER, M.M.B., J.C. VAN SWIETEN, M.L. BOTS, D.E. GROBBEE, J.J. CLAUS, J.H.W. VAN DEN HOUT, F. VAN HARSKAMP, H.L.J. TANGHE, P.T.V.M. DE JONG, J. VAN GIJN & A. HOFMAN. 1994. Cerebral white matter lesions, vascular risk factors and cognitive function in a population-based study. Neurology **44:** 1246–1252.

8. HOFMAN, A., F. BOOMSMA, M.A.D.H. SCHALEKAMP & H.A. VALKENBURG. 1979. Raised blood pressure and plasma noradrenaline concentrations in teenagers and young adults selected from an open population. BMJ **1:** 1536–1538.

9. BRETELER, M.M.B., J.J. CLAUS, D.E. GROBBEE & A. HOFMAN. 1994. Cardiovascular disease and the distribution of cognitive function in an elderly population: the Rotterdam Study. BMJ **308:** 1604–1608.

10. KALMIJN, S., L.J. LAUNER, J. LINDEMANS, J.L. BOTS, A. HOFMAN & M.M.B. BRETELER. 1999. Total homocysteine and cognitive decline in a community-based sample of elderly subjects: the Rotterdam Study. Am. J. Epidemiol. **150:** 283–289.

11. HOFMAN, A., A. OTT, M.M.B. BRETELER, M.L. BOTS, A.J.C. SLOOTER, F. VAN HARSKAMP, C.M. VAN DUIJN, C. VAN BROECKHOVEN & D.E. GROBBEE. 1997. Atherosclerosis, apolipoprotein E and the prevalence of dementia and Alzheimer's disease in the Rotterdam Study. Lancet **349:** 151–154.

12. SLOOTER, A.J.C., M. CRUTS, A. OTT, M.L. BOTS, J.C.M. WITTEMAN, A. HOFMAN, C. VAN BROECKHOVEN, M.M.B. BRETELER & C.M. VAN DUIJN. 1999. The effect of APOE on dementia is not through atherosclerosis: the Rotterdam Study. Neurology **53:** 1593–1595.

13. OTT, A., A.J.C. SLOOTER, A. HOFMAN, F. VAN HARSKAMP, J.C.M. WITTEMAN, C. VAN BROECKHOVEN, C.M. VAN DUIJN & M.M.B. BRETELER. 1998. Smoking and risk of dementia and Alzheimer's disease in a population-based cohort study: the Rotterdam Study. Lancet **351:** 1840–1843.

14. VAN DUIJN, C.M., L.M. HAVEKES, C. VAN BROECKHOVEN, P. DE KNIJFF & A. HOFMAN. 1995. Apolipoprotein E genotype and association between smoking and early onset Alzheimer's disease. BMJ **310:** 627–631.

15. POIRIER, J., M.-C. DELISLE, R. QUIRION et al. 1995. Apolipoprotein E4 allele as a predictor of cholinergic deficits and treatment outcome in Alzheimer disease. Proc. Natl. Acad. Sci. USA **92:** 12260–12264.

16. OTT, A., R.P. STOLK, A. HOFMAN, F. VAN HARSKAMP, D.E. GROBBEE & M.M.B. BRETELER. 1996. Association of diabetes mellitus and dementia: the Rotterdam Study. Diabetologia **39:** 1392–1397.

17. OTT, A., R.P. STOLK, F. VAN HARSKAMP, H.A.P. POLS, A. HOFMAN & M.M.B. BRETELER. 1999. Diabetes mellitus and the risk of dementia: the Rotterdam Study. Neurology **53:** 1937–1942.

18. OTT, A., M.M.B. BRETELER, M.C. DE BRUYNE, F. VAN HARSKAMP, D.E. GROBBEE & A. HOFMAN. 1997. Atrial fibrillation and dementia in a population-based study: the Rotterdam Study. Stroke **28:** 316–321.

19. KOSTER, T., F.R. ROSENDAAL, H. RONDE, E. BRIET, J.P. VANDENBROUCKE & R.M. BERTINA. 1993. Venous thrombosis due to poor anticoagulant response to activated protein C: Leiden Thrombophilia Study. Lancet **342:** 1503–1506.

20. SVENSSON, P.J. & B. DAHLBACK. 1994. Resistance to activated protein C as a basis for venous thrombosis. N. Engl. J. Med. **330:** 517–522.

21. BERTINA, R.M., B.P.C. KOELEMAN, T. KOSTER, F.R. ROSENDAAL, R.J. DIRVEN, H. DE RONDE, P.A. VAN DER VELDEN & P.H. REITSMA. 1994. Mutation in blood coagulation factor V associated with resistance to activated protein C. Nature **369:** 64–67.

22. KONTULA, K., A. YLIKORLALA, H. MIETTINEN, A. VUORIO, R. KAUPPINEN-MÄKELIN, L. HÄMÄLÄINEN, H. PALOMAKI & M. KASTE. 1995. Arg506Gln factor V mutation in patients with ischemic cerebrovascular disease and survivors of myocardial infarction. Thromb. Haemost. **73:** 558–560.

23. RIDKER, P.M., C.H. HENNEKENS, K. LINDPAINTER, M.J. STAMPFER, P.R. EISENBERG & J.P. MILETICH. 1995. Mutation in the gene coding for coagulation factor V and the risk of myocardial infarction, stroke and venous thrombosis in apparently healthy men. N. Engl. J. Med. **332:** 912–917.

24. Bots, M.L., F. van Kooten, M.M.B. Breteler, P.E. Slagboom, A. Hofman, F. Haverkate, P. Meijer, P.J. Koudstaal, D.E. Grobbee & C. Kluft. 1998. Response to activated protein C in subjects with and without dementia: the Dutch vascular factors in dementia study. Haemostasis 28: 209–215.
25. Bots, M.L., M.M.B. Breteler, F. van Kooten, F. Haverkate, P. Meijer, P.J. Koudstaal, D.E. Grobbee & C. Kluft. 1998. Coagulation and fibrinolysis markers and risk of dementia: the Dutch vascular factors in dementia study. Haemostasis 28: 216–222.
26. Kalmijn, S., L.J. Launer, A. Ott, J.C.M. Witteman, A. Hofman & M.M.B. Breteler. 1999. Dietary fat intake and the risk of dementia in a population-based study: the Rotterdam Study. Ann. Neurol. 42: 776–782.
27. McGeer, P.L. & E.G. McGeer. 1995. The inflammatory response system of brain: implications for therapy of Alzheimer and other neurodegenerative diseases. Brain Res. Rev. 21: 195–218.
28. Eikelenboom, P. & R. Veerhuis. 1996. The role of complement and activated microglia in the pathogenesis of Alzheimer's disease. Neurobiol. Aging 17: 673–680.
29. Thomas, T., M. Mullan et al. 1996. beta-Amyloid-mediated vasoactivity and vascular endothelial damage. Nature 380: 168–171.
30. Andersen, K., L.J. Launer, A. Ott, A.W. Hoes, M.M.B. Breteler & A. Hofman. 1995. Do nonsteroidal anti-inflammatory drugs decrease the risk for Alzheimer's disease? The Rotterdam Study. Neurology 45: 1441-1445.
31. in 't Veld, B.A., L.J. Launer, A.A.W. Hoes, A. Ott, A. Hofman, M.M.B. Breteler & B.H.C. Stricker. 1998. NSAIDs and incident Alzheimer's disease: the Rotterdam Study. Neurobiol. Aging 19: 607–611.
32. de Groot, J.C., F.E. de Leeuw & M.M.B. Breteler. 1998. Cognitive correlates of cerebral white matter changes. J. Neural Transm. Suppl. 53: 41–67.
33. Bots, M.L., J.C. van Swieten, M.M.B. Breteler, P.T.V.M. de Jong, J. van Gijn, A. Hofman & D.E. Grobbee. 1993. Cerebral white matter lesions and atherosclerosis in the Rotterdam Study. Lancet 341: 1232–1237.
34. Breteler, M.M.B., N.M. van Amerongen, J.C. van Swieten, J.J. Claus, D.E. Grobbee, J. van Gijn, A. Hofman & F. van Harskamp. 1994. Cognitive correlates of ventricular enlargement and cerebral white matter lesions on MRI: the Rotterdam Study. Stroke 25: 1109-1115.
35. de Leeuw, F.E., J.C. de Groot, M. Oudkerk, J.C.M. Witteman, A. Hofman, J. van Gijn & M.M.B. Breteler. 1999. A follow-up study of blood pressure and cerebral white matter lesions. Ann. Neurol. 46: 827–833.
36. de Groot, J.C., F.E. de Leeuw, M. Oudkerk, J. van Gijn, A. Hofman, J. Jolles & M.M.B. Breteler. 2000. Cerebral white matter lesions and cognitive function: the Rotterdam Scan Study. Ann. Neurol. 47: 145–151.

Relevance of White Matter Changes to Pre- and Poststroke Dementia

FLORENCE PASQUIER,[a,c] HILDE HÉNON,[a,b] AND DIDIER LEYS[b]

Department of Neurology, [a]Memory and [b]Stroke Units, EA 2691 MENRT, University Hospital of Lille, F-59037 Lille, France

ABSTRACT: White matter changes are often associated with stroke, risk factors for stroke, and dementia. From a theoretical point of view, they may be associated with an increased risk of pre- or poststroke dementia because (i) they are linked with subtle cognitive decline, which may add to the consequences of the stroke lesions and of associated Alzheimer pathology; and (ii) they indicate an increased risk of stroke recurrence. The aim of this study was to evaluate the contribution of white matter changes to pre- and poststroke dementia. The relationship between preexisting dementia and white matter changes was evaluated in the Lille stroke–dementia cohort. We assessed the cognitive functioning prior to stroke in 202 consecutive patients with ischemic or hemorrhagic stroke, by means of the Informant Questionnaire on Cognitive Decline in the Elderly (IQCODE). We classified in the dementia group patients with IQCODE scores of 104 or more. White matter changes were rated on CT with the Blennow's rating scale. Thirty-three of 202 patients were demented before stroke (16.3%; 95% confidence interval: 11.2–21.4); the logistic regression analysis found that female sex, family dementia, white matter changes, and cerebral atrophy were independently associated with prestroke dementia. White matter changes were also associated with an increased risk of poststroke dementia, 2 years after stroke onset. Thus, white matter changes contribute to dementia occurring in stroke patients.

INTRODUCTION

White matter abnormalities are often associated with stroke and with risk factors for stroke such as age, arterial hypertension, cardiac diseases, and diabetes mellitus (for review see Leys *et al.*[1]). They can be associated with subtle neuropsychological and behavioral changes: patients with white matter hyperintensities perform worse in tests measuring executive functions, mental speed, attention, and delayed verbal recall,[2] at least above a threshold in healthy elderly individuals.[3] Therefore, the contribution of white matter changes to pre- and poststroke dementia should be considered.

White matter changes are more frequent in so-called vascular dementia (VaD) than in Alzheimer's disease (AD).[4] They are an independent predictor of poststroke dementia.[5] Among stroke patients, leukoaraiosis is more frequent in those who have lacunes or deep cerebral hemorrhages than in those who have territorial infarcts or superficial hemorrhages.[6,7] Stroke patients who have the highest risk to have white

[c]Address for correspondence: Florence Pasquier, M.D., Ph.D., Clinique Neurologique, Centre Hospitalier et Universitaire, 59037 Lille, France. Tel.: +33 320 44 57 85; fax: +33 320 44 60 28. e-mail: pasquier@chru-lille.fr

matter changes are patients with presumed small-vessel diseases.[1] The consequences of the cognitive impairment are more prominent in patients with lacunar infarcts and with no or mild physical disability. Therefore, multiple lacunar infarcts in both hemispheres and in strategic areas are one main cause of VaD.

Besides age, previous stroke, cerebral atrophy, left side of infarcts, and total infarction area, extent of white matter changes are a risk factor of poststroke dementia.[1,8] White matter changes are associated with a higher risk of stroke recurrence after adjustment to age and to other vascular risk factors.[9,10] However, stroke can be considered the cause of only one-half of poststroke dementia.[9] Alzheimer pathology and white matter changes may also contribute to cognitive decline, and in most patients these mechanisms may be combined.[11]

The aim of this study was to evaluate the contribution of white matter changes to pre- and poststroke dementia.

METHOD

The link between preexisting dementia and white matter changes was evaluated in the Lille stroke–dementia cohort.[12] We assessed the cognitive status before stroke in 202 consecutive patients aged over 40 years with ischemic or hemorrhagic stroke by means of the Informant Questionnaire on Cognitive Decline in the Elderly (IQ-CODE)[13] within the first 48 hours after stroke onset. We classified patients with IQ-CODE scores ≤104 as having preexisting dementia. At admission, CT scan were performed without contrast, on an Elscint 2004 Elite Plus machine by means of 5-mm contiguous slices. Leukoaraisis was defined according to the criteria of Inzitari *et al.*[14] and scored by means of the 0–3 point rating scale of Blennow *et al.*[15] It was assessed on the hemisphere contralateral to the focal vascular lesion, if any. Cerebral atrophy was scored on the Leys *et al.*[16] 0–3 point rating scale. We determined the number and location of old infarcts and silent infarcts. At 6 months, 1 year, and 2 years post stroke, survivors underwent a battery of neuropsychological tests. A structured interview for psychiatric symptoms and a questionnaire of activity of daily living were performed. Dementia was determined according to the DSM-IV criteria. Criteria for AD were those of the NINCDS-ADRDA work group, and criteria for VaD were those of the NINDS-AIREN group.

RESULTS

Of the 202 patients (105 women, 97 men; median age 75 years, range: 42–101 years; 25 deep hemorrhages; 177 ischemic strokes); 33 (16.3%; 95% CI, 11.2–21.4) had a prestroke dementia. Only one was recognized before stroke. Leukoaraiosis was a significant ($p = 0.0002$) independent variable of prestroke dementia according to the logistic regression analysis, besides female sex ($p = 0.0002$), family history of dementia ($p = 0.0016$), and cerebral atrophy score ($p = 0.01$). Of the 33 patients with prestroke dementia, 22 died within 2 years; 11 were seen at least one time; 7 had AD and 4 had VaD. All of these 11 demented patients had leukoaraiosis, except one patient with AD.

Of the 169 remaining patients, 58 died within 2 years; 104 were seen at least one time; 29 had dementia. Of the 29 patients with poststroke dementia (AD=10, VaD=17, others=2), 22 (76%) had leukoaraiosis at stroke onset, whereas 24 (32%) of the 75 patients without dementia 2 years post stroke had leukoaraiosis at onset ($p < 0.0001$).

DISCUSSION

This study showed that leukoaraisosis was associated with pre- and poststroke dementia. Extent of white matter changes was found to be one risk factor of poststroke dementia.[8] In our study, AD was the cause of two-thirds of prestroke and of one-third of poststroke dementia, and VaD was the cause of one-third of prestroke and of two-thirds of poststroke dementia. There is some overlap between AD and VaD. Wallin suggested that leukoaraiosis could be one feature implicated in this overlap,[17] especially in subtypes of AD. Less pronounced Alzheimer pathology is required for the development of dementia if there is also vascular involvement such as white matter changes.[18] White matter lesions are linked with hypertension and hypotension,[19,20] diabetes mellitus, and coronary artery disease[21] and would be more extensive in patients with the ApoE ε4-ε4 than in others.[22] These factors are risk factors for AD and for cerebrovascular disease.

White matter changes seem to be a risk factor for pre- and poststroke dementia. This could be related to Alzheimer as well as to vascular pathology and could be mediated through several different pathogenic pathways.[23]

REFERENCES

1. LEYS, D., H. HÉNON & F. PASQUIER. 1998. White matter changes and poststroke dementia. Dement. Geriatr. Cogn. Disord. 9(Suppl. 1): 25–29.
2. BRETELER, M.M.B., J.C. VAN SWIETEN, M.L. BOTS et al. 1994. Cerebral white matter lesions, vascular risk factors, and cognitive function in a population-based study: The Rotterdam study. Neurology 44: 12466–1252.
3. BOONE, K.B., B.L. MILLER, C.M. MEHRINGER et al. 1992. Neuropsychological correlates of white-matter lesions in healthy elderly subjects: a threshold effect. Arch. Neurol. 49: 549–554.
4. SCHMIDT, R. 1992. Comparison of magnetic resonance imaging in Alzheimer's disease, vascular dementia and normal aging. Eur. Neurol. 32: 164–169.
5. TATEMICHI, T.K., M. PAIK, E. BAGLIELLA et al. 1994. Risk of dementia after stroke in a hospitalized cohort: results of a longitudinal study. Neurology 44: 1885–1891.
6. HIJDRA, A., B. VERBEETEN, JR. & J.A.P.M. VERHULST. 1990. Relation of leukoaraiosis to lesion type in stroke patients. Stroke 21: 890–894.
7. LEYS, D., J.P. PRUVO, Ph. SCHELTENS et al. 1992. Leukoaraiosis: relationship with the types of focal lesions occuring in acute cerebrovascular disorders. Cerebrovasc. Dis. 2: 169–176.
8. LIU, C.K., B.L. MILLER, J.L. CUMMINGS et al. 1992. A quantitative MRI study of vascular dementia. Neurology 42: 138–143.
9. TATEMICHI, T.K., M.A. FOULKES, J.P. MOHR et al. 1990. Dementia in stroke survivors in the stroke data bank cohort: prevalence, incidence, risk factors and computed tomographic findings. Stroke 21: 858–866.
10. INZITARI, D., A. DiCARLO, M. MASCHALCHI et al. 1995. The cardiovascular outcome of patients with motor impairment and extensive leukoaraiosis. Arch. Neurol. 52: 687–681.

11. PASQUIER, F. & D. LEYS. 1997. Why are stroke patients prone to develop dementia? J. Neurol. **244:** 135–142.
12. HÉNON, H., F. PASQUIER, I. DURIEU *et al.* 1997. Preexisting dementia in stroke patients. Baseline frequency, associated factors, and outcome. Stroke **28:** 2429–2436.
13. JORM, A.F. & A.E. KORTEN. 1988. Assesment of cognitive decline in the elderly by informant interview. Br. J. Psychiatry **152:** 209–213.
14. INZITARI, D., G.P. GIORDANO, A.L. ANCONA *et al.* 1990. Leuko-araiosis, intracerebral hemorrhage and arterial hypertension. Stroke **21:** 1419–1423.
15. BLENNOW, K., A. WALLIN, C. UHLEMANN & C.G. GOTTFRIES. 1991. White-matter lesions on CT in Alzheimer patients: relationship to clinical symptomatology and vascular factors. Acta Neurol. Scand. **83:** 187–193.
16. LEYS, D., J.P. PRUVO, H. PETIT *et al.* 1989. Maladie d'Alzheimer: analyse statistique des résultats du scanner X. Rev. Neurol. (Paris) **145:** 134–139.
17. WALLIN, A. 1998. The overlap between Alzheimer's disease and vascular dementia: the role of white matter changes. Dement. Geriatr. Cogn. Disord. **9**(Suppl. 1): 30–35.
18. SNOWDON, D.A., L.H. GREINER, J.A. MORTIMER *et al.* 1997. Brain infarction and the clinical expression of Alzheimer disease: The Nun Study. JAMA **227:** 813–817.
19. SKOOG, I. 1998. A review on blood pressure and ischaemic white matter lesions. Dement. Geriatr. Cogn. Disord. **9**(Suppl. 1): 13–19.
20. VELDINK, J.H., PH. SCHELTENS, C. JONKER & L.J. LAUNER. 1998. Progression of cerebral white matter hyperintensities on MRI is related to diastolic blood pressure. Neurology **51:** 319–320.
21. GUPTA, S.R., M.H. NAHEEDY, J.C. YOUNG *et al.* 1988. Periventricular white matter changes and dementia. Clinical, neuropsychological, radiological, and pathological correlation. Arch. Neurol. **45:** 637–641.
22. BRONGE, L., S.E. FERNAEUS, M. BLOMBERG *et al.* 1999. White matter lesions in Alzheimer patients are influenced by apolipoprotein E genotype. Dement. Geriatr. Cogn. Disord. **10:** 89–86.
23. VAN GIJN, J. 1998. Leukoaraiosis and vascular dementia. Neurology **51**(Suppl. 3): S3–S8.

Corpus Callosum Measurement as an *in Vivo* Indicator for Neocortical Neuronal Integrity, but not White Matter Pathology, in Alzheimer's Disease

HARALD HAMPEL,[a,b,c] STEFAN J. TEIPEL,[a,b] GENE E. ALEXANDER,[b] BARRY HORWITZ,[b] PIETRO PIETRINI,[b] HANNS HIPPIUS,[a] HANS-JÜRGEN MÖLLER,[a] MARK B. SCHAPIRO,[b] AND STANLEY I. RAPOPORT[b]

[a]*Dementia and Neuroimaging Section, Department of Psychiatry, Ludwig-Maximilian University, 80336 Munich, Germany*

[b]*Laboratory of Neurosciences, National Institute on Aging, National Institutes of Health, Bethesda, Maryland 20892, USA*

The primary neocortical histopathologic changes of Alzheimer's disease (AD) are found predominately in layer 3 and 5 large pyramidal neurons within association cortex.[1–4] These neurons give rise to long-reaching intracortical projections.[5–10] Their selective loss has been proposed as the substrate of a progressive neocortical disconnection syndrome in AD.[11] Until now, the question has been unresolved as to what extent subcortical fiber degeneration contributes to cortical disconnection in AD. In a histopathologic study on postmortem brain tissue from patients with AD, Brun and Englund (1986) described white matter lesions which markedly differed in quantity from subcortical lesions in nondemented controls and in quality from lesions found in multi-infarct dementia.[12] Several investigators later used T2-weighted magnetic resonance imaging (MRI) to visualize subcortical lesions as areas of increased signal intensity (white matter hyperintensities [WMH])[13–15] when investigating subcortical pathology in AD compared with cognitively healthy age-matched controls. WMH, however, have commonly been found in T2-weighted MRI scans of older subjects, correlating with age, cerebrovascular disease, and hypertension.[16–21] They occur both in cognitively unimpaired subjects[22] and in dementia.[18,23] A disease-specific difference between AD patients and healthy elderly subjects with regard to the quantity of WMH is still controversial.[23–26] Even less is known about possible regional differences in the distribution of white matter lesions in AD compared to controls.[27]

To elucidate possible topological differences in the distribution of WMH between AD patients and age-matched healthy control subjects, we used a previously reported rating scale which provides semiquantitative measures for lobar and periventricular WMH load. A relatively high inter-rater reliability has been reported for this scale.[28] To assess the contribution of subcortical pathology to neocortical disconnec-

[c]Address for correspondence: Harald Hampel, M.D., Dementia and Neuroimaging Section, Department of Psychiatry, Ludwig-Maximilian University, Nussbaumstr. 7, 80336 Munich, Germany. Tel.: +01149-89-5160-5822; fax: +49-89-5160-5856.
e-mail: hampel@psy.med.uni-muenchen.de

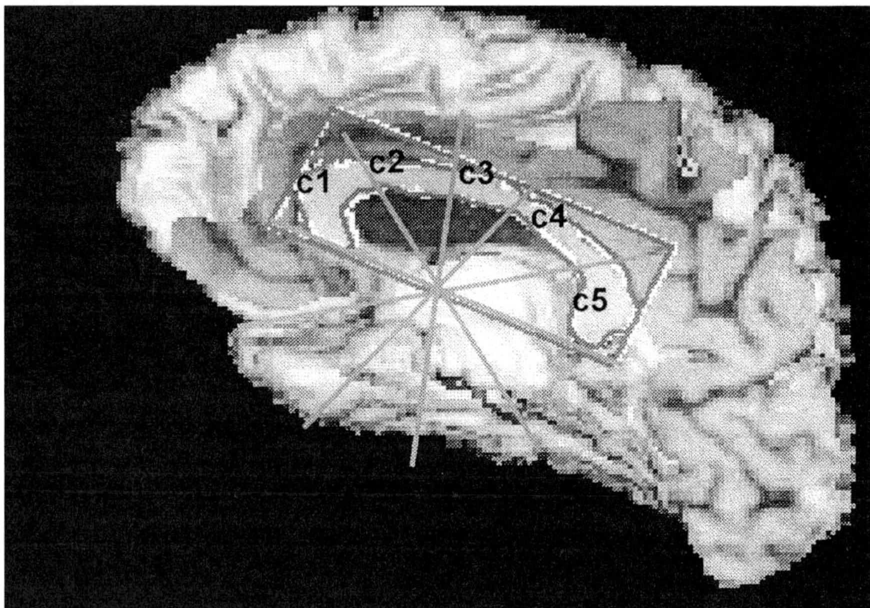

FIGURE 1. Corpus callosum measurement method as described elsewhere:[35] midsagittal view of regions c1 (anterior/rostrum) to c5 (posterior/splenium).

tion, we correlated corpus callosum atrophy and WMH load on a regional basis in healthy aging and in AD. Studies of the corpus callosum are particulary interesting, because corpus callosum atrophy can reflect subcortical fiber degeneration, as shown in multiple sclerosis or vascular dementia,[29–34] as well as primary loss of callosally projecting large pyramidal neurons of neocortical layers 3 and 5. Using a newly developed method to measure total and regional areas of corpus callosum in MRI (FIG. 1) in a previous study, we reported a region-specific pattern of corpus callosum atrophy in AD patients having minimal subcortical hyperintensities compared to healthy age matched controls.[35] Both groups were not hypertensive and had minimal cerebrovascular risk factors. The pattern of corpus callosum atrophy in these patients indicated a cell-type-specific loss of interhemispheric projecting neurons, due to primary neocortical pathology in AD. This was further supported by a statistically significant correlation between regional corpus callosum atrophy and the regional pattern of cortical metabolic decline in [18]FDG-PET within the AD group.[36] In another recently published study, we investigated 20 AD patients and 21 healthy age-matched controls with a relatively wide range of subcortical hyperintensities. We did not find any statistically significant difference in total or regional WMH load between both groups.[37] Consistent with our previous findings on AD patients with only minimal white matter changes, we found atrophy in the patients of the anterior and posterior corpus callosum with a relative preservation of the callosal body. In healthy controls, frontal lobe WMH load was significantly correlated with anterior corpus callosum size (FIG. 2). No significant correlation, however, was observed be-

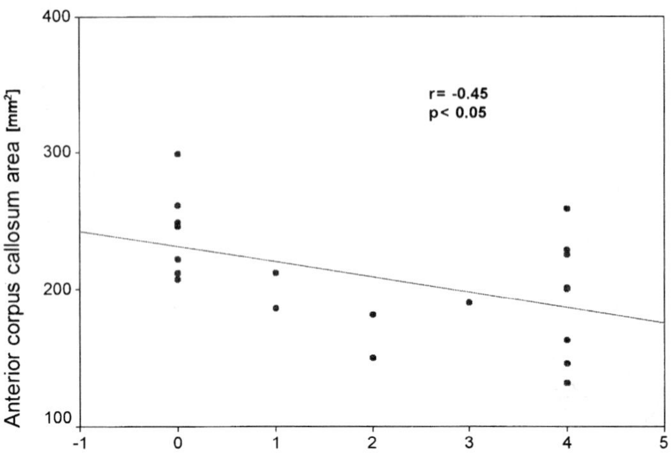

FIGURE 2. Correlation between anterior corpus callosum area and frontal lobe white matter hyperintensity load in 21 healthy elderly control subjects.

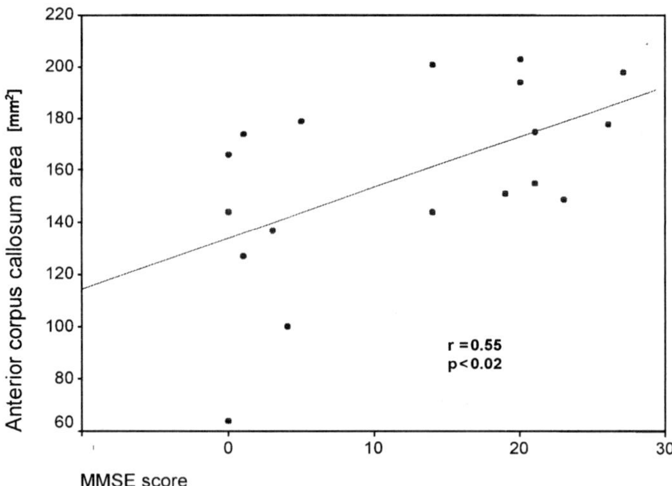

FIGURE 3. Correlation between anterior corpus callosum area and degree of cognitive impairment (MMSE-Score) in 20 patients with AD.

tween corpus callosum subregions and lobar WMH load in the AD group. Corpus callosum size was significantly correlated with the degree of cognitive impairment (MMSE score) in AD subjects (FIG. 3) and with age in healthy controls (FIG. 4). WMH load, however, was correlated only with age in both groups.

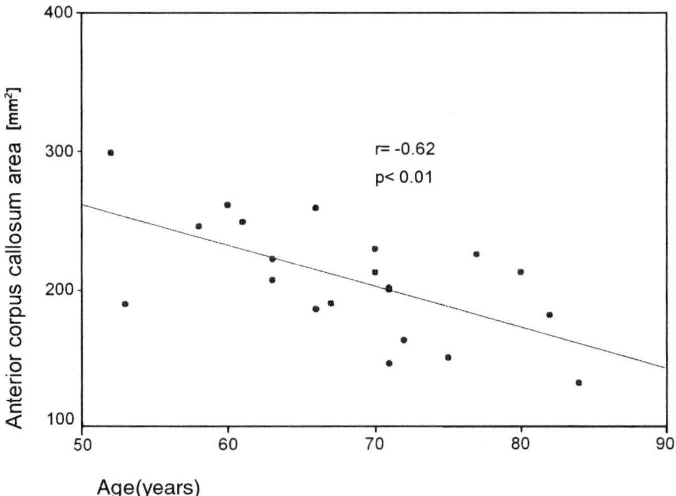

FIGURE 4. Correlation between anterior corpus callosum area and age in 21 healthy elderly control subjects.

In conclusion, no difference in the quantity and regional distribution of subcortical hyperintensities could be found between AD patients and healthy controls, who were carefully screened to exclude cerebrovascular risk factors. This supports the notion that WMH in both groups may result predominately from nonspecific age-related vascular changes.[38] A significant age-related correlation between frontal corpus callosum size and frontal lobe white matter load in the healthy controls is in agreement with reported data of frontal lobe involvement in healthy aging.[39,40] In AD, however, corpus callosum size appears to be related to disease severity, but not to the extent of subcortical fiber degeneration as measured by WMH load. The uncoupling between WMH and corpus callosum atrophy suggests that subcortical changes have only marginal effects on the neocortical disconnection in AD patients who do not have cerebrovascular risk factors.

It seems important, therefore, to investigate the relation of subcortical hyperintensities to the pattern of regional corpus callosum atrophy, particulary in patients with vascular dementia. While corpus callosum atrophy in nonhypertensive AD patients seems to primarily reflect abnormal cortical neuronal integrity, examining corpus callosum fibers, which traverse the subcortical white matter in an anterior-posterior topography, may allow us to identify effects of subcortical hyperintensities on cortical connectivity in vascular dementia. Quantitative changes in the corpus callosum therefore may be a valuable tool to assess neocortical integrity in different diseases on a regional basis.

To further establish the potential of the corpus callosum as an *in vivo* marker of cell-type-specific neocortical neuron loss in AD, the temporal sequence of hippocampal and corpus callosum atrophy in patients with early AD should be examined. A study on the strength of correlations between regional corpus callosum atrophy and regional pattern of cortical metabolic impairment in relation to dementia progression would further validate measures of corpus callosum area as a parameter of neocortical neuron loss.

Furthermore, it is of interest to establish a reliable *in vivo* marker for neuronal loss and neuronal integrity in AD, because it can be used in combination with PET in clinical drug trials in AD.[41] Metabolic impairment in PET reflects a continuum of AD pathology from reversible functional downregulation of neuronal metabolism to final and irreversible neuronal death.[42–44] The corpus callosum as potential *in vivo* marker for loss of cortical neurons may permit reversible functional impairment, where corpus callosum atrophy in spite of significant metabolic decline has not yet occurred, to be discriminated from disease stages with considerable irreversible neuronal loss. This would help to select promising groups of AD patients with at least partially reversible deficits for clinical intervention studies. Finally, measures of corpus callosum atrophy may serve as a valuable substitute for PET to assess neocortical functional integrity in clinical centers where PET is not available.

ACKNOWLEDGMENTS

This work was supported by a stipend from the Ernst Jung Foundation, Hamburg, Germany, to Dr. H. Hampel, connected to the Ernst Jung Medal in gold won by Prof. H. Hippius.

The authors thank Dr. P. Herscovitch for the excellent organization of the NIH PET program, the PET Department technologists, headed by Dr. P. Baldwin, as well as the MRI Department technologists for their assistance with scanning. We also thank the LNS medical and nursing staff for valuable support.

Part of the presented results have been read at scientific meetings and published, as indicated, in scientific journals.

REFERENCES

1. MANN, D.M. 1996. Pyramidal nerve cell loss in Alzheimer's disease. Neurodegeneration **5**: 423–427.
2. HOF, P.R. *et al.* 1991. Neocortical neuronal subpopulations labeled by a monoclonal antibody to calbindin exhibit differential vulnerability in Alzheimer's disease. Exp. Neurol. **111**: 293–301.
3. LEWIS, D.A. *et al.* 1987. Laminar and regional distributions of neurofibrillary tangles and neuritic plaques in Alzheimer's disease: a quantitative study of visual and auditory cortices. J. Neurosci. **7**: 1799–1808.
4. MORRISON, J.H. *et al.* 1987. A monoclonal antibody to non-phosphorylated neurofilament protein marks the vulnerable cortical neurons in Alzheimer's disease. Brain Res. **416**: 331–336.
5. ARENDT, T. *et al.* 1998. Cortical distribution of neurofibrillary tangles in Alzheimer's disease matches the pattern of neurons that retain their capacity of plastic remodelling in the adult brain. Neuroscience **83**: 991–1002.
6. MORRISON, J.H. *et al.* 1997. Life and death of neurons in the aging brain. Science **278**: 412–419.
7. ARMSTRONG, R.A. 1993. Is the clustering of neurofibrillary tangles in Alzheimer's patients related to the cells of origin of specific cortico-cortical projections? Neurosci. Lett. **160**: 57–60.

8. JONES, E.G. 1984. Laminar distribution of cortical efferent cells. *In* Cerebral Cortex: Cellular Components of the Cerebral Cortex. A. Peters & E.G. Jones, Eds.: 521–553. Plenum. New York.

9. TIGGES, J. *et al.* 1981. Areal and laminar distribution of neurons interconnecting the central visual cortical areas 17, 18, 19 and MT in squirrel monkey (saimiri). J. Comp. Neurol. **202:** 539–560.

10. GLICKSTEIN, M. *et al.* 1976. Degeneration of layer III pyramidal cells in area 18 following destruction of callosal input. Brain Res. **104:** 148–151.

11. MORRISON, J.H. *et al.* 1986. The laminar and regional distribution of neocortical somatostatin and neuritic plaques: implications for Alzheimer's disease as a global neocortical disconnection syndrome. *In* The Biological Substrates of Alzheimer's Disease. A.B. Scheibel & A.F. Weschler, Eds.: 115–131. Academic Press. New York.

12. BRUN, A. *et al.* 1986. A white matter disorder in dementia of the Alzheimer type: a pathoanatomical study. Ann. Neurol. **19:** 253–262.

13. AWAD, I.A. *et al.* 1986. Incidential subcortical lesions identified on magnetic resonance imaging in the elderly. II. Postmortem pathological correlations. Stroke **17:** 1090–1097.

14. BRAFFMAN, B. *et al.* 1988. Brain MR: pathologic correlation with gross and histopathology. 1. Lacunar infarction and Virchow-Robin spaces. Am. J. Neuroradiol. **9:** 621–628.

15. BRAFFMAN, B. *et al.* 1988. Brain MR: pathologic correlation with gross and histopathology. 2. Hyperintense white matter foci in the elderly. Am. J. Neuroradiol. **9:** 629–636.

16. SCHMIDT, R. *et al.* 1998. Prevalence and risk factors for white matter damage. *In* Uncommon Causes of Dementia. Current Issues in Neurodegenerative Disorders. F. Fazekas, R. Schmidt & A. Alavi, Eds.: 11–25. ICG Publications. Dordrecht.

17. PADOVANI, A. *et al.* 1997. Correlates of leukoaraiosis and ventricular enlargement on magnetic resonance imaging: a study in normal elderly and cerebrovascular patients. Eur. J. Neurol. **4:** 15–23.

18. BRETELER, M.M. *et al.* 1994. Cerebral white matter lesions, vascular risk factors, and cognitive function in a population-based study: the Rotterdam Study. Neurology **44:** 1246–1252.

19. AWAD, I.A. *et al.* 1986. Incidential subcortical lesions identified on magnetic resonance imaging in the elderly. I. Correlations with age and cerebrovascular risk factors. Stroke **17:** 1084–1089.

20. BRADLEY, W.G. *et al.* 1984. Patchy periventricular white matter lesions in the elderly: a common observation during NMR imaging. Noninvasive Med. Imag. **1:** 35–41.

21. YLIKOSKI, A. *et al.* 1995. White matter hyperintensities on MRI in the neurologically nondiseased elderly: analysis of cohorts of consecutive subjects aged 55 to 85 years living at home. Stroke **26:** 1171–1177.

22. ALMKVIST, O. *et al.* 1992. White-matter-hyperintensity and neuropsychological functions in dementia and healthy aging. Arch. Neurol. **49:** 626–532.

23. SCHMIDT, R. 1992. Comparison of magnetic resonance imaging in Alzheimer's disease, vascular dementia and normal aging. Eur. Neurol. **32:** 164–169.

24. SCHELTENS, P. *et al.* 1992. White matter lesions on magnetic resonance imaging in clinically diagnosed Alzheimer's disease. Brain **115:** 735–748.

25. BOWEN, B.C. *et al.* 1990. MR signal abnormalities in memory disorder and dementia. Am. J. Neuroradiol. **11:** 283–290.

26. ERKINJUNTTI, T. *et al.* 1994. Lack of difference in brain hyperintensities between patients with early Alzheimer's disease and control subjects. Arch Neurol. **51:** 260–268.

27. HAMPEL, H. *et al.* 1997. Strukturelle Magnetresonanztomographie in der Diagnose und Erforschung der Demenz vom Alzheimer-Typ. Nervenarzt **68:** 365–378.

28. SCHELTENS, P. *et al.* 1993. A semiquantitative rating scale for the assessment of signal hyperintensities on magnetic resonance imaging. J. Neurol. Sci. **114:** 7–12.

29. YAMANOUCHI, H. *et al.* 1990. Loss of nerve fibres in the corpus callosum of progressive subcortical vascular encephalopathy. J. Neurol. **237:** 39–41.

30. BARKHOF, F.J. *et al.* 1998. Functional correlates of callosal atrophy in relapsing-remitting multiple sclerosis patients. A preliminary MRI study. J. Neurol. **245:** 153–158.
31. LAISSY, J.P. *et al.* 1993. Midsagittal MR measurements of the corpus callosum in healthy subjects and diseased patients: a prospective survey. Am. J. Neuroradiol. **14:** 145–154.
32. LYOO, K. *et al.* 1997. Regional atrophy of the corpus callosum in subjects with Alzheimer's disease and multi-infarct dementia. Psychiatry Res. Neuroimaging **74:** 63–72.
33. POZZILLI, C. *et al.* 1991. Anterior corpus callosum atrophy and verbal fluency in multiple sclerosis. Cortex **27:** 441–445.
34. GEAN-MARTON, A.D. *et al.* 1991. Abnormal corpus callosum: a sensitive and specific indicator of multiple sclerosis. Radiology **180:** 215–221.
35. HAMPEL, H. *et al.* 1998. Corpus callosum atrophy is a possible indicator for region and cell type specific neuronal degeneration in Alzheimer disease: an MRI analysis. Arch. Neurol. **55:** 193–198.
36. TEIPEL, S.J. *et al.* 1999. Region specific corpus callosum atrophy correlates with regional pattern of cortical glucose metabolism in Alzheimer's disease. Arch. Neurol. **56:** 467–473.
37. TEIPEL, S.J. *et al.* 1998. Dissociation between white matter pathology and corpus callosum atrophy in Alzheimer's disease. Neurology **51:** 1381–1385.
38. FAZEKAS, F. *et al.* 1998. Pathophysiologic mechanisms in the development of age-related white matter changes of the brain. Dementia **9**(Suppl.): 2–5.
39. COWELL, P.E. *et al.* 1994. Sex differences in aging of the human frontal and temporal lobes. J. Neurosci. **14:** 4748–4755.
40. SALMON, E. *et al.* 1991. Decrease of frontal metabolism demonstrated by positron emission tomography in a population of healthy elderly volunteers. Acta Neurol. Belg. **91:** 288–295.
41. TEIPEL, S.J. *et al.* 1999. Positron emission tomography in Alzheimer's disease—from resting-state to activation studies. Drug News Perspect. **12**(2): 83–90.
42. RAPOPORT, S.I. 1983. Brain Metabolism in Aging and Dementia. Publication # 83-2625. National Institutes of Health Publication. U.S. Department of Health and Human Services, Public Health Service. Bethesda, MD.
43. RAPOPORT, S.I. & C.L. GRADY. 1993. Parametric *in vivo* brain imaging during activation to examine pathological mechanisms of functional failure in Alzheimer disease. Int. J. Neurosci. **70:** 39–56.
44. RAPOPORT S.I. 1991. Positron emission tomography in Alzheimer's disease in relation to disease pathogenesis: a critical review. Cerebrovasc. Brain Metab. Rev. **3:** 297–335.

Contrast-enhanced MRI of White Matter Lesions in Patients with Blood-Brain Barrier Dysfunction

LARS-OLOF WAHLUND[b,c] AND LENA BRONGE[a]

Departments of [a]Radiology and [b]Clinical Neuroscience, NEUROTEC,
Division of Geriatric Medicine, Huddinge University Hospital, Huddinge, Sweden

ABSTRACT: White matter lesions (WMLs) and blood-brain barrier (BBB) dysfunction are common in dementia. Both conditions may be a consequence of small-vessel disease, in which case the BBB damage could be suspected to be located to the WMLs. Magnetic resonance imaging (MRI) can be used to show WMLs as well as to detect BBB damage when using an intravenous contrast agent, gadolinium. We examined 10 demented patients with WMLs, including 5 cases with BBB (elevated CSF/serum albumin ratios). Results showed no significant changes in MR signal in the WMLs after contrast administration. We conclude that WMLs are not related to BBB damage to such a degree that is detectable with this method and that the elevated CSF albumin might have another origin.

INTRODUCTION

Nonspecific white matter lesions (WMLs) are commonly seen in magnetic resonance imaging (MRI) of the brains of the elderly. The etiology and clinical significance of WMLs have been the subject of some debate, with the more extensive WMLs being considered a result of chronic low-grade ischemia or malnutrition due to small-vessel disease in the watershed areas.[1,2]

A number of authors have reported a higher CSF/serum albumin ratio in patients with WMLs as compared to controls, indicating a blood-brain barrier (BBB) damage. This has been seen in both Alzheimer's disease (AD)[3] and vascular dementia (VaD),[4] as well as in non-demented patients with WMLs.[5] The fact that the increased albumin ratio seen in these patients was unrelated to cerebral infarcts suggests that the BBB impairment occurs as a consequence of a diffuse small-vessel disease.[4–7]

MRI is sensitive at detecting WMLs. Together with an intravenous paramagnetic contrast agent, such as gadolinium (Gd), MRI can also detect and quantify BBB damage.[8–10] There are indications that BBB dysfunction observed in some dementia patients may be due to the same microvascular pathology that causes WMLs.

In an attempt to further characterize the nature and significance of WMLs, we examined a group of demented patients who had WMLs and elevated CSF/serum albu-

[c]Address for correspondence: Dr. L.O. Wahlund, Department of Clinical Neuroscience, NEUROTEC, Karolinska Institute, Huddinge Hospital, S-141 86 Huddinge, Sweden. Tel.: +46 8 58585419; fax: +46 8 58585482.
e-mail: lars-olof.wahlund@neurotec.ki.se

TABLE 1. Demographic and clinical data

Patient No.	Age	Sex	Diagnosis	No. of Cerebro-Vascular Risk Factors	BBB Damage	CSF/Serum Albumin Ratio
1	69	M	AD	0	no	4.0
2	73	F	MCI	1	no	5.0
3	74	F	SCI	1	no	5.0
4	78	M	VaD	0	no	6.7
5	72	M	AD	0	no	9.1
6	74	M	VaD	2	yes	12.1
7	73	M	VaD	3	yes	15.0
8	73	F	VaD	1	yes	15.9
9	76	F	AD	0	yes	16.3
10	63	M	FLD	0	yes	16.7

VaD, vascular dementia; AD, Alzheimer's disease; FLD, frontal lobe dementia; MCI, mild cognitive impairment; SCI, subjective cognitive impairment (could not be verified in neuropsychological tests).

NOTE: The patients were diagnosed according to DSM-IV, NINCDS-ADRDA and NINDS-AIREN criteria. The table shows how many of the following cerebro-vascular risk factors each patient had; History of stroke/TIA, hypertension, diabetes mellitus, coronary artery disease and claudicatio intermittens. Patient no 4 had none of the above mentioned cerebrovascular risk-factors but still fulfilled the NINDS-AIREN criteria for vascular dementia. CSF/serum albumin ratios <10.2 are considered normal. [12]

min ratios, as well as a control group who had WMLs but normal albumin ratios. The aim of the study was to investigate whether an increased BBB permeability could be shown in the WML areas using an optimized, Gd-enhanced, MRI technique.

MATERIALS AND METHODS

Patients

The study included 10 patients with cognitive impairment who had previously been examined with either CT or MRI and been shown to have WMLs. Five of the patients had signs of BBB damage, as indicated by elevated CSF/serum albumin ratios (>10.2), whereas the other 5 had values within the normal range (≤10.2). The demographic and clinical data as well as the albumin ratios are shown in TABLE 1.

The study was approved by the local ethical committee and was conducted with the understanding and informed consent of each patient.

Magnetic Resonance Imaging

All MRI examinations were performed on a 1.5 T system (Magnetom SP, Siemens). A coronal plane was used. A routine PD/T2 W fast SE sequence (TR/TE 3500/19-93) was performed to identify the WMLs. To measure contrast enhancement, each patient was imaged with a T1 W SE sequence (TR/TE: 600/14 ms, FoV:

173 × 230 mm, matrix: 192 × 256, NEX = 2) to obtain 19 five-mm-thick slices with 1.5-mm interslice gap. In addition, we performed a T1 W 3D gradient echo (GE), using a magnetization prepared rapid GE, (MPRAGE) (TR/TE: 10/4 ms, FA: 10, FoV: 191 × 255 mm, matrix: 192 × 256) with 64 slices and 2.8-mm slice thickness.

The contrast medium used was GdDTPA-BMA (Omniscan®, Nycomed).

All three sequences, PD/T2 FSE, T1 SE, and T1 3D GE, were performed before the contrast medium was injected. The patient received a double standard dose of GdDTPA-BMA (0.2 mmol/kg body weight) and images were repeated during 30 minutes with the T1 W SE sequence starting at times 5, 15, and 25 minutes post injection and the T1 W GE sequence starting at 10 and 20 minutes post injection.

Evaluation of the images obtained was performed on a separate workstation. The WMLs were identified as hyperintensities on the T2 W images and the same areas were thereafter identified on the corresponding preinjection T1 W images. Corresponding to every lesion measured, a ROI was placed in the same image slice over an area of normal appearing white matter. The MR signal was then measured in all ROIs, the lesions, as well as in the apparently normal areas, in all T1 W sequences (SE and GE), both before and after contrast injection. The signal change over time was analyzed separately for the two MR sequences and curves of contrast enhancement over time were drawn. Ratios between the signal in the lesions and the signal in the corresponding normal white matter areas were calculated so as to discover different enhancement patterns in the two types of areas and to compensate for possible signal variation in the different images.

Statistics

Analysis of variance (ANOVA) for repeated measures was used for significance testing. Significant changes were looked for in the MR signal or signal ratio, compared to the signal in the preinjection image. The *p* values were adjusted according to the Huynh-Feldt procedure. Adjusted *p* values less than 0.05 were considered statistically significant.

RESULTS

No visually detectable contrast enhancements were seen in any lesion in any patient. We also found no convincing contrast enhancement in any patient when analyzing the measured signals and the calculated signal ratios.

When statistically evaluating the mean values from all 10 patients we found no significant changes in either signal (SE: p <0.90, GE: p <0.95) nor signal ratio (SE: p <0.99, GE: p <0.36) over time in the group as a whole.

The group of 5 patients with suspected BBB damage showed no increases in either mean MR signal or signal ratio over time. The 5 patients without signs of BBB damage showed a slight, but nonsignificant, mean increase in MR signal and signal ratio, 5 minutes post contrast. Grouping the patients according to diagnosis showed no statistically significant changes in MR signal or signal ratio over time.

DISCUSSION

The presence and significance of BBB dysfunction in dementia remains controversial. A number of studies have indicated increased BBB leakage in VaD,[4,11] whereas there have been disparate results regarding AD. Blennow *et al.*[12] reported that AD patients had increased CSF/serum albumin ratios, indicative of BBB impairment; this was, however, related to coexisting vascular factors, such as hypertension, diabetes, or ischemic heart disease, rather than to the condition of AD.

Since the BBB dysfunction seen in some demented patients also is suspected to be due to diffuse small-vessel pathology,[4,7] BBB damage might be expected in the WML areas. The BBB dysfunction caused by microvascular ischemic injury is probably caused by defective tight junctions and basal membranes,[13] giving a general increase in permeability. Cerebrovascular conditions such as chronic hypertension and impaired autoregulation of cerebral perfusion can also open up the tight junctions.[13]

The present MRI study, which failed to detect any significant contrast enhancement, is to our knowledge the first to investigate possible BBB damage in patients selected as being known to have extensive WMLs. Even patients with an elevated CSF/serum albumin ratio indicative of BBB damage failed to show a detectable contrast enhancement in the WMLs.

Our results indicate that the WMLs are not related to BBB damage. There might be several different other explanations for this finding. For instance, impaired BBB might be located to other areas in the CNS, such as cortical or medullar structures, and as such may be caused by mechanisms other than small-vessel disease of the white matter. Furthermore the primary source of protein in the CSF is the choroid plexus,[14] and it is therefore feasible that elevated CSF albumin levels could be due to a dysfunction in these areas resulting in an increased leakage or decreased reabsorption of proteins.

In summary, this small pilot study, using contrast-enhanced dynamic MR imaging, failed to detect any BBB leakage in WMLs of demented patients with or without indications of BBB dysfunction. Our findings suggest a true integrity of the BBB in WMLs, although there is also a possibility that any leakage is of such low grade or appears in such small areas at the same time that it is not detectable with this method.

REFERENCES

1. MEYER, J.S., J. KAWAMURA & Y. TERAYAMA. 1992. Review article: white matter lesions in the elderly. J. Neurol. Sci. **110:** 1–7.
2. GOLOMB, J., A. KLUGER, J. GIANUTSOS *et al.* 1995. Nonspecific leukoencephalopathy associated with aging. Neuroimaging Clin. N. Am. 5(1): 33–44.
3. BLENNOW, K., A. WALLIN, C. UHLEMANN & C.G. GOTTFRIES. 1991. White-matter lesions on CT in Alzheimer patients: relation to clinical symptomatology and vascular factors. Acta Neurol. Scand. **83:** 187–193.
4. MECOCCI, P., L. PARNETTI, G.P. REBOLDI *et al.* 1991. Blood-brain barrier in a geriatric population: barrier function in degenerative and vascular dementias. Acta Neurol. Scand. **84:** 210–213.
5. PANTONI, L., D. INZITARI, G. PRACUCCI *et al.* 1993. Cerebrospinal fluid proteins in patients with leucoaraiosis: possible abnormalities in blood-brain barrier function. J. Neurol. Sci. **115:** 125–131.
6. ERKINJUNTTI, T., R. SULKAVA, J. PALO & L. KETONEN. 1989. White matter low attenuation on CT in Alzheimer's disease. Arch. Geront. Geriatr. **8:** 95–104.

7. WALLIN, A., K. BLENNOW, P. FREDMAN *et al.* 1990. Blood brain barrier function in vascular dementia. Acta Neurol. Scand. **81**(4): 318–322.
8. SCHMIEDL, U., J. KENNEY & K. MARAVILLA. 1991. MRI of blood-brain barrier permeability in astrocytic gliomas: application of small and large molecular weight contrast media. Magn. Res. Med. **22**: 288–292.
9. HAYAKAWA, K., K. YAMASHITA, M. MITSUMORI & Y. NAKANO. 1990. *In vivo* quantification of the blood-brain barrier injury using magnetic resonance enhancement. Invest. Radiol. **25**: S80–S81.
10. RHINE, W., D. BENARON, D. ENZMAN *et al.* 1993. Gd-DTPA MR detection of blood-brain barrier opening in rats after hyperosmotic shock. J. Comp. Assoc. Tomogr. **17**(4): 563–566.
11. TOMIMOTO, H., I. AKIGUCHI, T. SUENAGA *et al.* 1996. Alterations of blood-brain barrier and glial cells in white matter lesions in cerebrovascular and Alzheimer's disease patients. Stroke **27**: 2069–2074.
12. BLENNOW, K., A. WALLIN, P. FREDMAN *et al.* 1990. Blood-brain barrier disturbance in patients with Alzheimer's disease is related to vascular factors. Acta Neurol. Scand. **81**: 323–326.
13. POLLAY, M. & P.A. ROBERTS. 1980. Blood-brain barrier: a definition of normal and altered function. Neurosurgery **6**(6): 675–685.
14. CASERTA, M., D. CACCIOPPO, G. LAPIN *et al.* 1998. Blood-brain barrier integrity in Alzheimer's disease patients and elderly control subjects. J. Neuropsychiatr. Clin. Neurosci. **10**(1): 78–84.

The Association between White Matter Lesions on Magnetic Resonance Imaging and Noncognitive Symptoms

JOHN O'BRIEN,[a] ROBERT PERRY, ROBERT BARBER, ANIL GHOLKAR, AND ALAN THOMAS

Institute for the Health of the Elderly, Newcastle General Hospital, Newcastle upon Tyne, UK

ABSTRACT: A number of studies have suggested that cerebral changes, particularly deep white matter lesions (WML) visualized on magnetic resonance imaging (MRI), may be involved in the genesis of late life depression. This has been confirmed in a prospective study which also found a relationship between the presence of WML and poor 3-year outcome in elderly depressed subjects. Most studies find these lesions to predominate in frontal lobe and basal ganglia, supporting the hypothesis of "fronto-striatal" dysfunction in depression. To investigate whether WML are associated with mood disturbance in dementia, proton density and T_2-weighted images were obtained in 80 subjects with dementia (dementia with Lewy bodies, $n = 27$; Alzheimer's disease, $n = 28$; vascular dementia, $n = 25$) and 26 age-matched normal controls. Periventricular lesions (PVL), white matter lesions (WML), and basal ganglia hyperintensities (BG) were visually rated blind to diagnosis using a semiquantitative scale. Frontal WML were associated with higher depression scores in patients with dementia, implying a common pathophysiology of depression irrespective of diagnosis. Further study of the neurobiological basis of WML is needed. This can best be achieved by serial clinical assessment combined with *in vivo* and *in vitro* MRI and neuropathological examination.

WHITE MATTER LESIONS IN DEPRESSION

Neuroimaging studies have shown evidence of structural changes in subcortical and frontal areas in both unipolar and bipolar affective disorder. Individual studies have shown ventricular enlargement, sulcal widening, a reduction in overall frontal lobe, and specifically left subgenual prefrontal cortex volume and caudate atrophy.[1–4] These findings are still controversial, though frontal and caudate abnormalities have also been demonstrated using functional imaging techniques.[5,6] However, the most consistent abnormality described in depression comes from studies which have repeatedly shown an increase in the number and/or severity of signal hyperintensities in the white matter visualized on magnetic resonance imaging (MRI).[1,2,7,8] Signal hyperintensities can be divided into those adjacent to the ventricular system

[a]Address for correspondence: Dr. John O'Brien, Wolfson Research Centre, Institute for the Health of the Elderly, Newcastle General Hospital, Westgate Road, Newcastle upon Tyne, NE4 6BE, UK. Tel.: +44 (0)191 256 3323; fax: +44 (0)191 219 5051.
e-mail: j.t.o'brien@ncl.ac.uk

(periventricular lesions or PVL) and those deep in the white matter (WML).[9] An increase in hyperintensities, particularly WML, has been described in both unipolar and bipolar disorder but is most marked in elderly depressed subjects, particularly those with late onset depression.[8]

Major depressive disorder in older individuals often has a poor prognosis, and cerebral organic factors may be predictive of poor outcome. Severe WML on MRI may predispose to the onset of first ever depressions in some elderly subjects and have been reported to be associated with poor initial treatment response.[10] An adverse effect of severe WML was recently demonstrated in a prospective follow-up study of 54 elderly subjects with depression, all of whom underwent MRI scans at baseline which were rated for the presence and severity of WML and PVL.[11] Outcome was rated in accordance with established practice[12] as i) continuously well, $n = 11$ (severe WML = 0); ii) well after relapse, $n = 8$ (1 with severe WML); iii) depressive invalid, $n = 13$ (5 with severe WML); iv) currently in relapse, $n = 2$ (1 with severe WML); v) continuously ill, $n = 5$ (0 with WML); vi) demented, $n = 7$ (3 with severe WML); and dead, $n = 8$ (3 with severe WML). Data were analyzed categorizing patients in group (i) as having a "good" outcome and those in groups (ii)–(vii) as having a "bad" one.

Subjects with severe WML had a significantly worse outcome than others, and none remained continuously well (Fishers exact probability test, $p = 0.048$). There was no association between PVL and outcome. Survival analysis confirmed the effects of severe lesions on poor outcome. Survival functions for the severe and non-severe lesion groups were significantly different (Log rank test statistic 3.63, df = 1, $p = 0.04$). Median survival time for the 13 subjects with severe lesions was only 136 days (95% CI 0,309) compared to 315 days (95% CI 0,813) for those without lesions.[11]

These results demonstrated a significant effect of WML on outcome and, in keeping with previous research, show that some elderly patients with depression have evidence of damage to deep white matter structures which may play a role in the initiation, maintenance, and outcome of late life depression. Studies of the basal ganglia have shown the existence of five parallel, segregated frontal-subcortical circuits.[13] Two of these are highly relevant to affective disorders, because they involve reciprocal links between the caudate nucleus and the dorsolateral prefrontal cortex and the cingulate cortex, the two main frontal areas identified as abnormal by imaging studies in depression.[16] There is also good clinical evidence from diseases affecting these structures to suggest that these regions are involved in mood regulation. These findings have led to the hypothesis that disruption of the frontal-subcortical pathways, probably related to white matter lesions visualized on MRI, underpins the pathophysiology of depression.

WHITE MATTER LESIONS IN DEMENTIA

Introduction

Dementia is know to be associated with a high prevalence of both WML on MRI and noncognitive symptoms, particularly depression and psychosis. Because of the recognized link between WML and depression discussed above, we wished to test the hypothesis that white matter changes in dementia are associated with noncognitive symptoms, in particular depression. Full results from this study are presented elsewhere.[14]

Methods

Eighty subjects over the age of 60 years who fulfilled DSM-IV criteria for dementia were recruited. Diagnosis was made after a detailed clinical assessment. This included an interview with the subject and the most knowledgeable informant using the Geriatric Mental State/History Aetiology Schedule, review of clinical records, full psychiatric and medical history, and mental state and physical examination.[14] A standard dementia screen was completed which included hematology and biochemistry analysis, thyroid function tests, syphilis serology, B_{12} and folate levels, and computer tomography (CT) scan.

Standardized clinical diagnostic criteria were used to characterize the type of dementia. Diagnoses of Alzheimer's disease (AD), vascular dementia (VaD), and dementia with Lewy bodies (DLB) were made in accordance with NINCDS/ADRDA,[15] NINDS/AIREN,[16] and DLB Consensus criteria[17] blind to MRI scan findings. Pathological confirmation of clinical diagnosis has since been acquired in four patients. Applying these criteria, 28 subjects had AD (definite $n = 2$, probable $n = 24$, and possible $n = 2$), 25 had VaD (probable $n = 15$ and possible $n = 10$), and 27 had DLB (definite $n = 2$, probable $n = 24$, and possible $n = 2$).

Within three months of completing an MRI scan all subjects underwent a further assessment. Cognitive function was measured using the Cambridge Cognitive Examination which incorporates the Mini Mental State Examination (MMSE).[18] Depressive symptoms were rated using the Montgomery and Asberg Depression Rating Scale (MADRS).[19]

Twenty-six age-matched controls (Con) were recruited from among spouses and friends of dementia subjects. A detailed history and examination was undertaken to include demographic data and physical and psychiatric status. All control subjects completed the same assessments as listed above. Exclusion criteria were evidence of current depression (from history or MADRS >10) or dementia (from history or score <80 on the CAMCOG) and a history of any other significant neurological, physical, or psychiatric disorder including drug and alcohol abuse.

All scans were performed on a 1.0 Tesla Siemens Magnetom Impact MRI Scanner. Whole brain axial images of 5 mm thickness (0.5 mm gap) were obtained using proton density weighted and T_2-weighted turbo/fast spin echo sequences to allow detailed visualization of white matter lesions (RARE technique-rapid acquisition with relaxation enhancement: TR = 2800 ms; TE 14/85 ms; matrix 256 × 256; field of view = 230 mm giving pixel size = 0.92 × 0.92 mm; acquisition time = 4 min, 13 sec).

White matter lesions were rated from hard copies of proton density and T_2-weighted axial images using an established scale which provided a semiquantitative measurement of the type, size, frequency, and location of PVL and WML.[9]

TABLE 1. Subject characteristics

	DLB ($n = 27$)	AD ($n = 28$)	VaD ($n = 25$)	Con ($n = 26$)	p Value
Age (mean (SD))	75.9 (7)	77.4 (5)	76.8 (7)	76.2 (5)	ns
Sex (M:F)	19:9	10:18	15:10	14:12	ns
Education (years (SD))	9.1 (1)	9.7 (3)	9.9 (1)	10.1 (2)	ns
Length of history (mo (SD))	38.2 (19)	42.4 (25)	39.7 (25)	na	ns
MMSE (mean (SD))	13.6 (7)	15.5 (5)	18.2 (4)	28.1 (2)	< 0.001[*]
CAMCOG (mean (SD))	46.1 (26)	55.5 (16)	62.0 (13)	97.2 (5)	< 0.001[*]
MADRS (mean)	8.0	7.6	7.7	3.4	< 0.05**

ABBREVIATIONS: ns, not significant; na, not applicable; SD, standard deviation; DLB, dementia with Lewy bodies; AD, Alzheimer's disease; VaD, vascular dementia; Con, controls.

*post hoc Scheffé test showed significant differences between Con and AD, Con and VaD, Con and DLB ($p < 0.001$) and between VaD and DLB ($p < 0.05$). **Significant differences between Con and DLB, AD and VaD.

Results

Subject characteristics are summarized in TABLE 1. Groups were well matched for age, sex, length of history, and years of education. As would be expected CAMCOG and MMSE scores were significantly lower in all dementia groups compared to controls ($p < 0.001$). Subjects with DLB were significantly more impaired than those with VaD on MMSE (13.6 vs 18.2; $p < 0.05$) and CAMCOG (46.1 vs 62.0; $p < 0.05$). There were no differences between dementia groups with regard to MADRS scores though all dementia groups had significantly more depressive symptoms than controls ($p < 0.05$). PVL were positively correlated with age in all subjects (total PVL score r = 0.41, $p < 0.001$) but were not associated with cognitive impairment or depressive symptoms.

A link between regional deep white matter changes and depression was observed. Those with frontal WML had significantly higher depression scores than those without lesions (mean MADRS score for subjects with frontal WML = 8.3 vs without = 3.4; $p < 0.05$).

Conclusion

Depression is a frequent and clinically important feature of all dementias. As previously discussed, frontal and subcortical WML are implicated in late-life depression and influence outcome, possibly by disruption of frontal-subcortical circuits. The findings of this study suggest frontal WML may also be relevant in understanding depression in dementia, and imply a common pathophysiology of depression irrespective of diagnosis.

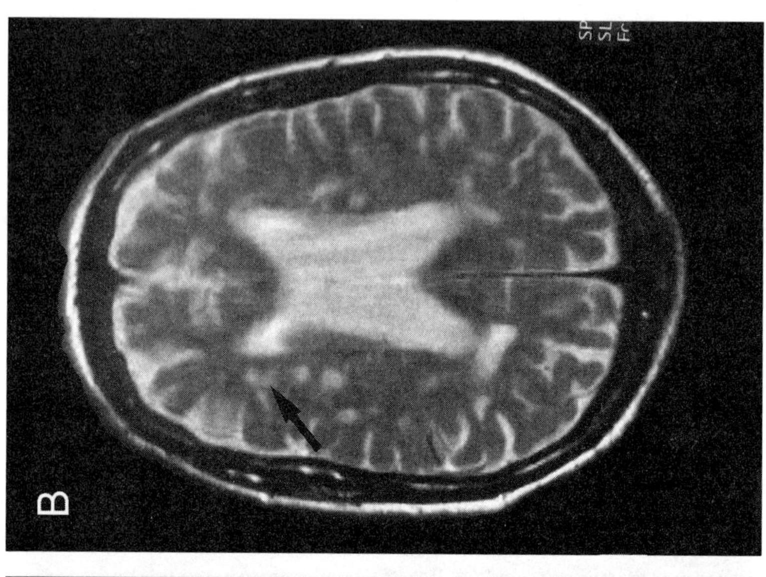
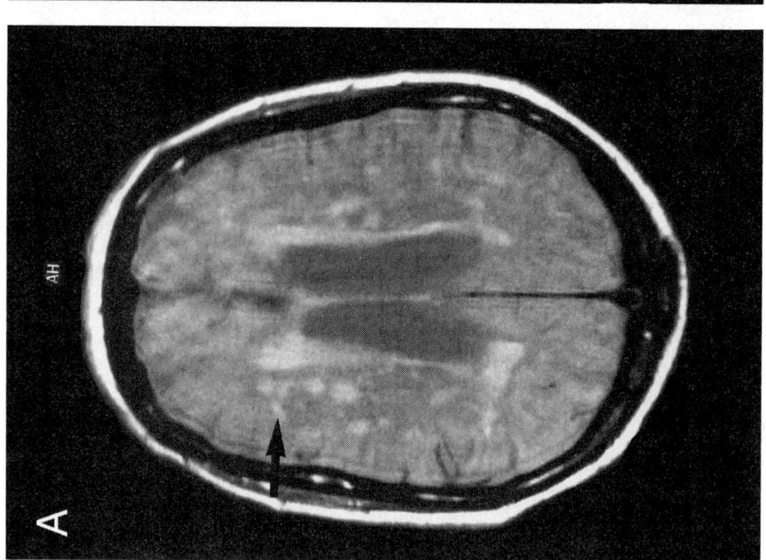

FIGURE 1. (A) Proton density (TR = 2800 ms, TE = 14 ms) and (B) T_2-weighted (TR = 2800 ms, TE = 85 ms) axial *in vivo* scans of elderly patient with depression. Note the presence of periventricular and scattered deep white matter lesions, especially in frontal lobe (*arrow*).

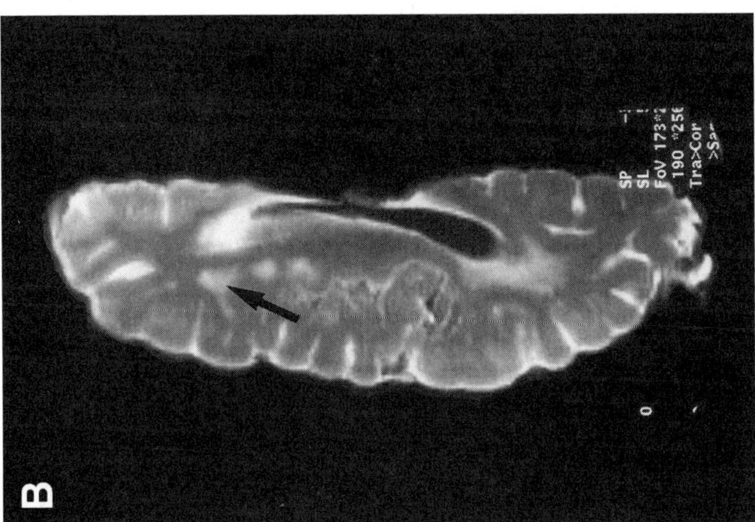

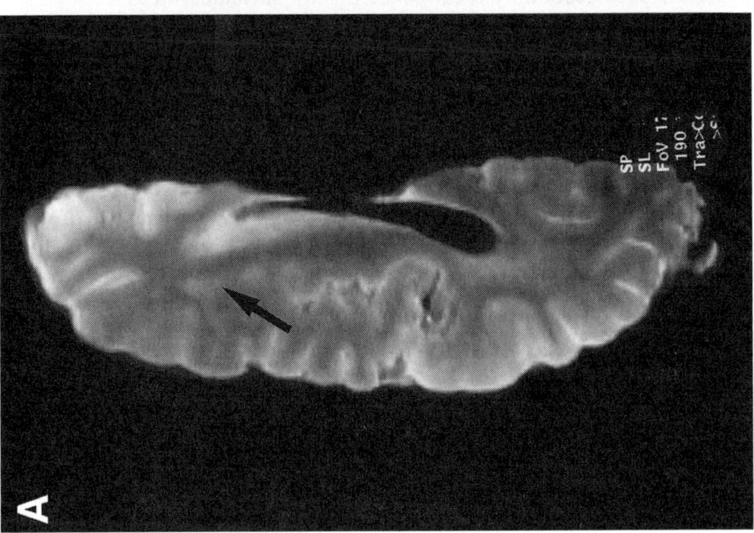

FIGURE 2. (**A**) Axial proton density postmortem scan (TR = 2800 ms, TE = 14 ms) of whole hemibrain of same patient after formalin fixation. Note that the same periventricular and deep white matter lesions can be visualized as seen on the *in vivo* scan. *Arrow* denotes same frontal lesion. (**B**) T_2-weigthed image (TR = 2800 ms, TE = 85 ms) of same slice.

NEUROPATHOLOGICAL BASIS OF LESIONS

Introduction

These clinical studies have demonstrated the potential importance of deep white matter changes in understanding important noncognitive symptoms like depression. However, our understanding of the neuropathology of such lesions is limited. Some studies have examined the pathology of hyperintensities seen on MRI, but none has included any patients with affective disorder.[20–25] WML can be found as punctate lesions (first degree) with reduced myelination and atrophy of the neuropil around fibrohyalinotic arterioles as well as confluent lesions (second and third degree) with gliosis and lacunar infarcts. They are associated with vascular risk factors. In contrast PVL (unless extensive) are probably not associated with vascular disease and usually represent areas of demyelination associated with discontinuity of the subependymal lining.[24]

To further investigate the neuropathological basis of white matter change in affective disorder we are currently undertaking longitudinal clinicopathological studies in depression and dementia combining *in vivo* and *in vitro* MRI with neuropathological analysis. *In vivo* scans are acquired as above on a 1.0 T Siemens scanner (FIG. 1). In cases where autopsy brain donation is achieved whole hemibrain MRI is acquired using the same imaging sequences, firstly in the axial plane to allow comparison with the *in vivo* scan (FIG. 2) and then coronally to facilitate accurate localization of lesions after coronal sectioning. Finally, after coronal sectioning slices are rescanned to determine that lesions are still present, to ensure artefacts have not appeared, and to accurately localize lesions to particular slices.

Conclusion

WML on MRI, particularly in frontal and subcortical areas, are associated with depressive disorder and depressive symptoms in dementia, implying a common pathophysiology of depression caused by disruption to fronto-striatal circuits. These lesions predict poor outcome in major depression, and understanding their pathogenesis will be important in terms of understanding the neurobiology of late life depression and may offer important new insights into therapeutic options for the treatment and prevention of depression.

REFERENCES

1. VIDEBECH, P. 1997. MRI findings in patients with affective disorder: a meta-analysis. Acta Psychiatr. Scand. **96:** 157–168.
2. RABINS, P.V., G.D. PEARLSON, E. AYLWARD, A.J. KUMA *et al.* 1991. Cortical magnetic resonance imaging changes in elderly inpatients with major depression. Am. J. Psychiatry **148:** 617–620.
3. DREVETS, W.C., J.L. PRICE, J.R. SIMPSON, R.D. TODD *et al.* 1997. Subgenal prefrontal cortex abnormalities in mood disorders. Nature **386:** 824–827.
4. COFFEY, C.E., W.E. WILKINSON, R.D. WEINER, L.A. PARASHOS *et al.* 1993. Quantitative cerebral anatomy in depression. Cereb. Anat. **50:** 7–16.
5. BEACH, C.J., K.J. FRISTON, R.G. BROWN, L.C. SCOTT *et al.* 1992. The anatomy of melancholia—focal abnormalities of cerebral blood flow in major depression. Psychol. Med. **22:** 604–615.

6. GOODWIN, G.M., M.P. AUSTIN, N. DOUGALL, M. ROSS *et al.* 1993. State changes in brain activity shown by the uptake of ^{99m}Tc-exametazine with single photon emission tomography in major depression before and after treatment. J. Affect. Disord. **29:** 243–253.

7. O'BRIEN, J.T., D. AMES & I. SCHWEITZER. 1996. White matter changes in depression and Alzheimer's disease: a review of magnetic resonance imaging studies. Int. J. Geriatr. Psychiatry **11:** 681–694.

8. O'BRIEN, J., P. DESMOND, D. AMES, I. SCHWEITZER, S. HARRIGAN & B. TRESS. 1996. A magnetic resonance imaging study of white matter lesions in depression and Alzheimer's disease. Br. J. Psychiatry **168:** 477–485.

9. SCHELTENS, P., F. BARKHOF, D. LEYS *et al.* 1993. A semiquantitative rating scale for the assessment of signal hyperintensities on magnetic resonance imaging. J. Neurol. Sci. **114:** 7–12.

10. SIMPSON, S., A. JACKSON, R.C. BALDWIN & A. BURNS. 1997. Subcortical hyperintensities in late-life depression: acute response to treatment and neuropsychological impairment. Int. Psychogeriatr. **9:** 257–275.

11. O'BRIEN, J.T., E. CHIU, I. SCHWEITZER, P. DESMOND & B. TRESS. 1998. Severe deep white matter lesions on MRI brain scan predict poor outcome in elderly patients with major depressive disorder. Br. Med. J. **317:** 982–984.

12. AMES, D. & N. ALLEN. 1991. The prognosis of depression in old age: good, bad or indifferent? Int. J. Geriatr. Psychiatry **6:** 477–481.

13. ALEXANDER, G.E. & M.D. CRUTCHER. 1990. Functional architecture of basal ganglia circuits neural substrates of parallel processing. TINS **13** (7): 266–271.

14. BARBER, R., A. GHOLKAR, C. BALLARD, P. SCHELTENS, I. MCKEITH, R. PERRY, P. INCE, D. BARER & J.T. O'BRIEN. 1999. White matter lesions on MRI in dementia with Lewy bodies, Alzheimer's disease, vascular dementia and normal ageing. J. Neurol. Neurosurg. Psychiatry **67:** 66–93.

15. MCKHANN, G., D. DRACHMAN, M. FOLSTEIN *et al.* 1984. Clinical diagnosis of Alzheimer's disease: report of the NINCDS-ADRDA Work Group under the auspices of Department of Health and Human Service Task Force on Alzheimer's Disease. Neurology **34:** 939–944.

16. ROMAN, G.C., T. TATEMISCHI, T. ERKINJUNTTI *et al.* 1993. Vascular dementia: diagnostic criteria for research studies. Report of the NINDS-AIRENS international workshop. Neurology **43:** 250–260.

17. MCKEITH, I.G., D. GALASKO & K. KOSAKA. 1996. Consensus guidelines for the clinical and pathological diagnosis of dementia with Lewy bodies (DLB): report of the consortium on DLB international workshop. Neurology **47:** 1113–1124.

18. ROTH, M., E. TYM, C. MOUNTJOY *et al.* 1986. CAMDEX. A standardised instrument for the diagnosis of mental disorder in the elderly with special reference to the early detection of dementia. Br. J. Psychiatry **149:** 698–709.

19. MONTGOMERY, S.A. & M. ASBERG. 1979. A new depression scale designed to be sensitive to change. Br. J. Psychiatry **134:** 382–389.

20. LEIFER, D., F.S. BUONANNO & E.P. RICHARDSON, JR. 1990. Clinicopathologic correlations of cranial magnetic resonance imaging of periventricular white matter. Neurology **40:** 911–918.

21. VAN SWIETEN, J.C., H.W. VAN DEN HOUT, B.A. VAN KETEL *et al.* 1991. Periventricular lesions in the white matter on magnetic resonance in the elderly. Brain **114:** 761–774.

22. WALDEMAR, G., P. CHRISTIANSEN, H.B.W. LARSSON *et al.* 1994. White matter resonance hyperintensities in dementia of the Alzheimer type: morphological and regional cerebral blood flow correlates. J. Neurol. Neurosurg. Psychiatry **57:** 1458–1465.

23. CHIMOWITZ, M.I., M.L. ESTES, A.J. FURLAN *et al.* 1992. Further observations on the pathology of subcortical lesions identified on magnetic resonance imaging. Arch. Neurol. **49:** 747–752.

24. FAZEKAS, F., R. KLEIMERT, H. OFFENBACHER *et al.* 1993. Pathologic correlates of incidential MRI white matter hyperintensities. Neurology **43:** 1683–1689.

25. SCHELTENS, P., F. BARKHOF, D. LEYS *et al.* 1995. Histopathologic correlates of white matter changes on MRI in Alzheimer's disease and normal aging. Neurology **45:** 883–888.

Neuropathological Findings in the Very Old

Results from the First 101 Brains of a Population-based Longitudinal Study of Dementing Disorders

J.H. XUEREB,[a] C. BRAYNE,[b,j] C. DUFOUIL,[c] H. GERTZ,[d] C. WISCHIK,[e]
C. HARRINGTON,[e] E. MUKAETOVA-LADINSKA,[f] M.A. McGEE, [g]
A. O'SULLIVAN,[h] D. O'CONNOR,[i] E.S. PAYKEL,[f] AND F.A. HUPPERT[f]

*Departments of [a]Pathology, [b]Community Medicine, and [f]Psychiatry,
University of Cambridge, Cambridge, UK*

[c]INSERM, Paris, France

[d]Department of Psychiatry, University of Leipzig, Leipzig, Germany

[e]Department of Psychiatry, University of Aberdeen, Aberdeen, Scotland

[g]MRC Biostatistics Unit, Cambridge, UK

[h]Cambridge Brain Bank, University of Cambridge, Cambridge, UK

[i]Department of Psychogeriatrics, Monash University, Melbourne, Australia

ABSTRACT: We report a unique longitudinal epidemiological study of cognitive decline in the elderly population of the city of Cambridge, UK. A population sample of people aged 75 and over was surveyed between 1984–1996 ($n = 2{,}616$) and followed 2.4, 6, and 9 years later. CAMDEX diagnostic criteria were used for clinical assessment, and the neuropathological protocol (in 101 cases) was based on the CERAD method, with additional features to allow Braak staging of neurofibrillary pathology. The main findings are of the heterogeneity of lesions to be found in very old populations, and the existence of considerable overlap in the pathologies found in the demented and nondemented. It seems that white matter (ischemic) pallor an amyloid angiopathy, as well as neuritic plaques, neurofibrillary tangles and Lewy body formation are all lesions that increase the likelihood of dementia.

INTRODUCTION

Dementia is a syndrome rather than a neuropathological diagnosis. It becomes increasingly common in old age, and by the age of 90 the prevalence of dementia is very high. In tandem with this, changes in the brains of older people show increasing numbers of the lesions associated with dementing conditions. It is important to link these parallel observations if progress is to be made in understanding dementia in extreme old age.

[j]Address for correspondence: C. Brayne, Department of Public Health and Primary Care, University of Cambridge, Institute of Public Health, Forvie Site, Robinson Way, Cambridge CB2 2SR, UK. Tel.: 00 44 1223 330334; fax: 00 44 1223 330330.
  e-mail: carol.brayne@medschl.cam.ac.uk

Clinicopathological studies up until relatively recently have concentrated on clinically clear-cut cases of Alzheimer's disease, collecting case series (as in CERAD),[1] with some controls in addition but not deriving from the same source population. Lately there have been two major changes to this approach. First, it has been recognized that vascular factors must be included, both within Alzheimer's disease and in their own right.[2] Second, the importance of prospective studies of both nondemented individuals and demented individuals is recognized in order to correlate changes observed during life with the pathological changes seen after death.[3] Several prospective cohort studies have used this second approach, with considerable success and important findings.

However, none of the studies published to date has combined these approaches with a genuinely population-based study. Such studies are essential if the finding from more selective studies are to be understood in their population context. The study described here is a unique longitudinal epidemiological study of cognitive decline and dementia in the city of Cambridge, and is linked to a brain donation program.

METHODS

Sample and Clinical Information

A population sample of people aged 75 and over in Cambridge was surveyed between 1984–1986 ($n = 2,616$) and followed 2.4 years, 6 years, and 9 years later ($n = 1,111, 628$, and 400).[4] At each stage a screening interview including the Mini Mental State Examination (MMSE) was included, as well as activities of daily living, physical health, social context, and contacts. In the baseline interview, all those scoring 24 or below on the MMSE and a third of those scoring 25 and 26 were selected for further diagnostic assessment using the Cambridge Examination for Mental Disorders in the Elderly. This interview is a structured standardized clinical interview, which includes an informant interview. In the 2.4 year interview, individuals were selected for diagnostic assessment if they scored below 22 on the MMSE, had a missing score or dropped 4 points or more; scored highly on the MMSE twice, or were aged 87 and over. Each diagnostic phase was followed by repeat diagnostic assessment, at least once. The CAMDEX diagnostic criteria functions operationally almost identically with ICD-10 and DSM-IV. A minimal category is similar to the questionable criteria used by the CERAD CDR scale.

All the individuals in the diagnostic assessment interview were approached by a liaison nurse (A 0'S) to request a statement of intention to donate their brains after death. After death the Brain Bank team was notified by family, carers or physicians, and permission for a limited postmortem requested. Whenever possible, a retrospective informant interview was carried out. Where available, the last diagnosis was used in the analysis; if the individual had not had diagnostic assessment, the screening records and the retrospective interview were scrutinized and a diagnosis based on the same criteria was made. A separate consensus process was carried out for the first 50 brains in which all clinical notes were reviewed, along with the retrospective informant interview. In relatively few cases was the diagnosis modified, as found by Thomas and colleagues.[5]

Postmortem Procedure

After death and notification of the Brain Bank, the brains were removed as soon as possible in the local mortuary. The brains were cut in the sagittal plane. One hemisphere was dissected, macroscopically examined, and frozen. The other half of the brain was formalin fixed for at least six weeks. For diagnostic purposes, blocks for paraffin embedding were taken from the hippocampus at the level of the lateral geniculate body and from the entorhinal cortex at the level of the mamillary body, from the frontal, temporal, parietal, and occipital lobe, from the basal ganglia, thalamus, and from two levels of the midbrain, pons, medulla, and cerebellum.

NEUROPATHOLOGICAL ASSESSMENT

Histological sections were stained with routine hematoxylin and eosin and congo red. Neurodegenerative pathology was assessed on immunohistochemical preparations; the antibodies were obtained from the Cambridge Brain Bank Laboratory. Anti-tau (monoclonal antibody 11/57) reacts with a phosphorylation-dependent epitope in the region of serine 396 of the tau molecule; it decorates neuritic plaques, neurofibrillary tangles, and neuropil threads. Antiubiquitin antibody (BR 251) is a polyclonal antibody directed against conjugated ubiquitin and was used to detect Lewy bodies. Ehrlich's hematoxylin was used as a counterstain and diaminobenzidine was the chromagen used. The silver method and immunohistochemistry with a monoclonal antibody against beta A4 peptide (donated by Dr. M. London, Nottingham University) were used to demonstrate beta A4 peptide deposits.

The CERAD protocol was followed for neuropathological assessment—Braak staging followed the procedure outlined previously.[6] These assessments were performed blind to clinical status.

Statistical Methods

Dementia status was taken as being minimally demented or nondemented. Burden of classical Alzheimer's lesions was estimated by taking the CERAD ratings for plaques, and tangles for the following areas: entorhinal hippocampal, frontal, temporal, parietal, and occipital areas. Microvascular burden was estimated by noting the presence or absence of microvascular lesions in hippocampal, frontal, temporal, parietal, occipital, deep grey and "other" areas. Macrovascular burden was assessed by the sum of such lesions noted in any area and their volume. Lewy bodies were assessed by their presence or absence in entorhinal, hippocampal, frontal, or temporal areas and, in addition, in substantia nigra, nucleus basalis, dorsal raphe nucleus, locus coeruleus, dorsal vagal nucleus, as well as neuronal loss in the substantia nigra. Vessel wall pathology was assessed according to detection of vascular amyloid in meningeal and parenchymal areas of hippocampus, occipital, frontal temporal, and parietal areas. White-matter pallor was checked in occipital, parietal, frontal, temporal, and deep white matter. Frequencies and Pearson correlations are presented for the 101 brains.

TABLE 1. The first 101 brains, age at death, dementia status, and gender

	Nondemented		Demented[a]	
	Men	Women	Men	Women
Age at death	(18)	(34)	(14)	(33)
<85	16.7	20.6	21.4	12.1
86–90	44.4	26.5	42.9	39.4
91–95	27.8	38.2	28.6	30.3
96+	11.1	14.7	7.1	18.2

NOTE: $n = 99$; two respondents could not be diagnosed due to extreme deafness.
[a]Minimally or above.

TABLE 2. Braak staging and CERAD scores

Braak Staging			CERAD Staging		
	Frequency	%		Frequency	%
0	1	(1.0)	None	49	(48.5)
1	7	(6.9)	Uncertain	27	(26.7)
2	20	(19.8)	Suggestion	19	(18.8)
3	32	(31.7)	Indicative	6	(5.9)
4	22	(21.8)			
5	18	(17.8)			
6	1	(1.0)			

RESULTS

Of the first 101 individuals who were neuropathologically assessed using CERAD and Braak, two had not received a premortem diagnosis and could not be assigned one later because of extreme deafness. Of the 99 with diagnoses, most were women with balanced numbers between those receiving a diagnosis and those not (TABLE 1). This was a reflection of the sampling strategy for an approach to donate brain tissue.

The Braak staging and CERAD scores are shown in TABLE 2. The modal Braak rating was 3 but "none" on CERAD, showing how differently these rating methods operate. The mean neurofibrillary tangle rating was 5.9, minimum 0 and maximum 14. The mean neuritic plaque rating was 3.5, minimum 0 and maximum 12.

Large numbers of individuals were found to have vascular amyloid with only 62% having no rating for meningeal, and 71% for parenchymal, measures; 60% had neither. A similar proportion had no white-matter pallor (59%) in any area.

Nearly half of the population had microinfarcts in at least one area (46%). Seventy-nine had no evidence of macroscopic infarction; in those affected, the infarct area ranged from 90 mm^2 to 900 mm^2.

Lewy bodies in substantia nigra were found in only six individuals, with a further 10 having Lewy bodies in the other areas examined. (Sixteen percent of Lewy bodies are found in any area.)

TABLE 3. Correlation between selected neuropathological variables

	Neuritic Plaques (NP)	Neurofibrillary Tangles (NFT)	White Matter Pallor (WMP)	Vascular Amyloid (VA)	Microvascular Infarcts (MVI)
NP	1	0.85***	0.27*	0.41***	−0.14
NFT		1	0.32**	0.44***	−0.09
WMP			1	0.21#	0.03
VA				1	−0.11

***p <0.0001. **p <0.005. *p <0.01. #p <0.05.

TABLE 4. Relationship between dementia and neuropathology

	No Dementia (%)	Dementia (%)	p
Braak stage			
0	1.9	0	0.007
1	3.9	10.6	
2	26.9	10.6	
3	42.3	21.3	
4	17.3	25.5	
5	7.7	29.8	
6	0	2.1	
CERAD			
None	61.5	34.0	0.003
Uncertain	26.9	25.5	
Suggestion	11.5	27.7	
Indicative	0	12.8	
NFT mean (s.d.)	5.0 (2.7)	7.0 (3.6)	0.003
NP mean (s.d.)	2.3 (2.5)	4.9 (3.9)	0.0002

	% Present		p
Vascular amyloid, meningeal	23.5	53.2	0.002
Vascular amyloid, parenchymal	15.7	42.6	0.003
Any vascular amyloid	25.5	55.3	0.003
White matter pallor	30.6	52.2	0.03
Vascular microinfarcts	33.3	40.5	0.5
Large macroinfarcts	14.6	14.0	0.93
Lewy bodies detected	9.6	23.4	0.06

The relationship between the variables examined is shown in TABLE 3. Tangles and neuritic plaques are highly intercorrelated, even in a sample where half the population is not demented. Strong correlations were also found, although weaker, between plaques, tangles, vascular amyloid, and white-matter pallor. Microvascular infarcts showed no relationship to any of these measures.

TABLE 4 gives the relationship between dementia and neuropathology, revealing the diversity of associates of dementia status. As expected, the distribution of plaques and tangles is clearly associated with dementia expression. The other associated variables, most particularly vascular amyloid, are also clearly associated. Microinfarcts were not associated with dementia expression at all, but Lewy body presence was markedly different in proportion, although not quite significant.

DISCUSSION

This study is one of a very few in which a cohort of individuals has been studied prospectively, irrespective of dementia status, with pathological examination of the brain. It is made more unique by the fact that it is population based, has accrued substantial numbers of brains, and is based on populations at greatest risk of dementia in the future. The main findings are of the heterogeneity of lesions to be found in very old populations. Considerable overlap exists in the pathologies found in the demented and nondemented, showing that none of the current unidemensional methods of viewing dementia accounts for its expression during life. This further confirms recent findings from an unselected postmortem series of dementia cases coming to the attention of services in London.[7]

A number of methodological issues should be considered before accepting the results presented here. Although population based, the individuals selected for request for brain donation were not randomly chosen. They were selected from those who come to clinical assessment (only after six years were all respondents approached). This sample was weighted toward dementia, and this is reflected in the 50:50 split on diagnosis. There was some loss of individuals when the teams were not notified of death although strenuous efforts were made to keep this to a minimum. This is in common with other similar studies.[8] This caution serves to highlight how much less representative samples from nonpopulation-based studies are likely to be. Methods of measurement and meaning of ratings are notoriously difficult.[8,9] In this study an attempt was made to quantify most dimensions considered to be important at present. These are unlikely to relate directly to measures employed in other studies, but the overall results should be robust.

The more recent clinicopathological studies and discussion are moving away from the assumption of a single dimension[10] to more complex models. It is already acknowledged that pure vascular dementia is rare[11] and that overlap exists between the nondemented and demented.[12] The results presented here show that if we are to understand dementia in the very old, its preventability, and relation to underlying pathology, we must measure many dimensions and increase our sample sizes to enhance the power. It seems that white-matter pallor and vascular amyloid, as well as plaques, tangles, and Lewy bodies are all lesions that increase the likelihood of expression of dementia during life.

ACKNOWLEDGMENTS

This cohort study has been supported by the Charles Woolfson Trust, the Medical Research Council, the Public Health and Operational Research Advisory Group of the East Anglian Regional Health Authority and Research into Ageing. We are grateful to Mrs. R. Hazleman for her assistance in liaison work with respondents. We are also indebted to the respondents, their families, their family doctors and practice staff.

REFERENCES

1. MIRRA, S.S., A. HEYMAN, D. MCKEEL, S.M. SUMI, B.J. CRAIN, L.M. BROWNLEE, F.S. VOGEL, J.P. HUGHES, G. VAN BELLE & L. BERG. 1991. The consortium to establish a registry for Alzheimer's disease. Neurology 41: 479–486.
2. GREINER, P.A. & W.R. MARKESBERY. 1997. Brain infarction and the clinical expression of Alzheimer's disease. JAMA 277: 813–817.
3. TRONCOSO, J.C., L.J. MARTIN, G. DAL FORNO & C.H. KAWAS. 1996. Neuropathology in controls and demented subjects from the Baltimore Longitudinal Study of Aging. Neurobiol. Aging 17: 365–371.
4. BRAYNE, C., F.A. HUPPERT, J.H. XUEREB, H.J. GERTZ, L.-Y. CHI, M.A. MCGEE, E.S. PAYKEL, C. HARRINGTON, E. MUKAETOVA-LADINSKA, A. O'SULLIVAN, T. DENING, C. FREER & C.M. WISCHIK. 1997. An epidemiological study of the dementias in Cambridge: from clinical progression to neuropathology. Proceedings of the 5th International Conference on Alzheimer's Disease, Osaka, Japan, 1996. Elsevier in Alzheimer's Disease: Biology, Diagnosis & Therapeutics. K. Iqbal, B. Winblad, T. Nishimura, M. Takeda & H.M. Wisniewski, Eds. John Wiley & Sons Ltd. Chichester, UK.
5. THOMAS, L.D., M.F. GONZALES, A. CHAMBERLAIN, K. BEYREUTHER, C.L. MASTERS & L. FLICKER. 1994. Comparison of clinical state, retrospective informant interview and the neuropathologic diagnosis of Alzheimer's disease. Int. J. Geriatr. Psychiatry 9: 233–236.
6. GERTZ, H.J., J. XUEREB, F.A. HUPPERT, et al. 1996. The relationship between clinical dementia and neuropathological staging (Braak) in a very elderly community sample. Eur. Arch. Psychiatry Clin. Neurol. Sci. 246:152–156.
7. HOLMES, C., N. CAIRNS, P. LANTOS & A. MANN. 1999. Validity of current clinical criteria for Alzheimer's disease, vascular dementia and dementia with Lewy bodies. Br. J. Psychiatry 174: 45–50.
8. COCHRAN, E.J., O.M. GOSTANIAN & S.S. MIRRA. 1995. Autopsy practices at CERAD and Alzheimer Disease Center sites: a survey of neuropathologists. Alzheimer's Dis. Assoc. 9: 203–207.
9. VAN BELLE, G., K. GIBSON, D. NOCHLIN, M. SUMI & E.B. LARSON. 1997. Counting plaques and tangles in Alzheimer's disease: concordance of technicians and pathologists. J. Neurol. Sci. 145: 141–146.
10. DUYKAERTS, C., M. BENNECIB, Y. GRIGNON, T. UCHIHARA, Y. HE, F. PIETTE & J.J. HAUN. 1997. Modelling the relation between neurofibrillary tangles and intellectual status. Neurobiol. Aging 3: 267–273.
11. HULETTE, C., D. NOCHLIN, D. MCKEEL, J.C. MORRIS, S.S. MIRRA, S.M. SUMI & A. HEYMAN. 1997. Clinical neuropathologic findings in multi-infarct dementia. Neurology 48: 668–672.
12. HAROUTUNIAN, V., D.P. PERL, D.P. PUROHIT, D. MARIN, K. KHAN, M. LANTZ, K.L. DAVIS & R. MOHS. 1998. Regional distribution of neuritic plaques in the nondemented elderly and subjects with very mild Alzheimer disease. Arch. Neurol. 55: 1185–1191.

Leukoaraiosis at Presentation and Disease Progression during Follow-up in Histologically Confirmed Cases of Dementia

R. CLARKE,[a,d] C. JOACHIM,[b] M. ESIRI,[b] J. MORRIS,[b] H. BUNGAY,[b]
A. MOLYNEUX,[b] M. BUDGE,[b] C. FROST,[c] E. KING,[b] L. BARNETSON,[b]
AND A.D. SMITH[b]

[a]Clinical Trial Service Unit and [b]Oxford Project to Investigate Memory and Ageing,
Radcliffe Infirmary, Oxford, and [c]London School of Hygiene & Tropical Medicine,
London, United Kingdom

INTRODUCTION

While Alzheimer's disease and vascular dementia have distinct histopathological features, the combination of both may result in more severe symptoms of dementia.[1,2] The effect of concomitant cerebrovascular disease or cerebrovascular risk factors on the clinical course of Alzheimer's disease is uncertain. Leukoaraiosis, the bilateral symmetrical white matter lucencies visible on computed tomography (CT), is common in very elderly people and in patients with vascular dementia and Alzheimer's disease.[3] Leukoaraiosis is more common among individuals with a prior history of stroke, or cardiovascular risk factors,[3] which has prompted many to consider that leukoaraioisis is a radiological correlate of small vessel disease. There is little histopathological evidence to substantiate this and, indeed, the pathological correlates of leukoaraiosis are by no means clear and may well reflect several different processes.[4,5] The aim of this longitudinal clinicopathological study was to examine the prevalence of leukoaraiosis on CT at presentation among histological subtypes of dementia and assess their relevance to clinical progression of dementia.

PATIENTS AND METHODS

Between July 1988 and April 1996, 198 patients with varying degrees of cognitive dysfunction were referred to the Oxford Project to Investigate Memory and Ageing[6,7]and were followed up until death, when a histopathological diagnosis of Alzheimer's disease (AD) was made using Consortium to Establish a Registry for Alzheimer's Disease (CERAD) criteria for definite or probable Alzheimer's disease.[8] All patients had an annual clinical examination, an assessment of cognitive function (MMSE), and a CT scan, as well as blood samples collected. The presence of leukoaraiosis on CT was determined independently by two radiologists, who were kept blind to the clinical and histological diagnosis. Blood homocysteine, folate, and

[d]Address for correspondence: Dr. Robert Clarke, Clinical Trial Service Unit, Radcliffe Infirmary, Oxford, OX2 6HE, UK. Tel.: 01865-557241; fax 01865-558817.
e-mail: robert.clarke@ctsu.ox.ac.uk

TABLE 1. Characteristics of cases with dementia by the presence of leukoaraiosis on CT at presentation

Mean Values (SD) or Percentage (%)	No. of Individuals	Leukoaraiosis on CT	
		−	+
No. of individuals	195	44%	56%
Males	84	57%	43%
Females	111	34%	66%
Mean (SD) age (years)	195	67 (9)	77 (8)
Current smoker, %	193	26%	26%
Clinical variables, mean (SD) or %			
Atrial fibrillation, %	195	3%	11%
Systolic blood pressure (mmHg)	195	141 (21)	154 (25)
Diastolic blood pressure (mmHg)	195	85 (11)	89 (14)
MMSE score (max 30)	195	19 (8)	15 (8)
Biochemical variables, mean (SD)			
Total homocysteine (μmol/l)	195	14 (9)	16 (7)
Serum folate (nmol/l)	195	9 (5)	7 (5)
Vitamin B12 (pmol/l)	195	325 (170)	316 (125)
ApoE ε4 allele frequency, %	195	38%	34%
Disease progression, mean (SD)			
Time to dependency (weeks)	195	145 (98)	104 (85)
Time to institutionalization (weeks)	114	110 (94)	79 (72)

vitamin B12 levels were measured using nonfasting samples that had been stored at −70°C as previously described.[9,10] Time to institutionalization and time to dependency were defined as the time intervals between the initial visit and admission to a nursing home and time to requirement of help with two or more of feeding, dressing or toilet functions, respectively. Differences in the probability of institutionalization or dependency during the follow-up period in the presence or absence of leukoaraiosis on CT at presentation were assessed using Kaplan Meier analysis and Cox proportional hazards ratio after adjusting for differences in age at presentation.

RESULTS

One hundred nine of 195 patients (56%) who had a CT scan performed had evidence of leukoaraiosis, and such individuals were on average 10 years older, and had higher mean sysytolic blood pressure and a shorter mean time to dependency and institutionalization than those without leukoaraiosis (TABLE 1). Leukoaraiosis was positively correlated with age at CT scan ($r = 0.51$, $p < 0.0001$), with systolic blood pressure (0.26, $p < 0.001$), and serum homocysteine ($r = 0.26$, $p < 0.001$); it inversely correlated with serum folate ($r = -0.19$, $p < 0.05$) and the initial MMSE score ($r = -0.22$, $p < 0.001$), but was unrelated to cigarette smoking or to blood levels of vitamin B12, total cholesterol or apo E ε4 alleles.

TABLE 2. Distribution of leukoaraiosis in subjects with dementia, clinical markers of disease severity, and progression by histological subtypes of Alzheimer's disease (AD) using CERAD criteria

	Histological Diagnosis of AD by CERAD		
	Negative[a]	Probable/Possible	Definite
No. of individuals	25	25	84
Mean (SD) age, (years)	71 (9)	81 (8)	74 (7)
Sex (% males)	48%	52%	42%
MMSE score, mean (SD) (maximum 30)	18 (7)	18 (8)	13 (8)
Leukoaraiosis (%)	46%	72%	68%
Time to dependency, median (weeks)	82	85	80
Time to institutionalization, median (weeks)	106	54	57

[a]Includes Parkinson's disease, vascular dementia and frontotemporal dementia.

TABLE 3. Relationship of leukoaraiosis to clinical progression of dementia when classified by severity of Alzheimer's pathology

		Probability of Institutionalization or Dependency			
		Probability of institutionalization by 3 years (%)		Probability of dependency by 3 years (%)	
		Leukoaraiosis on CT		Leukoaraiosis on CT	
Histological Diagnosis of AD by CERAD	No. of Individuals	− ($n = 45$)	+ ($n = 69$)	− ($n = 47$)	+ ($n = 86$)
Negative	25	50	63	52	81
Probable/possible	25	17	40	33	74
Definite	84	54	59	66	62
All	134	40	54*	39	62**

*$p = 0.055$.
** $p = 0.017$.

There was a high prevalence of leukoaraiosis in all histological subtypes of dementia among the 134 cases with available histological data (TABLE 2). Twenty-three of the 31 cases (74%) who had an infarct on CT had leukoaraioisis on CT, but most of these had probable or definite Alzheimer's disease. All the histological types of dementia had a high probability of dependency by three years, but those with leukoaraiosis had a higher probability of dependency than those without it ($p = 0.017$), but differences in the probability of institutionalization by three years were not statistically significant (TABLE 3). However, after adjustment for differences in age at presentation, the Cox proportional hazard ratios associated with leukoaraiosis at presentation for dependency was 1.44 (95% CI: 0.9 to 2.3; $p = 0.08$) and for institutionalization was 1.45 (95% CI: 0.8 to 2.5; $p = 0.23$).

CONCLUSION

Leukoaraiosis was strongly correlated with age, systolic blood pressure, and blood total homocysteine levels, as previously reported.[3] The prevalence of leukoaraiosis was higher in those with definite or probable Alzheimer's disease compared with the mixed category that included Parkinson's disease, frontotemporal dementia, and vascular dementia. Those cases with leukoaraiosis had a shorter median time to dependency than those without it, but these differences were no longer significant after adjustment for differences in age at presentation. These results suggest that leukoaraiosis, which is strongly correlated with age and cardiovascular risk factors, is common in all histological types of dementia, particularly in those with probable or definite Alzheimer's disease. More work is required to characterize the histopathological correlates of leukoaraiosis. Larger studies or a meta-analysis of similar studies is required to determine the prognostic significance of cardiovascular risk factors to disease progression in dementia. Reliable estimates of the epidemiologically predicted differences in disease progression associated with differences due to leukoaraiosis or to other cardiovascular risk factors in age and sex-specific groups are required to provide realistic expectation of treatment effects and thereby help in the design of clinical trials of vascular risk factor modification in patients with dementia.[11] A meta-analysis of similar longitudinal clinical studies has been initiated to resolve these issues.

REFERENCES

1. SNOWDEN, D.A., L.H. GREINER, J.A. MORTIMER, K.P. RILEY, P.A. GREINER & W.R. MARKESBERY. 1997. Brain infarction and the clinical expression of Alzheimer's disease: the Nun Study. JAMA **277:** 813–817.
2. NAGY, Z.S., M.M. ESIRI, K.A. JOBST, *et al.* 1997. The effects of additional pathology on the cognitive deficit of Alzheimer's disease. J. Neuropathol. Exp. Neurol. **56:** 165–170.
3. INZITARI, D., F. DIAZ, A. FOX, V.C. HACKINSKI, A. STEINGART, C. LAU, A. DONALD, *et al.* 1987. Vascular risk factors and leuko-araiosis. Arch. Neurol. **44:** 42–44.
4. BRUN, A. & E. ENGLAND. 1986. A white matter disorder in dementia of the Alzheimer type: a pathoanatomical study. Ann. Neurol. **19:** 253–262.
5. PANTONI, L. & J.H. GARCIA. 1997. Pathogenesis of leukaraiosis: a review. Stroke **28:** 652–659.
6. JOBST, K.A., A.D. SMITH, M. SZATMARI, *et al.* 1994. Rapidly progressing atrophy of medial temporal lobe in Alzheimer's disease. Lancet **343:** 829–830.
7. JOBST, K.A., A.D. SMITH, M. SZATMARI, *et al.* 1992. Detection in life of confirmed Alzheimer's disease using a simple measurement of medial temporal lobe atrophy by computed tomography. Lancet **340:** 1179–1183.
8. MIRRA, S.S., A. HEYMAN, D. MCKEEL, *et al.* 1991. The Consortium to Establish a Registry for Alzheimer's Disease (CERAD). 2. Standardization of the neuropathologic assessment of Alzheimer's disease. Neurology **41:** 479–486.
9. CLARKE, R., A.D. SMITH, K.A. JOBST, H. REFSUM, L. SUTTON & P.M. UELAND. 1998. Folate, vitamin B-12 and serum total homocysteine levels in confirmed Alzheimer's disease. Arch. Neurol. **55:** 1449–1455.
10. CLARKE, R., P. WOODHOUSE, A. ULVIK, *et al.* 1998. Variability and determinants of plasma total homocysteine levels in an elderly population. Clin. Chem. **44:** 102–107.
11. CLARKE, R., C. FROST, V. LEROY & R. COLLINS for the Homocysteine Lowering Trialist's collaboration. 1998. Lowering blood homocysteine with folic acid based supplements: meta-analysis of randomised trials. Homocysteine Lowering Trialist's Collaboration. Br. Med. J. **316:** 894–898.

Vascular Actions of Estrogen and Alzheimer's Disease

T. THOMAS[a,b,c] AND J. RHODIN[b]

[a]*Woodlands Medical and Research Center, Oldsmar, Florida 34677, USA*

[b]*Department of Anatomy College of Medicine, University of South Florida, Tampa, Florida 33612, USA*

ABSTRACT: Women are two to three times more likely to develop late-onset Alzheimer's disease (AD) than age-matched men. A large number of observational reports and a few randomized clinical trials have indicated that estrogen replacement therapy (ERT) may retard the development and severity of dementia in postmenopausal women. A chronic inflammatory reaction mediated by abnormal deposition of proteins such as amyloid-β (Aβ) is central to the pathology of AD. We investigated the effect of low doses of conjugated estrogen (Premarin) in an animal model of Aβ-induced vascular disruption and inflammatory reaction. Estrogen prevented vascular deposition of Aβ, endothelial and vessel wall disruption with plasma leakage, platelet and mast cell activation, and characteristic features of an inflammatory reaction: adhesion and transmigration of leukocytes. The beneficial effect was lost when estrogen treatment was discontinued. This novel protective effect of estrogen against Aβ-induced vascular dysfunction may contribute to the therapeutic efficacy of estrogen in AD and coronary vascular disease.

INTRODUCTION

Women have two- to threefold higher age-specific prevalence rates of AD and usually perform worse than men in tests of cognitive function.[1] Estrogen replacement therapy (ERT) in postmenopausal women accords protection against a number of degenerative diseases associated with aging such as cardiovascular illness,[2] osteoporosis,[3] and possibly AD.[4] A number of reports have indicated that estrogen therapy may retard the development and severity of dementia in postmenopausal women.[5] The beneficial reports of estrogen therapy are based mainly on retrospective studies and a small number of controlled clinical trials.[6] Because of the discrepancies in some of the findings and the potential for adverse events (endometrial hyperplasia, breast cancer, and thromboembolic events), we need further proof of a direct protective action of estrogen before ERT can be advocated for AD.

There is increasing evidence that chronic inflammation might contribute to the degenerative changes observed in AD brain. Several markers of inflammatory activity are significantly elevated in the brains of AD patients.[7,8] Several factors, includ-

[c]Address for correspondence: Tom Thomas, M.D., Ph.D., Woodlands Medical and Research Center, 3150 Tampa Road, Suite 16, Oldsmar, Florida 34677. Tel.: (727) 786-5587, Ext. 26; fax: (727) 785-3254.

e-mail: tthomas1@tampabay.rr.com

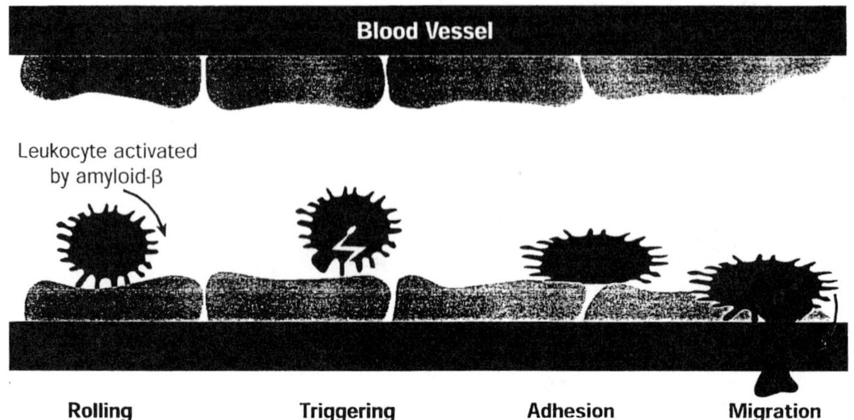

FIGURE 1. Schematic diagram of Aβ-induced inflammatory reaction. Aβ was used as a trigger to initiate the rolling, adhesion and transmigration of leukocytes. The inflammatory cascade involves the concerted action of oxygen radicals, cytokines, and adhesion molecules.

ing the Alzheimer peptide amyloid-β (Aβ), can initiate the classic complement cascade leading to the recruitment and activation of microglia that are of monocyte/macrophage lineage. A large number of epidemiological studies and few controlled clinical studies support the contention that nonsteroidal antiinflammatory drugs (NSAIDS) delay the incidence of AD.[8] The transient improvement in cognition produced by currently available acetylcholine esterase inhibitors and the toxic side effects of NSAIDS points to the need for further evaluating clinically useful agents, such as estrogens, which may be of therapeutic value in neurodegenerative diseases such as AD.

There is ample evidence indicating that progressive cerebral deposition of Aβ is central to the pathology of AD.[9] Recent reports from our laboratory and others indicate that Aβ-mediated vascular dysfunction may subject the neurons to oxidative and inflammatory damage.[10–13]

In view of the reports showing a protective role for estrogen in AD, we examined the *in vivo* effect of Premarin (the most widely prescribed form of estrogen) using an animal model of AD-like vascular pathology developed in our laboratory (FIG. 1).

METHODS

Animals

Adult male Sprague-Dawley rats weighing 200–250 g were divided into four groups ($n = 8$ or more per group). The control group received physiologic saline solution. The second group received Aβ alone. The third group was given Premarin orally for two weeks and then received Aβ. In the fourth group, Premarin treatment was discontinued for one week before administration of Aβ.

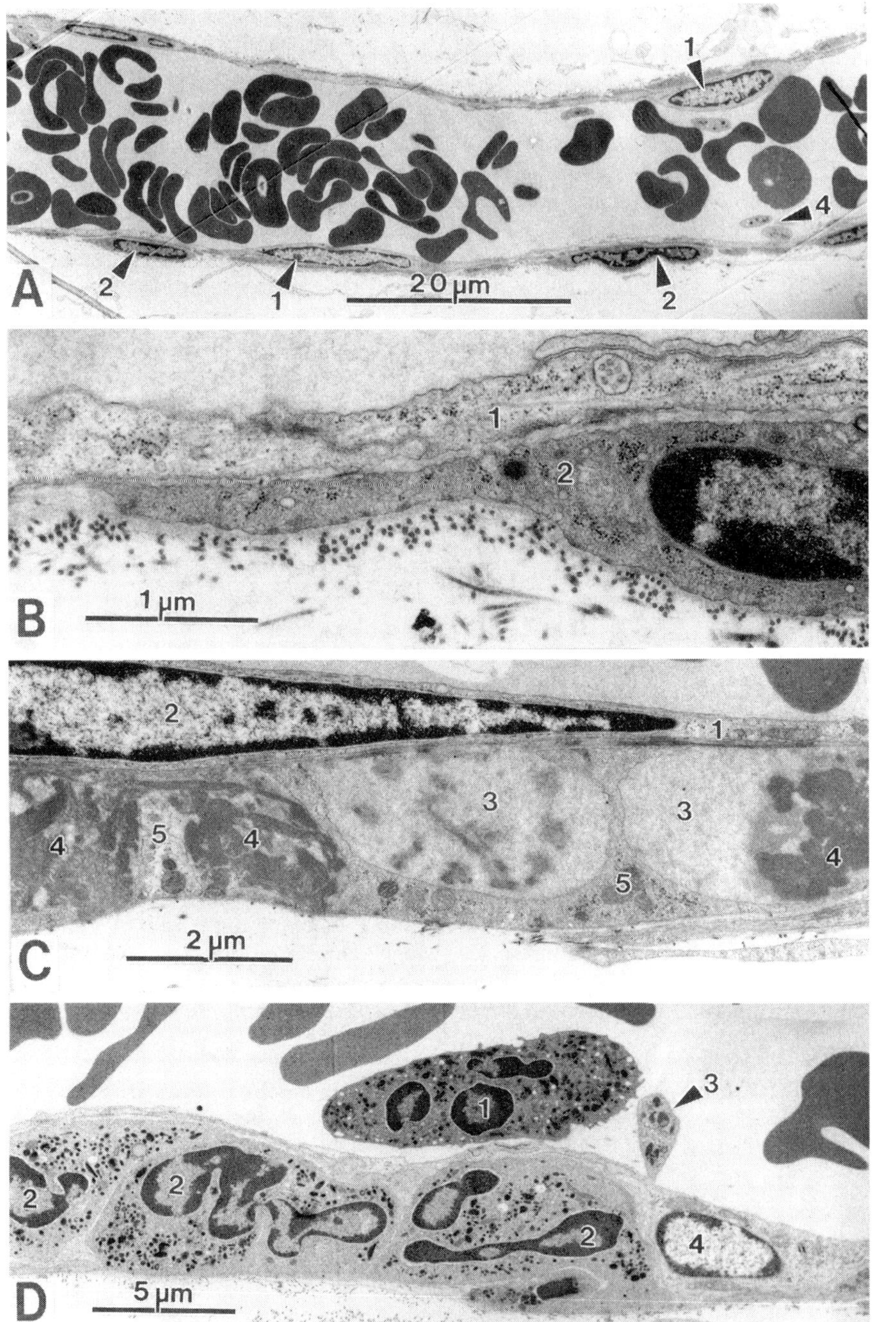

FIGURE 2. *Caption on following page.*

Rat Mesenteric Preparation

The rats were anesthetized with pentobarbital, 60 mg/kg body weight, administered intraperitoneally; and a cannula was introduced proximal to one of the mesenteric arteries. The pharmacologic agents were introduced via this cannula. A midline incision of the abdominal wall was made, and part of the small intestine together with its mesentery was pulled out and held flat on the lucite surface of a cradle. The plastic cradle was mounted on the stage of an Olympus BH-1 light microscope equipped with five objective lenses (4×, 10×, 32×, 40×, and 100× oil immersion). The mesenteric field was observed and video recorded throughout the entire experiment. The blood vessels in this preparation were transparent, enabling video recording under the light microscope so that the blood flow and the morphology of the vessel and its interaction with the various formed blood elements could be monitored in the live animal. The mesenteric surface was kept moist by superfusion of a warm saline solution. At the end of the experiment, the mesentery was superfused for 15 min with glutaraldehyde solution, and for an additional 15 min by osmic acid solution. Subsequently, the observed field was dehydrated and cut out for processing for transmission electron microscopy.

RESULTS

Intravital Observations

Aβ Alone

Serum Aβ levels averaged 1.6 ng/ml before Aβ infusion. The rats were infused with 0.25 ml of $A\beta_{1-40}$ in saline (100 ng Aβ/g body weight) for 2 min. At 30 min after Aβ infusion, there was an eightfold increase of Aβ levels and 99% of the administered Aβ was cleared within one hour. An average segment of at least 1000 μm of arterioles was video recorded for 60 min. There was an average of 20–25 leukocytes ($n = 15$) marginating and adhering to the endothelial lining (FIG. 2).

At certain points in an arteriole, there would be a distinct margination of platelets. In most instances, they would tumble, some attaching to the endothelium, others reaching the subendothelial space. The thickness of the arteriolar wall was increased at these specific points. Erythrocytes often became attached to the endothelial lining, usually anchored to it with part of the cell, fluttering in the rapid blood

---

FIGURE 2. (A) Premarin + Aβ. This demonstrates a perfectly normal 25-mm-wide precapillary arteriole. There is no leukocyte or platelet margination. Structures are the following: endothelial cell nuclei (1), smooth muscle cell nuclei (2), erythrocytes (3), platelets (4). Magnification: 1450×. **(B)** Premarin + Aβ. Wall of precapillary arteriole. The ultrastructure is completely normal. The endothelial cytoplasm (1) is not vacuolated or disrupted. There is no subendothelial plasma leakage distorting the smooth muscle cell (2). Magnification: 21,500×. **(C)** Aβ alone. The cytoplasm (1) and the nucleus (2) of the endothelial cell are normal. The subendothelial space is filled with plasma leakage (3) and fibrillar amyloid (4) which distort the smooth muscle cells (5). Magnification: 10,600×. **(D)** Premarin discontinued + Aβ. Wall of postcapillary venule. There is one marginated leukocyte (1) in the lumen. Several leukocytes (2) have reached the subendothelial space. A platelet (3) is attached to the endothelial cell (4). Magnification: 3800×.

flow. Electron microscope analysis demonstrated an abundance of red blood cells lodged in the subendothelial space. Many mast cells were activated, indicated by pronounced degranulation.

Premarin + Aβ

Rats received a daily oral administration of 200 μg Premarin per kg body weight for two weeks followed by a 2-min infusion of $A\beta_{1-40}$ in 0.25 ml saline (100 ng/g body weight). They were then subjected to the same routine video recording of the mesenteric arterioles as rats receiving Aβ alone. During an observation time of 60 min, there was an average of 2–4 leukocytes ($n = 8$) marginating and adhering to the endothelial lining. Invariably, however, they would all become detached. Platelets and erythrocytes were not observed to marginate or penetrate the endothelial lining. This video recording was identical to the controls. No activation or degranulation of mast cells was observed during this period.

Premarin Discontinued + Aβ

In rats that had received a daily oral administration of 200 μg Premarin per kg body weight for two weeks, the Premarin treatment was discontinued for one week, followed by a 2-min perfusion of 100 ng Aβ per gram of body weight. Again, the mesenteric arterioles were subjected to the same routine video recording as rats receiving Premarin + Aβ. There was an average of 15–20 leukocytes ($n = 8$) adhering to or transmigrating the endothelial lining. Platelets were marginating, tumbling, and penetrating the endothelial lining in certain areas of mostly precapillary arterioles. Erythrocytes were observed to adhere to the arteriolar wall.

Electron Microscope Observations

Controls and Premarin + Aβ

The structure of the arterioles was completely normal in both the control animals and those that were treated with Premarin for 2 weeks followed by a 2-min Aβ infusion (FIG. 3).

Aβ Alone and Premarin Discontinued + Aβ

The vascular disruption observed on discontinuation of Premarin was identical to the damage induced by Aβ treatment alone. Margination and adherence of leukocytes/monocytes was the initial event. The leukocytes then proceeded to penetrate the endothelial lining and either became lodged in the subendothelial space or reached the perivascular connective tissue, where they become macrophages.

Blood plasma and amyloid accumulated in the subendothelial space, separating and distorting the smooth muscle cells. The amyloid appeared as interwoven fibrillar bundles (FIG. 3). Platelets and erythrocytes were also trapped in the subendothelial space. The platelets were often degranulated and some appeared as empty, membrane-bound vacuoles. Most mast cells were degranulated.

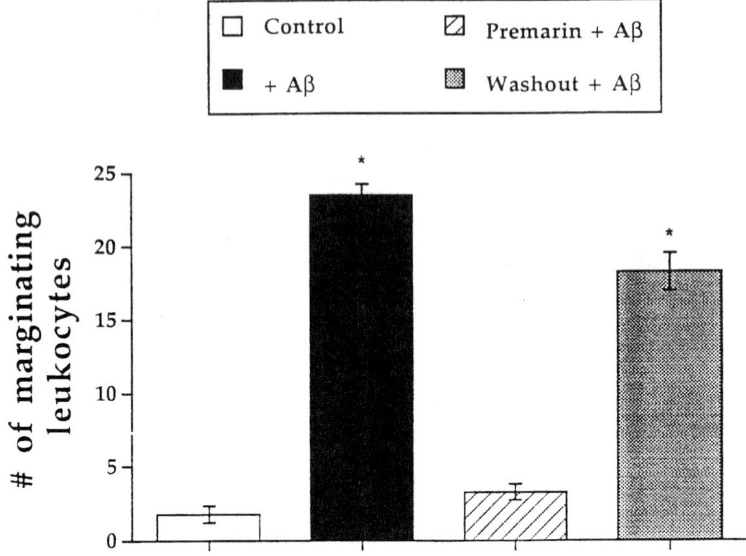

FIGURE 3. The number of leukocytes marginating under various treatment conditions. After intravital microscopy, the videotape was reviewed. The number of leukocytes marginating per 1000 μm length of the arteriole for a 60-min period were counted ($n \geq 8$ per group). Premarin treatment significantly reduced the number of marginating leukocytes.

DISCUSSION

Increasing life expectancy for women has led to the added risk of cognitive decline after menopause, possibly due to an estrogen deficiency state. There has been abundant data on the benefits of estrogen replacement for osteoporosis, heart disease, and even AD. This report illustrates novel actions of conjugated estrogens in protecting against Aβ-induced vascular damage and inflammatory response that might contribute to the reported efficacy of estrogen in AD therapy.

Currently available animal models for AD, including transgenic mice overexpressing amyloid precursor protein or presenelin genes, have focused exclusively on the neuropathological correlates of AD and have not proved to be satisfactory, as they rarely exhibit neuronal damage, inflammation, or cognitive deficits that are hallmarks in the AD brain. We recently developed an animal model that displays many of the typical characteristics of vascular pathology seen in AD.[12] The Aβ used in these studies is freshly prepared nonaggregated $A\beta_{1-40}$, which is typically associated with vascular deposits in AD brain and is the predominant form of circulating Aβ. The more fibrillar $A\beta_{1-42}$ predominantly found in senile plaques also produces vascular dysfunction.[14] Recent evidence from our laboratory and others have shown that peripheral vascular dysfunction may contribute to AD pathology.[12,15] A similar

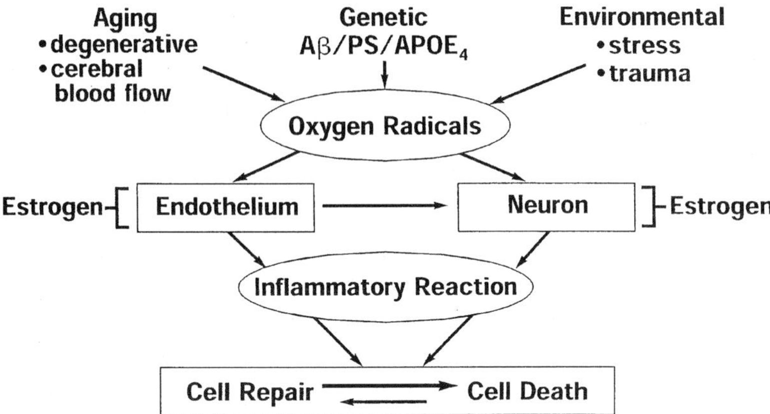

FIGURE 4. Schematic diagram of the etiology of AD and the protective action of estrogen. Aβ = amyloid-β, PS = presenelin, APOE = apolipoprotein E. Estrogen protects the endothelium and neuron from the deleterious effects of oxygen radicals and inflammatory reaction.

reaction in the cerebral vasculature is feasible because the architecture of the cerebral arterial wall is similar to the peripheral vessels except for the presence of endothelial tight junctions and a reduced number of pinocytic vesicles in the endothelium. In addition, all of the following peripheral actions of estrogen may contribute to the protective effect of estrogen against Alzheimer's disease. The vascular actions of estrogen include the following: improved lipid profile, enhancement of nitric oxide-mediated endothelial function, increased vasodilation and blood flow, inhibition of vascular smooth muscle proliferation, reduction of coagulation factors and platelet adhesiveness, and antioxidant actions such as inhibition of LDL oxidation. Estrogen, by protecting the endothelial cells from Aβ-induced damage, will also ensure the integrity of blood–brain barrier. Endothelial damage by Aβ, primarily due to oxidant stress within the endothelium, can lead to a cascade of events beginning with activation of vascular cytokines and proceeding to expression of adhesion molecules on the cell surface, which attracts monocytes and other leukocytes to adhere to the endothelial surface. Leukocyte extravasation from the blood into the tissues is a well orchestrated, multistep event involving a series of interactions between leukocytes and endothelial cells.[16] The antiinflammatory action of estrogen has been further supported by the recent observation that estrogen reduced markers of vascular inflammation in postmenopausal women.[17]

Interventions targeted at Aβ-mediated vascular dysfunction and inflammatory reactions may provide significant therapeutic utility in AD. But the toxic side effects of nonsteroidal antiinflammatory drugs (NSAIDS) point to the need to explore novel agents to prevent an Aβ-induced inflammatory cascade. In this regard estrogens might provide an alternative. The challenge is to balance the beneficial outcomes on osteoporosis, cardiovascular disease, and dementia against the risk of estrogen-dependent tumors.

The infiltration of leukocytes, as seen in our study, has been implicated as a mediator of injury in numerous inflammatory disorders.[16] The amelioration of this effect by estrogen may contribute to some of the beneficial effects attributed to ERT. A protective effect of estrogen on amyloid toxicity in cerebral blood vessels (FIG. 4) further supports a role for estrogen therapy in AD.

AD is considered to be a neurodegenerative disorder confined to the brain, particularly restricted to neuronal tissue. There is increasing evidence[14,15] that Aβ may contribute to vascular dysfunction in the CNS and peripheral tissues, and we demonstrate that estrogen has the capacity to protect the vasculature from the deleterious effects of Aβ. Inhibition of amyloid deposition is considered to be a prime target of AD therapy.[18,19] This report proves that estrogen therapy prevents the vascular deposition of Aβ with attendant inhibition of the toxic reaction of Aβ.

ACKNOWLEDGMENTS

This study was supported in part by a grant from Wyeth-Ayerst Pharmaceuticals. The authors acknowledge the excellent technical assistance of Margaret Bryant, Linda Clark, and Amanda Garces.

REFERENCES

1. RIPICH, D.N., S.A. PETRILL, P.J. WHITEHOUSE & E.W. ZIOL. 1995. Gender differences in language of AD patients: a longitudinal study. Neurology **45:** 299–301.
2. WENGER, N.K. 1998. Postmenopausal hormone therapy: is it useful for coronary prevention? Cardiol. Clin. **16:** 17–25.
3. GRADY, D., S.M. RUBIN, D.B. PETITTI *et al.* 1992. Hormone therapy to prevent disease and prolong life in postmenopausal women. Ann. Intern. Med. **117:** 1016–1037.
4. TANG, M-X., D. JACOBS, Y. STERN *et al.* 1996. Effect of estrogen during menopause on risk and age at onset of Alzheimer's disease. Lancet **348:** 429–432.
5. KAWAS, C., S. RESNIK, A. MORRISON *et al.* 1997. A prospective study of estrogen replacement therapy and the risk of developing Alzheimer's disease: the Baltimore longitudinal study of aging. Neurology **48:** 1517–1521.
6. HENDERSON, V.W., A. PAGANINI-HILL, C.K. EMANUEL *et al.* 1994. Estrogen replacement therapy in older women: comparisons between AD cases and non-demented control subjects. Arch. Neurol. **51:** 896–900.
7. PASIMETTI, G.M. 1996. Inflammatory mechanisms in neurodegeneration and Alzheimer's disease: the role of the complement system. Neurobiol. Aging **17:** 707–7168.
8. MCGEER, P.I., M. SCHULZER & E.G. MCGEER. 1996. Arthritis and anti-inflammatory agents as possible protective factors for Alzheimer's disease: a review of 17 epidemiologic studies. Neurology **47:** 425–4329.
9. SELKOE, D.J. 1994. Cell biology of the amyloid β protein precursor and the mechanism of Alzheimer's disease. Ann. Rev. Cell Biol. **10:** 373–403.
10. THOMAS, T., G. THOMAS, C. MCLENDON *et al.* 1996. β-Amyloid-mediated vasoactivity and vascular endothelial damage. Nature **380:** 168–171.
11. THOMAS, T., C. MCLENDON, E.T. SUTTON & G. THOMAS. 1997. Cerebrovascular endothelial dysfunction mediated by β-amyloid. NeuroReport **8:** 1387–1391.
12. THOMAS, T., E.T. SUTTON, M.W. BRYANT & J.A.G. RHODIN. 1997. In vivo vascular damage, leukocyte activation and inflammatory response induced by β-amyloid. J. Submicrosc. Cytol. Pathol. **29:** 293–304.
13. IADECOLA, C., F. ZHANG, K. NIWA *et al.* 1999. SOD1 rescues cerebral endothelial dysfunction in mice overexpressing amyloid precursor protein. Nat. Neurosci. **2:** 157–1611.

14. THOMAS, T., C. MCLENDON, A. TUGERTIMUR & K. THOMAS. 1998. Amyloid β-peptides, $A\beta_{1-40}$ and $A\beta_{1-42}$ induce cerebrovascular endothelial dysfunction. Alzheimer's Rep. **1:** 17–24.
15. HOFMAN, A., A. OTT, M.M.B. BRETELER *et al.* 1997. Atherosclerosis, apolipoprotein E, and prevalence of dementia and Alzheimer's disease in the Rotterdam study. Lancet **349:** 151–154.
16. LUSTER, A.D. 1998. Chemokines—chemotactic cytokines that mediate inflammation. N. Engl. J. Med. **338:** 436–445.
17. KOH, K.K., C. CARDILLO, M.N. BUI *et al.* 1999. Vascular effects of estrogen and cholesterol-lowering therapies in hypercholesteremic postmenopausal women. Circulation **99:** 354–360.
18. GEULA, C., C-K. WU, D. SAROFF *et al.* 1998. Aging renders the brain vulnerable to amyloid β-protein neurotoxicity. Nat. Med. **4:** 827–831.
19. XU, H., G.K. GOURAS, J.P. GREENFIELD *et al.* 1998. Estrogen reduces neuronal generation of Alzheimer's β-amyloid peptides. Nat. Med. **4:** 447–451.

Subcortical Vascular Dementia as a Specific Target for Clinical Trials

DOMENICO INZITARI,[a] TIMO ERKINJUNTTI,[b] ANDERS WALLIN,[c] TEODORO DEL SER,[d] MARCO ROMANELLI,[a] AND LEONARDO PANTONI[a,e]

[a]*Department of Neurological and Psychiatric Sciences, University of Florence, Florence, Italy*

[b]*Department of Clinical Neurosciences, Helsinki University Central Hospital, Helsinki, Finland*

[c]*Institute of Clinical Neuroscience, Götenberg University, Molndal, Sweden*

[d]*Section of Neurology, "Severo Ochoa" Hospital, Madrid, Spain*

ABSTRACT: Vascular cognitive impairment is considered the second most common form of mental deterioration in the elderly after degenerative dementias. Therapeutic approaches to vascular dementia mainly rely on the identification and treatment of risk factors. A number of drugs have also been tested with the aim of improving or slowing cognitive decline in patients affected by various forms of cerebrovascular disease. Most of these trials have yielded unsatisfactory results. We hypothesize that some of these failures depend on the inclusion of patients with pathophysiologically heterogeneous types of vascular cognitive decline. In this paper, we review some of the most important trials that tested drugs with a preventive or therapeutic aim in vascular dementia patients. Preliminary results suggest that some beneficial effects can be detected only when the trial population is homogeneous on a clinical and pathogenic basis. In particular, subcortical vascular dementia, a form with a rather univocal clinical, radiological, and pathological picture, seems a particularly apt choice as a target for future clinical studies. At present, only one therapeutic trial is being conducted in patients affected by this specific form of vascular dementia.

INTRODUCTION

At present, no drug has been definitively accepted as effective in vascular dementia (VaD). We suggest that this mainly depends on the current definition of VaD itself. As the term VaD is now commonly used, it, in fact, encompasses different clinical–pathological subtypes, linked with selective pathophysiological mechanisms, which are considered and listed in the most recent classifications.[1-3] Chui *et al.* classify the disorder into subtypes with the disclaimer, however, that their classification should serve only for research purposes. Different subtypes of VaD are defined according to location (cortical, deep or periventricular white matter, basal ganglia, thalamus), size (volume), distribution (large, small, or microvessel), sever-

[e]Address for correspondence: Leonardo Pantoni, M.D., Ph.D., Department of Neurological and Psychiatric Sciences, University of Florence, Viale Morgagni 85, 50134 Firenze, Italy. Tel.: #39-055-4277 995; fax: #39-055-4298 461.
e-mail: pantoni@neuro.unifi.it

ity (chronic ischemia vs. infarction), and etiology (embolism, atherosclerosis, arteriolosclerosis, cerebral amyloid angiopathy, and hypoperfusion) of the lesions. The National Institute of Neurological Disorders and Stroke and Association Internationale pour la Recherche et l'Enseignement en Neurosciences (NINDS-AIREN) criteria listed the following pathophysiological causes that may be associated with VaD syndromes: (1) multiple large complete infarcts; (2) strategic single infarcts; (3) small-vessel disease; (4) hypoperfusion; (5) hemorrhage; and (6) other mechanisms. A definitive systematization has not yet been reached because, according to Nyenhuis and Gorelick,[4] there has been little research comparing VaD subgroups on important variables such as the pattern and severity of cognitive or functional impairment, the relationship to stroke risk factors, demographic variables, and course of dementia. In fact, different VaD types share common risk factors, neurological findings, and clinical course. Moreover, different lesion types (for example, cortical territorial and small, deep infarcts, strategic infarcts, and hypoperfusion changes) may frequently occur in combination in the same patient. Modern imaging techniques have proved strongly supportive for a more detailed characterization of these subtypes. It has become more and more apparent that subcortical VaD, which is consistent with the NINDS-AIREN subtyping for both small-vessel and Binswanger's dementia and is so recognized in the 10th revision of the *International Classification of Disease* (ICD-10), is probably one the most frequent forms of VaD. Neuroimaging and clinical studies have indicated that this type of VaD has rather univocal radiological and clinical characteristics,[5,6] although a clinical–pathological correlation has not yet been established with precision.[7–11]

Finally, there are forms where vascular changes are combined with Alzheimer's disease or other types of pathologic degeneration (mixed dementia). Unfortunately for these last cases, neither clinical nor laboratory tools exist that are sensitive enough to permit a unequivocal identification.

Understanding the pathophysiological mechanism that causes cognitive impairment in individual cases is an essential step for choosing the proper treatments. Unlike what has been done so far, clinical trials should address a univocal pathophysiological setting, ascertain that a particular treatment has a rationale that fits with this setting, and include in the study patients homogeneously presenting a definite clinical–pathological condition. In this paper, treatments that have been proposed and tested in VaD are reviewed with the aim of disclosing clues to support the theory that failure of therapeutic trials in VaD, and lack of evidence for any effective treatment, may depend at least in part on the fact that these trials have not taken into account different subtypes of VaD.

PREVENTIVE TREATMENTS IN VASCULAR DEMENTIA

Ideally, cognitive impairment of vascular origin should be treated in its earliest phase, at a time when the mental deficit has not achieved its most severe degree (i.e., dementia). Dementia is ultimately caused by more or less severe loss of brain tissue, which can be either extensive or very selective affecting crucial areas or circuits. In both cases, at present, we have no means to regenerate the damaged tissue. Unlike primary degenerative dementias in which the cause of the process is unknown, however, in VaD we know enough about risk factors and pathogenic mechanisms to take preventive measures. Accordingly, the aim should be to identify subjects at risk, and, by treating their risk factors, to slow or even arrest the dementing process. Control of risk factors has a twofold objective: (a) prevention of cerebrovascular events; (b) slowing of the progression of underlying pathology. Blood hypertension (probably the main risk factor), diabetes mellitus, smoking, and hyperlipidemia, can all be effectively controlled.

Several large therapeutic trials have been carried out over the last decades with different types of treatments, including interventions for risk-factor control, antithrombotic agents (antiplatelet or anticoagulant), or even surgery, with the aim of stroke prevention. It is quite surprising, and in some ways unexplainable, that these trials have omitted to include, among preventable outcomes, cognitive decline. It is suggested that future trials avoid this omission. Moreover, therapeutic trials for stroke prevention have not classified different stroke types (for example, large cortical vs. lacunar infarct, linked with the multiinfarct or the subcortical VaD forms, respectively) on entry or as outcome events. Consequently, it is impossible to evaluate, even if indirectly, the impact of selective treatments on VaD subtypes. For example, given the association of lacunar stroke with VaD (lacunar state, subcortical VaD), it would be interesting to know whether antiplatelet agents are specifically able to prevent recurrence in patients with this stroke type. Actually, only two trials provided evidence regarding the possible preventive effect of antiplatelet agents in patients presenting with lacunar infarcts. The Accidents Ischemic Cerebraux Lies a l'Atherosclerose (AICLA) trial examined the effect of aspirin, aspirin plus dypiradomole, or placebo in patients with lacunar stroke only, showing that these treatments also reduced the stroke recurrence in this subgroup.[12] A significant benefit of ticlopidine for stroke prevention in patients with lacunar stroke was shown by the Canadian American Ticlopidine Study (CATS).[13]

Considering studies specifically addressing VaD, only small studies and hints are available. Meyer *et al.*, following a small number of patients, showed that control of vascular risk factors, such as arterial hypertension and smoking, was able to stabilize or improve the cognitive status of patients diagnosed with multi-infarct dementia.[14] The same authors observed that a too marked reduction in systolic blood pressure levels was associated with progression of mental deterioration.[14] More recently, the Syst-Eur trial, a randomized, double-blind, placebo-controlled trial for treating systolic hypertension, has provided the first clear-cut evidence that controlling hypertension reduces the incidence of dementia.[15] Using a treatment regimen consisting of nitrendipine, with the possible addition of enalapril, hydroclorothiazide, or both drugs titrated or combined to reduce the systolic blood pressure by at least 20 mmHg to reach a value <150 mmHg, reduced the incidence of dementia by 50% (from 7.7 to 3.8 cases per 1000 patients/year). The results of this study left several questions open, however, especially regarding the mechanisms by which hypertension control reduces the risk of dementia. Outcomes to be prevented included either Alzheimer's, mixed, or VaD. Diagnosis of dementia relied on a Mini-Mental Status Examination score of 23 or less, followed by the application of diagnostic criteria for dementia of the Diagnostic and Statistical Manual of Mental Disorders (DSM-III-R). The original and the modified Hachinski ischemic score, when a brain CT scan was available, served in the Syst-Eur trial to differentiate vascular from degenerative dementia in some of cases. Nowadays, these definitions appear broad and completely inadequate for any evaluation of mechanisms by which hypertension control reduces the risk of dementia and, in the light of the modern classification of VaD subtypes, on which subtype hypertension control may exert the highest impact. Another large therapeutic trial in hypertension, the Systolic Hypertension in the Elderly Program (SHEP) trial,[16] using as antihypertensive treatment a tyazide diuretic and a beta-blocker, failed to demonstrate a protective effect against cognitive impairment, suggesting that dementia cannot be prevented simply by lowering the blood pressure. In the early report of the Syst-Eur trial, the authors suggest that calcium channel blockers used in this study may have a direct neuroprotective effect or may alter production of β–amyloid or neurotransmission. However, calcium antagonists have also been shown to prevent age-related changes in the small vessels of experimental animals[17,18] and increase perfusion in the cerebral microcirculation.[19] The NUN study has demonstrated that small vessel disease has a major role in the clinical expression of dementia in subjects of old age and with pathological changes typical of Alzhemeir's disease.[20] Therefore, it could be suspected that small vessel VaD might be the most prone to bencfit from hypertension treatment. The prevention of the vascular component in mixed dementia may result in a delayed expression of the Alzheimer's pathology as well. Future studies taking into account different VaD subtypes will better clarify the impact of hypertension treatment in preventing VaD.

The role of antiplatelet or anticoagulant agents used for either primary or secondary prevention of stroke in preventing VaD is also not conclusively demonstrated. A survey carried out among Canadian neurologists and geriatricians regarding the use of antithrombotic treatments in subcortical VaD showed that the most commonly employed treatment was aspirin, although the majority of the specialists pointed out the need for a randomized clinical trial to assess the efficacy of aspirin in VaD. They also felt that neuroimaging would be required for participants in such trials.[21]

TREATING ESTABLISHED VASCULAR DEMENTIA

A number of drugs have been tested in patients diagnosed with VaD. Many of these trials, particularly the earlier ones, have included patients broadly defined as affected by multi-infarct dementia. Although the terms VaD and multi-infarct dementia may somehow overlap, they do not completely coincide, and it should be borne in mind that the target study population may be somehow different.

Once VaD occurs, control of risk factors for stroke and use of antithrombotic drugs may still be useful. In a small, placebo-controlled trial, Meyer and co-workers showed that aspirin given at a daily dose of 325 mg had a beneficial effect on cognitive performances of multi-infarct dementia patients.[22] In another preliminary report, men at risk of cardiovascular disease (defined on the basis of a positive family history and on the presence of risk factors) and treated with antiplatelet or anticoagulant agents scored higher on neuropsychological testing than those on placebo.[23] Although in this study cognitive function was not tested at baseline, its randomized, double-blind nature should have prevented an unbalanced selection of patients. It remains to be settled whether these compounds have an advantageous effect in VaD because they can reduce stroke recurrence, which in studies of cognitive decline in stroke patients was proven to be a major determinant of dementia progression,[24–26] although other effects have been proposed. Activation of platelets is also present in patients with cerebrovascular disease in the chronic stage.[27] Aspirin also has an antiinflammatory effect and reduces the production of cytokines that may have a harmful effect on neuronal and glial cells.[28]

Although oral anticoagulants are definitely effective in preventing cerebral infarcts of cardio-embolic origin and therefore may presumably prevent or ameliorate multi-infarct dementia on this basis, one recent trial, comparing the safety and efficacy of oral anticoagulants and aspirin in the secondary prevention of stroke, disclosed the former to be associated with an increased risk of cerebral hemorrhage in patients with white matter changes (leukoaraiosis) on computed tomography scan, consistent with small vessel subcortical disease and chronic ischemia.[29,30] This result may indicate that drugs potentially beneficial in some VaD subtype may be harmful in others.

Among the drugs intended to treat established VaD, ergot alcaloids have been the most investigated. The possible beneficial effect of these compounds seems to rely on their vasodilatatory action, mediated by α-1-receptor antagonism (this mechanism is disputed), and on a number of effects on cerebral parenchyma mediated by modulation of nitric oxide synthase, dopaminergic and cholinergic effects, increased cell glucose uptake, and O_2 utilization, leading to augmented resistance of neuronal and glial cells to ischemia.[31] Hydergine is the prototype of this class of drugs. In 1994 Schneider and Olin[32] overviewed clinical trials of hydergine in patients with possible dementia. One hundred and fifty-one reports of hydergine were initially identified, of which 47 fulfilled the predefinite selection criteria. Only in seven studies patients had symptoms consistent with VaD for a total of 227 treated and 209 control patients. These studies were largely variable in age range, sample size, rating scales, enrollment setting, and duration of observation. Quite broad definitions were used for entering patients. Owing to the very scarce comparability, no conclusion was judged possible from the meta-analysis of studies in VaD, although overall the effect of hydergine turned out to be superior to placebo.

Another agent of this class of drugs is nicergoline. In a randomized, double-blind study conducted with 136 patients (out of 252 originally screened) diagnosed as affected by mild to moderate multi-infarct dementia according to DSM-III criteria, nicergoline (30 mg) given orally b.i.d. for as long as 6 months, was found more effective than placebo for both the Sandoz Clinical Assessment Geriatric Scale and the Mini-Mental Status Examination.[33] The data do not provide any hint about which VaD subtype was the most prone to being beneficially altered by this drug. In fact, DSM-III criteria are obviously unable to distinguish among different VaD subtypes.

The prototypes of the xantine-derivative family of drugs are pentoxifylline and propentofylline. Among the mechanisms of action of this compound are: (1) reduction of phosphodiesterase activity; (2) adenosine antagonism; (3) reduction of Ca^{2+} intracellular influx. These may result in effects on blood components (diminished platelet aggregation and fibrinogen level, increased red blood cell deformability) and diminished blood viscosity, with a presumably beneficial effect in subcortical VaD through the improvement of microcirculation. At the parenchyma level, they have neuroprotective effects, diminish astrocyte reactivity, and increase mitochondrial function. Propentofylline has been preliminarily shown to increase cerebral glucose metabolism (as measured by positron emission tomography), to improve selective neuropsychological function, and to slow cognitive deterioration in patients with VaD, diagnosed according to DSM-III-R criteria.[34] In a 12-month, randomized, placebo-controlled trial in patients affected by Alzheimer's disease or VaD, the subgroup analysis restricted to VaD patients showed a positive effect in favor of propentofylline on scales evaluating global deterioration and a small, but statistically significant, difference on the Mini-Mental Status Examination score (+ 0.6 for active drug, − 0.6 for placebo).[35]

Early phase-III trials with propentofylline have shown effect both on cognition and on global impression of change, but also in progression of VaD.[36–39] Preliminary results of a European and Canadian double-blind, placebo-controlled, randomized, parallel group trial on the efficacy and safety of long-term treatment with propentofylline (300 mg t.i.d., 1 hour before meals) compared with placebo in patients with mild-to-moderate VaD according to NINDS-AIREN criteria were recently shown as a poster.[40] The study involved 2 segments, a 24-week, traditional parallel group design and a 24-week, combined randomized delayed-start/withdrawal design. The primary efficacy variables were the Alzheimer's Disease Assessment Scale–cognitive subscale (ADAS-Cog) and the Clinician's Interview Based Impression of Chance (CIBIC-Plus). The study showed significant symptomatic improvement and long-term efficacy in ADAS-Cog and CIBIC-Plus up to 48 weeks. In addition, sustained treatment effects for at least 12 weeks after withdrawal indicating an effect on disease progression could be shown. Propentofylline was well tolerated, with no negative effects after withdrawal (Barbara Kittner, personal communication).

An international study group has compared the efficacy of pentoxifylline (400 mg t.i.d.) with that of placebo over a period of 9 months.[41] The intention-to-treat analysis for those patients who completed the study ($n = 239$) showed a difference of 3.5 points ($p = 0.028$) on the Gottfries-Bråne-Steen (GBS) scale in favor of active treatment.[41] Post-hoc subgroup classification, carried out after the conclusion of the study, showed that 75% of patients included in this study had imaging characteristics consistent with subcortical VaD.[42]

Dihydropyridinic calcium antagonists have a double action on vascular bed and brain parenchyma. In the experimental animal, they reduce the age-related microvascular changes[17,18] and, acting on L-type Ca^{2+} receptors and nitric oxide metabolism, have a vasodilatatory effect with amelioration of blood supply in hypoperfused areas by dilating small vessels. Calcium antagonists also reduce pathological Ca^{2+} intracellular influx and nitric oxide-free radical interaction via the block of NMDA-mediated nitric oxide synthase induction. The Cochrane Collaboration Dementia Group has performed a meta-analysis of trials that tested nimodipine against placebo in demented patients, but an analysis restricted to VaD patients was not conducted and, therefore, no definitive conclusions can be drawn for this type of dementia.[43]

Thirty-one patients presenting with cognitive impairment, progressive bilateral motor dysfunction, and white matter changes (leukoaraiosis) on computed tomography, were treated in an open-label design with 90-mg daily dose of the dihydropyridinic calcium antagonist nimodipine to evaluate safety and possible beneficial effect.[44] A significant improvement in all the items of the Sandoz Clinical Assessment Geriatric (SCAG) scale over a 12-month period and no severe collateral effect, particularly hypotensive crises, were recorded in this trial.[44] These results suggest that nimodipine may be beneficial in patients with a subcortical form of VaD. This preliminary trial led to conduct a subgroup analyses on patients enrolled in the randomized, double-blind Scandinavian Multi-Infarct Dementia trial and whose CT scan was consistent with the diagnosis of subcortical VaD. The analysis indicates that nimodipine has a beneficial effect on attention and psychomotor performances in the subcortical group, while no clear advantage was shown in the general sample (Pantoni *et al.*, personal communication). These preliminary results are currently being tested in an international, multicentric, randomized, double-blind trial enrolling patients with subcortical VaD.

Posatirelin, a TRH analogue that interferes with cholinergic and monoaminergic systems, has been preliminarily shown to have a beneficial effect on the cognitive functions, attention, and motivation of patients suffering from probable VaD according to the NINDS-AIREN criteria when given i.m. at a daily dosage of 10 mg for as long as 12 weeks.[45]

EGb761 is a particular extract of ginkgo biloba used in Europe to alleviate symptoms associated with cognitive disorders. The mechanism of action of Egb761 in the central nervous system is only partially understood. The main effect seems to be related to its antioxidant properties through compounds acting as scavengers for free radicals with possible beneficial effects on excessive lipid peroxidation and cell damage in Alzheimer's and multi-infarct dementia. A placebo-controlled, double-blind, randomized trial of EGb761 was carried out in Alzheimer's disease (236 patients) and multi-infarct dementia (73 patients).[46] Patients were subclassified by DSM-III-R and ICD-10 criteria. The Alzheimer's Disease Assessment Scale (ADAS) cognitive subscale and the Geriatric Evaluation by Relatives Rating Instrument (GERRI) were used as primary outcome measures. The conclusions were that Egb761 was safe and appeared capable of stabilizing and, in a substantial number of cases, improving the cognitive performances and the social functioning of demented patients for six months to one year. The analysis was performed separately for the Alzheimer's disease subgroup, which formed the majority of the total sample, and in the combined multi-infarct dementia plus Alzheimer's disease groups. There was no difference in the effect between the two groups, but no conclusion can be drawn for the smaller multi-infarct subset of patients.

Memantine, a low-affinity, voltage-dependent, noncompetitive NMDA receptor antagonist, has raised expectations in both symptomatic and neuroprotective treatment of dementia.[47] In a first double-blind, placebo-controlled trial in severe dementia of mixed etiology, memantine (20 mg × 1) was well tolerated and showed functional improvement and reduction of care dependency as compared to placebo in severely demented patients.[48,49] Currently, two pivotal trials in mild-to-moderate VaD are ongoing in Europe and one trial in moderate-to-severe Alzheimer's disease in the USA (Hans-Jörg Moebius, personal communication).

SUBCORTICAL VASCULAR DEMENTIA AS A POSSIBLE SPECIFIC TARGET FOR CLINICAL TRIALS

The results of clinical trials so far conducted, often showing a nonspecific effect on global cognitive functions irrespective of the dementia type (vascular or degenerative), is barely convincing. Most of the trials are small and do not measure functional benefit. Attempts at meta-analyses have been started only very recently.

Thanks to advances in the knowledge of clinical and radiological characteristics distinctive of the different VaD subtypes, we think that a novel approach can be tried for testing treatments in VaD. After having identified a drug with a proper rationale, a trial should include patients homogeneous for fulfilling clinical and radiological criteria consistent with the current knowledge about specific VaD subtypes. Subcortical VaD seems the most suitable setting to be successfully approached in this way.

Clinically, subcortical VaD is characterized by the following:[7–11,50] (a) cognitive impairment: memory disturbances, particularly in recalling, impairment and slowness in thinking and processing time, deficient strategy and planning; this cognitive picture is presumably consequent to damage of frontal–subcortical circuits;[51] (b) personality and mood disorders: depression, abulia, irritability; (c) gait disturbances: short-stepped, wide-based, apraxic gait with tendency to fall; (d) motor deficits: focal weakness, dysarthria, dysphagia, tremor, and rigidity; and (e) urinary disorders: incontinence, urgency.

Upon neuroimaging, the hallmark of subcortical VaD is the presence of white matter changes. White matter changes appear as patchy or diffuse areas of bilateral hypodensity on computed tomography, and as punctuate, confluent, or diffuse hyperintense areas on magnetic resonance T_2-weighted images. In association with these images, discrete areas of cavitated or noncavitated focal lesions with the location (basal ganglia, internal capsule, corona radiata), size, and shape typical of lacunar infarction are very frequently seen.[52]

The basic mechanism is damage of the small parenchyma vessels (<500 μm) due to aging, arterial hypertension, and diabetes mellitus, acting singularly or in combination (arteriolosclerosis). The pathological process is characterized by progressive replacement of the smooth muscle cells in the vessel wall by lipidic, hyaline, and fibrous material, eventually leading to marked narrowing of the vessel lumen and loss of the physiological ability to modify the lumen diameter in relation to variations in perfusion or metabolism. This could lead to ischemia in the terminal distribution territories of these vessels (corresponding to the deep border-zone areas).[53] The structural and physiological alterations of small vessels may also cause a breakdown of the blood–brain barrier. The effect of ischemia can be either acute, severe, and localized, leading to small areas of veritable necrosis (lacunar infarction), or chronic, less severe, and diffuse, with histological alterations consistent with the definition of incomplete infarct.[54] In the white matter, incomplete infarction is characterized by rarefaction of the myelin sheaths, moderate loss of oligodendrocytes, and reactive gliosis.[55] An increased content of water and secondary rarefied appearance of the myelin bundles is also commonly found.

Despite the rather well-defined clinical, radiological, and (possibly) pathological pictures,[5,6] a few questions regarding subcortical VaD remain unanswered, the most crucial of which are: (1) Which lesions of the complex pathological picture, including lacunar infarct, status cribrosus, white matter changes, and of the frequently associated ventricular dilatation and cortical atrophy, are more directly involved in the clinical expression (particularly the cognitive deficits) and outcome? and (2) What is the role of vascular risk factors and co-morbid conditions?

Currently, designing and running a clinical trial with these patients may present some difficulties:

(a) Despite the rather univocal clinical and radiological features, as outlined above, there are not yet widely agreed upon and validated criteria;

(b) Criteria and cut-offs conventionally used for separating demented from non-demented patients may be difficult to apply in this setting: common criteria for definition of dementia and traditional tools, such as the Mini Mental State Examination, both focusing on abnormalities of the cortical functions, may be scarcely sensitive in this context.

(c) Outcome measures (cognitive): A global multi-domain cognitive scale, like the Alzheimer's Disease Assessment Scale (ADAS), which has been designed and validated specifically for the use in Alzheimer's disease patients, seem hardly applicable in patients with subcortical VaD, because they are focused on cortical rather than subcortical cognitive functions. Tests selectively assessing subcortical functions seem warranted, but which marker can be regarded as the most reproducible, sensitive, and specific one of the disease or its progression is unclear. A combination of multiple tests could be considered.

(d) Outcome measures (functional): Which functional scale is more apt to measure deficits in this setting is controversial. Due to difficulties in executive functions Instrumental Activities in Daily Living (IADL) may be more sensitive than Activities in Daily Living (ADL). Obviously there is a need for developing new instruments that measure executive functions more in detail.

(e) Length of follow-up observation: The clinical course may be variable, although in the majority of these patients the progression is slow and there may be long plateau periods. Predictors of type of course are not known.

CONCLUSIONS

Despite the common feeling that the treatment of VaD still rests on prevention, we have no firm data demonstrating any treatment known to be effective in either primary or secondary prevention of vascular diseases to be equally effective in preventing VaD. Moreover, no study has up until now selectively examined the impact of vascular risk factor control or other treatments for stroke prevention on selected VaD subtypes. Future perspectives in the treatment of VaD include actions on delayed neuronal death, on neurotransmission (e.g., cholinergic), and Alzheimer's disease type strategies, such as actions to decrease beta-protein expression and amyloid accumulation.

Existing evidence does not indicate any definitive treatment for established VaD. Apart from the impossibility of recovering irreversibly damaged brain tissue, the results of the many clinical trials that have examined the efficacy of several drugs with a promising rationale have not yet indicated a satisfactory, univocal treatment. In our opinion, this is partly the result of the heterogeneity of study patients, enrolled using too broad and nonspecific clinical definitions of VaD. Moreover, many studies are small, or did not use definitive endpoints, that is, functional rather than cognitive outcome measures. Combination therapies, based on drugs with complementary mechanisms of action, have not been considered.

We propose that, owing to the rather advanced knowledge and valid laboratory aids now available for distinguishing rather reliably among different subtypes of VaD, treatments should be tested in groups of patients who are homogeneous in clinical and pathological presentation. There are initial examples of such an approach. Among different VaD subtypes, subcortical VaD seems to be the one about which the most is known about the clinical syndromes, the radiological features, and the pathophysiological background, thus warranting the homogeneity of the study population.

This notwithstanding, designing and running clinical trials in this setting still appear difficult: the natural determinants of clinical expression and outcome are not completely elucidated, there are not agreed upon and validated entry criteria, and uncertainties exist about the choice of outcome measures, lengthiness of follow-up, and other issues. A consensus is needed to try to define these issues.

REFERENCES

1. CHUI, H.C., J.I. VICTOROFF, D. MARGOLIN *et al.* 1992. Criteria for the diagnosis of ischemic vascular dementia proposed by the State of California Alzheimer's Disease Diagnostic and Treatment Centers. Neurology **42:** 473–480.
2. ROMÁN, G.C., T.K. TATEMICHI, T. ERKINJUNTTI *et al.* 1993. Vascular dementia: diagnostic criteria for research studies. Report of the NINDS-AIREN International Workshop. Neurology **43:** 250–260.
3. WORLD HEALTH ORGANIZATION. 1993. ICD-10 Classification of Mental and Behavioural Disorders: Diagnostic Criteria for Research. WHO. Geneva. pp. 36–40.
4. NYENHUIS, D.L. & P.B. GORELICK. 1998. Vascular dementia: a contemporary review of epidemiology, diagnosis, prevention, and treatment. J. Am. Geriatr. Soc. **46:** 1437–1448.
5. WALLIN, A. & K. BLENNOW. 1991. The pathogenetic basis of vascular dementia. Alzheimer Dis. Assoc. Disord. **5:** 91–102.
6. WALLIN, A. & K. BLENNOW. 1994. The clinical diagnosis of vascular dementia. Dementia **5:** 181–184.
7. ERKINJUNTTI, T. 1987. Types of multi-infarct dementia. Acta Neurol. Scand. **75:** 391–399.
8. MAHLER, M.E. & J.L. CUMMINGS. 1991. The behavioural neurology of multi-infarct dementia. Alzheimer Dis. Assoc. Disord. **5:** 122–130.
9. ROMAN, G.C. 1987. Senile dementia of the Binswanger type: a vascular form of dementia in the elderly. JAMA **258:** 1782–1788.
10. BABIKIAN, V. & A.H. ROPPER. 1987. Binswanger's disease: a review. Stroke **18:** 2–12.
11. ISHII, N., Y. NISHIHARA & T. IMAMURA. 1986. Why do frontal lobe symptoms predominate in vascular dementia with lacunes? Neurology **36:** 340–345.
12. BOUSSER, M.G., E. ESCHWEGE, M. HAGUENAU *et al.* 1983. "AICLA" controlled trial of aspirin and dipyridamole in the secondary prevention of athero-thrombotic cerebral ischemia. Stroke **14:** 5–14.
13. GENT, M., J.A. BLAKELY, J.D. EASTON *et al.* 1989. The Canadian American Ticlopidine Study (CATS) in thromboembolic stroke. Lancet **i:** 1215–1220.
14. MEYER, J.S., B.W. JUDD, T. TAWAKLNA *et al.* 1986. Improved cognition after control of risk factors for multi-infarct dementia. JAMA **256:** 2203–2209.
15. FORETTE, F., M.L. SEUX, J.A. STAESSEN *et al.* 1998. Prevention of dementia in randomised double-blind placebo-controlled systolic hypertension in Europe (Syst-Eur) trial. Lancet **352:** 1347–1351.
16. SHEP COOPERATIVE RESEARCH GROUP. 1991. Prevention of stroke by antihypertensive drug treatment in older persons with isolated systolic hypertension. Final results of the Systolic Hypertension in the Elderly Program (SHEP). JAMA **265:** 3255–3264.
17. DE JONG, G.I., J. TRABER & P.G.M. LUITEN. 1992. Formation of cerebrovascular anomalies in the ageing rats is delayed by chronic nimodipine application. Mech. Ageing Dev. **64:** 255–272.

18. DE JONG, G.I., A.S. JANSEN, E. HORVATH *et al.* 1992. Nimodipine effects on cerebral microvessels and sciatic nerve in aging rats. Neurobiol. Aging **13:** 73–81.

19. LANGLEY, M.S. & E.M. SORKIN. 1989. Nimodipine. A review of its pharmacodynamic and pharmacokinetic properties and therapeutic potential in cerebrovascolar disease. Drugs **37:** 669–699.

20. SNOWDON, D.A., L.H. GREINER, J.A. MORTIMER *et al.* 1997. Brain infarction and the clinical expression of Alzheimer disease. The Nun Study. JAMA **277:** 813–817.

21. MOLNAR, F.J., M. MAN-SON-HING, P. ST JOHN *et al.* 1998. Subcortical vascular dementia: survey of treatment patterns and research considerations. Can. J. Neurol. Sci. **25:** 320–324.

22. MEYER, J.S., R.L. ROGERS, K.L. MCCLINTIC *et al.* 1989. Randomized clinical trial of daily aspirin therapy in multi-infarct dementia: a pilot study. J. Am. Geriatr. Soc. **37:** 549–555.

23. RICHARDS, M., T.W. MEADE, S. PEART *et al.* 1997. Is there any evidence for a protective effect of antithrombotic medication on cognitive function in men at risk of cardiovascular disease? Some preliminary findings. J. Neurol. Neurosurg. Psychiatry **62:** 269–272.

24. MIYAO, S., A. TAKANO, J. TERAMOTO & A. TAKAHASHI. 1992. Leukoaraiosis in relation to prognosis for patients with lacunar infarction. Stroke **23:** 1434–1438.

25. LOEB, C., C. GANDOLFO, R. CROCE & M. CONTI. 1992. Dementia associated with lacunar infarction. Stroke **23:** 1225–1229.

26. VAN ZAGTEN, M., J. BOITEN, F. KESSELS & J. LODDER. 1996. Significant progression of white matter lesions and small deep (lacunar) infarcts in patients with stroke. Arch. Neurol. **53:** 650–655.

27. IWAMOTO, T., H. KUBO & M. TAKASAKI. 1995. Platelet activation in the cerebral circulation in different subtypes of ischemic stroke and Binswanger's disease. Stroke **26:** 52–56.

28. PANTONI, L., C. SARTI & D. INZITARI. 1998. Cytokines and cell adhesion molecules in cerebral ischemia: experimental bases and therapeutic perspectives. Arterioscler. Thromb. Vasc. Biol. **18:** 503–513.

29. THE STROKE PREVENTION IN REVERSIBLE ISCHEMIA TRIAL (SPIRIT) STUDY GROUP. 1997. A randomized trial of anticoagulants versus aspirin after cerebral ischemia of presumed arterial origin. Ann. Neurol. **42:** 857–865.

30. PANTONI, L., D. INZITARI, FOR THE EUROPEAN TASK FORCE ON AGE-RELATED WHITE MATTER CHANGES. 1998. New clinical relevance of leukoaraiosis [letter]. Stroke **29:** 543.

31. VENN, R.D. 1980. Review of clinical studies with ergots in gerontology. Adv. Biochem. Psychopharmacology **23:** 363–377.

32. SCHNEIDER, L.S. & J.T. OLIN. 1994. Overview of clinical trials of hydergine in dementia. Arch. Neurol. **51:** 787–798.

33. HERRMANN, W.M., K. STEPHAN, K. GAEDE & M. APECECHE. 1997. A multicenter randomized double-blind study on the efficacy and safety of nicergoline in patients with multi-infarct dementia. Dement. Geriatr. Cogn. Disord. **8:** 9–17.

34. MIELKE, R., B. KITTNER, M. GHAEMI *et al.* 1996. Propentofylline improves regional cerebral glucose metabolism and neuropsychological performance in vascular dementia. J. Neurol. Sci. **141:** 59–64.

35. MARCUSSON, J., M. ROTHER, B. KITTNER *et al.* 1997. A 12-month, randomized, placebo-controlled trial of propentofylline (HWA 285) in patients with dementia according to DSM III-R. Dement. Geriatr. Cogn. Disord. **8:** 320–328.

36. ROTHER, M., T. ERKINJUNTTI, M. ROESSNER, B. KITTNER, J. MARCUSSON & I. KARLSSON. 1998. Propentofylline in the treatment of Alzheimer's disease and vascular dementia. Dement. Geriatr. Cogn. Disord. **9**(Suppl. 1): 36–43.

37. MIELKE, R., H.-J. MÖLLER, T. ERKINJUNTTI, B. ROSENKRANZ, M. ROTHER & B. KITTNER. 1998. Propentofylline in the treatment of vascular dementia and Alzheimer-type dementia: overview of phase I and phase II clinical trials. Alzheimer Dis. Assoc. Disord. **12**(Suppl. 2): S29–S35.

38. KITTNER, B., M. ROSSNER & M. ROTHER. 1997. Clinical trials in dementia with propentofylline. Ann. N.Y. Acad. Sci. **826:** 307–316.

39. ROTHER, M., B. KITTNER, K. RUDOLPHI, M. ROSSNER & K.H. LABS. 1996. HWA 285 (propentofylline)—a new compound for the treatment of both vascular dementia and dementia of the Alzheimer type. Ann. N.Y. Acad. Sci. **777:** 404–409.
40. PISCHEL, T. 1998. Long-term efficacy and safety of propentofylline in patients with vascular dementia: results of a 12 months placebo-controlled trial [abstract]. Neurobiol. Aging **19**(Suppl. 4): S182.
41. THE EUROPEAN PENTOXIFYLLINE MULTI-INFARCT DEMENTIA STUDY GROUP. 1996. European pentoxifylline multi-infarct dementia study. Eur. Neurol. **36:** 315–321.
42. KITTNER, B. 1998. Presented at the Osaka Conference on Vascular Dementia, October 7–9. Osaka, Japan. Personal communication.
43. QIZILBASH, N., J. LOPEZ ARRIETA & J. BIRKS. 1997. Nimodipine in the treatment of primary degenerative, mixed and vascular dementia. *In* Dementia and Cognitive Module of the Cochrane Database of Systematic Reviews. [updated 03 June 1997]. H. Beppu, F. Huppert, J. Kaye *et al.*, Eds. Available in The Cochrane Library [database on disk and CDROM]. The Cochrane Collaboration; Issue 3. Update Software; updated quarterly. Oxford. Oxfore, U.K.
44. PANTONI, L., M. CAROSI, S. AMIGONI *et al.* 1996. A preliminary open trial with nimodipine in patients with cognitive impairment and leukoaraiosis. Clin. Neuropharmacol. **19:** 497–506.
45. PARNETTI, L., L. AMBROSOLI, G. AGLIATI *et al.* 1996. Posatirelin in the treatment of vascular dementia: a double-blind multicentre study vs. placebo. Acta Neurol. Scand. **93:** 456–463.
46. LE BARS, P.L., M.M. KATZ, N. BERMAN *et al.* 1997. A placebo-controlled, double-blind, randomized trial of an extract of ginkgo biloba for dementia. North American EGb Study Group. JAMA **278:** 1327–1332.
47. PEARSONS, C.G., W. DANYSZ & G. QUACK. 1999. Memantine is a clinically well tolerated NMDA receptor antagonist—a review of preclinical data. Neuropharmacology. In press.
48. WINBLAD, B. & N. PORITIS. 1998. Clinical improvement in a placebo-controlled trial with memantine in care-dependent patients with severe dementia [abstract]. Neurobiol. Aging **19**(Suppl. 4): S303.
49. WINBLAD, B. & N. PORITIS. 1999. Memantine in severe dementia. J. Geriatr. Psychiatry Neurol. In press.
50. CUMMINGS, J.L. 1994. Vascular subcortical dementia: clinical aspects. Dementia **5:** 177–180.
51. CUMMINGS, J.L. 1993. Frontal-subcortical circuits and human behavior. Arch. Neurol. **50:** 873–880.
52. PANTONI, L. & J.H. GARCIA. 1995. The significance of cerebral white matter abnormalities 100 years after Binswanger's report. A review. Stroke **26:** 1293–1301.
53. PANTONI, L. & J.H. GARCIA. 1997. Pathogenesis of leukoaraiosis. A review. Stroke **28:** 652–659.
54. GARCIA, J.H., N.A. LASSEN, C. WEILLER *et al.* 1996. Ischemic stroke and incomplete infarction. Stroke **27:** 761–765.
55. BRUN, A. & E. ENGLUND. 1986. A white matter disorder in dementia of the Alzheimer type: a pathoanatomical study. Ann. Neurol. **19:** 253–262.

The Diagnosis of "Mixed" Dementia in the Consortium for the Investigation of Vascular Impairment of Cognition (CIVIC)

K. ROCKWOOD,[a,i] C. MACKNIGHT,[a] C. WENTZEL,[a] S. BLACK,[b]
R. BOUCHARD,[c] S. GAUTHIER,[d] H. FELDMAN,[e] D. HOGAN,[f] A. KERTESZ,[g]
AND P. MONTGOMERY[h] FOR THE CIVIC INVESTIGATORS

[a]*Division of Geriatric Medicine, Dalhousie University, Halifax, Nova Scotia, Canada*

[b]*Division of Neurology, University of Toronto, Toronto, Ontario, Canada*

[c]*Division of Neurology, Laval University, McGill University, Quebec, Canada*

[d]*Divisions of Neurology and Neurosurgery, Psychiatrics, and Medicine, McGill University, Quebec, Canada*

[e]*Division of Neurology, University of British Columbia, Vancouver, British Columbia, Canada*

[f]*Division of Geriatric Medicine, University of Calgary, Calgary, Alberta, Canada*

[g]*Division of Neurology, University of Western Ontario, London, Ontario, Canada*

[h]*Division of Geriatric Medicine, University of Manitoba, Winnipeg, Manitoba, Canada*

ABSTRACT: If vascular risk factors are risks for Alzheimer's disease (AD), and if "pure" vascular dementia (VaD) is less common than has been thought, what do we make of the diagnosis of mixed dementia? We report characteristics of those with mixed dementia in a prospective, seven center, clinic-based Canadian study.

Of 1,008 patients, 372 were diagnosed with AD, 149 with vascular cognitive impairment (VCI) including 76 with mixed AD/VaD, and 82 with other types of dementia. The mean age of patients with mixed AD/VaD was 78.0 ± 7.6 years; 49% were female. These proportions differed significantly between dementia diagnosis subgroup ($p < 0.001$) showing a trend which is evident in all comparisons—AD/VaD patients fall in between AD and VaD.

Vascular risk factors were present significantly more often in mixed AD/VaD than in AD ($p < 0.001$). More mixed AD/VaD (20%) than AD patients (4%) had focal signs, compared with 38% of those with vascular dementia and 12% with other types of dementia. Between the initial clinical diagnosis and the final diagnosis (which utilized neuroimaging and neuropsychological data) AD/VaD was the least stable diagnosis. Neuroimaging of ischemic lesions was the most common reason for reassignment from AD to the mixed AD/VaD diagnosis (17 cases).

These data suggest that an operational definition of mixed AD/VaD can be proposed on presentation and clinical/radiographic findings, but indifferent to vascular risk factors. The concept of mixed dementia should be extended to include vascular dementia in combination with dementias, other than Alzheimer's disease.

[i]Address for correspondence: Dr. Kenneth Rockwood, Division of Geriatric Medicine, Dalhousie University, QEII Health Sciences Centre, 5955 Jubilee Road, Halifax, Nova Scotia, Canada, B3H 2E1. Tel.: (902) 473-8687; fax: (902) 473-1050.
e-mail: rockwood@is.dal.ca

INTRODUCTION

The diagnosis of vascular dementia is in transition.[11,18,20,4,26,1,27,10] At one time "multiinfarct dementia" was believed to be the second most common cause of dementia, after Alzheimer's disease (AD), with a mixture of the two holding an ambiguous position.[18,21,4] The picture has become less clear, and the many definitions of what is now more commonly called "vascular" dementia reflect current uncertainty.[26]

The distinction between vascular dementia (VaD) and AD has become increasingly blurred,[18] and cases of pure VaD may be less common than had been widely assumed.[12,15,7] Furthermore, it has been argued that, alone or in combination with AD, a vascular cause is present in up to 50% of cases of dementia.[3] Consequently, the diagnosis of mixed dementia is being adopted with greater frequency.[18] For example, in the Canadian Study of Health and Aging (CSHA) the prevalence of mixed dementia was approximately 10 times the rate expected.[19] Mixed dementia nevertheless remains an unclear diagnosis, with significant variability between the various consensus-based criteria.[18] In consequence, empirical studies are needed. In this paper we describe vascular risk factors, clinical features, and radiographic characteristics of patients diagnosed with VaD, mixed dementia, AD, and other types of dementia.

METHODS

The Consortium for the Investigation of Vascular Impairment of Cognition (CIVIC) study is a 7-center cohort study designed to define the syndrome and subtypes of vascular cognitive impairment (VCI) including coincident ("mixed") AD and VaD. We report the proportion with mixed AD/VaD in our series, and their clinical and neuroradiographic characteristics, with a view to proposing diagnostic criteria.

Patients were recruited from Memory Clinics and ambulatory care clinics in geriatric medicine and neurology and received standard clinical assessments and, where indicated, neuropsychologic and radiographic procedures. The CIVIC study is based on usual clinical care, and takes an empirical approach to the diagnosis of vascular cognitive impairment. Measurements in the standard assessment included demographic data, the Mini-Mental State Examination (MMSE),[8] the Cumulative Illness Rating Scale (CIRS),[13] the Global Deterioration Scale (GDS),[16] the Functional Assessment Staging Tool (FAST),[17] and the Functional Rating Scale (FRS).[5] Each of these inventories provides a global score; in the case of the CIRS, the total score was calculated without the neurologic item (item #11).

The dementia syndrome was diagnosed according to DSM-III-R criteria.[2] The Modified Hachinski Score[22] was recorded. NINCDS-ADRDA criteria[14] were used to diagnose AD. VaD was defined according to clinical and radiographic features, using a checklist which combines all presently proposed criteria. The clinical features included sudden onset, stepwise progression, prolonged plateaus, periods of spontaneous improvement, onset or worsening in relation to stroke or to episode of hypoperfusion (e.g., dysrhythmia, intraoperative hypotension), focal neurological signs or symptoms, and evidence of "patchy" cognitive deficits during formal cognitive testing. Radiographic characteristics of vascular dementia included cortical or subcortical strokes or hemorrhages, lacunar infarction, and/or white matter ischemic changes. The criteria for a diagnosis of mixed AD/VaD were that the course was suggestive of AD, and the patient had focal neurologic symptoms or brain imaging suggestive of ischemia. The presence of vascular risk factors alone, in a patient with otherwise clinically typical AD, would not be enough to support a diagnosis of mixed AD/VaD. While the absence of neuroradiographic features was considered strong evidence against the diagnosis of a vascular component to the diagnosis, it did not rule it out.

We compared the distribution of demographic and clinical characteristics between four groups: AD, mixed AD/VaD, VaD, and other dementias. For categorical data, the significance of difference in proportions was tested with chi-square; for interval data, these differences were tested using analysis of variance. The limit of the chance of a type I error was set at $p < 0.05$. The presence of patchy cognitive deficits was quantitated by calculating Cronbach's alpha using the six cognitive items of the FRS, for each of the four diagnostic groups.

RESULTS

Of 1,008 patients presenting to the seven clinics, 603 were enrolled in the dementia cohort. Of these, 372 were diagnosed with AD, 149 with VCI (VaD, $n = 73$; mixed AD/VaD, $n = 76$), and 82 with other dementias (including dementia with Lewy bodies, $n = 16$ and frontotemporal dementia, $n = 18$).

For each of the analyses considered below, comparison of vascular risk factors, and clinical and radiographic features indicates a relatively consistent trend: VaD demonstrates the highest rates, AD the lowest, with AD/VaD falling somewhere between the two groups. TABLE 1 reports selected characteristics of patients, including vascular risk factors, by diagnostic group. History of stroke, diabetes, and elevated cholesterol occurred more frequently in subjects diagnosed with VaD than mixed AD/VaD, and more often for mixed AD/VaD than AD. A history of angina was more commonly observed in mixed AD than VaD; AD and other dementias demonstrated comparably low rates of angina.

TABLE 2 compares the clinical features of the four groups. The rate of sudden onset and focal signs was highest for VaD and lowest for AD, with the rate for mixed AD/VaD falling between these two groups. The frequency of stepwise deterioration was markedly higher for VaD than mixed AD/VaD.

TABLE 3 reports the radiographic features of the groups. VaD showed the greatest frequency of strokes. The rate of white matter changes was similar for VaD and AD/VaD, and markedly lower for both AD and other types of dementia. Of note, many patients with VaD features clinically have radiographic features which do not completely correlate: for example, of the 19 patients with single cortical strokes, only six had so-called "single strategic strokes" such as strokes in the angular gyrus. Evidence of patchy cognitive deficits followed the expected direction in that the cognitive items of the FRS demonstrated greatest internal consistency for AD ($\alpha = 0.85$) and other dementias ($\alpha = 0.85$), and lower consistency for VaD ($\alpha = 0.78$) and mixed AD/VaD ($\alpha = 0.80$).

TABLE 1. Selected characteristics of patients: demographic and vascular risk factors

Characteristics and Risk Factors	VaD $n = 73$	AD/VaD $n = 76$	AD $n = 372$	Other Dementia $n = 82$	p
Mean age, years	76.4 (7.9)	78.0 (7.6)	76.0 (8.2)	71.6 (10.7)	<0.001
Female, %	34.2	48.9	64.0	49.4	<0.001
Mean education, years	11.1 (3.9)	10.7 (4.0)	10.5 (3.8)	10.7 (3.8)	ns
Stroke, %	38.4	31.6	2.2	4.9	<0.001
Hypertension, %	54.8	56.8	50.9	36.2	<0.001
Diabetes, %	20.6	14.7	9.4	17.1	0.02
Hypercholesterolemia, %	19.0	14.3	12.0	18.4	<0.001
Angina comorbidity, %	32.9	37.3	12.6	13.4	<0.001

NOTE: Standard deviations are in parentheses.

In general, there was a marked consistency within etiologic categories, between the initial and final diagnoses, of patients with dementia. Of patients with dementia, 14% had a difference between their initial and final diagnoses. The proportion with a change was highest (71%) for those with a final diagnosis of mixed dementia, compared to 4% of those with a diagnosis of AD.

DISCUSSION

It is now time to move from consensus based to empirical criteria in the diagnosis of vascular dementia and its variants. The CIVIC study is an attempt to do this, through a multicenter investigation of patients presenting with memory problems. The study uses current criteria for defined dementia types, such as AD, and dementia with Lewy bodies, and collects data from all existing proposals for vascular dementia. The strategy, following Hachinski's recommendation,[11] is to collect careful descriptions of large numbers of cases. In so doing, we hope to be able to understand the validity of the constructs which emerge.

Four factors point to so-called "mixed" dementia as a useful starting place. Vascular risk factors seem to be risks for all types of dementia, not just vascular dementia.[24] For example, treatment of hypertension decreases the risk of dementia.[9] Disease expression in Alzheimer's is related to concomitant cerebrovascular lesions.[25] The prevalence of "pure" vascular dementia, without concomitant AD neuropathological lesions, may be less common than previously believed.[12,15,7] Finally, some treatments appear to be equally effective in Alzheimer's disease and vascular dementia.[23,6] These considerations have the potential to result in an increased prevalence of mixed AD/VaD.

Our data support the validity of the AD/VaD construct. On most of the clinical, radiographic, and even demographic features which we examined, mixed AD/VaD falls on a spectrum between AD and VaD. Three presentations appear in the experience of our clinics to give rise to a diagnosis of vascular dementia. Most commonly, patients present clinically with AD, but are found to have focal lesions, either on clinical examination, or, more often, on computerized tomography (CT) scan, or

TABLE 2. Comparison of clinical features

Clinical Features	VaD $n = 73$	AD/VaD $n = 76$	AD $n = 372$	Dementia $n = 82$	p
MMSE score, $\bar{x}$	19.7	17.0	17.2	20.0	0.002
CIRS score, $\bar{x}$	6.3	5.4	3.6	4.4	<0.001
FAST score, $\bar{x}$	4.3	4.4	4.2	4.0	ns
Sudden onset, %	17.8	2.6	0.5	2.4	<0.001
Stepwise deterioration, %	12.3	6.6	0	1.2	<0.001
Focal signs, %	38.4	19.7	3.8	12.2	<0.001
Focal symptoms, %	20.5	19.7	3.0	3.7	<0.001
Early gait abnormality, %	34.2	15.8	4.8	20.7	<0.001
Seizures, %	4.1	1.3	0.3	2.4	0.026
Hallucinations, %	9.6	3.9	4.3	9.8	ns
Fluctuating course, %	13.7	10.5	2.2	6.1	<.001

magnetic resonance imaging (MRI). Finally, some patients have evident features of both AD and VaD at presentation, or by a picture of patchy deficits on formal cognitive testing.

Our study has important limitations. As the protocol builds on usual clinical care, not all tests that might be desirable from a research standpoint are performed on all patients. Nevertheless, no single site variation importantly contributed to our overall results. The data are not population based. Importantly, while the concept of patchy cognitive deficits was useful in the clinical diagnosis, no formal measure of this construct exists. The differences revealed in internal consistency are more modest than expected, likely reflecting imprecision within the individual domains of the FRS, which is how cognitive testing by clinicians was recorded. Further work, using neuropsychological test data, will be needed to clarify this concept.

On the positive side, our data parallel much of the data collected in the second phase of the Canadian Study of Health and Aging, so that comparisons with population-based data are possible. In addition, by adopting an "all comers" strategy of tertiary care clinics across the country, we can profile the sorts of cases which come to detailed attention.

A more detailed look at the cases in our database shows that several patients with types of dementia other than AD and VaD may also have a vascular component. For example, vascular dementia was thought to be present in patients who also had cognitive impairment arising from multiple systems atrophy, progressive supranuclear palsy, dementia with Lewy bodies, or alcoholic dementia.

In summary, our study suggests that an operational definition of mixed AD/VaD can be proposed based on presentation and clinical/radiographic findings, but indifferent to vascular risk factors. Further studies should investigate whether, as appears likely, the concept of mixed dementia should be extended to include vascular dementia in combination with dementias other than Alzheimer's disease.

TABLE 3. Comparison of radiographic features of the groups

Radiographic Features	VaD $n = 73$ $n(\%)$	AD/VaD $n = 76$ $n(\%)$	AD $n = 372$ $n(\%)$	Other Dementia $n = 82$ $n(\%)$	p
Multiple cortical strokes,%	5 (7)	4 (5)	0 (0)	1 (1)	<0.001
Multiple subcortical strokes, %	12 (16)	6 (8)	0 (0)	1 (1)	<0.001
Single cortical strokes, %	19 (26)	10 (13)	4 (1)	0 (0)	<0.001
Single subcortical storke, %	11 (15)	10 (13)	5 (1)	0 (0)	<0.001
White matter changes, %	24 (33)	24 (32)	31 (8)	5 (6)	<0.001
Multiple lesions, %	11 (15)	12 (17)	0 (0)	0 (0)	<0.001
No identified lesions, %	2 (3)	3 (4)	331 (90)	75 (92)	<0.001

NOTE: Some radiographic features are not mutually exclusive. One AD patient had multiple intracerebral hemorrhages, not included in TABLE 3.

REFERENCES

1. AMAR, K., G.K. WILCOCK & M. SCOTT. 1996. The diagnosis of vascular dementia in the light of the new criteria. Age Ageing **25:** 51–55.
2. American Psychiatric Association. 1987. Diagnostic and Statistical Manual of Mental Disorders. 3rd edit., revised. American Psychiatric Association. Washington, DC.
3. BRUST, J.C.M. 1993. Vascular dementia reconsidered. Cerebrovasc. Dis. **3:** 26.
4. BOWLER, J.V., M. ELIASZIW, R. STEENHUIS, D.G. MUNOZ, R. FRY, H. MERSKEY & V.C. HACHINSKI. 1997. Comparative evolution of Alzheimer disease, vascular dementia, and mixed dementia. Arch. Neurol. **54:** 697–703.
5. CROCKETT, D., H. TUOKKO, W. KOCH & R. PARKS. 1989. The assessment of everyday functioning using the Present Functioning Questionnaire and the Functional Rating Scale in elderly samples. Clin. Gerontol. **8:** 3–25.
6. CUCINOTTA, D., M.A. AVENI-CASUCCI, F. PEDRAZZI, O. PONARI, M. CAPODAGLIO, P. VALDINA, I. TOXIRI, L. BARTORELLI, Q. GRANATA, C. FRANZINI *et al.* 1992. Multicentre clinical placebo-controlled study with buflomedil in the treatment of mild dementia of vascular origin. J. Int. Med. Res. **20:** 136–149.
7. ESIRI, M.M., G.K. WILCOCK & J.H. MORRIS. 1997. Neuropathological assessment of the lesions of significance in vascular dementia. J. Neurol. Neurosurg. Psychiatry **63:** 749–753.
8. FOLSTEIN, M.F., S.E. FOLSTEIN & P.R. McHUGH. 1975. "Mini-mental state": a practical guide for grading the cognitive state of patients for the clinician. J. Psychiatry Res. **12:** 189–198.
9. FORETTE, F., M.L. SEUX, J.A. STAESSEN, L. THIJS, W.H. BIRKENHAGER, M.R BABARSKIENE *et al.* 1998. Prevention of dementia in randomized double-blind placebo-controlled Systolic Hypertension in Europe (Syst-Eur) trial. Lancet **352:** 1347–1352.
10. GOLD, G., P. GIANNAKOPOULOS, C. MONTES-PAIXAO, F.R. HERRMANN, R. MULLIGAN, J.P. MICHEL & C. BOURAS. 1997. Sensitivity and specificity of newly proposed clinical criteria for possible vascular dementia. Neurology **49:** 690–694.
11. HACHINSKI, V. 1994. Vascular dementia: a radical redefinition. Dementia **5:** 130–132.
12. HULETTE, C., D. NOCHLIN, D. McKEEL, J.C. MORRIS, S.S. MIRRA, S.M. SUMI *et al.* 1997. Clinical-neuropathologic findings in multi-infarct dementia: a report of six autopsied cases. Neurology **48:** 668–672.
13. LINN, B.S., M.W. LINN & L. GUREL. 1968. Cumulative Illness Rating Scale. J. Am. Geriatr. Soc. **16:** 622–626.
14. McKHANN, G., D. DRACHMAN, M. FOLSTEIN, R. KATZMAN, D. PRICE & E.M. STADIAN. 1984. Clinical diagnosis of Alzheimer's disease: report of the NINCDS-ADRDA Work Group under the auspices of Department of Health and Human Services Task Force on Alzheimer's disease. Neurology **34:** 939–944.

15. NOLAN, K.A., M.M. LINO, A.W. SELIGMANN & J.P. BLASS. 1998. Absence of vascular dementia in an autopsy series from a dementia clinic. J. Am. Geriatr. Soc. **46:** 597–604.
16. REISBERG, B., S.H. FERRIS, M.J. DE LEON & T. CROOK. 1982. The Global Deterioration Scale for assessment of primary degenerative dementia. Am. J. Psychiatry **139:** 1136–1139.
17. REISBERG, B. 1988. Functional assessment staging (FAST). Psychoparmacol. Bull. **24:** 653–659.
18. ROCKWOOD, K. 1997. Lessons from mixed dementia. Int. Psychogeriatr. **9:** 245–249.
19. ROCKWOOD, K., E. EBLY, V. HACHINSKI & D. HOGAN. 1997. Presence and treatment of vascular risk factors in patients with vascular cognitive impairment. Arch. Neurol. **54:** 33–39.
20. ROCKWOOD, K., J. BOWLER, T. ERKINJUNTTI, V. HACHINSKI & A. WALLIN. 1999. Subtypes of vascular dementia. Alzheimer's Dis. Assoc. Disord. **13**(Suppl. 3): S59–S65.
21. ROCKWOOD, K., K. HOWARD, C. MACKNIGHT & S. DARVESH. 1999. Spectrum of disease in vascular cognitive impairment. Neuroepidemiology **18:** 248–254.
22. ROSEN, W.G., R.D. TERRY, P.A. FOULD, R. KATZMAN & A. PECK. 1980. Pathological verification of ischemic score in differentiation of dementias. Ann. Neurol. **7:** 486–488.
23. ROTHER, M., T. ERKINJUNTTI, M. ROESSNER, B. KITTNER, J. MARCUSSON & I. KARLSSON. 1998. Propentofylline in the treatment of Alzheimer's disease and vascular dementia: a review of phase III trials. Dement. Geriatr. Cognit. Disord. **9:** 36–43.
24. SKOOG, I. 1998. Status of risk factors of vascular dementia. Neuroepidemiology **17:** 2–9.
25. SNOWDON, D.A., L.H. GREINER, J.A. MORTIMER, K.P. RILEY, P.A. GREINER & W.R. MARKESBERY. 1997. Brain infarction and the clinical expression of Alzheimer disease. JAMA **277:** 813–817.
26. VERHEY, F.R.J., J. LODDER, N. ROZENDAAL & J. JOLLES. 1996. Comparison of seven sets of criteria used for the diagnosis of vascular dementia. Neuroepidemiology **15:** 166–172.
27. WETTERLING, T., R.-D. KANITZ & K.-J. BORGIS. 1996. Comparison of different diagnostic criteria for vascular dementia: (ADDTC, DSM-IV, ICD-10, NINDS-AIREN). Stroke **27:** 30–36.

Glial Modulating and Neurotrophic Properties of Propentofylline and Its Application to Alzheimer's Disease and Vascular Dementia

GARTH E. RINGHEIM[a]

Department of Neuroscience, Aventis Pharmaceuticals, Inc., Bridgewater, New Jersey 08807, USA

INTRODUCTION

Alzheimer's disease (AD) and vascular dementia (VaD) are two of the most common forms of dementia in the elderly. Together they represent one of the largest unmet medical needs of the Western industrialized nations where population demographics indicate a trend towards declining birth rates along with an increase in life expectancy. Alzheimer's disease is a progressive neurodegenerative condition that is associated with plaque deposits of beta amyloid (Aβ), tangled appearing dystrophic neurons, and pronounced cellular loss consisting primarily of neurons and glia. Vascular dementia, in contrast, is most often associated with stroke, lacunar infarcts, and associated white matter lesions. Though distinct in their pathological characteristics, it is not uncommon to find the white matter lesions associated with VaD occurring in clinically diagnosed AD patients.[1,2] It is likely, therefore, that therapeutic treatments targeted primarily for either VaD or AD will have therapeutic benefit on the other condition depending on the extent to which the two pathologies coexist in an individual. It is also likely that a therapeutic agent will have benefit in both diseases if common underlying disease mechanisms are being addressed. For example, neuronal cell death resulting from stress conditions associated with VaD may differ from that associated with AD, yet cell loss from either might be prevented if expression of a particular neuronal support factor such as nerve growth factor is upregulated.

Therapeutic approaches to treating dementia can be categorized into two main groups: symptomatic and disease modifying. Symptomatic treatments focus primarily on compensating for neuronal cell loss or functional impairment most often by seeking to enhance activity of the remaining neuronal cell populations. Examples of symptomatic treatments are acetylcholinesterase inhibitors that elevate the neurotransmitter acetylcholine or muscarinic agonists that enhance neurotransmitter receptor signaling. Disease modifying agents approach treatment as a matter of delaying disease progression by any one of several mechanisms that aim to ameliorate AD or VaD pathology. Treatment of the pathology would then result in the subsequent halting or slowing of further cognitive decline. One such approach is the

[a]Address for correspondence: Garth E. Ringheim, Department of Neuroscience, Aventis Pharmaceuticals, Inc., Route 202-206, Bridgewater, NJ 08807. Tel.: (908) 231-4928; fax: (908) 231-4335.
e-mail: garth.ringheim@Aventis.com

529

treatment with drugs that increase the production of endogenous factors supporting neuronal survival and synapse formation like fibroblast growth factor or nerve growth factor. Downregulation of brain immune activation has also been postulated to delay disease progression as has been reducing glutamate receptor function to prevent potential stress related excitatory amino acid-induced cell death. Lastly, treatment with nootropic (metabolic enhancing) compounds or inhibitors of apoptosis have all also been proposed to address neurodegenerative disease progression.

PROPENTOFYLLINE

Propentofylline is a pharmacological agent in late stage clinical development for both AD and VaD that has been shown to improve cognition and global function as well as conditions of daily living.[3,4] It is proposed that propentofylline achieves this by targeting the underlying mechanisms leading to the observed clinical manifestations of the two diseases. Evidence for this is based on data gathered from clinical trials with propentofylline as well as from *in vitro* and *in vivo* experiments demonstrating glial modulatory and neuronal supportive effects. The following is a short summation of experimental studies supporting the mechanism and mode of action proposed for propentofylline.

MECHANISM OF ACTION

Propentofylline is a novel xanthine derivative [1-(5′-oxohexyl)-3-methyl-7-propylxanthine] with inhibitory effects on the type I, II, and IV phosphodiesterases[5] and the transporters of extracellular adenosine.[6,7] The observed pharmacological effects of propentofylline are thus mediated by the elevation of intracellular cyclic nucleotides by phosphodiesterase inhibition. In the case of intracellular cyclic adenosine-5′,3′-monophosphate (cAMP), this is further reinforced by the elevation of extracellular adenosine and the subsequent activation of adenylate cyclase-coupled adenosine receptors.[8] It is this combined action of phosphodiesterase inhibition and adenosine receptor stimulation by propentofylline that provides for the unique pharmacological profile of propentofylline. In particular, the combined action of these two systems provides for the downregulation of activated glia, restoration of glutamate and calcium homeostasis, reduction of inflammatory cytokine and free radical production, and preservation of neuronal viability observed for this compound.

GLIAL MODULATION

The combined pharmacological effects of phosphodiesterase inhibition and adenosine receptor stimulation leads to a homeostatic modulation of glial function, particularly in the production of proinflammatory cytokines and free radicals. *In vitro*, propentofylline reduces the proliferation of microglia as well as the endotoxin-induced production of the proinflammatory cytokines interleukin-1β (IL-1β) and tumor necrosis factor-α (TNF-α)[9,10] and the generation of reactive oxygen species.[11] More specific to AD and plaque formation, propentofylline suppresses the production of inflammatory cytokines like TNF-α from cultured microglia activated by Aβ peptide with an affinity similar to that observed for endotoxin-stimulated TNF-α production.[12] Propentofylline has also been described as restoring the differentiated state of activated astrocytes as defined by morphology and K$^+$ and Cl$^-$ channel expression.[13,14] This is also evident *in vivo* where propentofylline treatment has been shown to inhibit astrocyte and microglia activation in both damaged and undamaged brain areas of gerbils after ischemia.[15] Taken together, the microglia and astrocyte suppressing effects of propentofylline that have been observed *in vitro* as well as *in vivo* make for a favorable pharmacological profile in therapies designed to delay or halt disease progression by regulating glial function.

NEUROPROTECTION

In addition to reducing the activation state of microglia and astrocytes, propentofylline has the added benefits of enhancing neuroprotection and inducing neurotrophic factor production. Neuroprotective effects have been shown in ischemic rat models where propentofylline significantly reduced infarct size in the affected brain areas.[15,16] Significant neuronal survival and reduction of neuronal intracellular accumulation of calcium has been shown with propentofylline treatment in ischemic gerbil brains.[15] This may be a result of a reduction in glutamate release observed in ischemic rats[17] and gerbils[18] pretreated with propentofylline. *In vitro*, propentofylline has been shown to suppress the neurotoxic effects of Aβ peptide on neuronal cell types.[19] It has also been shown that propentofylline induces astrocytes to secrete the neurotrophic factor NGF[20] and *in vivo*, to partially reverse the age-associated reduction of NGF in rats.[21] In AD and VaD, where neurons are in an environment of toxic stress, the neuroprotective and NGF-inducing properties of propentofylline would be expected to have an added therapeutic value that complements downregulation of glial activation.

LEARNING AND MEMORY

Learning and memory difficulties define the clinically observable measures of dementia. The clinical improvement in these parameters for patients treated with propentofylline has been described elsewhere.[1,2] Preclinical evidence for improvement of learning and memory are derived from several lines of experiments. As a model of AD, rats given ibotenic acid to induce cholinergic neuronal deficits in the basal forebrain followed by a 28 d treatment regimen with propentofylline showed marked improvement in dark avoidance, Morris water maze, and habituation tests.[22] Although noncholinergic neurons are also lost in this type of lesion, partial recovery of choline acetyltransferase activity was observed in the hippocampus of the rats from the previous study suggesting a partial protection or repair of cholinergic neurons. VaD animal models using spontaneously hypertensive rats that exhibit severe deficits in learning and memory also exhibit improvement in active avoidance tests after 15 d of propentofylline treatment.[23]

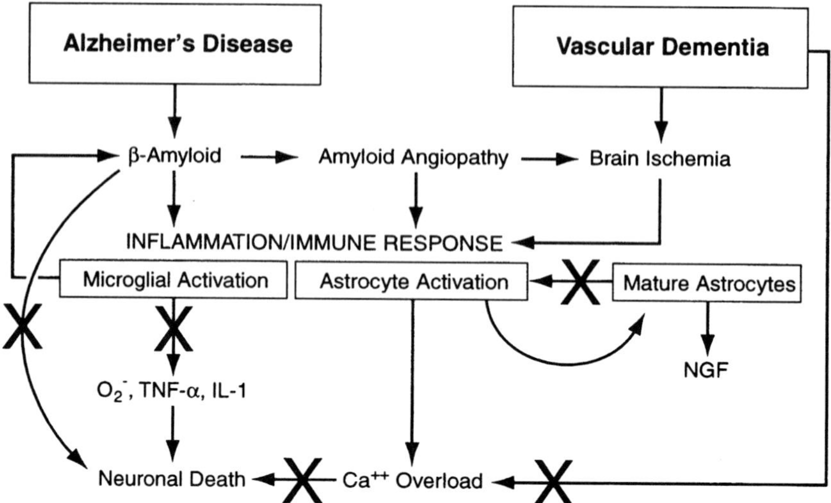

FIGURE 1. Effects of propentofylline. Propentofylline is an adenosine reuptake and phosphodiesterase inhibitor whose pharmacologic effects are mediated by elevation of the intracellular cyclic nucleotides cAMP and cGMP. Its actions include downregulation of activated glia, reduction of inflammatory cytokine and free radical production, restoration of glutamate and calcium homeostasis, and preservation of neuronal viability.

CONCLUSION

In summary, propentofylline is a compound with pharmacological properties that addresses the pathology associated with AD and VaD, which profoundly distinguishes this compound from symptomatic approaches that alter neurotransmitter levels in the brain. It has the combined effects of the following: 1) suppression of astrocyte and microglia activation and the subsequent production of proinflammatory cytokines and free radicals; 2) neuronal support via elevation of nerve growth factor levels; 3) neuroprotection for neurons under toxic stress; and 4) enhancement of learning and memory. With the above-mentioned biological effects, propentofylline would be anticipated to have an effect of halting or slowing the rate of AD or VaD patient decline by addressing the pathology of the disease (see FIG. 1). This is in contrast to symptomatic approaches that would be expected to have an expanded initial benefit due to cognition enhancement, but then continue to deteriorate with time until observable benefit has all but disappeared. Propentofylline as an agent that treats disease pathology would, on the other hand, be expected to show mild positive differences in cognition and activities of daily living versus placebo early with treatment that would continue to expand with time as a reflection of the extent to which the pathology is being treated. This differentiates propentofylline from symptomatic approaches currently in use and as such is representative of the next generation of compounds aimed at preserving cognition by affecting disease pathology. This category represents new challenges in the design and assessment of clinical trials distinct from symptomatic treatments and will require a careful assessment as to the expectations held in treating patients on these drugs over extended times.

REFERENCES

1. MIRSEN, T.R., D.H. LEE, C.J. WONG, J.F. DIAZ, A.F. FOX, V.C. HACHINSKI & H. MERSKEY. 1991. Clinical correlates of white-matter changes on magnetic resonance imaging scans of the brain. Arch. Neurol. **48:** 1015–1021.
2. SCHELTENS, P.H., F. BARKHOF, J. VALK, P.R. ALGRA, R. GERRITSEN VAN DER HOOP, J. NAUTA & C.H. WOLTERS. 1992. White matter lesions on magnetic resonance imaging in clinically diagnosed Alzheimer's disease. Evidence for heterogeneity. Brain **115:** 735–748.
3. KITTNER, B. 1996. Propentofylline (HWA 285): a subgroup analysis of phase III clinical studies in Alzheimer's disease and vascular dementia. *In* Alzheimer Disease: From Molecular Biology to Therapy. Robert Becker & Ezio Giacobini, Eds.: 361–365. Birkhauser. Boston.
4. ROTHER, M., B. KITTNER, K. RUDOLPHI, M. ROBNER & K.H. LABS. 1996. HWA 285 (propentofylline)—a new compound for the treatment of both vascular dementia and dementia of the Alzheimer type. Ann. N.Y. Acad. Sci. **777:** 404–409.
5. MESKINI, N., G. NEMOZ, I. OKYAYUZ-BAKLOUTI, M. LAGARD & A.F. PRIGENT. 1994. Phosphodiesterase inhibitory profile of some related xanthine derivatives pharmacologically active on the peripheral microcirculation. Biochem. Pharmacol. **47:** 781–788.
6. PARKINSON, F.E., A.R. PATERSON, J.D. YOUNG & C.E. CAS. 1993. Inhibitory effects of propentofylline on [^{3}H]adenosine influx. A study of three nucleoside transport systems. Biochem. Pharmacol. **46:** 891–896.
7. OHKUBO, T., Y. MITSUMOTO & T. MOHRI. 1991. Characterization of the uptake of adenosine by cultured rat hippocampal cells and inhibition of the uptake by xanthine derivatives. Neurosci. Lett. **133:** 275–278.
8. FREDHOLM, B.B. & K. LINDSTROM. 1986. The xanthine derivative 1-(5′-oxohexyl)-3-methyl-7-propyl xanthine (HWA 285) enhances the actions of adenosine. Acta Pharmacol. Toxicol. **58:** 187–192.
9. SI, Q.-S., Y. NAKAMURA, P. SCHUBERT, K. RUDOLPHI & K. KATAOKA. 1996. Adenosine and propentofylline inhibit the proliferation of cultured microglial cells. Exp. Neurol. **137:** 345–349.
10. SI, Q.-S., Y. NAKAMURA, T. OGATA, K. KATAOKA & P. SCHUBERT. 1999. Differential regulation of cytokine- and free radical-release from microglia by propentofylline. Brain Res. **812:** 97–104.
11. BANATI, R., P. SCHUBERT, G. ROTHE, J. GEHRMANN, K. RUDOLPHI, G. VALET & G.W. KREUTZBERG. 1994. Modulation of intracellular reactive oxygen intermediates in peritoneal macrophages and microglia/brain macrophages by propentofylline. J. Cereb. Blood Flow Metab. **14:** 145–149.
12. RINGHEIM, G.E., A.M. SZCZEPANIK, W. PETKO & S. FUNES. 1998. Effect of propentofylline on suppressing cytokine and free radical production from microglia activated by beta amyloid peptide 1–42. Soc. Neurosci. Abstr. **24:** Part 2, No. 689.10, p.1752.
13. SCHUBERT, P., T. OGATA, C. MARCHINI, S. FERRONI & K. RUDOLPHI. 1997. Protective mechanisms of adnosine in neurons and glial cells. Ann. N.Y. Acad. Sci. **825:** 1–10.
14. SCHUBERT, P. & K. RUDOLPHI. 1998. Interfering with the pathologic activation of microglial cells and astrocytes in dementia. Alzheimer Dis. Assoc. Disord. **12**(Suppl. 2): S21–S28.
15. DELEO, J., L. TÓTH, P. SCHUBERT, K. RUDOLPHI & G.W. KREUTZBERG. 1987. Ischemia-induced neuronal cell death, calcium accumulation and glial response in the hippocampus of the Mongolian gerbil and protection by propentofylline (HWA 285). J. Cereb. Blood Flow Metab. **7:** 745–752.
16. PARK, C.K. & K. RUDOLPHI. 1994. Antiischemic effects of propentofylline (HWA 285) against focal cerebral infarction in rats. Neurosci. Lett. **178:** 235–238.

17. ANDINE, P., K.A. RUDOLPHI, B.B. FREDHOLM & H. HAGBERG. 1990. Effect of propentofylline (HWA 285) on extracellular purines and excitatory amino acids in CA1 of rat hippocampus during transient ischemia. Br. J. Pharmacol. **100:** 814–818.
18. MIYASHITA, K., T. NAKJIMA, A. ISHIKAWA & T. MIYATAKE. 1992. An adenosine uptake blocker, propentofylline, reduces glutamate release in gerbil hippocampus following transient forebrain ischemia. Neurochem. Res. **17:** 147–150.
19. GIOVANNI, A. & F. WIRTZ-BRUGGER. 1998. Amyloid-induced and NGF withdrawal-induced apoptosis in differentiated PC12 cells: relation to cell-cycle. Soc. Neurosci. Abstr. **24:** Part 2, No. 573.16, p.1463.
20. SHINODA, I., Y. FURUKAWA & S. FURUKAWA. 1990. Stimulation of nerve growth factor synthesis/secretion by propentofylline in cultured mouse astroglial cells. Biochem. Pharmacol. **39:** 1813–1816.
21. NABESHIMA, T., A. NITTA, K. FUJI, T. KAMEYAMA & T. HASEGAWA. 1994. Oral administration of NGF synthesis stimulators recovers reduced brain NGF content in aged rats and cognitive dysfunction in basal-forebrain-lesioned rats. Gerontology **40**(Suppl. 2): 46–56.
22. FUJI, K., M. HIRAMATSU & T. NABESHIMA. 1993. Effects of repeated administration of propentofylline on memory impairment produced by basal forebrain lesion in rats. Eur. J. Pharmacol. **236:** 411–417.
23. GOTO, M., N. DEMURA & T. SAKAGUCHI. 1987. Effects of propentofylline on disorder of learning and memory in rodents. Jpn. J. Pharmacol. **45:** 373–378.

Investigating the Natural Course and Treatment of Vascular Dementia and Alzheimer's Disease

Parallel Study Populations in Two Randomized, Placebo-Controlled Trials

BARBARA KITTNER,[a,d] PETER PAUL DE DEYN,[b] AND TIMO ERKINJUNTTI[c]

[a]*European/Canadian Propentofylline Study Group, Aventis Pharmaceuticals, Route 202-206, Bridgewater, New Jersey 08807, USA*

[b]*Department of Neurology, Middleheim Hospital, Born-Bunge Foundation, University of Antwerp, Antwerp, Belgium*

[c]*Department of Neurology, University of Helsinki, Memory Research Unit, Helsinki, Finland*

INTRODUCTION

Propentofylline is a glial cell modulator that has been shown to interfere with neuroinflammatory processes linked to the pathologic activation of microglial cells and reactive astrocytes — common elements in the pathophysiology of Alzheimer's disease (AD) and vascular dementia (VaD).[1] Propentofylline has been efficacious in both dementia subtypes, as seen in early Phase II studies,[2] and its mechanism of action suggests that it may interfere with the underlying disease process rather than simply providing symptomatic relief. Two recent studies, one in AD and one in VaD, confirmed propentofylline's efficacy; in addition, randomized withdrawal and delayed onset of treatment segments of these trials indicated a potential effect on disease progression.[3] Most of the 37 study centers in Europe and Canada participated in both trials, providing a data set that could be used for comparisons between the AD and the VaD populations without concerns regarding intercenter variability. NINCDS/ADRDA[4] and NINDS/AIREN criteria[5] were used for defining probable AD and possible/probable VaD patients, respectively. Due to the long treatment periods of 72 (AD) and 48 (VaD) weeks, the severity of the disease was limited to baseline MMSE scores of 18 to 26 for AD patients and 15 to 26 for VaD patients. Centralized ratings of CT and MRI scans were performed prior to enrollment to enhance the homogeneity of the patient populations (particularly the VaD population).[6]

RESULTS

The two study populations were comprised of 486 AD (study 304) and 444 VaD (study 305) patients. The ITT populations, which excluded only a few patients with

[d]Corresponding author.

TABLE 1. Patient population demographics: study 304 (AD) and 305 (VaD)

	VaD	AD
Patients randomized	444	486
ITT patients	434	478
Mean age	70.2 ± 9.0	71.2 ± 7.8
Mean age at onset	67.0 ± 9.4	68.2 ± 8.0
Duration	3.8 ± 3.2	3.7 ± 2.2
Women	195	296
Men	239	182
Baseline MMSE	21.4 ± 2.8	21.3 ± 2.4

TABLE 2. Concomitant illnesses:[a] study 304 (AD) and 305 (VaD)

	VaD ($n = 434$)		AD ($n = 478$)	
	Patients	Mentions	Patients	Mentions
Total number	410	1382	375	921
Diabetes mellitus	80	90	46	47
Hypertension	274	276	113	113
Ischemic heart disease	105	110	69	72
Other heart disease	99	103	53	56
Musculoskeletal system	133	181	130	157
Symptoms	93	122	70	80

[a]On the basis of the International Classification of Diseases (ICD).

no post-baseline assessment, were comparable at baseline with respect to age, age at onset of dementia, and duration and severity of dementia as defined by the MMSE score. The distribution of men and women differed between studies, with a greater percentage of women in the AD study (study 304) and a greater percentage of men in the VaD study (study 305) (TABLE 1). Baseline scores of the cognitive tests (the cognitive subscale of the Alzheimer's Disease Assessment Scale [ADAS-cog], the Syndrome Short Test [SKT]) were also comparable. Assessments of activities of daily living (ADL) or assessments that included ADL (Disability Assessment in Dementia [DAD], Gottfries-Bråne-Steen scale [GBS], Caregiver's Activity Survey [CAS]) indicated more pronounced impairment of the VaD patients than the AD patients, most likely due to prior strokes. A higher percentage of the VaD patients (94.5%) reported a concomitant disease compared with the AD patients (78.5%). The mean number of reported concomitant diseases for VaD patients was also greater than that of AD patients; VaD patients averaged 3.4 diseases compared with only 2.5 for AD patients. This discrepancy is primarily due to a higher frequency of hypertension, ischemic and other heart disease, and diabetes mellitus in the VaD population (TABLE 2). Consequently, more VaD patients took concomitant medications than did AD patients (95.6% compared with 78.2%). However, the mean number of drugs taken per patient on concomitant medications was similar for the two populations. VaD patients on concomitant medications took, on average, 3.9 drugs, com-

TABLE 3. Concomitant medications:[a] study 304 (AD) and 305 (VaD)

	VaD (*n* = 434)		AD (*n* = 478)	
	Patients	Mentions	Patients	Mentions
Total Number	415	1623	374	1357
Alimentary tract	286	445	196	314
Antithrombotic agents	255	283	91	100
Cardiovascular system	319	678	212	386
Musculoskeletal system	72	80	76	94
Nervous system	298	397	196	300

[a]Based on World Health Organization (WHO) classification.

pared with 3.6 drugs for AD patients on concomitant medications. The most prevalent medications in both populations were for treatment of the cardiovascular system, the alimentary tract, and the nervous system. The latter category included short-acting benzodiazepines and neuroleptics for inducing sleep; these drugs were not permitted for daytime use during the studies, nor were antidepressants. VaD patients took more antithrombotic agents, primarily acetylsalicylic acid for prophylaxis. Percentages were similar for the AD and VaD populations with respect to the other most common concomitant medications, although somewhat higher for the VaD patients. The distribution of concomitant agents for the musculoskeletal system was roughly equivalent for the two populations (TABLE 3).

Both NINCDS and NINDS criteria require documented dementia with deficits in memory and at least two other areas of cognition. The criteria distinguish probable AD and VaD on the basis of the course of the dementia and, for VaD, the presence of cerebrovascular disease (CVD). The latter is defined by focal neurologic signs, evidence of CVD on neuroradiologic examination, and a relationship between CVD and dementia as determined by the onset or course of the cognitive impairment. The CVD criteria are also captured in the Hachinski ischemia score, which was an inclusion criterion in the AD study, but was only included for description of the patients in the VaD study to allow patients with possible VaD. Possible VaD was diagnosed in patients presenting with deficits in at least two areas of cognition, not necessarily including memory, and two of the criteria for evidence of CVD. Investigators were asked to provide detailed information on the diagnostic criteria in order to permit further analyses/dialogue regarding the validity of the criteria.

Almost all of the AD patients fulfilled the NINCDS/ADRDA criteria; only two patients had no documented cognitive deficit for more than a year or no gradual progression during the year before enrollment. Six AD patients had no documented memory impairment, whereas all of the VaD patients, including those with possible VaD, had memory impairments. On the basis of the NINDS/AIREN criteria as defined for study 305, 175 (40.3%) of the VaD patients had probable VaD, 242 (55.8%) had possible VaD, and 17 (3.9%) could not be classified because they presented with only one of the three criteria for CVD. Most of the possible VaD patients had a clinical course compatible with a diagnosis of VaD; 76.0% had an abrupt onset, and 81.8% had at least one episode of worsening of their cognitive deficits. Focal signs were present in 65.3% of the possible VaD patients during their neurologic exami-

TABLE 4. Hachinski ischemia scores: study 304 (AD) and 305 (VaD)

	VaD		AD	
	n	*%*	*n*	*%*
Total number	434	100.0	478	100.0
Abrupt onset	315	72.6	0	0.0
Stepwise deterioration	323	74.4	1	0.0
Fluctuating course	263	60.6	11	2.3
Nocturnal confusion	66	15.2	26	5.4
Preservation of personality	330	76.0	248	51.9
Depression	47	10.8	16	3.3
Somatic complaints	182	41.9	53	11.1
Emotional incontinence	111	25.6	59	12.3
History of hypertension	292	67.3	133	27.8
History of strokes	283	65.2	6	1.3
Associated atherosclerosis	246	56.7	52	10.9
Focal signs	336	77.4	28	5.9
Focal symptoms	337	77.6	3	0.6
Total score: mean ± SD	10.4 ± 2.7	—	1.4 ± 1.1	—

TABLE 5. Cognitive impairments: study 304 (AD) and 305 (VaD)

	Possible VaD *n* = 242		Probable VaD *n* = 175		AD *n* = 478	
	n	*%*	*n*	*%*	*n*	*%*
Memory	242	100.0	175	100.0	472	98.7
Orientation	198	81.8	146	83.4	426	89.1
Language	97	40.1	63	36.0	143	29.9
Praxis	106	43.8	87	49.7	175	36.6
Attention	175	72.3	119	68.0	279	58.4
Visual-spatial	112	46.3	87	49.7	235	49.2
Problem solving	189	78.1	157	89.7	330	69.0
Social function	163	67.4	119	68.0	209	43.7

nation. Evidence of relevant CVD on neuroradiologic assessment, as defined in the NINDS/AIREN criteria, could only be found in 27.7% of the possible VaD patients. This percentage may be lower than what might typically be expected due to the involvement of a central rater (because the presence of ischemic lesions and the severity of white matter changes may be judged differently by different investigators). Hachinski ischemia score findings reflected the information collected for the diagnostic criteria for AD and VaD. The AD patients had a mean score of 1.4, whereas the VaD patients had a mean score of 10.4. Very few AD patients had a history of stroke, stepwise deterioration, or focal signs and symptoms (TABLE 4).

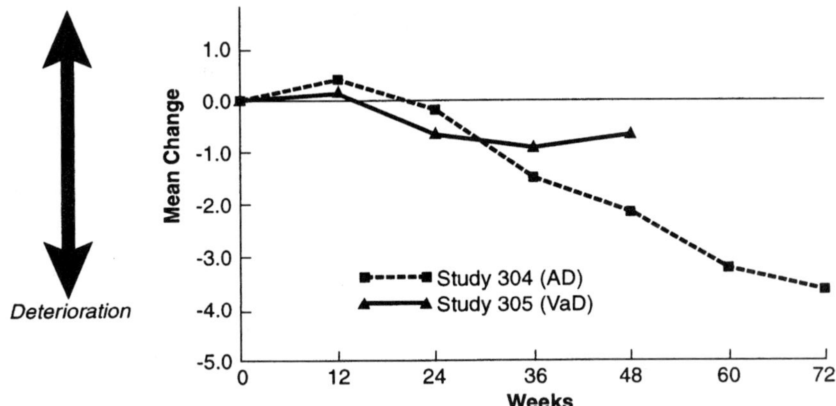

FIGURE 1. Placebo data demonstrate a typical decline in cognitive function (as assessed by ADAS-cog scores) for AD patients in study 304 compared with the relatively stable performance of VaD patients in study 305.

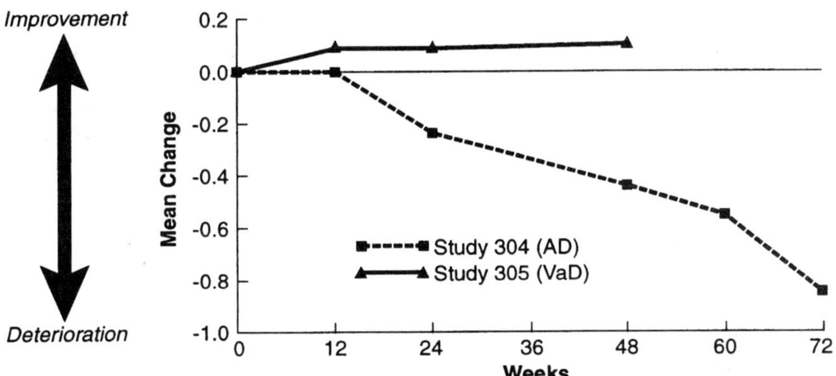

FIGURE 2. Global function (CIBIC-Plus) data for placebo patients in study 304 (AD) and study 305 (VaD) demonstrate a steep decline for AD patients compared with a slight improvement in VaD patients.

A comparison of baseline cognitive impairment profiles for both studies showed that a majority of the patients in both populations suffered from impairments in memory, orientation, and problem solving. Prevalence figures for other impairments were lower for both populations overall, but were typically higher for VaD patients compared with AD patients for individual categories (TABLE 5). Although these differences did not translate to different baseline scores for the cognitive tests, a comparison of the course of the placebo patients from both studies over the observation period of 48 weeks clearly showed that the VaD patients deteriorated more slowly or not at all. By contrast, the AD patients on placebo progressed steadily after a period of stability of 12–24 weeks (FIGS. 1 and 2).

CONCLUSIONS

Increased knowledge about AD, and the development of specific drugs for its treatment, have led to a large number of studies and to wide use of the NINCDS/ADRDA criteria in clinical studies. Studies in VaD have been less common, because vascular factors or vascular disease were considered to be of lesser importance as an underlying cause of cognitive deficits; in fact, the latter issue has been a source of considerable controversy and debate regarding the definition and diagnosis of VaD. However, many recent observations have led to the acknowledgment that vascular disease may not only coincide with the cognitive impairments, but may also actually contribute to or cause the dementia. The NINDS/AIREN criteria are based on a clinical history of stroke, the presence of ischemic lesions on neuroradiologic examination, and the assumption that the two are related. Both the NINCDS/ADRDA and the NINDS/AIREN criteria use the same definition for dementia, but they distinguish their intended patient populations according to the clinical course and the absence or presence of CVD.

Studies 304 and 305 were conducted mostly at the same study sites and thus may provide new insights into the discussion regarding the overlap of AD and VaD. Rigorous application of the diagnostic criteria led to a relatively "clean" AD population in study 304. The subgroup of possible VaD as defined in study 305 may include patients with AD, particularly if one considers the low percentage of patients with evidence of CVD on the neuroradiologic examination in the central rating. A steady progression of disease would be expected if the possible VaD patients in study 305 were actually AD patients; however, a separate, preliminary analysis of these patients indicated a similar course to that of the probable VaD patients. The fact that the concept of dementia used for both AD and VaD in these studies included impairment in memory plus two additional areas of cognition may have skewed the VaD population towards the characteristics of an AD population. Further confounding the interpretation of these data on disease progression are findings from previous studies, which indicate that disease course may vary among AD populations, sometimes producing relatively little progression over time in placebo patients.[7] Additional analyses of the combined data from the current studies may shed new light on these and other questions surrounding the diagnosis, natural history, and treatment possibilities for both the AD and VaD patient populations.

REFERENCES

1. RINGHEIM, G.E. 2000. Glial modulating and neurotrophic properties of propentofylline: applications to Alzheimer's disease and vascular dementia. Ann. N.Y. Acad. Sci. This volume.
2. KITTNER, B., M. RÖSSNER & M. ROTHER. 1997. Clinical trials in dementia with propentofylline. Ann. N.Y. Acad. Sci. **826:** 307–316.
3. BODICK, N., F. FORETTE, D. HADLER et al. 1997. Protocols to demonstrate slowing of Alzheimer disease progression. Position paper from the International Working Group on Harmonization of Dementia Drug Guidelines. The Disease Progression Sub-Group. Alzheimer Dis. Assoc. Disord. **11**(Suppl 3): 50–53.
4. MCKHANN, G., D. DRACHMANN, M. FOLSTEIN et al. 1984. Clinical diagnosis of Alzheimer's disease: report of the NINCDS-ADRDA Working Group under the auspices of the Department of Health and Human Services Task Force on Alzheimer's Disease. Neurology **34:** 939–949.

 5. ROMÁN, G.C., T.K. TATEMICHI, T. ERKINJUNTTI *et al.* 1993. Vascular dementia: diagnostic criteria for research studies: report of the NINDS-AIREN International Workshop. Neurology **43:** 250–260.
 6. SCHELTENS, P. & B. KITTNER. 2000. Preliminary results from an MRI/CT-based database for vascular dementia and Alzheimer's disease. Ann. N.Y. Acad. Sci. This volume.
 7. Data on file, Hoechst Marion Roussel, 1999.

Preliminary Results from an MRI/CT-Based Database for Vascular Dementia and Alzheimer's Disease

PHILIP SCHELTENS[a,c] AND BARBARA KITTNER[b]

[a]*European/Canadian Propentofylline Study Group, Department of Neurology, Academisch Ziekenhuis VU, PO Box 7057, 1007 MB Amsterdam, The Netherlands*

[b]*Hoechst Marion Roussel, Bridgewater, New Jersey, USA*

INTRODUCTION

The value of magnetic resonance imaging (MRI) and computerized tomography (CT) for the diagnosis of Alzheimer's disease (AD) and vascular dementia (VaD) has been the subject of numerous studies. Characteristic findings have been defined for each dementia type, including atrophy of specific brain areas (for example, medial temporal lobe atrophy [MTA][1] for AD or ischemic lesions in particular regions for VaD[2]). However, these findings may not be exclusive to either AD or VaD, respectively.[3–6] Furthermore, assessments of atrophy and vascular lesions, particularly white matter changes, may be subjective, potentially yielding a high degree of heterogeneity when used as a screening procedure for clinical studies.

The purpose of this study was to assess atrophy and white matter changes objectively and independently through the use of a central rating system and to use these findings to verify and support individual investigators' diagnoses of patients participating in two parallel studies of dementia: study 304, which involved probable AD patients according to NINCDS/ADRDA criteria,[7] and study 305, which involved possible and probable VaD patients according to NINDS/AIREN criteria.[2]

This is the first time, to our knowledge, that central CT/MRI rating was applied in large, international, multicenter studies. Because the two trials were performed as companion studies, the central rating permits subgroup analyses across study populations on the basis of scan parameters.

METHODS

The central rating system involved a team of two raters. The scans were sent as hard copies by courier from the investigators to the rating team before the patient was enrolled in the study. Although the study design had included a scanning proto-

[c]Address for Correspondence: Philip Scheltens, MD, Dept. of Neurology, Academisch Ziekenhuis VU, PO Box 7057, 1007 MB Amsterdam, The Netherlands. Tel.: +31 20 444 4444 (ext. 552); fax: +31 20 444 0715.

e-mail: p.scheltens@azvu.nl

TABLE 1. CT/MRI finding in AD patients (study 304)

	AD Patients (NINCDS-ADRDA)	
	n	%
Randomized patients	486	100
Cortical atrophy	393	81
Ventricular dilatation	363	75
Mass lesion	—	—
Focal lucency or high signal intensity		
White matter	194	40
Grey matter	61	13

TABLE 2. CT/MRI findings[a] in VaD patients (study 305)

	VaD Patients (NINDS-AIREN)	
	n	%
All randomized patients	440	100
Evidence of cerebrovascular disease		
Large-vessel strokes	101[b]	23
Small-vessel disease		
Multiple basal ganglia and white matter lacunae	94	21
Bilateral thalamic lesions	6	1
Large-vessel lesions of dominant hemisphere	37	8
Bilateral large-vessel hemispheric strokes	6	1
Extensive periventricular white matter lesions[c]	223	51
Atrophy	350	80

[a] According to NINDS criteria.
[b] Number of strokes, not patients.
[c] Also considered evidence of small-vessel disease.

col, many scans had not been performed according to its specifications. The rating team filled out a case report for each patient that included specific forms for AD and VaD patients as well as a common form for rating scales and linear measures independent of the AD/VaD diagnosis. The scans were returned to the investigators with the diagnosis-specific forms within a 2-week window. The case report for the VaD patients used the published NINDS/AIREN criteria for relevant cerebrovascular disease.[2] The following items were rated: global cortical atrophy and ventricular enlargement according to Scheltens *et al.*[8]; medial temporal atrophy on MRI according to Scheltens *et al.*[1] and on CT according to the method of De Leon *et al.*[9]; and white matter changes on CT (leuko-araiosis) according to Blennow *et al.*[10] and on MRI using the scale by Scheltens *et al.*[11]

TABLE 3. Mean rating of atrophy in study 304 (AD) and study 305 (VaD)

Location (Score)	AD			VaD		
	n	Mean	SD	*n*	Mean	SD
Sulcal widening (0–18)	485	5.5	3.5	433	5.1	3.3
Ventricular widening (0–21)	485	6.0	4.9	433	6.7	4.9
Medial temporal atrophy (0–4)	198	2.2	2.0	177	2.5	1.9

TABLE 4. Linear measures of atrophy (Indices) in Study 304 (AD) and Study 305 (VaD)

Location (Score)	AD Patients			VaD Patients		
	n	Mean	SD	*n*	Mean	SD
Frontal horn index	480	33.7	5.0	428	33.7	5.3
Bicaudate index	481	15.4	3.8	426	15.8	4.1
Third ventricle index	481	5.8	2.3	427	6.5	3.1
Cella media index	482	28.8	6.0	427	29.7	6.4

TABLE 5. Number of lacunar infarcts in study 304 (AD) and study 305 (VaD)

No. lacunar infarcts	1	2	3	4	5	6	7	8
No. AD patients	40	16	3	1	—	1	—	—
No. VaD patients	69	24	13	6	7	1	—	1

RESULTS

Of the 486 randomized patients enrolled in study 304 (AD), 393 had CT scans and 93 had MRI images available for central rating. The corresponding numbers for the 444 patients in study 305 (VaD) were 296 for CT and 144 for MRI scans. Within the AD population, atrophy was found as cortical atrophy in 393 patients (81%) and as ventricular dilatation in 363 patients (75%) (TABLE 1). Focal lucencies were detected in the white matter in 194 patients (40%) and in the grey matter in 61 patients (13%). Mass lesions were not found in any of the AD patients, because this type of lesion was excluded by the AD study protocol. Atrophy, however, was a common finding in the VaD patients; 350 patients (80%) showed signs of atrophy on CT scan or MRI (TABLE 2).

Evidence of relevant cerebrovascular disease on neuroradiologic examination is defined by NINDS/AIREN criteria as large-vessel strokes in relevant areas of the brain and small-vessel disease, both being of a specific distribution or severity. Overall, 101 large-vessel strokes were found on the scans of the VaD patients; 94 patients had multiple lacunae in the basal ganglia and the white matter; and 6 patients had bilateral thalamic lesions (TABLE 2). Severe lesions were found in 37 patients with large-vessel strokes of the dominant hemisphere and in 6 patients with bilateral large-vessel strokes. In addition, 223 patients had extensive (defined by the NINDS

TABLE 6. Leukoaraiosis (CT) and white matter changes (MRI) in study 304 (AD) and study 305 (VaD)

	AD			VaD		
Leuko-Araiosis on CT scan						
N (%) of patients	*n*	%		*n*	%	
Total	389	100		294	100	
Score >0	153	39		224	76	
Score = 3	18	5		46	16	
White matter changes on MRI						
	n	Mean	SD	*n*	Mean	SD
Periventricular	92	3.1	1.7	135	3.5	1.5
Deep white matter	92	4.0	5.7	139	7.98	6.9

criteria[2] as involving $\geq 25\%$ of the white matter) periventricular white matter lesions. Since the criterion of relevant cerebrovascular disease on neuroradiologic examination was met in 242 of the VaD patients, lesions involving the white matter contributed to the diagnosis in a great majority of these individuals.

Measurements of atrophy indices showed only minor differences between the AD and VaD populations with respect to sulcal and ventricular widening and medial temporal atrophy (TABLE 3). Other linear measures yielded similar results (TABLE 4).

VaD patients had more lacunar infarcts overall compared with AD patients, although 56 AD patients had one or two infarcts (TABLE 5). More VaD than AD patients (76% versus 39%) had signs of leukoaraiosis on CT scans; moreover, a greater percentage of VaD patients (16% versus 5%) had a score of 3 (TABLE 6). VaD patients also scored higher with respect to deep white matter hyperintensities on MRI, but not with respect to periventricular hyperintensities.

Preliminary analysis of the correlation between CT/MRI findings and age or severity of cognitive impairment showed a mild-to-moderate correlation between atrophy and white matter changes with age and atrophy (cognition was assessed by the cognitive tests, e.g., ADAS-cog).

CONCLUSIONS

The current study confirmed that central rating of CT and MRI examinations is feasible within the context of large clinical studies, even when many countries and a wide variety of scanners are involved. Although AD and VaD may be clinically distinct and were considered as such by the investigators in studies 304 and 305, analysis of the neuroradiologic data revealed considerable overlap between them. This was particularly true for the presence of atrophy (including medial temporal atrophy) in both patient populations. Moreover, although the VaD population was generally characterized by white matter involvement on CT/MRI, 40% of the AD population also showed white matter changes.

These findings require further analysis across the two study populations for subgroups presenting with and without white matter changes and with and without medial temporal atrophy in order to determine whether these subgroups differ clinically. However, the concepts of dementia utilized in these studies (NINCDS/ADRDA for study 304 [AD] and NINDS/AIREN for study 305 [VaD]) may limit the conclusions that can be drawn from such subgroup analyses.

REFERENCES

1. SCHELTENS, P., D. LEYS, F. BARKHOF *et al.* 1992. Atrophy of medial temporal lobes on MRI in "probable" Alzheimer's disease and normal aging: diagnostic value and neuropsychological correlates. J. Neurol. Neurosurg. Psychiatry **55:** 967–972.
2. ROMÁN, G.C., T.K. TATEMICHI, T. ERKINJUNTTI *et al.* 1993. Vascular dementia: diagnostic criteria for research studies. Report of the NINDS-AIREN International Work Group. Neurology **43:** 250–260.
3. TIERNEY, M.C., R.H. FISHER, A.J. LEWIS *et al.* 1988. The NINCDS-ADRDA Work Group criteria for the clinical diagnosis of probable Alzheimer's disease: a clinico-pathological study of 57 cases. Neurology **38:** 359–364.
4. SCHELTENS, P., F. BARKHOF, J. VALK *et al.* 1992. White matter lesions on magnetic resonance imaging in Alzheimer's disease: evidence for heterogeneity. Brain **115:** 735–743.
5. SNOWDON, D.A., L.H. GREINER, J.A. MORTIMER *et al.* 1997. Brain infarction and the clinical expression of Alzheimer's disease: the Nun Study. JAMA. **277:** 813–817.
6. PASQUIER, F., D. LEYS & P.H. SCHELTENS. 1998. The influence of coincidental vascular pathology on symptomatology and course of Alzheimer's disease. J. Neural. Transm. **54:** 117–129.
7. MCKHANN, G., D. DRACHMAN, M. FOLSTEIN *et al.* 1984. Clinical diagnosis of Alzheimer's disease: report of the NINCDS-ARDRA work group under the auspices of Department of Health and Human Services Task Force on Alzheimer's Disease. Neurology **34:** 939–944.
8. SCHELTENS, P., F. PASQUIER, J.G. WEERTS *et al.* 1997. Qualitative assessment of cerebral atrophy on MRI: inter- and intra-observer reproducibility in dementia and normal aging. Eur. Neurol. **37:** 95–99.
9. DE LEON, M.J., A.E. GEORGE, L.A. STYLOPOULOS *et al.* 1989. Early marker for Alzheimer's disease: the atrophic hippocampus. Lancet **II:** 672–673.
10. BLENNOW, K., A. WALLIN, C. UHLEMANN *et al.* 1991. White-matter lesions on CT in Alzheimer's patients: relation to clinical symptomatology and vascular factors. Acta Neurol. Scand. **83:** 187–193.
11. SCHELTENS, P., F. BARKHOF, D. LEYS *et al.* 1993. A semiquantitative rating scale for the assessment of signal hyperintensities on magnetic resonance imaging. J. Neurol. Sci. **114:** 7–12.

Alzheimer's Disease and Vascular Dementia

Some Points of Confluence

HEDDA AGÜERO-TORRES[a,b] AND BENGT WINBLAD[a,b]

[a]*Stockholm Gerontology Research Center and* [b]*Department of Clinical Neuroscience, Occupational Therapy, and Elderly Care Research, Division of Geriatric Medicine, Karolinska Institute, S-11382 Stockholm, Sweden*

ABSTRACT: The lack of biologic markers for Alzheimer's disease and vascular dementia, the controversy regarding the definition of vascular dementia, and the new evidence of vascular risk factors for Alzheimer's disease suggest that the traditional differentiation between Alzheimer's disease and vascular dementia is no longer very clear. We believe that both vascular and degenerative mechanisms contribute to the development of dementia, especially in very old age. The question of whether they are two independent parallel processes or interacting pathologies needs to be clarified.

INTRODUCTION

Because of the dramatic increase in the elderly population, the morbidity and disability of this group are becoming more and more relevant for researchers and for those who provide health care and social services. Dementia is an emerging public health problem, as it is one of the most common diseases in the elderly and a major cause of disability and mortality.[1,2] Alzheimer's disease (AD) and vascular dementia (VaD) are the most common dementing disorders, accounting for 90–95% of all dementias.[3] However, the traditional clear differentiation between them has become blurred.

DIAGNOSTIC CRITERIA AND DEFINITIONAL ISSUES IN DEMENTING DISORDERS

Among the many disorders known to cause dementia, AD and VaD are the most common, especially in elderly populations. Because of the lack of biologic markers for these conditions, the differential diagnosis is essentially clinical, based on diagnostic criteria. Therefore, a brief description of these criteria is needed in order to understand the difficulties in classification.

[a]Address for correspondence: Hedda Agüero-Torres, MD, PhD, Stockholm Gerontology Research Center, 'The Kungsholmen Project', Box 6401, S-11382 Stockholm, Sweden. Tel.: +46 8 6905854; fax: +46 8 6905954.

e-mail: Hedda.Aguero-Eklund@neurotec.ki.se

Diagnostic Criteria for Alzheimer's Disease

The diagnosis of Alzheimer's disease is essentially clinical, because until now no specific biologic markers have been identified. However, some diagnostic criteria have been created to facilitate the medical diagnosis. Two main sets of diagnostic criteria include criteria for AD, the one given by the *Diagnostic and Statistical Manual* (DSM-III-R and DSM-IV)[4,5] and the one given by the *International Classification of Disease* (ICD-10).[6] A third set of diagnostic criteria by The National Institute for Neurological Disorders and Stroke and the Alzheimer's Disease and Related Disorders Association (NINCDS-ADRDA),[7] which is specific for AD, has been created. These three sets of criteria share many common features. To make a diagnosis of AD, all three require (1) insidious onset of dementia, (2) a gradually progressive deteriorating course, and (3) exclusion of all other specific causes of dementia. In ICD-10, the presence of apoplectic onset or focal neurologic signs early in the illness are exclusion criteria. The NINCDS-ADRDA criteria take a somewhat different approach by grading the level of diagnostic certainty. Differences between definite, probable, and possible AD diagnosis reflect the available information and how closely the patient's syndrome resembles "classic" AD. A definite diagnosis can be reached when pathologic evidence of AD is added to a diagnosis of clinical probable AD. Probable AD is characterized by deficits in two or more areas of cognition. Possible AD is diagnosed when only one cognitive area is affected in the absence of any other identifiable cause, when the clinical course is atypical, or when a second disease potentially related to dementia is present but is not considered the cause of dementia.

The validity of an AD diagnosis has been studied in terms of reproducibility and confirmation at autopsy. The agreement between different clinicians in making an AD diagnosis expressed as kappa index was 0.49,[8] 0.72,[9] and 0.63[10] when NINCDS-ADRDA criteria were used. The reproducibility of DSM III-R resulted in a kappa value of 0.55[11] and 0.67.[12] The accuracy rate of clinically based diagnoses, when compared with pathologic findings, varies from 0.62 to 0.92.[13]

Diagnostic Criteria for Vascular Dementia

The definition of VaD has been changing over time. In 1955, Roth[14] proposed the term "artherosclerotic psychosis" for dementing disorders in the elderly which, regarding survival and progression, differed from senile psychosis. In 1969, this clinical syndrome was described. The investigators pointed out that hypertension occurred in about 50% of the cases and that symptoms generally started after a number of strokes.[15] In support of the theory that strokes, rather than generalized ischemia, are the cause of dementia associated with cardiovascular disease, Hachinski and collaborators[16] introduced the term "multi-infarct dementia" (MID) in 1974. After this initial definition of MID as a poststroke dementia, a broader term, "vascular dementia" (VaD), was introduced to identify the acquired intellectual impairment resulting from cerebrovascular lesions of the brain.[17] The term VaD was questioned because it included dementia caused by both ischemic and hemorrhagic cerebrovascular damage, when it is known that ischemic vascular dementia is far more common than that caused by hemorrhage or hypoxia.[18,19] Recently, the definition of dementia itself was criticized by Hachinski.[20] In 1995, Bowler and Hachinski[21] proposed a new term, "vascular cognitive impairment," in which all cognitive disturbances related to cerebrovascular disorders are included, regardless of the degree of severity.

As a consequence of the variation in the definition of VaD, different diagnostic criteria have been proposed. Among the many operational criteria,[4–6,22–26] only three have been used in epidemiologic research.[4,5,26]

Traditional criteria such as the DSM[4,5] or the Hachinski ischemic scale (HIS)[22] have been strongly criticized.[27] However, recent results of a meta-analysis of the HIS in pathologically verified dementia[28] confirmed the utility of this instrument for the detection of MID. Using the standard cut-off of the scale (a score of 7 or higher), the discrimination between MID and AD was very accurate, with a sensitivity of 89% and a specificity of 89%. Recently, two new sets of criteria, one proposed by the State of California Alzheimer's Disease Diagnostic and Treatment Centers (AD-DTC)[25] and one reported by The National Institute for Neurological Disorders and Stroke and Association Internationalle pour la Recherche et l'Enseignement en Neurosciences (NINDS-AIREN),[26] have also been validated against neuropathology.[29] The investigators concluded that the sensitivity of both NINDS-AIREN and ADDTC criteria is unexpectedly low (60%). Although the two systems were able to exclude patients with AD, they failed to diagnose one third of the neuropathologically confirmed cases of VaD. Both ADDTC and NINDS-AIREN criteria rely for their diagnosis on neuroimaging, which is not often available in population-based surveys. These criteria require that other types of dementia are excluded; however, AD diagnostic criteria include the same requirement.

All clinicians trying to differentiate between vascular and degenerative dementia in both clinical and research settings are aware that elderly people are often affected by more than one disease. Therefore, an elderly subject who has both dementia and any vascular disease may present many difficulties in being classified as an AD or a VaD case. No single system of diagnostic criteria available at the moment can be accepted as definitive.

VAD AND AD: POINTS OF CONFLUENCE

It is well established that cardiovascular risk factors are the main causes of cerebrovascular disease. The presence of cardiovascular risk factors has traditionally been used to make a clinical differentiation between AD and VaD, because the diagnosis of AD is a diagnosis of exclusion, particularly with regard to vascular disease. The clinical differentiation between these conditions has improved, thanks to more detailed diagnostic criteria for AD and to the consideration in the VaD diagnosis of the temporal sequence of events, which aims to recognize the cause/effect relationship. However, the problem of subclinical disease complicates the assessment not only of the dementia type, but also of the cardiovascular disease.

Evidence is emerging from pathologic and etiologic studies of overlap between degenerative and vascular dementing disorders. In the elderly, multimorbidity is extremely common. Among subjects aged 75 and older included in the Kungsholmen Project,[30] the prevalence of dementia, heart disease, cerebrovascular disease, cancer, and hip fracture was 12%, 17%, 9%, 12%, and 11%, respectively. Twenty-eight percent of the participants had at least one disease, and 14% had more than one. This multimorbidity increases the probability of a subject being affected at the same time by two diseases without any causal relation. However, this does not preclude the possibility that these two diseases may contribute to the same syndrome (i.e., dementia) through different mechanisms (such as degenerative and vascular).

Some epidemiologic studies have suggested an overlap between AD and VaD. Cognitive impairment has been associated with cardiovascular disease and atherosclerotic index[31] and cardiovascular risk factors such as diabetes,[32,33] hypertension,[34] obesity, smoking, and hypertriglyceridemia,[35] and atrial fibrillation.[36] Recent reports have also found an association between some cardiovascular risk factors and AD. Hypertension, which is the most powerful risk factor for VaD,[37] has also been found to increase the risk of AD.[38] In the Kungsholmen Project, a longitudinal population-based study of people aged 75+, blood pressure reduction was associated with an increased incidence of dementia and AD[39] and with cognitive decline.[40] The relationship between blood pressure and dementia is complicated. Both high and low blood pressure may play a role in the pathogenesis of dementia. In addition, dementia itself may alter the blood pressure level.[41] Other reported vascular factors related to the risk of AD are atherosclerosis index,[42] atrial fibrillation,[43] and diabetes mellitus.[44–46]

At autopsy, vascular lesions are frequently associated with AD, and they have been related to the presence and severity of the symptoms.[47,48] Moreover, some authors have suggested that pure vascular dementia is uncommon at brain necropsy.[49,50] Additionally, cerebral amyloid angiopathy is common in AD, but it is also associated with cerebral atherosclerosis.[51] These findings stress the need for valid neuropathologic criteria for vascular dementia,[52] but they also suggest that perhaps it is important to recognize a broader spectrum of disease between pure VaD and AD.

CONCLUSION

Finally, we believe that it is currently possible to identify two groups of subjects affected by typical AD or typical VaD. However, mixed and/or unclear cases are more common than expected, and they need to be studied separately. This new strategy has begun only recently in epidemiologic research.[53]

The study of cardiovascular risk factors for dementia or AD has great relevance for prevention and treatment. Epidemiologic data give the basis for planning primary prevention and clinical trials. However, there is still the need for a general consensus on disease definition and diagnostic criteria.

ACKNOWLEDGMENTS

We thank all members of the Kungsholmen Project group for their collaboration. We also thank the Swedish Society for Medical Research, the "Gamla Tjänarinnor" Foundation, the Swedish Council for Social Research, the Einar Belvéns Foundation, and the SHMF-90.

REFERENCES

1. AGÜERO-TORRES, H. *et al.* 1998. Prognostic factors in very old demented adults: a seven-year follow-up from a population-based survey in Stockholm. J. Am. Geriatr. Soc. **46:** 444–452.
2. AGÜERO-TORRES, H. *et al.* 1998. Dementia is the major cause of functional dependence in the elderly: 3-year follow-up data from a population-based study. Am. J. Public Health **88:** 1452–1456.
3. FRATIGLIONI, L. 1998. Epidemiology. *In* Health Economics of Dementia. B. Winblad, A. Wimo, B. Jonsson & G. Karlsson, Eds: 13–31. John Wiley & Sons. New York.
4. AMERICAN PSYCHIATRIC ASSOCIATION. 1987. Diagnostic and Statistical Manual of Mental Disorders, 3rd ed, revised (DSM III-R). :97–163. American Psychiatric Association. Washington, DC.
5. AMERICAN PSYCHIATRIC ASSOCIATION. 1994. Diagnostic and Statistical Manual of Mental Disorders, 4th ed (DSM IV). :133–155. American Psychiatric Association. Washington, DC.
6. WORLD HEALTH ORGANIZATION. 1990. ICD-10 draft of chapter V: Categories F00-F99, Mental and Behavioral Disorders (Including Disorders of Psychological Development): Diagnostic Criteria for Research. Geneva, Switzerland. World Health Organization, Division of Mental Health. Document WHO/MNH/MEP/89.2, REV 1.
7. MCKHANN, G. *et al.* 1984. Clinical diagnosis of Alzheimer's disease: report of the NINCDS-ADRDA Work Group under the auspices of Department of Health and Human Services Task force on Alzheimer's disease. Neurology **34:** 939–944.
8. LOPEZ, O.L. *et al.* 1990. Reliability of NINCDS-ADRDA criteria for the diagnosis of Alzheimer's disease. Neurology **40:** 1517–1522.
9. BALDERESCHI, M. *et al.* 1994. Cross-national interrater agreement on the clinical diagnostic criteria for dementia. Neurology **44:** 239–249.
10. FARRER, LA. *et al.* 1995. Consistency of clinical diagnostic in a community-based longitudinal study of dementia and Alzheimer's disease. Neurology **45:** 2159–2164.
11. KUKULL, W.A. *et al.* 1990. The validity of 3 clinical diagnostic criteria for Alzheimer's disease. Neurology **40:** 1364–1369.
12. FRATIGLIONI, L. *et al.* 1992. Clinical diagnosis of Alzheimer's disease and other dementias in a population survey. Agreement and causes of disagreement in applying DSM III-R criteria. Arch. Neurol. **49:** 927–932.
13. KLATKA, L.A. *et al.* 1996. Incorrect diagnosis of Alzheimer's disease. Arch. Neurol. **53:** 35–42.
14. ROTH, M. 1955. The natural history of mental disorders in old age. J. Ment. Sci. **101:** 281–301.
15. MAYER-GROSS, W. *et al.* 1969. Clinical Psychiatry, 3rd ed. Tindal & Carsell. London.
16. HACHINSKI, V.C. *et al.* 1974. Multi-infarct dementia: a cause of mental deterioration in the elderly. Lancet **ii:** 207–210.
17. LOEB, B. 1985. Vascular dementia. *In* Handbook of Clinical Neurology, Vol. 2. Neurobehavioral Disorders. J.A.M. Frederiks, Ed. : 353–369. Elsevier. Amsterdam.
18. DRACHACMAN, D.A. 1993. New criteria for the diagnosis of vascular dementia: do we know enough yet? Neurology **43:** 243–245.
19. TATEMICHI, T.K. *et al.* 1994. Dementia associated with cerebrovascular disease, other degenerative diseases and metabolic disorders. *In* Alzheimer's Disease. R.T. Terry, R. Katzman & K.L. Bick, Eds. :123–166. Raven Press. New York.
20. HACHINSKI, V.C. 1992. Preventable senility: a call for action against the vascular dementias. Lancet **340:** 645–647.
21. BOWLER, J.B. & V.C. HACHINSKI. 1995. Vascular cognitive impairment: a new approach to vascular dementia. *In* Cerebrovascular Disease. V. Hachinski, Ed. :357–376. Ballière Tindall. London.
22. HACHINSKI, V.C. *et al.* 1975. Cerebral blood flow in dementia. Arch. Neurol. **32:** 632–637.
23. ROSEN, W.G. *et al.* 1980. Pathological verification of ischemic score in differentiation of dementias. Ann. Neurol. **7:** 486–488.
24. LOEB, C. & C. GANDOLFO. 1983. Diagnostic evaluation of degenerative and vascular dementia. Stroke **14:** 399–401.

25. CHUI, H.C. *et al.* 1992. Criteria for the diagnosis of ischemic vascular dementia proposed by the state of California Alzheimer's disease diagnostic and treatment centers. Neurology **42:** 473–480.
26. ROMAN, G.C. *et al.* 1993. Vascular dementia: diagnostic criteria for research studies. Report of the NINDS-AIREN International Workshop. Neurology **43:** 243–245.
27. O'BRIEN, M.D. 1988. Vascular dementia is underdiagnoed. Arch. Neurol. **45:** 797–798.
28. MORONEY, J.T. *et al.* 1997. Meta-analysis of the Hachinski Ischemic score in pathologically verified dementias. Neurology **49:** 1096–1105.
29. GOLD, G. *et al.* 1997. Sensitivity and specificity of newly proposed clinical criteria for possible vascular dementia. Neurology **49:** 690–694.
30. AGÜERO-TORRES, H. *et al.* 1998. Dementia is the major cause of functional dependence in the elderly. Three-year follow-up data from a population-based study. Am. J. Public Health **88:** 1452–1456.
31. BRETELER, M.M.B. *et al.* 1994. Cardiovascular disease and the distribution of cognitve function in elderly people: the Rotterdam study. Brit. Med. J. **308:** 1604–1608.
32. KALMIJN, S. *et al.* 1995. Glucose in tolerance, hyperinsulinaemia and cognitive function in a general population of elderly men. Diabetologia **38:** 1096–1102.
33. STOLK, R.P. *et al.* 1997. Insulin and cognitive function in an elderly population. The Rotterdam Study. Diabetes Care **20:** 792–795.
34. ELIAS, M.F. *et al.* 1993. Untreated blood pressure level is inversely related to cognitive functioning: the Framinghan study. Am. J. Epidemiol. **138:** 353–364.
35. KILANDER, L. *et al.* 1997. Cognitive function, vascular risk factors and education. A cross-sectional study based on a cohort of 70-year-old men. J. Intern. Med. **242:** 313–321.
36. KILANDER, L. *et al.* 1998. Atrial fibrillation is an independent determinant of low cognitive function: a cross-sectional study in elderly men. Stroke **29:** 1816–1820.
37. FORETTE, F. & F. BOLLER. 1991. Hypertension and risk of dementia in the elderly. Am. J. Med. **90:** 14S–19S.
38. SKOOG, I. *et al.* 1996. 15-year longitudinal study of blood pressure and dementia. Lancet **347:** 1141–1145.
39. GUO, Z. *et al.* 1999. Blood pressure and dementia in persons over 75 years old: follow-up results from the Kungsholmen Project. Submitted.
40. ZHU, L. *et al.* 1998. Blood pressure reduction, cardiovascular diseases, and cognitive decline in the Mini-mental State Examination in a community population of normal very old people: a three-year follow-up. J .Clin. Epidemiol. **51:** 385–391.
41. GUO, Z. *et al.* 1997. Blood pressure and dementia in the elderly: epidemiologic perspectives. Biomed. Pharmacother. **51:** 68–P73.
42. HOFMAN, A. *et al.* 1997. Atherosclerosis, apolipoprotein E, and prevalence of dementia and Alzheimer's disease in the Rotterdam study. Lancet **349:** 151–154.
43. OTT, A. *et al.* 1997. Atrial fibrillation and dementia in a population-based study. The Rotterdam study. Stroke **28:** 316–321.
44. LEIBSON, C.L. *et al.* 1979. Risk of dementia among persons with diabetes mellitus: a population-based cohort study. Am. J. Epidemiol. **45:** 301–308.
45. OTT, A. *et al.* 1996. Association of diabetes mellitus and dementia: the Rotterdam study. Diabetologia **39:** 1392–1397.
46. BRAYNE, C. *et al.* 1998. Vascular risks and incident dementia: results from a cohort study of the very old. Dementia & Geriatric Cognit. Dis. **9:** 175–180.
47. SNOWDOW, D.A. *et al.* 1997. Brain infarction and the clinical expression of Alzheimer's disease. The Nun study. J.A.M.A. **277:** 813–817.
48. PASQUIER, F. & D. LEYS. 1997. Why are stroke patients prone to develop dementia? J. Neurol. **244:** 135–142.
49. TOMLINSON, B.E. *et al.* 1970. Observations of the brains of demented old people. J. Neurol. Sci. **11:** 205–242.
50. HULETTE, C. *et al.* 1997. Clinical-neuropathological findings in multi-infarct dementia: a report of 6 autopsy cases. Neurology **48:** 668–672.
51. ELLIS, R.J. *et al.* 1996. Cerebral amyloid angiopathy in the brains of patients with Alzheimer's disease: the CERAD experience, part XV. Neurology **46:** 592–596.
52. GORELICK, P.B. *et al.* 1996. Is vascular dementia really Alzheimer's disease or mixed dementia? Neuroepidemiology **15:** 286–290.
53. ROCKWOOD, K. 1997. Lessons from mixed dementia. Int. Psychogeriatrics **9:** 245–249.

Index of Contributors

Agüero-Torres, H., 547–552
Alafuzoff, I., 244–251
Alexander, G.E., 470–476
Amouyel, P., 437–441
Apró, E., 72–82
Asthana, S., 222–228

Baker, L., 222–228
Ballard, C., 442–445
Barber, B., 442–445
Barber, R., 482–489
Bardenheuer, H.J., 299–306
Barnetson, L., 407–410, 497–500
Beach, T.G., 366–373
Belardinelli, N., 164–166
Berr, C., 437–441
Bertoni-Freddari, C., 164–166 , 451–456
Black, S., 522–528
Blank, C., 293–298
Blass, J.P., 204–221
Bouchard, R., 522–528
Boyt, A.A., 222–228
Brayne, C., 490–496
Breteler, M.M.B., 457–465
Bronge, L., 477–481
Brown, W.R., 39–45
Brulin, P., 285–292
Bryant, M., 345–352
Bu, G., 167–175
Budge, M., 407–410, 497–500
Bungay, H., 497–500
Burgermeister, P., 307–316
Burn, D., 293–298
Bushby, K., 293–298

Calhoun, M.E., 307–316
Calingasan, N.Y., 353–356
Carstens, M.E., 150–155
Caselli, U., 451–456
Casoli, T., 164–166, 451–456
Challa, V.R., 39–45

Cherrier, M., 222–228
Cho, H.-S., 144–149
Chung, S.-Y., 357–365
Clarke, R., 497–500
Coulthard, A., 293–298
Craft, S., 222–228
Crawford, F., 156–163
Crawford, K., 411–423

David-Fromentin, I., 437–441
Davis, J., 89–96
De Deyn, P.P., 535–541
de Jager, C., 407–410
De Jong, G.I., 72–82
de la Monte, S.M., 61–71
de la Torre, J.C., 424–436
De Lange, R., 293–298
De Villiers, J.N.P., 200–203
De Vos, R.A.I., 72–82
de Waal, R.M.W., 187–199
del Ser, T., 510–521
Desmond, D.W., 262–272
Di Stefano, G., 164–166
Dufouil, C., 490–496
Durham, R.A., 366–373

Emery, V.O., 229–238
Emmerling, M.R., 118–122, 366–373
Erkinjuntti, T., 262–272, 510–521, 535–541
Esiri, M.M., 239–243, 497–500
Etienne, D., 61–71
Evans, L.M., 118–122

Fagan, A.M., 167–175
Farkas, E., 72–82
Farlow, M.R., 387–393
Fattoretti, P., 164–166, 451–456
Feldman, H., 522–528
Ferrier, I.N., 83–88
Ferroni, S., 24–33

Frackowiak, J., 6–18
Frangione, B., 129–137
Friedland, R.P., 123–128
Frost, C., 497–500
Fujise, N., 46–54

Galeazzi, L., 164–166, 451–456
Gauthier, S., 522–528
Ge, Y.-W., 387–393
Gertz, H., 490–496
Getz, G.S., 167–175
Ghiso, J., 129–137
Gholkar, A., 482–489
Gibson, G.E., 204–221, 353–356
Gillie, E.X., 229–238
Giunta, S., 451–456
Gracciotti, N., 451–456
Grammas, P., 55–60
Greenberg, S.M., 144–149
Greiner, L.H., 34–38

Hachinski, V., 1–5
Hampel, H., 470–476
Han, S.-H., 357–365
Hansen, L.A., 138–143
Haque, A., 411–423
Harkany, T., 374–386
Harrington, C., 490–496
Hatazawa, J., 252–261
Helbecque, N., 437–441
Helisalmi, S., 244–251
Hénon, H., 466–469
Hippius, H., 470–476
Hirata, S., 46–54
Hirata, Y., 252–261
Hofstetter, C.R., 138–143
Hogan, D., 522–528
Hogervorst, E., 407–410
Holtzman, D., 167–175
Honer, W.G., 366–373
Horwitz, B., 470–476
Hoyer, S., 299–306
Humphrey, J., 97–109, 156–163, 446–450
Huppert, F.A., 490–496

Ince, P.G., 293–298
Inzitari, D., 262–272, 510–521
Ishizuka, K., 46–54
Iversen, S.D., 407–410

Joachim, C., 497–500
Johansson, J., 293–298
Johnston, C., 407–410
Jucker, M., 307–316

Kalaria, R.N., 83–88, 293–298
Kalimo, H., 273–284
Kato, H., 252–261
Katzman, R., 138–143
Kenny, R.A., 442–445
Kertesz, A., 522–528
Kimura, T., 46–54
King, E., 407–410, 497–500
Kittner, B., 535–541, 542–546
Kossmann, T., 118–122
Kotze, M.J., 200–203
Kraft, J., 61–71
Kundtz, A., 156–163
Kuo, Y.-M., 110–117, 118–122, 335–344, 366–373

Lacombe, P., 317–323, 394–406
LaDu, M.J., 167–175
Lahiri, D.K., 387–393
LaManna, J.C., 123–128
Lee, J.H., 138–143
Leteurtre, E., 285–292
Leys, D., 466–469
Lin, C., 317–323
Luiten, P.G.M., 72–82, 374–386
Lukas, R.J., 335–344

MacKnight, C., 522–528
Mannermaa, A., 244–251
Marchini, C., 24–33
Markesbery, W.R., 34–38
Martin, E., 299–306
Martin, T., 335–344
Martins, R.N., 222–228

Maruya, H., 252–261
Masliah, E., 317–323
Massey, A., 110–117
Maurage, C.A., 285–292
Mazur-Kolecka, B., 6–18
McCarron, M.O., 176–179
McGee, M.A., 490–496
McKeith, I., 442–445
Mead, S., 129–137
Mehta, P.D., 118–122
Melchor, J., 89–96
Meyer, J.S., 411–423
Milwain, E., 407–410
Mito, Y., 252–261
Miyakawa, T., 46–54
Miyazaki, H., 24–33
Möller, H.-J., 470–476
Molyneux, A., 497–500
Montgomery, P., 522–528
Moody, D.M., 39–45
Morganti-Kossmann, M.C., 118–122
Morino, T., 24–33
Morris, C.M., 83–88, 293–298
Morris, J., 497–500
Mucke, L., 317–323
Mukaetova-Ladinska, E., 490–496
Mullan, M., 97–109, 156–163, 446–450
Munoz, D.,1–5

Nagata, K., 252–261
Nakabayashi, J., 46–54
Nakamura, Y., 24–33
Nicoll, J.A.R., 176–179, 293–298

O'Brien, J., 442–445, 482–489
O'Connor, D., 490–496
O'Donnell, H.C., 144–149
O'Sullivan, A., 490–496
Ogata, T., 24–33
Olichney, J.M., 138–143
Ono, T., 46–54
Otte-Höller, I., 187–199

Pantoni, L., 262–272, 510–521

Paris, D., 97–109, 446–450
Parker, T., 97–109, 446–450
Pasquier, F., 466–469
Paykel, E.S., 490–496
Penke, B., 374–386
Perry, G., 123–128
Perry, R., 482–489
Peruzzi, P., 394–406
Peskind, E., 222–228
Pietrini, P., 470–476
Placzek,, A., 156–163
Plant, G., 129–137
Plaschke, K., 299–306
Pluta, R., 324–334
Plymate, S., 222–228
Potocnik, F.C.V., 150–155, 200–203
Potter, P.E., 366–373
Prior, R., 180–186
Pucci, E., 164–166

Raby, C.A., 118–122
Rapoport, S.I., 470–476
Raskind, M., 222–228
Rauch, G.M., 411–423
Rauch, R.A., 411–423
Reardon, C., 167–175
Rebeck, G.W., 144–149
Reimann-Philipp, U., 55–60
Révész, T., 129–137
Rhodin, J., 345–352, 501–509
Richard, F., 437–441
Ringheim, G.E., 529–534
Rockwood, K., 262–272, 522–528
Roher, A.E., 110–117, 118–122, 335–344, 366–373
Román, G.C., 19–23
Romanelli, M., 510–521
Rosand, J., 144–149
Rossor, M., 293–298
Rostagno, A., 129–137
Ruchoux, M.M., 285–292

Sato, M., 252–261
Satoh, Y., 252–261
Scaravilli, F., 293–298

Schapiro, M.B., 470–476
Schellenberg, G., 222–228
Scheltens, P., 262–272, 442–445, 542–546
Schubert, P., 24–33
Segal, A.Z., 144–149
Shaw, F., 442–445
Sheu, R.K.-F., 204–221
Shi, J., 123–128
Signorino, M., 164–166
Smith, A.D., 407–410, 497–500
Smith, J.A., 229–238
Smith, M.A., 123–128
Snowdon, D.A., 34–38
Sohn, Y.K., 61–71
Soininen, H., 244–251
Sparks, D.L., 335–344
Spiegel, K., 118–122
St Clair, D., 293–298
Stahel, P.F., 118–122
Steur, E.N.H.J., 72–82
Su, G., 156–163
Sue, L.I., 366–373
Suo, Z., 156–163
Sutton, E.T., 345–352

Taljaard, J.J.F., 150–155, 200–203
Teipel, S.J., 470–476
Terashi, H., 252–261
Thal, L.J., 138–143
Thomas, A., 482–489
Thomas, A.J., 83–88
Thomas, N.J., 293–298
Thomas, T., 345–352, 501–509
Thore, C.R., 39–45
Town, T., 97–109, 446–450

Urmoneit, B., 180–186

Van Eldik, L., 167–175
Van Nostrand, W.E., 89–96, 187–199
Van Rensburg, S.J., 150–155, 200–203
Verbeek, M.M., 187–199
Vidal, R., 129–137
Viitanen, M., 273–284
Von Euw, D., 317–323, 394–406
Vorbrodt, A.W., 6–18

Wagner, M., 89–96
Wahlund, L.-O., 477–481
Walker, D.G., 366–373
Wallin, A., 262–272, 510–521
Wands, J.R., 61–71
Watahiki, Y., 252–261
Watson, M.D., 118–122
Wegiel, J., 6–18
Weigel, P.H., 55–60
Weller, R.O., 110–117
Wentzel, C., 522–528
Wesseling, P., 187–199
Wihl, G., 180–186
Winblad, B., 547–552
Winkler, D.T., 307–316
Wischik, C., 490–496
Wisniewski, H.M., 6–18
Wyss-Coray, T., 317–323

Xuereb, J.H., 490–496

Yokoyama, E., 252–261
Younkin, L.H.., 144–149
Younkin, S.G., 144–149
Yun, S.-W., 299–306
Yuya, H., 252–261